SELECTED CHAPTERS FROM

CONTEMPORARY

Nutrition

A Functional Approach

Third Edition

Gordon M. Wardlaw PH.D.
Formerly of Department of Human Nutrition,
College of Education and Human Ecology
The Ohio State University

Anne M. Smith PH.D., R.D., L.D.
Department of Human Nutrition,
College of Education and Human Ecology
The Ohio State University

Angela L. Collene M.S., R.D., L.D.
Dietetics Program
Department of Family and Consumer Sciences
Ashland University

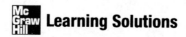 **Learning Solutions**

Boston   Burr Ridge, IL   Dubuque, IA   New York   San Francisco   St. Louis
Bangkok   Bogotá   Caracas   Lisbon   London   Madrid
Mexico City   Milan   New Delhi   Seoul   Singapore   Sydney   Taipei   Toronto

Selected Chapters from
Contemporary Nutrition: A Functional Approach
Third Edition

2 3 4 5 6 7 8 9 0 DIG DIG 14 13 12

ISBN-13: 978-0-07-766233-2
ISBN-10: 0-07-766233-4

Learning Solutions Consultant: Jill Albracht
Production Editor: Janie Larsen
Printer/Binder: Digital Impressions

CONTEMPORARY

Nutrition

A Functional Approach Third Edition

Gordon M. Wardlaw PH.D.
Formerly of Department of Human Nutrition,
College of Education and Human Ecology
The Ohio State University

Anne M. Smith PH.D., R.D., L.D.
Department of Human Nutrition,
College of Education and Human Ecology
The Ohio State University

Angela L. Collene M.S., R.D., L.D.
Dietetics Program
Department of Family and Consumer Sciences
Ashland University

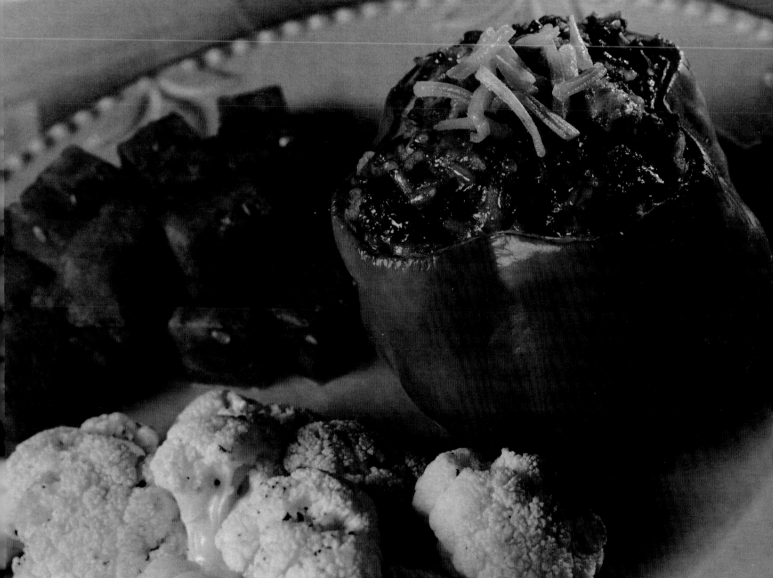

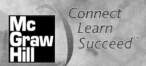

Connect
Learn
Succeed™

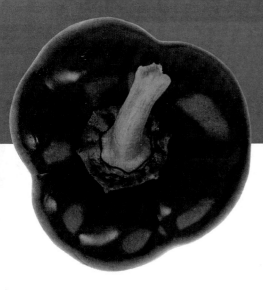

About the Authors

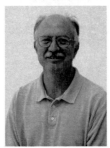

GORDON M. WARDLAW, Ph.D., has taught introductory nutrition courses to students in the Department of Human Nutrition at The Ohio State University and at other colleges and universities. Dr. Wardlaw is the author of many articles that have appeared in prominent nutrition, biology, physiology, and biochemistry journals and was the 1985 recipient of the American Dietetic Association's Mary P. Huddleson Award. Dr. Wardlaw is a member of the American Society for Nutritional Sciences and is certified as a Specialist in Human Nutrition by the American Board of Nutrition. Dr. Wardlaw is currently retired from academia.

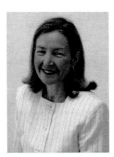

ANNE M. SMITH, Ph.D., R.D., L.D., currently teaches nutrition majors and nonmajors at The Ohio State University and was the recipient of the 1995 Outstanding Teacher Award from the College of Human Ecology. Dr. Smith is the Director of the Didactic Program in Dietetics in the Department of Human Nutrition, College of Education and Human Ecology, of The Ohio State University and received the 2008 Outstanding Dietetic Educator Award from the Ohio Dietetic Association and the 1998 Emerging Dietetic Leader Award from the American Dietetic Association. She also was the recipient of the 2006 Outstanding Faculty Member Award from the Department of Human Nutrition for her commitment to undergraduate education in nutrition and the 2011 Distinquished Service Award from the College of Education and Human Ecology. Dr. Smith has conducted research in the area of vitamin and mineral metabolism and was awarded the 1996 Departmental Research Award from the Ohio Agricultural Research and Development Center. Dr. Smith's research articles have appeared in prominent nutrition journals. She is a member of the American Nutrition Society and the American Dietetic Association.

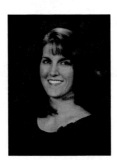

ANGELA L. COLLENE, M.S., R.D., L.D., currently teaches dietetics majors and non-majors as adjunct faculty at Ashland University, Department of Family and Consumer Sciences. During her graduate studies at The Ohio State University, where she received the Graduate Student Award in 2003, she had the privilege of learning from both Dr. Wardlaw and Dr. Smith. Her career began in clinical human nutrition research at O.S.U., where she served as a Registered Dietitian and Clinical Studies Coordinator for research studies related to diabetes and aging. Other professional experiences include community nutrition lecturing and counseling, owner of a personal chef business, and many diverse and rewarding science writing and editing projects. Her interests include novel approaches to glycemic control, weight management, and—quite predictably for the mother of three little girls—maternal and child nutrition. Mrs. Collene is a member of the American Dietetic Association.

Brief Contents

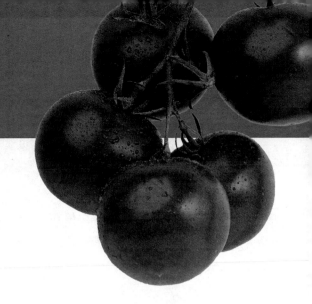

Preface

Dear Students,

Welcome to the fascinating world of nutrition! We are all nutrition experts, in a sense, because we all eat—several times a day. At the same time, though, nutrition can seem a bit confusing. One reason for all the confusion is that it seems like "good nutrition" is a moving target: different authorities have different ideas of how we should eat and nutrition recommendations are subject to change! Are eggs good for us or not? Should we model our diets after a pyramid or a plate? Second, there are so many choices. Did you know that the average supermarket carries about 40,000 food and beverage products? Food manufacturers and grocery chains have one purpose—to make as large a profit as possible. Typically, the most aggressively marketed items are not the healthiest. This has made shopping very complicated. In addition, as a nation, we eat out a lot. When we eat foods that someone else has prepared for us, we surrender control over how much salt and fat is in our food and how much food goes on our plates. There is a lot yet to learn, and you are undoubtedly interested in what you personally should be eating and how the food you eat affects you.

Contemporary Nutrition: A Functional Approach is designed to accurately convey changing and seemingly conflicting messages to all kinds of students. Our students commonly have misconceptions about nutrition, and many have a limited background in biology or chemistry. We teach complex scientific concepts at a level that will enable you to meaningfully apply the material to your own life. Contemporary Nutrition: A Functional Approach, is organized somewhat differently than the traditional nutrition textbook in that Part Three presents information on vitamins, minerals and water using "a functional approach". Instead of describing these nutrients in their traditional categories (e.g., water soluble vitamins), we discuss them in groups based on their functions in either fluid and electrolyte balance, bone health, energy metabolism, or bone health, and as antioxidants. Learning about these nutrients in this format will enable you to immediately understand how they interact in food and in our bodies and how they work together to support these key functions that sustain our health.

We have written Contemporary Nutrition: A Functional Approach to help you make informed choices about the food you eat. We will take you through explanations of the nutrients in food and their relationship to health, but will also make you aware of the multitude of other factors that drive food choices. To guide you, we refer to many reputable research studies, books, policies, and web sites throughout the book. With this information at your fingertips, you will be well equipped to make your own informed choices about what and how much to eat. There is much to learn, so let's get started!

-Anne Smith

-Angela Collene

Connecting Students to Course Concepts

Introducing McGraw-Hill ConnectPlus™ Nutrition

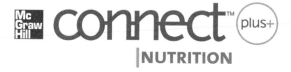

McGraw-Hill Connect® is a web-based assignment and assessment platform that gives students the means to better connect with coursework, instructors, and important concepts that they will need to know for success now and in the future. Connect Nutrition includes high quality interactive questions and tutorials, LearnSmart, digital lecture capture, eBook, and more!

Save time with auto-graded assessments and tutorials.

You can easily create customized assessments that will be automatically graded. All Connect content is created by nutrition instructors so it is pedagogical, instructional, and at the appropriate level. Interactive questions using high-quality art from the textbook, animations and videos from a variety of sources, take you way beyond multiple choice.

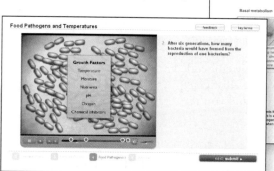

Connect Assessment: Classification Interactive

Connect Assessment: Animation Tutorial

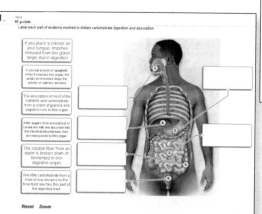

Connect Assessment: Labeling Interactive

> "... I and my adjuncts have reduced the time we spend on grading by 90 percent and student test scores have risen, on average, 10 points since we began using Connect!"
>
> —William Hoover, Bunker Hill Community College

Gather assessment information

All Connect questions are tagged to learning outcome, specific topics, level of difficulty, and allow you to tag your own learning outcomes—so you can easily track assessment data!

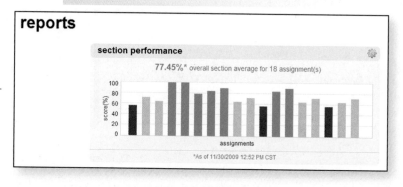

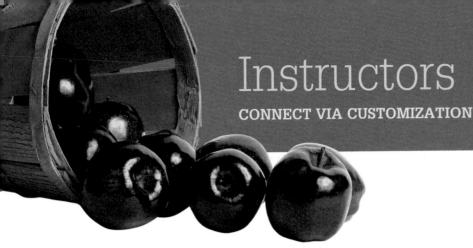

Instructors

CONNECT VIA CUSTOMIZATION

Presentation Tools allow you to customize your lectures.

Enhanced Lecture Presentations contain lecture outlines, art, photos, tables, and animations embedded where appropriate. Fully customizable, complete and ready to use, these presentations will streamline your work and let you spend less time preparing for lecture!

Editable Art   Fully editable (labels and leaders) line art from the text.

Animations   Over 50 animations bringing key concepts to life, available for instructors *and* students.

Animation PPTs   Animations are truly embedded in PowerPoint® for ultimate ease of use! Just copy and paste into your custom slideshow and you're done!

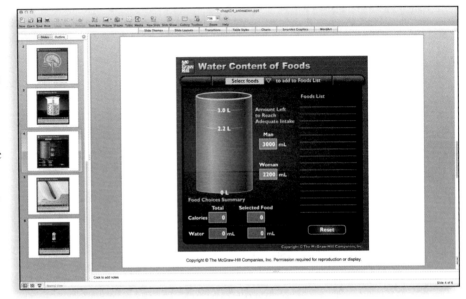

Take your course online—*easily and quickly* with one-click Digital Lecture Capture.

McGraw-Hill Tegrity® records and distributes your lectures with just a click of a button. Students can view them anytime/anywhere via computer, iPod, or mobile device. Tegrity® indexes and records your slideshow presentations, and anything shown on your computer, so **students can use keywords to find exactly what they want to study.**

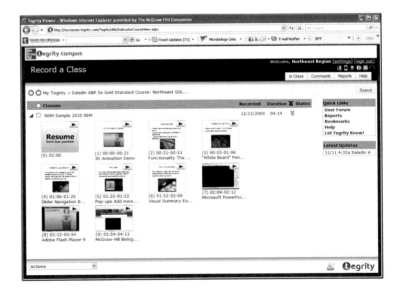

Students

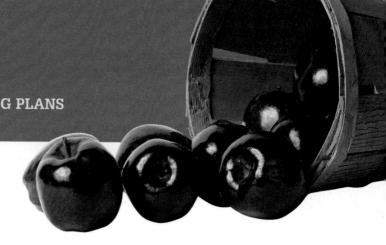

Access content anywhere, any time, with a customizable, interactive eBook.

McGraw-Hill ConnectPlus eBook takes digital texts beyond a simple PDF. With the same content as the printed book, but optimized for the screen, ConnectPlus has embedded animations and videos, which bring concepts to life and provide "just in time" learning for students. Fully integrated self-study questions allow students to interact with the questions in the text and determine if they're gaining mastery of the content.

> **"Use of technology, especially LEARNSMART, assisted greatly in keeping on track and keeping up with the material."**
>
> —*student, Triton College*

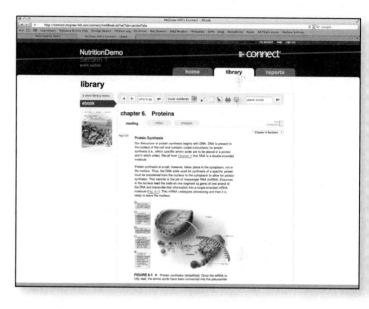

McGraw-Hill LearnSmart™ A Diagnostic, Adaptive Learning System

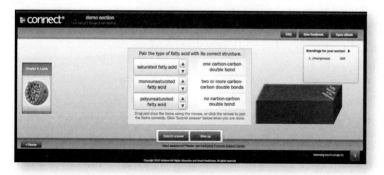

McGraw-Hill *LearnSmart* is an adaptive learning system designed to help students learn faster, study more efficiently, and retain more knowledge for greater success.

LearnSmart effectively assesses students' skill levels to determine which topics students have mastered and which require further practice. A personalized learning path based upon student strengths and weaknesses gives students exactly the help they need, when they need it.

Self-study resources are also available at www.mhhe.com/wardlawcont9.

> **"I love LearnSmart. Without it, I would not be doing as well."**
>
> —*student, Triton College*

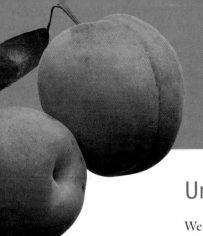

Understanding Our Audience

We have written *Contemporary Nutrition* assuming that our students have a limited background in college-level biology, chemistry, or physiology. We have been careful to include the essential science foundation needed to adequately comprehend certain topics in nutrition, such as protein synthesis in Chapter 6. The science in this text has been presented in a simple, straightforward manner so that undergraduate students can master the material and apply it to their own lives. The Concept Maps that provide a visual depiction of macronutrient functions and characteristics are an additional aid to help students grasp nutrition science.

Featuring the Latest Guidelines and Research

The vast amount of published research is constantly reshaping our knowledge of nutritional science. The ninth edition has been carefully updated to reflect current scientific understanding, as well as the latest health and nutrition guidelines. Students will learn about the Dietary Guidelines for Americans, 2010, MyPlate, and Healthy People 2020.

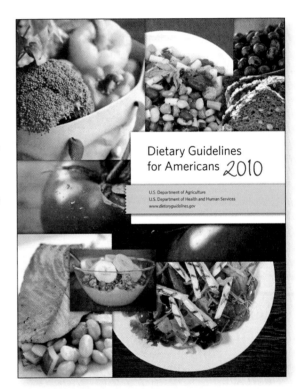

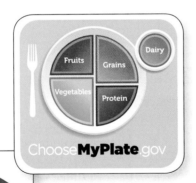

Connecting with a Personal Focus

Applying Nutrition on a Personal Level

Throughout the ninth edition we reinforce the fact that each person responds differently to nutrients. To further convey the importance of applying nutrition to their personal lives, we include many examples of people and situations that resonate with college students. We also stress the importance of learning to intelligently sort through the seemingly endless range of nutrition messages to recognize reliable information and to sensibly apply it to their own lives. Our goal is to provide students the tools they need to eat healthy and make informed nutrition decisions after they leave this course.

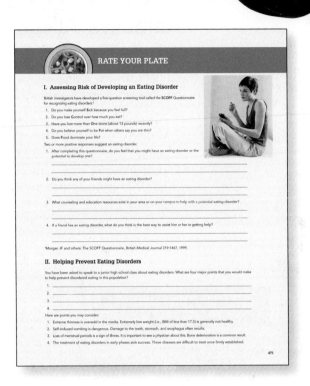

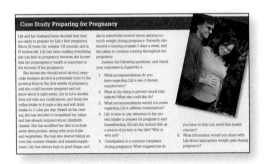

Challenging Students to Think Critically

The pages of *Contemporary Nutrition* contain numerous opportunities for students to learn more about themselves and their diet and to use their new knowledge of nutrition to improve their health. In the ninth edition, pedagogical elements, such as Making Decisions, Critical Thinking, Case Studies, and Nutrition and Your Health, are further enhanced by the addition of What Would You Choose? and Newsworthy Nutrition. Many of the thought-provoking topics highlighted in these features are expanded upon in the online resources found in Connect Nutrition.

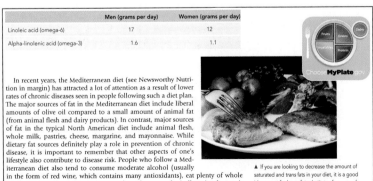

	Men (grams per day)	Women (grams per day)
Linoleic acid (omega-6)	17	12
Alpha-linolenic acid (omega-3)	1.6	1.1

In recent years, the Mediterranean diet (see Newsworthy Nutrition in margin) has attracted a lot of attention as a result of lower rates of chronic diseases seen in people following such a diet plan. The major sources of fat in the Mediterranean diet include liberal amounts of olive oil compared to a small amount of animal fat (from animal flesh and dairy products). In contrast, major sources of fat in the typical North American diet include animal flesh, whole milk, pastries, cheese, margarine, and mayonnaise. While dietary fat sources definitely play a role in prevention of chronic disease, it is important to remember that other aspects of one's lifestyle also contribute to disease risk. People who follow a Mediterranean diet also tend to consume moderate alcohol (usually in the form of red wine, which contains many antioxidants), eat plenty of whole grains and few refined carbohydrates, and are also more physically active than typical North Americans.

An alternative plan for reduction of cardiovascular disease is Dr. Dean Ornish's purely vegetarian (**vegan**) diet plan (see Further Reading 12). This diet is very low in fat, including only a scant quantity of vegetable oil used in cooking and the small amount of oils present in plant foods. Individuals restricting fat intake to 20% of

▲ If you are looking to decrease the amount of saturated and trans fats in your diet, it is a good idea to opt for lower-fat substitutes for some of your current high-fat food choices. How do you think this meal compares with the fried meal on p. 179? How does it compare to MyPlate recommendations?

What Would You Choose?

Your brother and his wife have asked you to watch your 18-month-old niece, Lila, while they enjoy a weekend getaway at the lake to celebrate their anniversary. Before they drop her off, you make a trip to the grocery store to pick up some kid-friendly foods. Lila does not have any food allergies, but your brother warned you that she has gotten into some picky eating behaviors. Which of the following snack foods would you choose for your little houseguest?

ⓐ Reduced-fat popcorn

ⓑ Raw baby carrots with ranch dressing

ⓒ Fat-free light yogurt

ⓓ Whole-grain crackers with sliced cheddar cheese

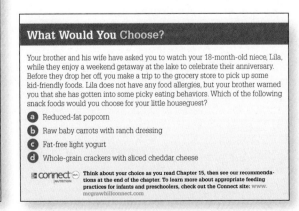

connect NUTRITION Think about your choice as you read Chapter 15, then see our recommendations at the end of the chapter. To learn more about appropriate feeding practices for infants and preschoolers, check out the Connect site: www. mcgrawhillconnect.com

xi

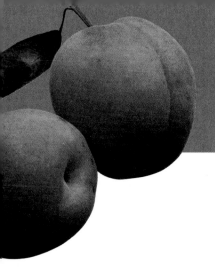

Making Visual Connections

Attractive, Accurate Artwork

More than 1000 drawings, photographs, and tables in the text were critically analyzed to identify how each could be enhanced and refined to help students more easily master complex scientific concepts.

- Many illustrations were updated or replaced to inspire student inquiry and comprehension and to promote interest and retention of information.
- Many illustrations were redesigned to use brighter colors and a more attractive, contemporary style. Others were fine-tuned to make them clearer and easier to follow. Navigational aids show where a function occurs and put it in perspective of the whole body.

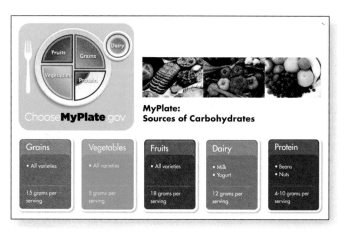

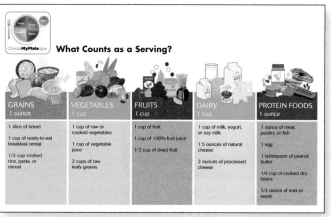

TABLE 2-5 Recommended Diet Changes Based on the Dietary Guidelines

If You Usually Eat This,	Try This Instead	Benefit
White bread	Whole-wheat bread	• Higher nutrient density, due to less processing • More fiber
Sugary breakfast cereal	Low-sugar, high-fiber cereal with fresh fruit	• Higher nutrient density • More fiber • More phytochemicals
Cheeseburger with French fries	Hamburger and baked beans	• Less saturated fat and trans fat • Less cholesterol • More fiber • More phytochemicals
Potato salad	Three-bean salad	• More fiber • More phytochemicals
Doughnuts	Bran muffin/bagel with light cream cheese	• More fiber • Less fat
Regular soft drinks	Diet soft drinks	• Fewer calories
Boiled vegetables	Steamed vegetables	• Higher nutrient density, due to reduced loss of water-soluble vitamins
Canned vegetables	Fresh or frozen vegetables	• Higher nutrient density, due to reduced loss of heat-sensitive vitamins • Lower in sodium
Fried meats	Broiled meats	• Less saturated fat
Fatty meats, such as ribs or bacon	Lean meats, such as ground round, chicken, or fish	• Less saturated fat
Whole milk	Low-fat or fat-free milk	• Less saturated fat • Fewer calories • More calcium
Ice cream	Sherbet or frozen yogurt	• Less saturated fat • Fewer calories
Mayonnaise or sour cream salad dressing	Oil-and-vinegar dressings or light creamy dressings	• Less saturated fat • Less cholesterol • Fewer calories
Cookies	Popcorn (air popped with minimal margarine or butter)	• Fewer calories and trans fat
Heavily salted foods	Foods flavored primarily with herbs, spices, lemon juice	• Lower in sodium
Chips	Pretzels	• Less fat

▲ Choose low-sugar, high-fiber cereal with fresh fruit instead of sugary breakfast cereal.

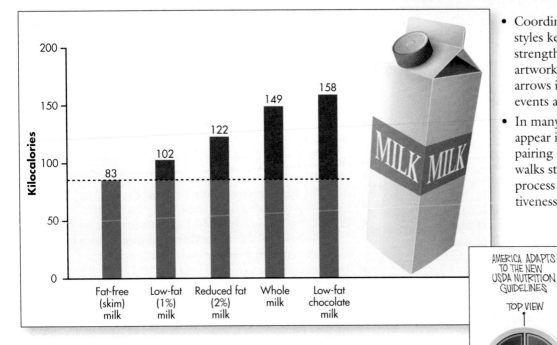

- Coordinated color schemes and drawing styles keep presentations consistent and strengthen the educational value of the artwork. Color-coding and directional arrows in figures make it easier to follow events and reinforce interrelationships.

- In many figures, process descriptions appear in the body of the figures. This pairing of the action and an explanation walks students step-by-step through the process and increases the teaching effectiveness of these figures.

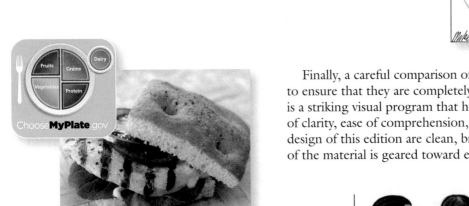

Finally, a careful comparison of artwork with its corresponding text was done to ensure that they are completely coordinated and consistent. The final result is a striking visual program that holds readers' attention and supports the goals of clarity, ease of comprehension, and critical thinking. The attractive layout and design of this edition are clean, bright, and inviting. This creative presentation of the material is geared toward engaging today's visually oriented students.

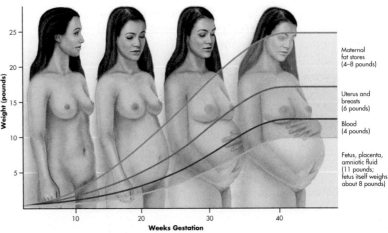

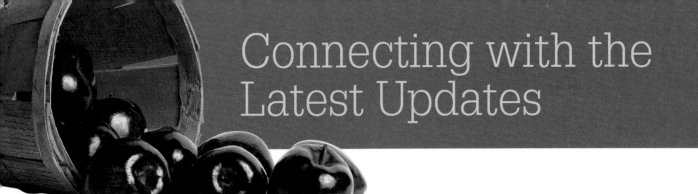

Connecting with the Latest Updates

Chapter-by-Chapter Revisions

Chapter 1: *Choosing What You Eat and Why*

- Chapter 1 has been reorganized beginning with a discussion of factors that influence our food choices and ending with a conversation about eating well in college.
- Chemical details of nutrients (e.g., dissacharides) have been moved to chapters on specific nutrients. Details on the hormonal control of appetite have been moved to Chapter 7.
- The newly released *Healthy People 2020* (HP2020) report is discussed, including its key "Nutrition and Weight Status" objectives.
- The new *What Would You Choose* feature focuses on time-saving breakfast options, especially for college students.
- Two *Newsworthy Nutrition* margin features are included in Chapter 1. One describes the link between TV food ads and childhood obesity and the other the link between a healthy diet and risk of sudden cardiac death.
- Causes of Death have been updated in Table 1-2.
- Added Figure 1-4 to illustrate the percentage of adults who are obese by state in 2009.

Chapter 2: *Guidelines for Designing a Healthy Diet*

- The *What Would You Choose* feature illustrates nutrient density and energy density.
- The new USDA food guide, MyPlate, released in June 2011, has been included with references to www.Choose MyPlate.gov and the Daily Food Plans that accompany MyPlate.
- The new Dietary Guidelines for Americans, 2010, released in January 2011, are fully discussed.
- Discussion of the scientific method, nutrient standards, and recommendations for healthy eating have been reorganized.
- New Figure 2-8 compares American intakes to current recommendations and Figure 2-11 shows what counts as a serving with MyPlate.
- New Figure 2-26 illustrates the concept of empty calories from solid fats and/or added sugars. *Newsworthy Nutrition* highlights the increasing costs of healthy eating.
- The new Rate Your Plate, "Are you putting health advice into practice?" reflects the 2010 Dietary Guidelines for Americans and 2008 Physical Activity Guidelines.

Chapter 3: *The Human Body: A Nutrition Perspective*

- Figure 3-7 is a new illustration of the pancreas and the function of endocrine cells secreting hormones into the bloodstream.

- *What Would You Choose* focuses on the best menu options to alleviate gastrointestinal complaints such as constipation.
- The *Newsworthy Nutrition* margin feature focuses on the link between gut bacteria and health and disease.

Chapter 4: *Carbohydrates*

- *What Would You Choose* focuses on the sugar content, including high-fructose corn syrup, of beverages.
- Figure 4-7 is now MyPlate: Sources of Carbohydrates.
- Table 4-2 now includes Stevia as an alternative sweetener.
- The *Newsworthy Nutrition* margin feature focuses on the link between high-fructose corn syrup and obesity.
- Recommendations from the new 2010 Dietary Guidelines regarding carbohydrate intake have been added.
- Figure 4-12 is a new illustration from the 2010 Dietary Guidelines of the sources of added sugars in U.S. diets.

Chapter 5: *Lipids*

- The new *What Would You Choose* feature focuses on the fat content of ground beef.
- Figure 5-5 has been revised to MyPlate: Sources of Fats.
- Peanut Butter: Is it "good fat?," has been included.
- Recommendations from the new 2010 Dietary Guidelines regarding fat intake have been added.
- Goals of Healthy People 2020 regarding reducing saturated fat intake, death from coronary heart disease, and total blood cholesterol are included.
- *Newsworthy Nutrition* focuses on research showing that a low-fat diet is not necessary for weight loss.

Chapter 6: *Proteins*

- The new *What Would You Choose* feature focuses on protein and amino acid intake and weight training.
- Figure 6-4 is now MyPlate: Sources of Protein.
- Recommendations from the new 2010 Dietary Guidelines regarding protein intake have been added.
- *Newsworthy Nutrition* focuses on the link between colon cancer and recent fat, protein, and red meat consumption.

Chapter 7: *Energy Balance and Weight Control*

- The new *What Would You Choose* feature focuses on the calorie content of frozen desserts.
- Figure 7-1 has been updated with obesity trends for 2009.
- New Weight Status Objectives from Healthy People 2020 are included.
- Recommendations from the new 2010 Dietary Guidelines regarding "Balancing Calories to Manage Weight," have been added.

- Two *Newsworthy Nutrition* features are included. One focuses on research indicating that small changes result in large weight changes and the other on a popular weight loss drug that has been withdrawn from the market.

Chapter 8: *Overview of the Micronutrients*

- The Overview of the Micronutrients is now a distinct chapter with useful and relevant pedagogical elements.
- The new *What Would You Choose* feature exemplifies factors to consider when choosing a dietary supplement.
- Figure 8-1 has been updated to include micronutrients that contribute to immune function.
- Tables summarizing vitamins and minerals include the recently revised recommendations for calcium and vitamin D.
- Food group sources of the vitamins are now illustrated using the MyPlate graphic (e.g., Figure 8-2, MyPlate: Sources of Vitamins and Choline).
- Table 8-3 provides tips for preserving the vitamin content of fruits and vegetables.
- The *Newsworthy Nutrition* margin feature reports on a link between multivitamin use and reduced heart attack risk.
- A completely new *Nutrition & Your Health* feature offers insights on the importance of choline in the human diet.
- The *Rate Your Plate* feature examines the nutritional contribution of breakfast cereals.

Chapter 9: *Nutrients Involved in Fluid and Electrolyte Balance*

- The new *What Would You Choose* feature focuses on the best choice of bottled water, especially when working out.
- A new Figure 9-10 shows the water content of foods as a bar chart.
- All figures illustrating food sources of nutrients involved in fluid and electrolyte balance have been updated to include the new MyPlate concept.
- Stronger recommendations for all population groups to reduce sodium intake are stressed throughout the chapter.
- The *Newsworthy Nutrition* feature presents the sodium-to-potassium ratio of the diet as a predictor of cardiovascular disease.

Chapter 10: *Nutrients that Function as Antioxidants*

- The new *What Would You Choose* feature examines uses of antioxidants as food additives.
- Discussions of how to convert International Units (IU) to milligrams for vitamin E and retinol activity equivalents (RAE) for vitamin A have been expanded.
- All figures illustrating food sources of nutrients that function as antioxidants have been updated to include the new MyPlate concept.
- The *Newsworthy Nutrition* feature presents results of SELECT, a large clinical trial examining the efficacy of antioxidant supplementation for cancer prevention.
- Figure 10-17 has been updated to show current supplement sales figures for 2009 and 2010, and the Top Five Dietary Supplements have been updated for 2010.

Chapter 11: *Nutrients Involved in Bone Health*

- The new *What Would You Choose* feature explores the amount and bioavailability of vitamin D from commonly consumed dairy products.
- All figures illustrating food sources of nutrients involved in bone health have been updated to include the new MyPlate concept.
- Statistics regarding prevalence and costs associated with osteoporosis have been updated.
- The new Figure 11-4 illustrates the projected economic burden of osteoporosis through 2025.
- The role of vitamin K in bone health is included in the text and Table 11-5.
- The Food and Nutrition Board's updated recommendations for calcium and vitamin D have been incorporated into the chapter.
- The *Newsworthy Nutrition* feature explores a potential drawback of widespread use of calcium supplements for osteoporosis prevention.
- Table 11-4 has been reorganized to more clearly present factors that impair vitamin D status.
- Updated recommendations from the American Academy of Pediatrics and the Dietary Guidelines regarding vitamin D supplementation for infants and children are presented.

Chapter 12: *Micronutrient Function in Energy Metabolism and Blood Health*

- The new *What Would You Choose* feature focuses on rich sources of folic acid, especially for pregnant women.
- All figures illustrating food sources of micronutrients involved in energy metabolism and blood health have been updated to include the new MyPlate concept.
- Iodide, chromium, manganese, and molybdenum are now discussed along with other micronutrients involved in energy metabolism.
- The *Newsworthy Nutrition* margin feature focuses on research showing that folic acid added to cereal reduces the number of neural-tube defects.
- Zinc is now discussed along with other micronutrients involved in blood health.

Chapter 13: *Nutrition: Fitness and Sports*

- The *What Would You Choose* feature compares and contrasts some popular sports nutrition products.
- Discussion of the 2008 Physical Activity Guidelines for Americans has been expanded.
- Table 13-5 has been updated with protein needs of athletes.
- New products have been added to Table 13-6, Popular Energy Drinks and Table 13-8, Popular Energy Bars and Gels. Table 13-6 now includes caffeine, energy, and sugar content of energy drinks.
- The *Newsworthy Nutrition* feature distinguishes between sports drinks and energy drinks for athletic performance.

Chapter 14: *Eating Disorders*

- The *What Would You Choose* feature addresses how to approach a friend with a suspected eating disorder.

- The upcoming revisions to the *Diagnostic and Statistical Manual of Mental Disorders* related to eating disorders have been discussed, including the probable reclassification of Binge-Eating Disorder as an eating disorder.
- Discussion of genetics and eating disorders has been enhanced.
- Information on Muscle Dysmorphia has been included.
- The *Newsworthy Nutrition* feature points out common threads between binge eating and binge drinking.

Chapter 15: *Undernutrition Throughout the World*
- The new *What Would You Choose* feature focuses on choices to help put an end to world hunger.
- The content has been updated with current statistics on food insecurity, homelessness, hunger, and malnutrition.
- Table 15-2 has been updated to include new federally subsidized programs that supply food for people in the U.S.
- A New section, "Access to Healthy Food," includes discussion of food deserts in low income neighborhoods.
- The global impact of HIV/AIDS has been updated and illustrated in Figure 15-4.
- The *Newsworthy Nutrition* margin feature focuses on whether HIV-positive women should choose to breastfeed.
- Prevalence of genetically modified crops is updated.

Chapter 16: *Safety of Our Food Supply*
- *What Would You Choose* focuses on choosing fruits and vegetables with the best nutritional value, fewest preservatives and pesticides, and lowest risk for foodborne illness.
- The content has been updated with information about the most recent outbreaks of foodborne illnesses.
- Discussion of the new FDA Food Safety Modernization Act, signed into law in 2011 is included.
- The Food Safety Danger Zone has been updated.
- *Newsworthy Nutrition* focuses on the *E. coli* outbreak that was linked to German organic sprouts.

Chapter 17: *Pregnancy and Breastfeeding*
- The *What Would You Choose* feature addresses food choices to meet the needs of a pregnant vegetarian.

- Physical Activity Guidelines for pregnancy are included.
- New figures have been added to illustrate how nutrient requirements for pregnancy and breastfeeding differ from those of the RDAs/AIs of adult women.
- The *Newsworthy Nutrition* feature explores a proposed increase in vitamin D recommendations during pregnancy.
- Recommendations from the new 2010 Dietary Guidelines pertinent to pregnancy and breastfeeding have been added.
- Advice on maternal dietary restrictions to prevent food allergies has been updated to reflect the updated position of the American Academy of Pediatrics.
- Discussion of Fetal Alcohol Syndrome has been updated with the updated Fetal Alcohol Spectrum Disorders.

Chapter 18: *Nutrition from Infancy through Adolescence*
- The *What Would You Choose* feature looks into healthy and age-appropriate food choices for children.
- Throughout the chapter, including the *Newsworthy Nutrition* feature, the importance of family meals is emphasized.
- The latest American Academy of Pediatrics (AAP) recommendations on infant feeding have been included.
- Revised recommendations from the AAP and National Institute of Allergy and Infectious Disease for preventing food allergies and atopic disease have been included.
- New Figure 18-3 shows examples of meals that comply with MyPlate for children, ages 2, 4, 8, and 16.

Chapter 19: *Nutrition During Adulthood*
- The *What Would You Choose* feature explores nutritional approaches for reducing cancer risk.
- Recommendations from the new 2010 Dietary Guidelines and the 2008 Physical Activity Guidelines pertaining to older adults have been included.
- Figures have been added comparing nutrient requirements for older adults with those of the young adults.
- The *Newsworthy Nutrition* feature focuses on research regarding caloric restriction and longevity.

Connections that Suit Your Needs

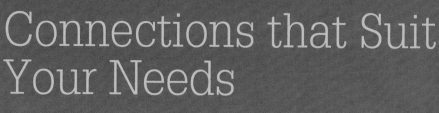
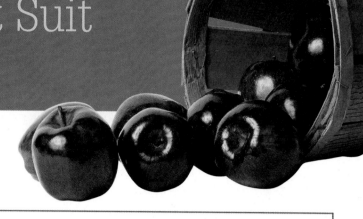

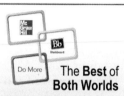 The **Best** of **Both Worlds**

McGraw-Hill Higher Education and Blackboard® have teamed up!

What does this mean for you?

- **Life simplified.** Now, all McGraw-Hill content (text, tools, & homework) can be accessed directly from within your Blackboard course. All with one sign-on.

- **Deep integration.** McGraw-Hill's content and content engines are seamlessly woven within your Blackboard course.

- **No more manual synching!** Connect® assignments within Blackboard automatically (and instantly) feed grades directly to your Blackboard grade center. No more keeping track of two gradebooks!

- **A solution for everyone.** Even if your institution is not currently using Blackboard, we have a solution for you. Ask your McGraw-Hill representative for details.

Customize your course materials to your learning outcomes!

Create what you've only imagined.

Introducing McGraw-Hill Create™—a new, self-service website that allows you to create custom course materials—print and eBooks—by drawing upon McGraw-Hill's comprehensive, cross-disciplinary content. Add your own content quickly and easily. Tap into other rights-secured third-party sources as well. Then, arrange the content in a way that makes the most sense for your course. Even personalize your book with your course name and information! Choose the best format for your course: color print, black-and-white print, or eBook. The eBook is now even viewable on an iPad! And, when you are done, you will receive a free PDF review copy in just minutes!

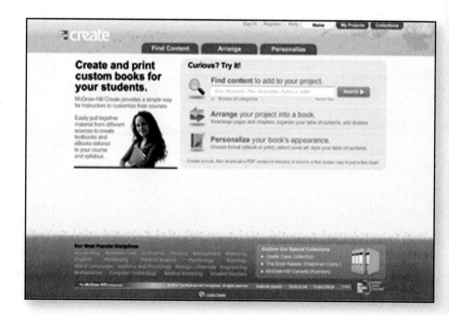

Finally, a way to quickly and easily create the course materials you've always wanted.

Imagine that.

Visit McGraw-Hill Create—www.mcgrawhillcreate.com—**today and begin building your perfect book.**

Acknowledgments

Special Acknowledgements

Writing a textbook requires much energy and constant support. We are indebted to several individuals for their creative abilities and generous interest in the production of this book. First, our deepest gratitude to our long-time editor Lynne Meyers, whose commitment, patience and encouragement has been extraordinary. She and her staff at McGraw-Hill have guided and assisted us through every phase of this and several previous revisions of Contemporary Nutrition. This edition is also much improved by the written contributions of our new author, Angela Collene, M.S., R.D. We thank her for her significant contributions to the "functional" chapters in Part Three and for her work on the recent updates to the Dietary Guidelines, MyPlate, and Healthy People 2020. Finally, we are grateful to Sheila Frank and her staff for the meticulous coordination of the many production efforts needed to produce the very appealing yet accurate third edition.

Thank you to reviewers

Our goal is to provide students and educators with the most accurate, up-to-date, and useful textbook possible. As with earlier editions, the quality of the ninth edition of *Contemporary Nutrition* is largely dependent on the thorough, professional assistance of nutrition educators from academic institutions across the nation. We are indebted to these colleagues who reviewed the eighth edition, evaluated new material for the ninth edition, participated in instructional symposia, and responded to surveys. The advice and suggestions from these colleagues have been used in every chapter and have resulted in a textbook that is current and inviting.

Gregory Avellana
Ohio University

Alena Clark
University of Northern Colorado

Robert DiSilvestro
The Ohio State University

Mary Jeanne Doyle
The University of Montana Missoula College of Technology

Keith M. Erikson
The University of North Carolina, Greensboro

Leslie Sisson Goudarzi
Kilgore College

Megan Govindan
West Virginia University

Charlene Harkins
University of Minnesota, Duluth

Maureen Baun Jamgochian
College of the Canyons

Gail L. Kaye
The Ohio State University

Molly Michelman
University of Nevada

Maria Montemagni
College of the Sequoias

Cheryl Neudauer
Minneapolis Community and Technical College

Janet Tou
West Virginia University

Ann M. Volk
Antelope Valley College

Mary Watson
University of Nebraska, Omaha

Contents

Part Four Nutrition: Beyond the Nutrients 460

Part Five Nutrition: A Focus on Life Stages 594

CONTEMPORARY *Nutrition*

A Functional Approach   **Third Edition**

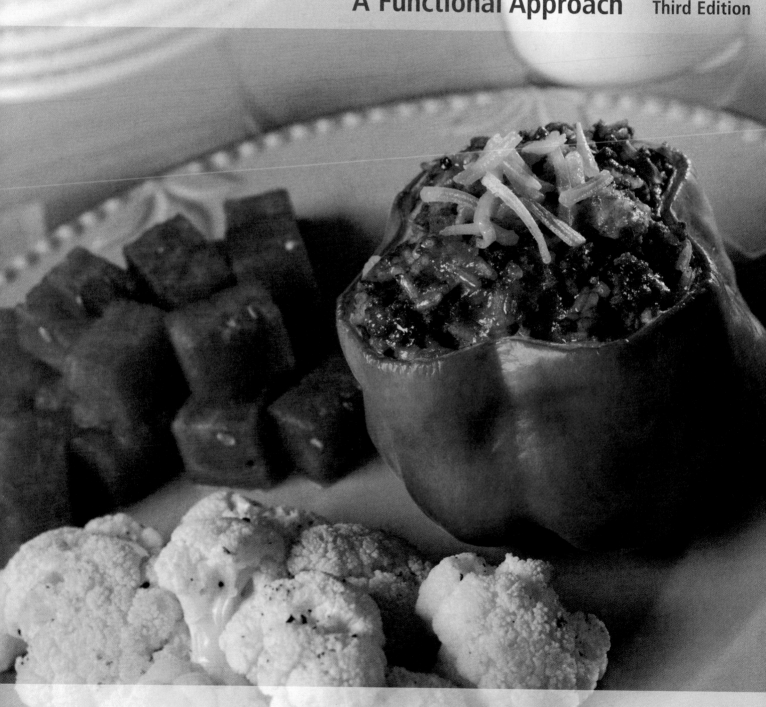

Chapter 1 Choosing What You Eat and Why

Rate Your Plate: We begin each chapter with a "What Would You Choose?" activity to get you thinking. We hope you will be able to make a choice that is right for you using the concepts discussed in the chapter. At the end of each chapter, we provide a discussion and summary of the logic behind what we would recommend. The "choice" aspect of this activity fits well with the new food guide tool, ChooseMy-Plate. You will learn more about this new tool in Chapter 2, and we will reinforce its guidelines in our "What Would You Choose?" activities.

Student Learning Outcomes

Chapter 1 is designed to allow you to:

1.1 Describe how our food habits are affected by the flavor, texture, and appearance of food; routines and habits; early experiences and customs; advertising; nutrition and health concerns; restaurants; social changes; and economic, as well as physiological processes affected by meal size and composition.

1.2 Identify diet and lifestyle factors that contribute to the 15 leading causes of death in North America.

1.3 Define the terms *nutrition, carbohydrate, protein, lipid (fat), alcohol, vitamin, mineral, water, kilocalorie (kcal),* and *fiber.*

1.4 Determine the total calories (kcal) of a food or diet using the weight and calorie content of the energy-yielding nutrients and use the basic units of the metric system to calculate percentages, such as percent of calories from fat in a diet.

1.5 List the major characteristics of the North American diet, the food habits that often need improvement, and the key "Nutrition and Weight Status" objectives of the *Healthy People 2020* report.

1.6 Describe a basic plan for health promotion and disease prevention and what to expect from good nutrition and a healthy lifestyle.

1.7 Identify food and nutrition issues relevant to college students.

What Would You Choose?

You were awake last night until 2:30 A.M. finishing a group project. Unfortunately, your Psychology 101 class meets at 9:00 this morning. When your alarm goes off at 7:30 A.M., you decide to sleep those extra 20 minutes it would take to sit down and enjoy breakfast at the dining hall. What's your best time-saving breakfast option?

a Skip breakfast, but plan to consume a few extra calories at lunch and dinner.

b Eat a low-fat granola bar and iced coffee from the vending machines in your dorm.

c Fix yourself a quick bowl of Wheaties with a banana and low-fat milk along with a yogurt, all from your dorm room "pantry."

d Pick up a ham, egg, and cheese bagel.

 Think about your choice as you read Chapter 1, then see our recommendations at the end of the chapter. To learn more about breakfast choices, check out the Connect site: www.mcgrawhillconnect.com

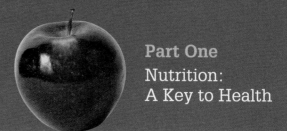

Research has clearly shown that a lifestyle that includes a diet rich in fruits, vegetables, and whole grains, coupled with regular exercise, can enhance our quality of life in the short term and keep us healthy for many years to come. Unfortunately, this healthy lifestyle is not always easy to follow. When it comes to "nutrition," it is clear that some of our diets are out of balance with our metabolism, physiology, and physical activity level.

We begin Chapter 1 with some questions. What influences your daily food choices? How important are factors such as taste, appearance, convenience, cost or value? Is nutrition one of the factors you consider? Are your food choices influencing your quality of life and long-term health? By making optimal dietary choices, we can bring the goal of a long, healthy life within reach. This is the primary theme of Chapter 1 and throughout this book.

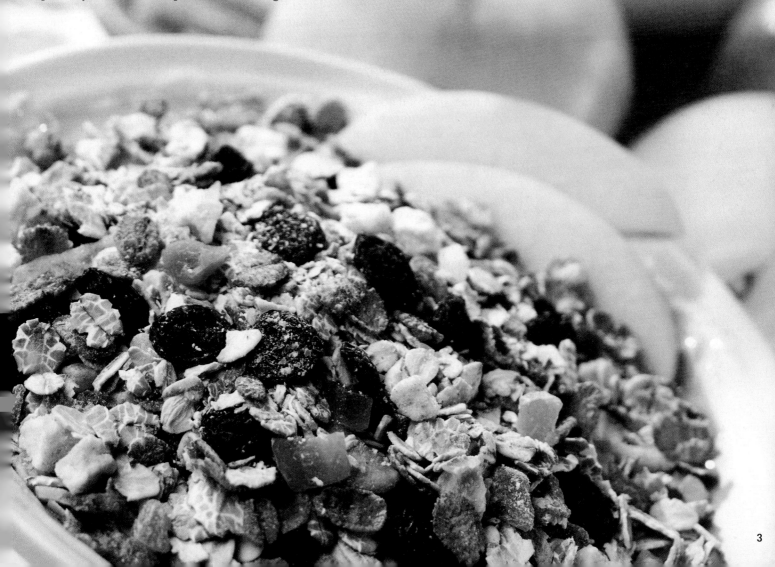

The ultimate goal of this book is to help you find the best path to good nutrition. The information presented is based on emerging science that is translated into everyday actions that improve health. After completion of your nutrition course you should understand the knowledge behind the food choices you make and recommend to others. We call this achievement of making food choices that are right for you "nutrition literacy."

 Refresh Your Memory

As you begin your study of choosing what you eat and why in Chapter 1, you may want to review:

- The metric system in Appendix I.

1.1 Why Do You Choose the Food You Eat?

In your lifetime, you will eat about 70,000 meals and 60 tons of food. Many factors influence our food choices including celebrations (see the comic below). Chapter 1 begins with a discussion of these factors and ends with a conversation specifically about eating well as a college student. In between, we examine the powerful effect of dietary habits in determining overall health and take a close look at the general classes of nutrients—as well as the calories—supplied by the food we eat, the major characteristics of the North American diet, the food habits that often need improvement, and the key "Nutrition and Weight Status" objectives in the *Healthy People 2020* report.

Understanding what drives us to eat and what affects food choice will help you understand the complexity of factors that influence eating, especially the effects of our routines and food advertising (Fig. 1-1). You can then appreciate why foods may have different meanings to different people and thus why food habits and preferences of others may differ from yours.

What Influences Your Food Choices?

Food means so much more to us than nourishment—it reflects much of what we think about ourselves. In the course of our lives, we spend the equivalent of 3 to 4 years eating. Yes, the Bureau of Labor Statistics estimated that in 2010 Americans spent the equivalent of 17 days eating and drinking. If we live to be 80 years old, that will add up to 3.7 years of eating and drinking. Overall, our daily food choices stem

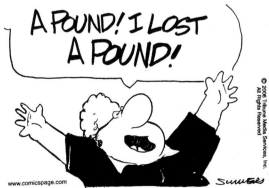
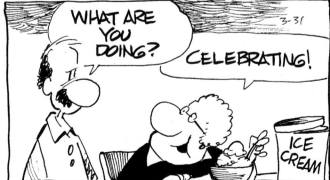

Copyright, 2002, Tribune Media Services. Reprinted with permission.

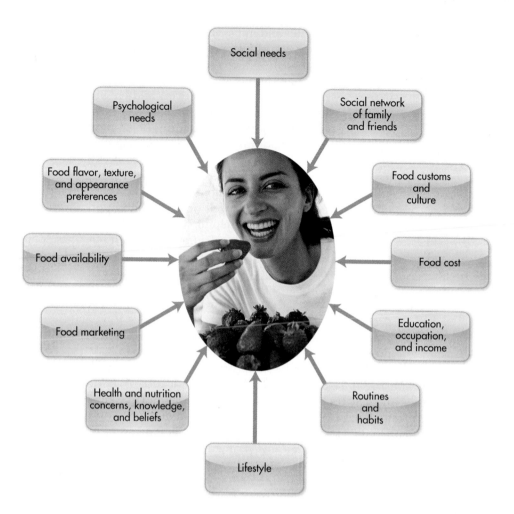

from a complicated mix of biological and social influences (see Fig. 1-1). Let's examine some of the key reasons we choose what we eat.

Flavor, texture, and *appearance* are the most important factors determining our food choices. Creating more flavorful foods that are both healthy and profitable is a major focus of the food industry. These foods are often referred to as "healthy" choices or "better for you" products. The challenge to the food industry is to match the "taste" of the foods we prefer with the nutrition and health characteristics of these products.

Early influences that expose us to various people, places, and events have a continuing impact on our food choices. Many ethnic diet patterns begin as we are introduced to foods during childhood. Developing healthy patterns during childhood, therefore, will go a long way to ensuring healthy preferences and choices when we are teenagers and adults. Food advertising and marketing have been shown to have a definite effect on weight gain in children and adolescents. Read more about the effect of television advertising and the development of obesity in childhood in the Newsworthy Nutrition margin note.

Routines and habits are tied to some food choices. Food habits, food availability, and convenience strongly influence choices. Most of us eat from a core group of foods with about 100 basic items accounting for 75% of an individual's total food intake. Recent surveys indicate that the most commonly purchased foods in America are milk (about 30 gallons yearly), ready-to-eat cereal, bottled water (about 25 gallons per year), soft drinks (nearly 50 gallons per year), and bread. It is no surprise that milk and cereal are both on the top-five list because they are eaten together as the daily breakfast for many Americans. Bottled water has become the drink of choice for business meetings and other large-group gatherings, including outdoor activities. Despite the

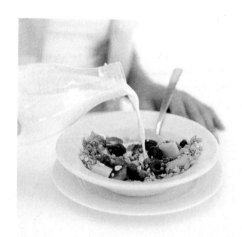

▲ Cereal and milk are two of the most commonly purchased foods in America largely because they are eaten together for breakfast every day by many.

popularity of water and milk, Americans still drink nearly twice as many carbonated soft drinks per year as either water or milk. The large amount of sugar in many soft drinks is of particular concern because studies have found an association between consumption of sugar-sweetened drinks and obesity in children. Bread is also on the list because it is typically consumed at every meal in America, making it one of the most common forms of grain eaten.

Advertising is a major media tool for capturing the food interest of the consumer. Consumers have more food choices than ever and these choices are well advertised in newspapers, magazines, billboards, radio, television, and now the Internet. The food industry in the United States spends well over $33 billion on advertising. Some of this advertising is helpful, as it promotes the importance of food components such as calcium and fiber in our diets. However, the food industry also advertises highly sweetened cereals, cookies, cakes, and soft drinks because they bring in the greatest profits. It is estimated that as much as $10 billion is spent on advertising food and beverages to America's children and youth. A 2008 Federal Trade Commission survey of 44 major food and beverage marketers in the United States found that they spent $1.6 billion to promote products to children and adolescents in 2006 (see Further Reading 6). Recent studies in several Western countries clearly indicate an association between TV advertising of foods and drinks and the prevalence of childhood obesity, especially in the United States. (Read about one of these studies in Newsworthy Nutrition.) Concern for the negative effect of advertising and marketing on the diets and health of children led the Center for Science in the Public Interest to publish *Guidelines for Responsible Food Marketing to Children* in 2005 (see Further Reading 2). These guidelines provide criteria for marketing food to children in a manner that does not undermine children's diets or harm their health.

Restaurant dining plays a significant role in our food choices, although the recession caused a 11.5 percent decline in food eaten away from home between 2006 and 2009 (Fig 1-2). Restaurant food is often calorie-dense, in large portions, and of poorer nutritional quality compared to foods made at home. Fast-food and pizza restaurant menus typically emphasize meat, cheese, fried foods, and carbonated beverages. I response to recent consumer demands, restaurants have placed healthier items on

FIGURE 1-2 ▶ This chart shows the total food expenditures adjusted for inflation from 1990 to 2009 including food eaten at home and away from home. Total food expenditures as well as food eaten away from home dipped declined during the recession from 2006 to 2009.

Source: http://www.ers.usda.gov/AmberWaves/September11/Features/FoodSpending.htm

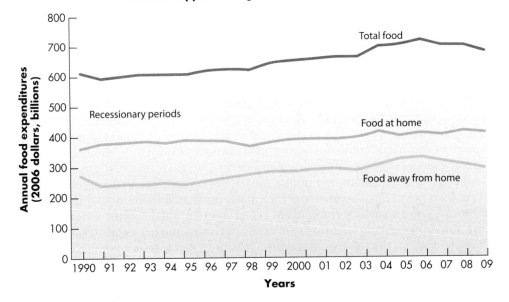

Total food expenditures adjusted for inflation dipped during the 2007–09 recession

their menus and many are listing nutritional content on their menus. Mandatory posting of the calorie content of restaurant items is expected to go into effect soon as a result of the health care reform bill that President Obama signed into law in March 2010. The law requires that chain restaurants with 20 or more locations post the calorie content of their offerings on menus or menu boards with other nutritional information available upon request.

Social changes are leading to a general time shortage for many of us. This creates the need for *convenience.* Supermarkets now supply prepared meals, microwavable entrees, and various quick-prep frozen products.

Economics play a minor role in our food choices. Increases in personal income have exceeded increases in dollars spent for food. This has resulted in the average North American spending only about 12% of after-tax income on food (greater for low-income people). However, as income increases, so do meals eaten away from home and preferences for foods such as cookies, chocolate, cheese, and meat. Also keep in mind that as calorie intake increases so does the food bill.

Last but not least, *nutrition*—or what we think of as "healthy foods"—also directs our food purchases. North Americans who tend to make health-related food choices are often well-educated, middle-class professionals. These same people are generally health-oriented, have active lifestyles, and focus on weight control. In the 2008 Health and Diet Survey (a snapshot of the nation's dietary habits), the Food and Drug Administration (FDA) found that more than half (54%) of consumers in the United States read the food label when buying a product for the first time. This number was an increase since 2002. Among those who are reading the Nutrition Facts, 67% use the label "often" to check how high or low a food is in calories and in substances such as salt, vitamins, and fat; 55% "often" use the label to get a general idea of the food's nutritional content; and 46% "often" use the calorie information on the label. Their key findings also indicate that consumers are increasingly aware of the link between diet and heart disease. Of those surveyed, 91% knew of this link, 81% knew that certain foods or drinks may help prevent heart disease or heart attacks, and 62% mentioned fats as a factor related to heart disease (see Further Reading 4).

Why Are You So Hungry?

Two drives, **hunger** and **appetite,** influence our desire to eat. These drives differ dramatically. Hunger is primarily our physical biological drive to eat and is controlled by internal body mechanisms. For example, as foods are digested and absorbed by the stomach and small intestine, these organs send signals to the liver and brain to reduce further food intake.

Appetite, our primarily psychological drive to eat, is affected by many of the external food choice mechanisms we discussed in the last section, such as environmental and psychological factors and social customs (see Fig. 1-1). Appetite can be triggered simply by seeing a tempting dessert or smelling popcorn popping at the movie theater. Fulfilling either or both drives by eating sufficient food normally brings a state of **satiety,** a feeling of satisfaction that temporarily halts our desire to continue eating.

A region of the brain helps regulate satiety. Imagine a game of tug-of-war in the brain. The *feeding center* and the *satiety center* work in opposite ways to promote adequate availability of nutrients at all times. When stimulated, cells in the feeding center signal us to eat. As we eat, cells in the satiety center are stimulated and we stop eating. For example, when we haven't eaten for a while, stimulation of the feeding center signals

hunger The primarily physiological (internal) drive to find and eat food, mostly regulated by internal cues to eating.

appetite The primarily psychological (external) influences that encourage us to find and eat food, often in the absence of obvious hunger.

satiety State in which there is no longer a desire to eat; a feeling of satisfaction.

MAKING DECISIONS

Putting Our Food Choices into Perspective

The next time you pick up a candy bar or reach for a second helping, remember the internal and external influences on eating behavior. You should now understand that daily food intake is a complicated mix of biological and social influences. Body cells, nutrients in the blood, hormones, brain chemicals, and our social and family customs all influence food choices. When food is abundant, appetite—not hunger—most likely triggers eating. Satiety associated with consuming a meal may reside primarily in our psychological frame of mind. Also, because satiety regulation is not perfect, body weight can fluctuate. We become accustomed to a certain amount of food at a meal. Providing less than that amount leaves us wanting more. One way to use this observation for weight-loss purposes is to train your eye to expect less food by slowly decreasing serving sizes to more appropriate amounts. Your appetite then readjusts as you expect less food. Keep track of what triggers your eating for a few days. Is it primarily hunger or appetite? The Rate Your Plate activity in this chapter also asks you to keep track of what influences your food intake on a daily basis.

nutrients Chemical substances in food that contribute to health, many of which are essential parts of a diet. Nutrients nourish us by providing calories to fulfill energy needs, materials for building body parts, and factors to regulate necessary chemical processes in the body.

essential nutrient In nutritional terms, a substance that, when left out of a diet, leads to signs of poor health. The body either cannot produce this nutrient or cannot produce enough of it to meet its needs. Then, if added back to a diet before permanent damage occurs, the affected aspects of health are restored.

us to eat. When the nutrient content in the blood rises after a meal, the satiety center is stimulated and we no longer have a strong desire to seek food. Admittedly, this concept of a tug-of-war between the feeding and satiety centers is an oversimplification of a complex process. The various feeding and satiety messages from body cells to the brain do not single-handedly determine what we eat. We often eat because food confronts us (see Further Reading 17). Almost everyone has encountered a mouthwatering dessert and devoured it, even on a full stomach. It smells, tastes, and looks good. We might eat because it is the right time of day, we are celebrating (see the cartoon in this section), or we are seeking emotional comfort to overcome the blues. After a meal, memories of pleasant tastes and feelings reinforce appetite. If stress or depression sends you to the refrigerator, you are mostly seeking comfort, not food calories. Appetite may not be a physical process, but it does influence food intake. We will discuss more about this mechanism, including the effect of meal size and composition on satiety, in Chapter 7 on energy balance and weight control.

CONCEPT CHECK

Hunger is the primarily physical or internal desire to find and eat food. Fulfilling it creates satiety—no further desire to eat exists. Satiety is influenced by hunger-related (internal) signals from the brain and other organs, as well as the content of the foods in the meal. Food intake is also affected by appetite-related (external) forces like social customs, time of day, and being with others. Factors such as flavor, appearance, and texture; early influences, routines, and habits; advertising and restaurant menus; economics and convenience; seeking emotional comfort; social changes; and hopefully, nutrition and health concerns, also greatly influence our food choices. North Americans probably respond more to external, appetite-related forces than to hunger-related ones in choosing when and what to eat.

1.2 How Is Nutrition Connected to Good Health?

Fortunately the foods we eat can support good health in many ways depending on their components. You just learned, however, that lifestyle habits and other factors may have a bigger impact on our food choices than the food components themselves. Unfortunately many North Americans suffer from diseases that could have been prevented if they had known more about the foods and, more importantly, had applied this knowledge to planning meals and designing their diet. We will now look at the effect these choices are having on our health both today and in the future.

What Is Nutrition?

Nutrition is the science that links foods to health and disease. It includes the processes by which the human organism ingests, digests, absorbs, transports, and excretes food substances.

Nutrients Come from Food

What is the difference between food and **nutrients**? Food provides the energy (in the form of calories) as well as the materials needed to build and maintain all body cells. Nutrients are the substances obtained from food that are vital for growth and maintenance of a healthy body throughout life. For a substance to be considered an **essential nutrient,** three characteristics are needed:

- First, at least one specific biological function of the nutrient in the body must be identified.

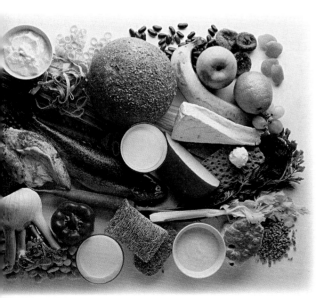

▲ Many foods are rich sources of nutrients.

- Second, omission of the nutrient from the diet must lead to a decline in certain biological functions, such as production of blood cells.
- Third, replacing the omitted nutrient in the diet before permanent damage occurs will restore those normal biological functions.

Why Study Nutrition?

Nutrition is a lifestyle factor that is a key to developing and maintaining an optimal state of health for you. A poor diet and a sedentary lifestyle are known to be **risk factors** for life-threatening **chronic** diseases such as **cardiovascular (heart) disease, hypertension, diabetes,** and some forms of **cancer** (Table 1-1). Together, these and related disorders account for two-thirds of all deaths in North America (Table 1-2)

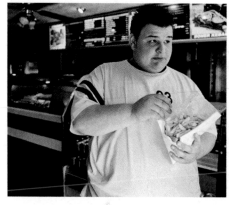

▲ Major health problems are largely caused by a poor diet, excessive calorie intake, and not enough physical activity.

TABLE 1-1 Glossary Terms to Aid Your Introduction to Nutrition*

Cancer	A condition characterized by uncontrolled growth of abnormal cells.
Cardiovascular (heart) disease	A general term that refers to any disease of the heart and circulatory system. This disease is generally characterized by the deposition of fatty material in the blood vessels (hardening of the arteries), which in turn can lead to organ damage and death. Also termed coronary heart disease (CHD), as the vessels of the heart are the primary sites of the disease.
Cholesterol	A waxy lipid found in all body cells; it has a structure containing multiple chemical rings. Cholesterol is found only in foods of animal origin.
Chronic	Long-standing, developing over time. When referring to disease, this term indicates that the disease process, once developed, is slow and lasting. A good example is cardiovascular disease.
Diabetes	A group of diseases characterized by high blood **glucose.** Type 1 diabetes involves insufficient or no release of the hormone insulin by the pancreas and therefore requires daily insulin therapy. Type 2 diabetes results from either insufficient release of insulin or general inability of insulin to act on certain body cells, such as muscle cells. Persons with type 2 diabetes may or may not require insulin therapy.
Hypertension	A condition in which blood pressure remains persistently elevated. Obesity, inactivity, alcohol intake, excess salt intake, and genetics may each contribute to the problem.
Kilocalorie (kcal)	Unit that describes the energy content of food. Specifically, a kilocalorie (kcal) is the heat energy needed to raise the temperature of 1000 grams (1 liter) of water 1° Celsius. Kcal refers to a 1000 calorie unit of measurement, but is commonly referred to as calories. It is a familiar term for the energy content of a food, so we will use it in this book.
Obesity	A condition characterized by excess body fat.
Osteoporosis	Decreased bone mass related to the effects of aging (including estrogen loss during menopause in women), genetic background, and poor diet.
Risk factor	A term used frequently when discussing the factors contributing to the development of a disease. A risk factor is an aspect of our lives—such as heredity, lifestyle choices (e.g., smoking), or nutritional habits.

glucose A six-carbon sugar that exists in a ring form; found as such in blood, and in table sugar bound to fructose; also known as *dextrose,* it is one of the simple sugars.

*Many bold terms are also defined in the page margins within each chapter and in the glossary at the end of this book.

TABLE 1-2 Fifteen Leading Causes of Death in the United States

Rank	Cause of Death	Percent of Total Deaths
	All causes	100
1	Heart disease*†#	24.6
2	Cancer*‡	23.3
3	Chronic lower respiratory diseases‡	5.6
4	Stroke (cerebrovascular diseases)*†#‡	5.3
5	Accidents (unintentional injuries)	4.8
6	Alzheimer's disease*	3.2
7	Diabetes mellitus*	2.8
8	Influenza and pneumonia	2.2
9	Kidney disease*‡	2.0
10	Intentional self harm (suicide)	1.5
11	Blood-borne infections (septicemia)	1.4
12	Chronic liver disease and cirrhosis†	1.2
13	Essential hypertension*	1.1
14	Parkinson's disease	0.8
15	Assault (homicide)	0.7

From Centers for Disease Control and Prevention, *National Vital Statistics Report*, Preliminary Data for 2009, March 16, 2011. Canadian statistics are quite similar.

*Causes of death in which diet plays a part.

†Causes of death in which excessive alcohol consumption plays a part.

‡Causes of death in which tobacco use plays a part.

#Diseases of the heart and cerebrovascular disease are included in the more global term "cardiovascular disease."

stroke A decrease or loss in blood flow to the brain that results from a blood clot or other change in arteries in the brain. This in turn causes the death of brain tissue. Also called a *cerebrovascular accident*.

NEWSWORTHY NUTRITION

Healthy diet lowers women's risk of sudden cardiac death

Sudden cardiac death (death occurring within 1 hour after symptom onset) is the cause of more than half of all heart-related deaths and usually occurs as the first sign of heart disease, especially in women. Lifestyle information from the Nurses' Health Study (81,722 women) was used to determine if adherence to a healthy lifestyle lowers the risk of sudden cardiac death among women. Low-risk lifestyle was considered as not smoking, not overweight, exercising 30 minutes/day or longer, and following the Mediterranean Diet. Risk of sudden cardiac death dropped by 92% with a combination of the four healthy lifestyles; and women who ate a diet most similar to the Mediterranean Diet with a high proportion of vegetables, fruits, nuts, omega-3 fats, and fish, along with moderate amounts of alcohol and small amounts of red meat, had a 40% less risk than women whose diets least resembled this diet. The conclusion is that a healthy diet along with other healthy lifestyle factors can protect women from sudden cardiac death.

Source: Chiuve SE, and others: Adherence to a low-risk, healthy lifestyle and risk of sudden cardiac death among women. *Journal of the American Medical Association*, 306:62, 2011 (see Further Reading 3).

connect NUTRITION **Check out the Connect site www.mcgrawhillconnect.com to further explore women's risk of sudden cardiac death.**

(see Further Reading 9). Not meeting nutrient needs in younger years makes us more likely to suffer health consequences, such as bone fractures from the disease **osteoporosis,** in later years. At the same time, taking too much of a nutrient—such as a vitamin A supplement—can be harmful. Another dietary problem, drinking too much alcohol, is associated with many health problems.

U.S. government scientists have calculated that a poor diet combined with a lack of sufficient physical activity contributes to hundreds of thousands of fatal cases of cardiovascular disease, cancer, and diabetes each year among adults in the United States. Thus, the combination of poor diet and too little physical activity may be the second leading cause of death in the United States. In addition, **obesity** is considered the second leading cause of preventable death in North America (smoking is the first). When they occur together, obesity and smoking cause even more health problems. Obesity and chronic diseases are often preventable. An important key to good health and more health care dollars in your pocket, is to realize that the cost of prevention, usually when we are children and young adults, is a small fraction of the cost of treating these diseases when we are older.

The good news is that the increased interest in health, fitness, and nutrition shown by Americans has been associated with long-term decreasing trends for heart disease, cancer, and stroke (the three leading causes of death) that continued in 2009. Mortality from heart disease, the leading cause of death, has been declining steadily since 1980. As you gain understanding about your nutritional habits and increase your knowledge about optimal nutrition, you will have the opportunity to dramatically reduce your risk for many common health problems. Read more about research on the link between eating a healthy diet and protection against death from heart disease in Newsworthy Nutrition. For additional help, the U.S. federal government provides two websites that contain links to many sources of health and nutrition information (www.healthfinder.gov and www.nutrition.gov). Other useful sites are www.webmd.com and www.eatright.org.

1.3 What Are the Classes and Sources of Nutrients?

To begin the study of nutrition, let's start with an overview of the six classes of nutrients. You are probably already familiar with the terms **carbohydrates, lipids** (fats and oils), **proteins, vitamins,** and **minerals.** These, plus **water,** make up the six classes of nutrients found in food.

Nutrients can then be assigned to three functional categories: (1) those that primarily provide us with calories to meet energy needs (expressed in **kilocalories [kcal]**); (2) those important for growth, development, and maintenance; and (3) those that act to keep body functions running smoothly. Some function overlap exists among these categories. The energy-yielding nutrients, carbohydrate, fat, and protein, make up a major portion of most foods (Table 1-3).

Let's now look more closely at these six classes of nutrients.

Carbohydrates

Chemically, carbohydrates can exist in foods as simple sugars and complex carbohydrates. **Simple sugars,** frequently referred to as *sugars,* are relatively small molecules. These sugars are found naturally in fruits, vegetables, and dairy products. Table sugar, sucrose, is an example of a simple sugar that is added to many foods we eat. Glucose, also known as blood sugar or dextrose, is an example of a simple sugar in your blood. **Complex carbohydrates** are formed when many simple sugars are joined together. For example, plants store carbohydrates in the form of **starch,** a complex carbohydrate made up of hundreds of sugar units. Breads, cereals, grains, and starchy vegetables are the main sources of complex carbohydrates.

TABLE 1-3 Major Functions of the Various Classes of Nutrients

Nutrient Classes That Provide Energy	Nutrient Classes That Promote Growth, Development, and Maintenance	Nutrient Classes That Regulate Body Processes
Most carbohydrates	Proteins	Proteins
Proteins	Lipids	Some lipids
Most lipids	Some vitamins	Some vitamins
	Some minerals	Some minerals
	Water	Water

Carbohydrates, proteins, lipids, and water are needed in relatively large amounts, so they are called **macronutrients.** Vitamins and minerals are needed in such small amounts in the diet that they are called **micronutrients.**

carbohydrate A compound containing carbon, hydrogen, and oxygen atoms. Most are known as *sugars, starches,* and *fibers.*

lipid A compound containing much carbon and hydrogen, little oxygen, and sometimes other atoms. Lipids do not dissolve in water, and include fats, oils, and cholesterol.

protein Food and body compounds made of amino acids; proteins contain carbon, hydrogen, oxygen, nitrogen, and sometimes other atoms, in a specific configuration. Proteins contain the form of nitrogen most easily used by the human body.

vitamin Compound needed in very small amounts in the diet to help regulate and support chemical reactions in the body.

mineral Element used to promote chemical reactions and to form body structures.

water The universal solvent; chemically, H_2O. The body is composed of about 60% water. Water (fluid) needs are about 9 (women) or 13 (men) cups per day; needs are greater if one exercises heavily.

kilocalorie (kcal) Heat energy needed to raise the temperature of 1000 grams (1 L) of water 1 degree Celsius; also written as *Calories.*

simple sugar Monosaccharide or disaccharide in the diet.

complex carbohydrate Carbohydrate composed of many monosaccharide molecules. Examples include glycogen, starch, and fiber.

macronutrient A nutrient needed in gram quantities in a diet.

micronutrient A nutrient needed in milligram or microgram quantities in a diet.

cell The structural basis of plant and animal organization. Cells contain genetic material and systems for synthesizing energy-yielding compounds. Cells have the ability to take up compounds from and excrete compounds into their surroundings.

bond A linkage between two atoms formed by the sharing of electrons, or attractions.

fiber Substances in plant foods not digested by the processes that take place in the human stomach or small intestine. These add bulk to feces. Fiber naturally found in foods is also called dietary fiber.

During digestion, complex carbohydrates are broken down into single sugar molecules (such as glucose), and absorbed via **cells** lining the small intestine into the bloodstream (see Chapter 3 for more on digestion and absorption). However, the **bonds** between the sugar molecules in certain complex carbohydrates, called **fiber,** cannot be broken down by human digestive processes. Fiber passes through the small intestine undigested to provide bulk for the stool (feces) formed in the large intestine (colon).

Aside from enjoying their taste, we need sugars and other carbohydrates in our diets primarily to help satisfy the calorie needs of our body cells. Carbohydrates provide a major source of calories for the body, on average 4 kcal per gram. Glucose, a simple sugar that the body can derive from most carbohydrates, is a major source of calories for most cells. When not enough carbohydrate is consumed to supply sufficient glucose, the body is forced to make glucose from proteins—not a healthy change. Chapter 4 focuses on carbohydrates.

Lipids

Lipids (mostly fats and oils) in the foods we eat also provide energy. Lipids yield more calories per gram than do carbohydrates—on the average, 9 kcal per gram—because of differences in their chemical composition. They are also the main form for energy storage in the body.

Lipids dissolve in certain chemical solvents (e.g., ether and benzene) but not in water. In this book, the more familiar terms *fats* and *oils* will generally be used, rather than lipids or triglycerides. Generally, fats are lipids that are solid at room temperature and oils are lipids that are liquid at room temperature. We obtain fats and oils from animal and plant sources. Animal fats, such as butter or lard, are solid at room temperature. Plant oils, such as corn or olive oil, tend to be liquid at room temperature. Solid fat should be limited in our diet because it can raise blood **cholesterol.** High blood cholesterol leads to clogged arteries and can eventually lead to cardiovascular disease (see Chapter 5).

Certain fats are essential nutrients that must come from our diet. These key fats that the body cannot produce, called essential fatty acids, perform several important functions in the body: they help regulate blood pressure and play a role in the synthesis and repair of vital cell parts. However, we need only about 4 tablespoons of a common plant oil (such as the canola or soybean oil) each day to supply these essential fatty acids. A serving of fatty fish, such as salmon or tuna, at least twice a week is another healthy source of essential fatty acids. The unique fatty acids in these fish complement the healthy aspects of common vegetable oils. This will be explained in greater detail in Chapter 5, which focuses on lipids.

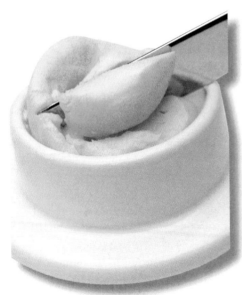

▲ Butter is an animal fat made from milk fat and is solid at room temperature.

enzyme A compound that speeds the rate of a chemical reaction but is not altered by the reaction. Almost all enzymes are proteins (some are made of genetic material).

amino acid The building block for proteins containing a central carbon atom with nitrogen and other atoms attached.

Proteins

Proteins are the main structural material in the body. For example, proteins constitute a major part of bone and muscle; they are also important components in blood, body cells, **enzymes,** and immune factors. Proteins can also provide calories for the body—on average, 4 kcal per gram. Typically, however, the body uses little protein for the purpose of meeting daily calorie needs. Proteins are formed when **amino acids** are bonded together. Some of these are essential nutrients.

Protein in our diet also comes from animal and plant sources. The animal products meat, poultry, fish, dairy products, and eggs are significant sources of protein in most diets. Beans, grains, and some vegetables are good plant protein sources. Plant protein is important to include in vegetarian diets.

Most North Americans eat up to two times as much protein as the body needs to maintain health. This amount of extra protein in the diet reflects the standard of living and the dietary habits of most North Americans and is generally not harmful for healthy persons with no evidence of heart or kidney disease, diabetes, or family history of colon cancer or kidney stones. The excess is used for calorie needs and carbohydrate production but ultimately can contribute to storage of fat. Chapter 6 focuses on proteins.

Vitamins

The main function of vitamins is to enable many **chemical reactions** to occur in the body. Some of these reactions help release the energy trapped in carbohydrates, lipids, and proteins. Remember, however, that vitamins themselves contain no usable calories for the body.

The 13 vitamins are divided into two groups: four are **fat-soluble** because they dissolve in fat (vitamins A, D, E, and K); nine are **water-soluble** because they dissolve in water (the B vitamins and vitamin C). The two groups of vitamins have different sources, functions, and characteristics. Water-soluble vitamins are found mainly in fruits and vegetables, whereas dairy products, nuts, seeds, oils, and breakfast cereals are good sources of fat-soluble vitamins. Cooking destroys water-soluble vitamins much more readily than it does fat-soluble vitamins. Water-soluble vitamins are also excreted from the body much more readily than are fat-soluble vitamins. Thus, the fat-soluble vitamins, especially vitamin A, are much more likely to accumulate in excessive amounts in the body, which then can lead to toxicity. Vitamins are introduced in Chapter 8.

Minerals

Minerals are structurally simple, **inorganic** substances, which do not contain carbon atoms. Minerals such as sodium and potassium typically function independently in the body, whereas minerals such as calcium and phosphorus function as parts of simple mineral combinations, such as bone mineral. Because of their simple structure, minerals are not destroyed during cooking, but they can still be lost if they dissolve in the water used for cooking and that water is then discarded. Minerals are critical players in nervous system functioning, water balance, structural (e.g., skeletal) systems, and many other cellular processes, but produce no calories as such for the body.

The 16 or more essential minerals required in the diet for good health are divided into two groups: **major minerals** and **trace minerals** because dietary needs vary enormously. If daily needs are less than 100 milligrams, the mineral is classified as a trace mineral; otherwise, it is a major mineral. Minerals that function based on their electrical charge when dissolved in water are also called **electrolytes;** these include sodium, potassium, and chloride. Many major minerals are found naturally in dairy products and fruits, whereas many trace minerals are found in meats, poultry, fish, and nuts. Minerals are introduced in Chapter 8.

Water

Water makes up the sixth class of nutrients. Although sometimes overlooked as a nutrient, water (chemically, H_2O) has numerous vital functions in the body. It acts as a **solvent** and lubricant, as a vehicle for transporting nutrients and waste, and as a medium for temperature regulation and chemical processes. For these reasons, and because the human body is approximately 60% water, the average man should consume about 3 liters—equivalent to 3000 grams or about 13 cups—of water and/or other fluids containing water every day. Women need closer to 2200 grams or about 9 cups per day.

Water is not only available from the obvious sources, but it is also the major component in some foods, such as many fruits and vegetables (e.g., lettuce, grapes, and melons). The body even makes some water as a by-product of **metabolism.** Water is examined in detail in Chapter 2.

Other Important Components in Food

Another group of compounds in foods from plant sources, especially within the fruit and vegetable groups, is what scientists call **phytochemicals.** Although these plant components are not considered essential nutrients in the diet, many of these substances provide significant health benefits. Considerable research attention is focused on various phytochemicals in reducing the risk for certain diseases. For example, evidence from animal and laboratory studies indicate that compounds in blueberries and

chemical reaction An interaction between two chemicals that changes both chemicals.

inorganic Any substance lacking carbon atoms bonded to hydrogen atoms in the chemical structure.

electrolytes Substances that separate into ions in water and, in turn, are able to conduct an electrical current. These include sodium, chloride, and potassium.

solvent A liquid substance in which other substances dissolve.

metabolism Chemical processes in the body by which energy is provided in useful forms and vital activities are sustained.

phytochemical A chemical found in plants. Some phytochemicals may contribute to a reduced risk of cancer or cardiovascular disease in people who consume them regularly.

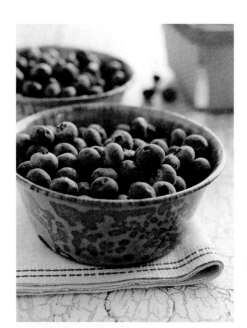

▲ Blueberries are among the fruits, vegetables, beans, and whole-grain breads and cereals that are typically rich in phytochemicals.

TABLE 1-4 Food Sources of Some Phytochemical Compounds under Study

Phytochemical	Food Sources
Allyl sulfides/organosulfurs	Garlic, onions, leeks
Saponins	Garlic, onions, licorice, legumes
Carotenoids (e.g., lycopene)	Orange, red, yellow fruits and vegetables (egg yolks are a source as well)
Monoterpenes	Oranges, lemons, grapefruit
Capsaicin	Chili peppers
Lignans	Flaxseed, berries, whole grains
Indoles	Cruciferous vegetables (broccoli, cabbage, kale)
Isothiocyanates	Cruciferous vegetables, especially broccoli
Phytosterols	Soybeans, other legumes, cucumbers, other fruits and vegetables
Flavonoids	Citrus fruit, onions, apples, grapes, red wine, tea, chocolate, tomatoes
Isoflavones	Soybeans, other legumes
Catechins	Tea
Polyphenols	Blueberries, strawberries, raspberries, grapes, apples, bananas, nuts
Anthocyanosides	Red, blue, and purple plants (blueberries, eggplant)
Fructooligosaccharides	Onions, bananas, oranges (small amounts)
Resveratrol	Grapes, peanuts, red wine

Some related compounds under study are found in animal products, such as sphingolipids (meat and dairy products) and conjugated linoleic acid (meat and cheese). These are not phytochemicals per se because they are not from plant sources, but they have been shown to have health benefits.

strawberries prevent the growth of certain cancer cells. Although certain phytochemicals are available as dietary supplements, research suggests that their health benefits are best obtained through the consumption of whole foods. Foods with high phytochemical content are sometimes called "superfoods" because of the health benefits they are thought to confer. There is no legal definition of the term superfood, however, and there is concern that it is being over-used in marketing certain foods. Table 1-4 lists some noteworthy phytochemicals with their common food sources. Tips for boosting the phytochemical content of your diet will be discussed in Chapter 2.

Sources of Nutrients

Now that we know the six classes of nutrients, it is important to understand that the quantities of the various nutrients that people consume in different foods vary widely. On a daily basis we consume about 500 grams, or about 1 pound, of protein, fat, and carbohydrate. In contrast, the typical daily mineral intake totals about 20 grams (about 4 teaspoons), and the daily vitamin intake totals less than 300 milligrams (1/15 of a teaspoon). Although we require a gram or so of some minerals, such as calcium and phosphorus, we need only a few milligrams or less of other minerals each day. For example, we need about 10 milligrams of zinc per day, which is just a few specks of the mineral.

The nutrient content of the foods we eat also differs from the nutrient composition of the human body. This is because growth, development, and later maintenance of the human body are directed by the genetic material (DNA) inside body cells. This genetic blueprint determines how each cell uses the essential nutrients to perform body functions. These nutrients can come from a variety of sources. Cells are not concerned about whether available amino acids come from animal or plant sources. The carbohydrate glucose can come from sugars or starches. The food that you eat provides cells with basic materials to function according to the directions supplied by the genetic material (**genes**) housed in body cells. Genetics and nutrition will be discussed in Chapter 3.

1.4 What Are Your Sources of Energy?

Calories

Humans obtain the energy we need for involuntary body functions and voluntary physical activity from various calorie sources: carbohydrates (4 kcal per gram), fats (9 kcal per gram), and proteins (4 kcal per gram). Foods generally provide more than one calorie source. Plant oils, such as soybean or canola oil are one exception; these are 100% fat at 9 kcal per gram.

Alcohol is also a source of calories for some of us, supplying about 7 kcal per gram. It is not considered an essential nutrient, however, because it has no required function. Still, alcoholic beverages, such as beer—also rich in carbohydrate—are a contributor of calories to the diet of many adults.

The body releases the energy from the chemical bonds in carbohydrate, protein, and fat (and alcohol) into other forms of energy in order to:

- Build new **compounds.**
- Perform muscular movements.
- Promote nerve transmissions.
- Maintain electrolyte balance within cells.

Chapters 7 and 12 describe how that energy is released from the chemical bonds in energy-yielding nutrients and then used by body cells to support the processes just described.

The energy in food is often expressed in terms of calories on food labels. As defined earlier, a calorie is the amount of heat energy it takes to raise the temperature of 1 gram of water 1 degree Celsius (1°C, centigrade scale). (Chapter 7 has a diagram of the bomb calorimeter that can be used to measure calories in foods.) A calorie is a tiny measure of heat, so food energy is more conveniently expressed in terms of the kilocalorie (kcal), which equals 1000 calories. (If the "c" in calories is capitalized, this also signifies kilocalories.) A kcal is the amount of heat energy it takes to raise the temperature of 1000 grams (1 liter) of water 1°C. The abbreviation *kcal* is used throughout this book. On food labels, the word *calorie* (without a capital "C") is also used loosely to mean *kilocalorie*. Any values given on food labels in calories are actually in kilocalories (Fig. 1-3). A suggested intake of 2000 calories per day on a food label is technically 2000 kcal.

genes A specific segment on a chromosome. Genes provide the blueprints for the production of all body proteins.

alcohol Ethyl alcohol or ethanol (CH_3CH_2OH) is the compound in alcoholic beverages.

compound A group of different types of atoms bonded together in definite proportion.

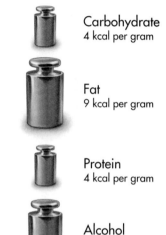

Carbohydrate
4 kcal per gram

Fat
9 kcal per gram

Protein
4 kcal per gram

Alcohol
7 kcal per gram

▲ Calorie content of energy nutrients and alcohol.

Nutrition Facts

Serving Size 1 slice (36g)   Servings Per Container 19

Amount Per Serving

Calories 80   Calories from Fat 10

	% Daily Value*			% Daily Value*
Total Fat 1g	**2%**	**Total Carbohydrate** 15g		**5%**
Saturated Fat 0g	**0%**	Dietary Fiber 2g		**8%**
Trans Fat less than 1g **				
Cholesterol 0mg	**0%**	Sugars less than 1g		
Sodium 200mg	**8%**	**Protein** 3g		
Vitamin A 0%	Vitamin C 0%	Calcium 0%		Iron 4%

HONEY WHEAT BREAD

*Percent Daily Values (DV) are based on a 2,000 calorie diet. Your daily values may be higher or lower depending on your calorie needs:

		Calories:	2,000	2,500
Total Fat	Less than		65g	80g
Sat Fat	Less than		20g	25g
Cholesterol	Less than		300mg	300mg
Sodium	Less than		2,400mg	2,400mg
Total Carbohydrate			300g	375g
Dietary Fiber			25g	30g

** Intake of *trans* fat should be as low as possible.

INGREDIENTS: WHOLE WHEAT, WATER, ENRICHED WHEAT FLOUR [FLOUR, MALTED BARLEY, NIACIN, REDUCED IRON, THIAMINE MONONITRATE (VITAMIN B1) AND RIBOFLAVIN (VITAMIN B2)], CORN SYRUP, PARTIALLY HYDROGENATED COTTONSEED OIL, SALT, YEAST.

FIGURE 1-3 ▶ Use the nutrient values on the Nutrition Facts label to calculate calorie content of a food. Based on carbohydrate, fat, and protein content, a serving of this food (Honey Wheat Bread) contains 81 kcal ([15 × 4] + [1 × 9] + [3 × 4] = 81). The label lists 80, suggesting that the calorie value was rounded down.

Calculating Calories

Use the 4-9-4 estimates for the calorie content of carbohydrate, fat, and protein introduced over the last few pages to determine calorie content of a food. Consider these foods:

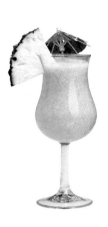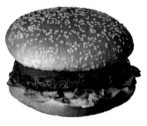

1 Large Hamburger

Carbohydrate	39 grams × 4 =	156 kcal
Fat	32 grams × 9 =	288 kcal
Protein	30 grams × 4 =	120 kcal
Alcohol	0 grams × 7 =	0 kcal
Total		**564 kcal**

8-ounce Piña Colada

Carbohydrate	57 grams × 4 =	228 kcal
Fat	5 grams × 9 =	45 kcal
Protein	1 gram × 4 =	4 kcal
Alcohol	23 grams × 7 =	161 kcal
Total		**438 kcal**

You can also use the 4-9-4 estimates to determine what portion of total calorie intake is contributed by the various calorie-yielding nutrients. Assume that one day you consume 290 grams of carbohydrates, 60 grams of fat, and 70 grams of protein. This consumption yields a total of 1980 kcal ([290 × 4] + [60 × 9] + [70 × 4]5 = 1980). The percentage of your total calorie intake derived from each nutrient can then be determined:

$$\% \text{ of kcal as carbohydrate} = (290 \times 4) \div 1980 = 0.59 \ (\times 100 = 59\%)$$
$$\% \text{ of kcal as fat} = (\ 60 \times 9) \div 1980 = 0.27 \ (\times 100 = 27\%)$$
$$\% \text{ of kcal as protein} = (\ 70 \times 4) \div 1980 = 0.14 \ (\times 100 = 14\%)$$

Check your calculations by adding the percentages together. Do they total 100?

MAKING DECISIONS

Percentages and the Metric System

You will use a few mathematical concepts in studying nutrition. Besides performing addition, subtraction, multiplication, and division, you need to know how to calculate percentages and convert English units of measurement to metric units.

Percentages

The term percent (%) refers to a part of the total when the total represents 100 parts. For example, if you earn 80% on your first nutrition examination, you will have answered the equivalent of 80 out of 100 questions correctly. This equivalent could be 8 correct answers out of 10; 80% also describes 16 of 20 (16/20 = 0.80 or 80%). The decimal form of percents is based on 100% being equal to 1.00. It is difficult to succeed in a nutrition course unless you know what a percentage means and how to calculate one. Percentages are used frequently when referring to menus and nutrient composition. The best way to master this concept is to calculate some percentages. Some examples follow:

Question	Answer
What is 6% of 45?	6% = 0.06 or 0.06 × 45 = 2.7
What percent of 99 is 3?	3/99 = 0.03 or 3% (0.03 × 100)

Joe ate 15% of the adult Recommended Dietary Allowance (RDA = 8 milligrams) for iron at lunch. How many milligrams did he eat?

$$0.15 \times 8 \text{ milligrams} = 1.2 \text{ milligrams}$$

The Metric System

The basic units of the metric system are the meter, which indicates length; the gram, which indicates weight; and the liter, which indicates volume. Appendix I in this textbook lists conversions from the metric system to the English system (pounds, feet, cups) and vice versa. Here is a brief summary:

A gram (g) is about 1/30 of an ounce (28 grams to the ounce).
5 grams of sugar or salt is about 1 teaspoon.
A pound (lb) weighs 454 grams.
A kilogram (kg) is 1000 grams, equivalent to 2.2 pounds.
To convert your weight to kilograms, divide it by 2.2.
A 154-pound man weighs 70 kilograms (154/2.2 = 70).
A gram can be divided into 1000 milligrams (mg) or 1,000,000 micrograms (μg or mcg).
   10 milligrams of zinc (approximate adult needs) would be a few grains of zinc.
Liters are divided into 1000 units called milliliters (ml).
One teaspoon equals about 5 milliliters (ml), 1 cup is about 240 milliliters, and 1 quart
   (4 cups) equals almost 1 liter (L) (0.946 liter to be exact).

If you plan to work in any scientific field, you will need to learn the metric system. *For now, remember that a kilogram equals 2.2 pounds, an ounce weighs 28 grams, 2.54 centimeters equals 1 inch, and a liter is almost the same as a quart.* In addition, know the fractions that the following prefixes represent: micro (1/1,000,000), milli (1/1000), centi (1/100), and kilo (1000).

CONCEPT CHECK

Nutrition is the study of food and nutrients—their digestion, absorption, and metabolism, and their effect on health and disease. Food contains the vital nutrients essential for good health: carbohydrates, lipids (fats and oils), proteins, vitamins, minerals, and water. Nutrients have three general functions in the body: (1) to provide materials for building and maintaining the body; (2) to act as regulators for key metabolic reactions; and (3) to participate in metabolic reactions that provide the energy necessary to sustain life. A common unit of measurement for this energy is the kilocalorie (kcal). On average, carbohydrates and protein provide 4 kcal per gram of energy to the body, while lipids provide 9 kcal per gram. Although not considered a nutrient, alcohol provides about 7 kcal per gram. The other classes of nutrients (vitamins, minerals, and water) do not supply calories but are essential for proper body functioning.

1.5 What Is the Current State of the North American Diet and Health?

Does Obesity Threaten Our Future?

In 2001, the U.S. Surgeon General issued a Call to Action about the obesity epidemic in America. Over the past 10 years, however, the problem has worsened. Whereas in 2001 61% of U.S. adults were overweight or obese, in 2010 the rates were even higher with 68%, or 190 million people, overweight or obese. A recent report from the Trust for America's Health and the Robert Wood Johnson Foundation indicated that between 2009 and 2010 the percentage of obese adults increased in 16 states and did not decline in any states. Their report, "F as in Fat: How Obesity Threatens America's Future 2011" (July 2011), also revealed that 12 states now have obesity rates above 30%, compared to 2006, when only one state was above 30%. This recent report (Fig. 1-4) is based on self-reported state-by-state obesity data from the Centers for Disease Control and Prevention (CDC) (see Further Reading 16). Because we tend to underreport our

FIGURE 1-4 ▶ Percentage of adults who are obese,* by state, 2009.

*Body mass index (BMI) ≥ 30, or about 30 pounds overweight for a 5' 4" person, based on self-reported weight and height.

Source: CDC, Behavioral Risk Factor Surveillance System.

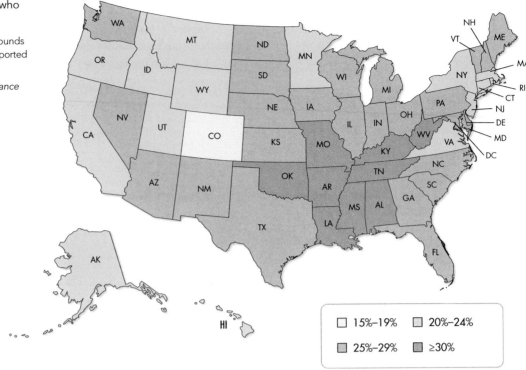

Legend: □ 15%–19% □ 20%–24% ■ 25%–29% ■ ≥30%

weight, the percentage of Americans who are obese is probably greater than reported. Even more alarming are the statistics for children. In 2001 nearly 12% of children and adolescents were overweight, whereas in 2010 nearly one-third of children and teens fell into these categories.

It is well documented that this extra weight of more than 4.5 billion extra pounds has and will continue to have dangerous consequences. In an earlier section of this chapter, we already pointed out that obesity plays a role in chronic illness, including heart disease, stroke, high blood pressure, high cholesterol, diabetes, arthritis, and certain cancers. It is estimated that obesity kills more than 110,000 Americans a year. Because of its role in so many chronic disorders, obesity is also an expensive condition. More than $150 billion is spent annually on health care related to obesity, and obesity costs U.S. employers $73 billion in lost productivity every year. It has become obvious that the answers to the obesity crisis are not simple. From a nutrition perspective, however, the problem can be clearly stated. Most of us continue to eat too much, especially foods with a high number of calories and a low number of nutrients, and we do not engage in enough physical activity.

Assessing the Current North American Diet

With the aim of finding out what North Americans eat, federal agencies conduct surveys to collect data about food and nutrient consumption, as well as connections between diet and health. In the United States, the U.S. Department of Health and Human Services monitors food consumption with the National Health and Nutrition Examination Survey (NHANES). In Canada, this information is gathered by Health Canada in conjunction with Agriculture and Agrifood Canada. Survey data indicate that North American adults consume about 15% of their calorie intake as proteins, 52% as carbohydrates, and 33% as fats. These percentages, which do not consider alcohol, fall within the ranges recommended by the Food and Nutrition Board (FNB) of the National Academy of Sciences. The FNB advocates that 10%

to 35% of calories come from protein, 45% to 65% from carbohydrate, and 20% to 35% from fat. These standards apply to people in both the United States and Canada.

Food-consumption data also indicate that animal sources supply about two-thirds of protein intake for most North Americans, whereas plant sources supply only about one-third. In many other parts of the world, it is just the opposite: plant proteins—from rice, beans, corn, and other grains and vegetables—dominate protein intake. About half the carbohydrate in North American diets comes from simple sugars; the other half comes from starches (such as in pastas, breads, and potatoes). About 60% of dietary fat comes from animal sources and 40% from plant sources.

Results from national nutrition surveys and other studies show that North Americans consume more calories than ever before and from a wide variety of foods. Individuals, however, often do not choose the foods that will meet all their nutrient needs. Food availability data from 1909 to 2007 confirm that the major contributors to increased energy intake over the last century are oils, shortening, meat, cheese, and frozen desserts. Since 1970 there has been an increase in added sweeteners, and carbonated beverage availability has increased at the expense of milk.

In the next section, we discuss recommendations to consume a variety of nutrient-dense foods within and across the food groups, especially whole grains, fruits, vegetables, low-fat or fat-free milk or milk products, and lean meats and other protein sources. These foods will provide nutrients that are often overlooked, including various B vitamins, vitamin C (especially for smokers), vitamin D, vitamin E, calcium, potassium, magnesium, iron, fiber, and many phytonutrients. Daily intake of a balanced multivitamin and mineral supplement is another strategy to help meet nutrient needs but does not make up for a poor diet, particularly for calcium, potassium, and fiber intake. Also keep in mind that taking numerous dietary supplements can lead to health problems (see Nutrition and Your Health in Chapter 10).

Routinely, experts also recommend that we pay more attention to balancing calorie intake with needs. An excess intake of calories is usually tied to overindulgence in sugar, fat, and alcoholic beverages. African-Americans and Hispanics have a greater chance of developing hypertension than do other ethnic groups in North America and therefore may need to decrease the amount of **salt** (sodium chloride) and alcohol in their diets. These substances are two of the many factors linked to hypertension. Moderation of salt and alcohol intake—along with certain fats, cholesterol, and total calorie intake—is a recommended practice for all adults.

Many North Americans would benefit from a healthier balance of food in their diets. Moderation is the key for some foods, such as sugared soft drinks and fried foods. For other foods, such as fruits and vegetables, increased quantity and variety are warranted. Few adults currently meet the new recommendation to "fill half your plate with fruits and vegetables" promoted in the new USDA MyPlate guidelines for total servings of vegetables and fruits.

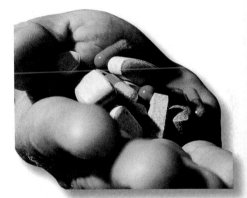

▲ Taking numerous nutrient supplements can lead to health problems. Nutrition and Your Health in Chapter 10 will explore the appropriate and safe use of nutrient supplements in detail.

salt Compound of sodium and chloride in a 40:60 ratio.

Health Objectives for the United States for the Year 2020

Health promotion and disease prevention have been public health strategies in North America for the past three decades. One part of this strategy is *Healthy People 2020*, a report issued in December 2010 by the U.S. Department of Health and Human Services' (DHHS) Public Health Service. Every 10 years, DHHS issues a collection of health objectives for the nation. These objectives are developed by experts in federal agencies and target major public health concerns, setting goals for the coming decade. *Healthy People 2020* sets forth more than 600 health objectives across 42 topic areas and outlines national standards to eliminate health disparities, improve access to health education and quality health care, and strengthen public health services. The vision for 2020 is a society in which all people live long, healthy lives. Important new features of *Healthy People 2020* include a focus on health equity and social determinants of health, and a move to an interactive, personalized website at www.HealthyPeople.gov.

The overarching goals of *Healthy People 2020* aim to:

- Attain high-quality, longer lives free of preventable disease, disability, injury, and premature death.
- Achieve health equity, eliminate disparities, and improve health of all groups.
- Create social and physical environments that promote good health for all.
- Promote quality of life, healthy development, and healthy behaviors across all life stages.

Healthy People 2020, like earlier versions, includes a topic area specific to nutrition. This topic is called Nutrition and Weight Status, and its objectives target individual behaviors, as well as the policies and environments that support these behaviors. Nutrition and weight status is important because a healthful diet helps us reduce our risks for numerous health conditions that burden the public health system, including heart disease, high blood pressure, diabetes, osteoporosis, and some cancers. Good nutrition for children is also emphasized in this report because of its importance for growth and development. The goal of this topic is to promote health and reduce chronic disease risk through the consumption of healthful diets and achievement and maintenance of healthy body weights. This goal also includes increasing household food security and eliminating hunger.

The Nutrition and Weight Status objectives are based on strong science that supports the health benefits of eating a healthful diet and maintaining a healthy body weight. A healthful diet is described as one that includes:

- Consuming a variety of nutrient-dense foods within and across the food groups, especially whole grains, fruits, vegetables, low-fat or fat-free milk or milk products, and lean meats and other protein sources
- Limiting intake of solid fats, cholesterol, added sugars, sodium (salt), and alcohol
- Limiting intake of calories to meet needs for calories

The objectives also emphasize that individual behaviors, as well as the policies and environments that support these behaviors in settings such as schools, worksites, health care organizations, and communities, should be addressed in any efforts to change diet and weight.

Table 1-5 is a list of the six categories of objectives for the Nutrition and Weight Status topic, along with the the 22 specific objectives. Table 1-6 provides a more detailed sample of nine of the specific Nutrition and Weight Status objectives along with the current status of these objectives and their targets for 2020.

Other new topic areas highlight changes in the health needs of specific segments of the population: Early and Middle Childhood, Adolescence, and Older Adults. Because young people develop habits, including eating and physical activity behaviors, which are likely to persist throughout life, new objectives promote strengthened health education in schools and communities and fostering an environment in which young people can develop healthy habits. Older adults are the fastest-growing segment of the American population and are at high risk for experiencing the chronic health problems that so severely impact our health care system. The objectives for Older Adults include improving access to health care, helping older adults to manage their own health conditions, and ensuring proper training and support of professionals and nonprofessionals who care for this population.

A scientifically exciting new topic area is **Genomics.** Nine of the ten leading causes of death have a strong genetic component. Genetic testing is becoming a

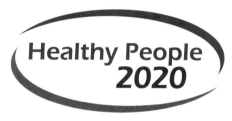

▲ Many nutrition-related objectives are part of the *Healthy People 2020* report. The report outlines health promotion and disease prevention objectives for the United States for the year 2020.

TABLE 1-5 *Healthy People 2020*: Nutrition and Weight Status Objectives

Category 1: Healthier Food Access

1. Increase the number of states with nutrition standards for child care.

2. Increase the proportion of schools that offer nutritious foods and beverages outside of school meals.

3. Increase the number of states that have incentive policies for food retail to provide foods that are encouraged by the 2010 Dietary Guidelines for Americans.

4. Increase the proportion of Americans who have retail access to foods recommended by the 2010 Dietary Guidelines for Americans.

Category 2: Health Care and Worksite Settings

5. Increase the proportion of primary care physicians who measure patients' body mass index (BMI).

6. Increase the proportion of physician office visits that include nutrition or weight counseling or education.

7. Increase the proportion of worksites that offer nutrition and weight-management classes and counseling.

Category 3: Weight Status

8. Increase the proportion of adults who are at a healthy weight.

9. Reduce the proportion of adults who are obese.

10. Reduce the proportion of children and adolescents who are considered obese.

11. Prevent inappropriate weight gain in youth and adults.

Category 4: Food Insecurity

12. Eliminate very low food security among children.

13. Reduce household food insecurity and in so doing reduce hunger.

Category 5: Food and Nutrient Consumption

14. Increase the contribution of fruits to the diets of the population ages 2 years and older.

15. Increase the variety and contribution of vegetables to the diets of the population ages 2 years and older.

16. Increase the contribution of whole grains to the diets of the population ages 2 years and older.

17. Reduce consumption of calories from solid fats and added sugars in the population ages 2 years and older.

18. Reduce consumption of saturated fat in the population ages 2 years and older.

19. Reduce consumption of sodium in the population ages 2 years and older.

Category 6: Iron Deficiency

20. Increase consumption of calcium in the population ages 2 years and older.

21. Reduce iron deficiency among young children and females of childbearing age.

22. Reduce iron deficiency among pregnant females.

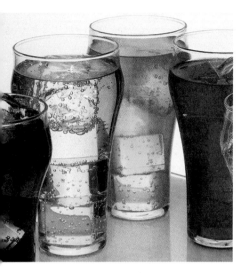

▲ Moderation in the intake of some foods, such as sugared soft drinks and fried foods, can lead to a healthier balance of food in the North American diet.

TABLE 1-6 A Sample of Nutrition and Weight Status Objectives from *Healthy People 2020* along with Details about the Current Status and Targets for 2020

	Target	Current Estimate
Increase the proportion of adults at a healthy weight.	33.9%	30.8%
Reduce the proportion of overweight or obese children and adolescents.	14.6%	16.2%
Increase the contribution of the following to the diets of the population ages 2 years and older (per 1000 calories).		
• Fruits	0.9 cup	0.5 cup
• Total vegetables	1.1 cups	0.8 cup
• Whole grains	0.6 ounce	0.3 ounce
Reduce consumption of calories from solid fats (of total calorie intake).	16.7%	18.9%
Reduce consumption of calories from added sugars (of total calorie intake).	10.8%	15.7%
Increase consumption of calcium in the population ages 2 years and older.	1300 mg	1118 mg
Reduce iron deficiency among females of childbearing age.	9.4%	10.4%

Note: In later chapters, we will explore additional nutrition-related objectives, such as those addressing osteoporosis, various forms of cancer, diabetes prevention and treatment, food allergies, cardiovascular disease, low birth weight, nutrition during pregnancy, breastfeeding, eating disorders, physical activity, and alcohol use.

valuable tool for improving diagnosis and treatment of chronic diseases, especially for cancers of the breast and colon. In combination with family history, genetic testing can help health care professionals guide patients in treatment options, including lifestyle changes. The relationship between genetics and nutrition will be discussed in Chapter 3.

1.6 What Can You Expect from Good Nutrition and a Healthy Lifestyle?

The obesity epidemic in the United States illustrates that something is not right with many of our diets and/or lifestyles. The strong association between obesity and poor health is clear. The reverse is also well documented—when an obese or overweight person loses just 5% to 10% of body weight, that person's risks of many chronic diseases are greatly reduced.

Because weight gain is one of the greatest lifelong nutrition challenges we face, we encourage you to seek a lifestyle that will make gaining weight more difficult and maintaining a healthy weight easier. Believe it or not, preventing obesity in the first place is the easiest approach. Unfortunately, many aspects of our society make it hard for us not to gain weight. The earlier (preferably in childhood) we develop lifestyle habits of good nutrition, regular physical activity, and the avoidance of addictions to salt, fat, sweets, high-calorie foods, and sedentary lifestyles, the better (see

Further Readings 14 and 15). As you enter the workforce, seek out employers who offer wellness programs that encourage weight management and weight loss among their employees. Aim to live in a city or town that has opportunities for physical activity such as bike paths, walking trails, and parks, as well as access to fresh fruits and vegetables through farmers' markets and community gardens. Seek out organizations that offer running or walking clubs. Make a habit of shopping at grocery stores that offer a good selection of fruits, vegetables, and other healthy foods. When dining out, choose restaurants that have tasty but healthy options on their menu. While we still are choosing foods with too many calories, many other dietary habits have improved during the past decade. Today we can choose from a tremendous variety of food products, the result of continual innovation by food manufacturers. We are eating more breakfast cereals, pizza, pasta entrees, stir-fried meats and vegetables served on rice, salads, tacos, burritos, and fajitas than ever before. Sales of whole milk are down, and sales of fat-free and 1% low-fat milk have increased. Consumption of frozen vegetables rather than canned vegetables is also on the rise. Despite the alarming problem of overweight and obesity, our cultural diversity, varied cuisines, and general lack of nutrient deficiencies should be points of pride for North Americans.

Today, North Americans live longer than ever and enjoy better general health. Many also have more money and more diverse food and lifestyle choices to consider. The nutritional consequences of these trends are varied. Deaths from cardiovascular disease, for example, have dropped dramatically since the late 1960s, partly because of better medical care and diets. Affluence, however, has also led to sedentary lifestyles and high intakes of animal fat, cholesterol, salt, and alcohol. This lifestyle pattern has led to problems such as cardiovascular disease, hypertension, diabetes, and, of course, obesity. Greater efforts are needed by the general public to lower intake of animal fat and cholesterol and to improve variety in our diets, especially from fruits, vegetables, and whole grains. With better technology and greater choices, we can have a much better diet today than ever before—if we know what choices to make.

Nutrition experts generally agree that there are no "good" or "bad" foods, but some foods provide relatively few nutrients in comparison to calorie content. In Chapter 2, you will learn that an individual's total diet is the proper focus in a nutritional evaluation. Health experts have prepared many reports and outlined numerous objectives to get us closer to being a *Healthy People* as soon as 2020. In Chapter 2, we will discuss the new "Dietary Guidelines" that were published in 2010, and the new interactive program called "ChooseMyPlate.gov" that was unveiled in 2011. As you reexamine your nutritional habits, remember your health is largely your responsibility. Your body has a natural ability to heal itself. Offer it what it needs, and it will serve you well. Confusing and conflicting health messages hinder diet change. Nutrition science does not have all the answers, but as you will see, enough is known to help you set a path to good health and put diet-related recommendations you hear in the future into perspective. Table 1-7 summarizes several diet, physical activity, and general lifestyle recommendations to promote your health and prevent chronic diseases in the future. In total, these contribute to maximal health and prevention of the diseases listed. The final section in Chapter 1, Nutrition and Your Health: Eating Well in College, elaborates on several nutrition issues very relevant to most college students, including the "freshman 15," vegetarianism, fuel for athletes, eating disorders, and alcohol and binge drinking. This section gives you a "sneak peek" at issues that will be covered more fully later in the book.

▼ A healthy diet benefits people of all ages.

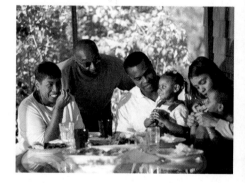

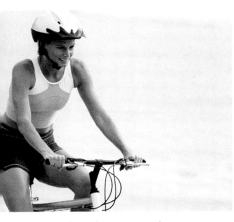

▲ Regular physical activity complements a healthy diet. Whether it is all at once or in segments throughout the day, incorporate 30 to 60 minutes or more of such activity into your daily routine.

TABLE 1-7 Recommendations for Health Promotion and Disease Prevention

Diet

Consuming enough essential nutrients, including fiber, while moderating energy, solid fat, cholesterol, added sugar, and alcohol intake can result in:

- Increased bone mass during childhood and adolescence
- Prevention of some adult bone loss and osteoporosis, especially in older adults
- Fewer dental caries
- Prevention of digestive problems, such as constipation
- Decreased susceptibility to some cancers
- Decreased degradation of the retina (intake of green and orange vegetables, in particular)
- Lower risk of obesity and related diseases, such as type 2 diabetes and cardiovascular disease
- Reduced risk for deficiency diseases, such as cretinism (lack of iodide), scurvy (lack of vitamin C), and anemia (lack of iron, folate, or other nutrients)

Physical Activity

Adequate, regular physical activity (at least 30 minutes on most or all days) helps reduce the risk of:

- Obesity
- Type 2 diabetes
- Cardiovascular disease
- Some adult bone loss and loss of muscle tone
- Premature aging
- Certain cancers

Lifestyle

Minimizing alcohol intake (no more than two drinks per day for men and one drink for both women and all adults age 65 years and older) helps prevent:

- Liver disease
- Accidents

Not smoking cigarettes or cigars helps prevent:

- Lung cancer, other lung disease, kidney disease, cardiovascular disease, and degenerative eye diseases

In addition, minimum use of medication, no illicit drug use, adequate sleep (7 to 8 hours), adequate water and related fluid intake (9 to 13 cups per day), and a reduction in stress (practice better time management, relax, listen to music, have a massage, and stay physically active) provide a more complete approach to good nutrition and health. Add to this maintaining close relationships with others and a positive outlook on life. Finally, consultation with health care professionals on a regular basis is important. This is because early diagnosis is especially useful for controlling the damaging effects of many diseases. Prevention of disease is an important investment of one's time, including during the college years.

CONCEPT CHECK

Surveys in the United States and Canada show that we generally have a variety of foods available to us. However, some of us could improve our diets by focusing on food sources rich in various vitamins, minerals, and fiber. In addition, many of us should reduce our consumption of calories, added sugar, protein, solid fat, cholesterol, salt, and alcoholic beverages. These recommendations are consistent with an overall goal to attain and maintain good health.

Eating Well in College

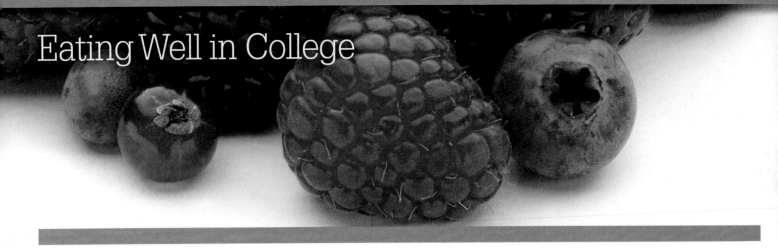

The college years are a time for freedom and a chance to make personal lifestyle decisions. Studies show that the diets of college students are not optimal. Typically, students fall short of diet recommendations for whole grains, vegetables, fruits, milk, and meat, opting instead to max out on fats, sweets, and alcohol. This information is disturbing because young adulthood is the time when many health behaviors are formed that will persist throughout life.

What is it about the college lifestyle that makes it so difficult to build healthy habits? In this section we will discuss several topics and provide possible solutions.

Food Choices

College students face changes in academic requirements, interpersonal relationships, and living environment. These stressful situations contribute to poor health behaviors. For example, when writing papers and cramming for exams, balanced meals are all-too-easily replaced by high-fat and

▼ Late-night pizza can add extra calories to the college student's daily intake.

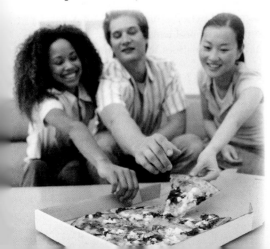

high-calorie fast-foods; convenience items; and sugary, caffeinated beverages. Physical activity is sacrificed in favor of study time.

Also consider that on campus, you are faced with a wide variety of dining choices. Dining halls, fast-food establishments, bars, and vending machines combine to offer food 24 hours per day. While it is certainly possible to make wise food choices at each of these outlets, the temptations of convenience, taste, and value (i.e., inexpensive, oversized portions) may persuade the college student to select unhealthy options.

Meals and snacks are also times to socialize. You may feel pressured to eat a big lunch at noon without regard to hunger if your peers are meeting in the dining hall to catch up. While chatting, it is easy to lose track of portions and to overeat. In addition, food may be a source of familiarity and comfort in a new and stressful place.

Weight Control and the "Freshman Fifteen"

Studies show that most college students gain weight during their first year (see Further Reading 5). The "freshman fifteen" is a term used to describe the weight gained by students during their first year of college. Although most freshman do not gain the fifteen pounds, a recent study of U.S. and Canadian college students found that students pack on 6 to 9 pounds their first year away from home. Although calorie intake does not increase significantly, dramatic increases in beer drinking and significant decreases in physical activity are key reasons for the weight gain (see Further Reading 8).

There are several reasons to maintain a healthy weight. Over the long term, risk of chronic diseases goes up as weight increases. In the short term, losing excess weight can improve how you feel and perform. Detecting "flab" around your midsection or feeling that your clothes are getting tighter are two good indicators that you are carrying excess weight. If weight loss is necessary, with some knowledge and perseverance, you can safely lose excess pounds.

Behavioral research clearly demonstrates that setting several small, achievable goals will spur motivation. As you will learn in Chapter 7, body weight is a balancing act between calories in and calories burned. Try keeping track of your calorie consumption for several days and comparing that to your energy needs, based on your age, gender, and activity level. You can use one of the equations presented in Chapter 7 or take advantage of the interactive tools on www.Choose MyPlate.gov to estimate your energy needs.

A healthy rate of weight loss is one to two pounds per week. Greater rates of weight loss will not likely be sustained over time. Remember that the numbers on the scale are not as important as your body composition—the amount of fat in relation to lean mass. One pound of weight loss requires a deficit of 3500 kilocalories. Thus, to lose one pound per week, you will need to cut back on food intake and/or increase your exercise routine to shift the energy balance equation by 500 kilocalories per day.

Although many students skip breakfast, breakfast is the *most* important meal of the day. Starting the day off with a fortified,

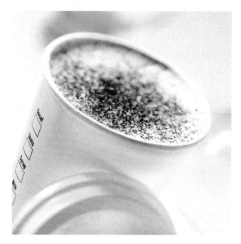

▲ Research (see Further Reading 13) has shown that gourmet coffee beverages, such as lattes and cappuccinos, can increase calorie consumption by about 200 kcal per day.

whole-grain breakfast cereal, skim milk, and a serving of fruit puts you on the right path for meeting recommendations for fiber, calcium, and fruit intake. Even though it may seem that coffee gets your brain going in the morning, your brain is fueled best by carbohydrates, not caffeine. Studies also show that eating breakfast prevents overeating later in the day. Read more about breakfast choices in the *What Would You Choose* recommendations at the end of this chapter.

One of the biggest contributors to weight gain for college students is consuming several hundred calories per day

▶ **Five Simple Tips to Avert Weight Gain**

- *Eat breakfast.* Rev up your metabolism with a protein source such as an egg or low-fat yogurt, at least one serving of whole grains such as a breakfast cereal, and a fruit such as a banana.

- *Plan ahead.* Eat a balanced meal or snack every 3 to 4 hours.

- *Limit liquid calories.* Drink water instead of high-calorie soft drinks, fruit juice, alcohol, or coffee; if you drink alcohol, limit it to 1 or 2 drinks per day.

- *Stock the fridge.* Keep a stash of low-calorie, nutritious snacks, such as pretzels, light microwave popcorn, fruit (fresh, canned, or dried).

- *Exercise regularly.* Find a friend to work out with you. Experts recommend 30 minutes of moderate exercise at least 5 days a week.

in sugary or alcoholic beverages. One 12-ounce can of regular cola contains about 140 kcal. A 12-ounce can of regular beer has 150 kcal. Consuming gourmet coffee beverages, such as lattes and cappuccinos can increase average calorie consumption by about 200 kilocalories per day (see Further Reading 13). Even fruit juices have at least 100 kcal per 8-ounce glass. Furthermore, a 24-ounce mug of a soft drink makes you feel no fuller than an equal volume of water, yet the soft drink adds 300 kcal more. A convenient stash of water is the best way to quench your thirst.

Exercise is very important to any weight loss and weight maintenance plan but sticking with it is hard to do. When you find yourself short on time, exercise is often the first thing we sacrifice. To ensure your success at boosting daily activity, choose activities you enjoy such as working out with friends at the campus recreation center, participating in intramural sports, or taking an activity class like dancing. Don't forget the brisk walking to and from classes. For more information on planning an exercise program, see Chapter 10.

Alcohol and Binge Drinking

Excessive alcohol consumption is a big problem on college campuses. Legal or not, many college students consider drinking alcohol to be a "rite of passage" into adulthood. On campuses, binge drinking—consuming five or more drinks in a row for men, or four drinks or more for women—has become an epidemic. A new level of "extreme drinking" goes far beyond binge drinking. For example, recent studies indicate that college students celebrate twenty-first birthdays with an average of 12 drinks for men and nine for women (see Further Reading 12).

The statistics on the impact of binge drinking on college campuses are sobering. An estimated two of every five students on college campuses participates in binge drinking. Each year, 1400 college students between the ages of 18 and 24 die from alcohol-related unintentional injuries, including motor vehicle crashes. In addition to deaths and injuries, other problems stemming from binge drinking include unsafe sex and its consequences, long-term health problems, suicides, academic problems, legal troubles, and

alcohol abuse or dependence. Thirty-one percent of college students meet the criteria for a diagnosis of alcohol abuse.

In addition alcohol consumption definitely contributes to weight gain—by virtue of its own calories and the increased food consumption at events where drinking occurs. If you choose to drink alcohol, do so in moderation—no more than two drinks per day for men and one drink per day for women. Be aware of the warning signs and dangers of alcohol poisoning shown in the margin. Excessive alcohol intake, has many long-term health and nutrition implications that are covered in Chapter 16.

Eating Disorders

As many as 30% of college students are at risk of developing an eating disorder. As you will learn in Chapter 13, disordered eating is a mild and short-term change in eating patterns that typically occurs in response to life stress, a desire to change appearance, or a bad habit. Sometimes, disordered eating habits may lead to an eating disorder, such as anorexia nervosa, bulimia nervosa, or binge-eating disorder. Chapter 13 includes advice on what to do if you suspect that your roommate or friend is suffering from an eating disorder.

Starving the body also starves the brain, limiting performance in academics and beyond, and the negative consequences of disordered eating may last a lifetime. Ultimately, eating disorders do not arise from problems with food but rather from problems with self-esteem, control, and abusive relationships. Frequently, what begins as a diet spirals into a much larger problem. Eating disorders are not just diets gone bad—they require professional intervention. Left unchecked, eating disorders lead to serious adverse effects, such as loss of menstrual periods, thinning of bones, gastrointestinal problems, kidney problems, heart abnormalities, and eventually death.

Choosing a Vegetarian Lifestyle

Many college students experiment with or adopt a vegetarian eating pattern. Plant-based diets can meet nutrition needs and decrease risk of many chronic diseases, but they require appropriate planning at all life stages.

Protein is not typically deficient, even with a vegan diet, which contains no animal products. However, vegetarians, and especially vegans, may be at risk for deficiencies of several vitamins and minerals. Consuming a ready-to-eat breakfast cereal is an easy and inexpensive way to obtain these nutrients. See Chapter 6 for more information on vegetarian food planning.

Restaurants and campus dining services have responded to the growing interest in vegetarian meals by offering a variety of vegetarian options. For optimal health benefits, choose foods that are baked, steamed, or stir-fried rather than deep-fried; select whole grains rather than refined carbohydrates; and consume food fortified with vitamins and minerals. Even if you do not follow a plant-based diet all the time, choosing several plant-based meals each week can help with weight control and boost intake of fiber and healthy phytochemicals. You will learn in Chapter 2 that the new ChooseMyPlate program recommends that the largest portion of your plate be filled with plant foods, including whole grains, fruits and vegetables.

Fuel for Competition: Student Athletes

Students who compete in sports such as intramural and intercollegiate athletics need to consume more calories and nutrients. Despite an emphasis on a lean physique athletes at all levels must take care not to severely restrict calories, as this could impact performance and health. Muscles require adequate carbohydrates for fuel and protein for growth and repair. Fat, as well, is an important source of stored energy for use during exercise. Low levels of body fat in women may lead to amenorrhea (cease menstruating), a condition costly to long-term bone health.

In addition to fueling the body with calories, fluids are essential for health and performance. While water is adequate for events lasting less than 60 minutes, sports drinks are ideal for longer events because they supply carbohydrates to fuel fatigued muscles as well as electrolytes to replenish those lost in perspiration. Intentional fluid losses to "make weight" for a competition are detrimental to health and performance.

Athletes also should take care not to be wooed by the supplement industry.

Increasing food intake to meet the energy demands of athletic training is usually sufficient to also meet vitamin and mineral needs. As an exception, athletes may be at risk for iron-deficiency anemia. Consuming a balanced multivitamin and mineral supplement is adequate for most people. Individual vitamin, mineral, amino acid, or herbal supplements are not advised, in spite of the hype of supplement makers.

Tips for Eating Well on a College Student's Budget

Because higher education can be hard on the wallet it is good to know that it is possible to eat well on campus on a budget. If you live on campus, participate in a prepaid campus meal plan (see Further Reading 1). These are generally designed to offer great food value with a variety of healthy foods. If you live off campus or have your own kitchen, plan ahead. Packing a lunch from home will save a lot of cash compared to grabbing lunch on the run and puts you more in control of healthy choices. For example, preparing a sandwich at home costs less than half as much as purchasing one at a fast-food restaurant or deli.

Never go grocery shopping on an empty stomach—everything will look good and you'll buy more. Also, go to the store with a list in hand and stick to it, because impulse buys tend to drain your wallet. Buy store-brand foods rather than name-brand items. Make use of canned and frozen fruits and vegetables—they are just as nutritious as fresh fruits and vegetables, particularly if you choose low-sodium and low-sugar varieties. Rather than buying cartons of fruit juice, select cans of fruit juice concentrate and mix with water at home. Likewise, preparing other drinks, such as iced tea, from store-brand powder (look for sugar-free) will save over gallon jugs or vending machine containers of drinks. Canned (fruits, tuna) and dry (oatmeal) foods can be nutritious and last a long time, so you can avoid throwing out spoiled items. Finally, eggs and peanut butter are inexpensive and simple sources of protein.

In conclusion, *The College Student's Guide to Eating Well on Campus* (see Further Reading 10) and *The Dorm Room Diet* (see Further Reading 11) are excellent books with more details on ways college students can plan a healthy diet and stay fit.

▶ **The warning signs and symptoms of alcohol poisoning**

- Semiconsciousness or unconsciousness
- Slow respiration of eight or fewer breaths per minute or lapses between breaths of more than 8 seconds
- Cold, clammy, pale, or bluish skin
- Strong odor of alcohol, which usually accompanies these symptoms

Some calorie traps for college students:

	Number of Calories
Six-pack of regular beer	900
Two handfuls of almonds	500
Two handfuls of granola	330
Personal-size pizza	500 to 600
1 cup of ice cream	300
Two handfuls of frosted cereal	250

Source: Ann Litt, The College Student's Guide to Eating Well on Campus

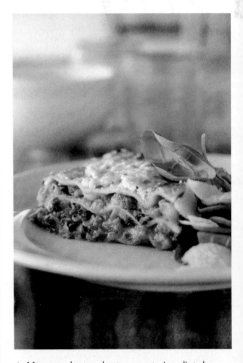

▲ Many students adopt a vegetarian diet during college. Guidelines for planning a nutritious vegetarian diet, with items such as this veggie lasagna, and spinach salad are presented in Chapter 6.

Case Study Typical College Student

Andy is like many other college students. He grew up on a quick bowl of cereal and milk for breakfast and a hamburger, French fries, and cola for lunch, either in the school cafeteria or at a local fast-food restaurant. At dinner, he generally avoided eating any of his salad or vegetables, and by 9 o'clock he was deep into bags of chips and cookies. Andy has taken most of these habits to college. He prefers coffee for breakfast and possibly a chocolate bar. Lunch is still mainly a hamburger, French fries, and cola, but pizza and tacos now alternate more frequently than when he was in high school. One thing Andy really likes about the restaurants surrounding campus is that, for less than a dollar more, he can make his hamburger a double or get extra cheese and pepperoni on his pizza. This helps him stretch his food dollar; searching out large-portion value meals for lunch and dinner now has become part of a typical day.

Provide some dietary advice for Andy. Start with his positive habits and then provide some constructive criticism, based on what you now know.

Answer the following questions, and check your responses in Appendix A.

1. **Start with Andy's positive habits:** What healthy choices are being made when Andy eats at local restaurants?

2. **Now provide some constructive criticisms:**

   a. What are some of the negative aspects of items available at fast-food restaurants?
   b. Why is ordering the "value meals" a dangerous habit?
   c. What healthier substitutions could he make at each meal?
   d. List some healthier choices he could make at fast-food restaurants on campus.

Summary (Numbers refer to numbered sections in the chapter.)

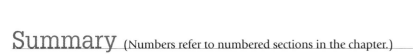

1.1 The flavor, texture, and appearance of foods primarily influence our food choices. Several other factors also help determine food habits and choices: food availability and convenience; early childhood experiences and ethnic customs; nutrition and health concerns; advertising; restaurants; social changes; and economics. A variety of external (appetite-related) forces affect satiety (feeling of satisfaction that halts our desire to continue eating). Hunger cues combine with appetite cues, such as easy availability of food, to promote food intake.

1.2 Nutrition is a lifestyle factor that is a key to developing and maintaining an optimal state of health. A poor diet and a sedentary lifestyle are known to be risk factors for life-threatening chronic diseases such as heart disease, hypertension, diabetes, and cancer. Not meeting nutrient needs in younger years makes us more likely to suffer health consequences in later years. Too much of a nutrient also can be harmful. Drinking too much alcohol is another dietary problem associated with many health problems.

1.3 Nutrition is the study of the food substances vital for health and the study of how the body uses these substances to promote and support growth, maintenance, and reproduction of cells. Nutrients in foods fall into six classes: (1) carbohydrates, (2) lipids (mostly fats and oils), (3) proteins, (4) vitamins, (5) minerals, and (6) water. The first three, along with alcohol, provide calories for the body to use.

1.4 The body transforms the energy contained in carbohydrate, protein, and fat into other forms of energy that in turn allow the body to function. Fat provides, on average, 9 kcal per gram, whereas both protein and carbohydrate provide, on average, 4 kcal per gram. Vitamins, minerals, and water do not supply calories to the body but are essential for proper body function.

1.5 The overweight and obesity problem has worsened with 68% of people in the United States (190 million people) reported to be overweight or obese in 2010. This increase is a result of eating too much, especially foods with a high number of calories and a low number of nutrients, and not engaging in enough physical activity. Results from large nutrition surveys in the United States and Canada suggest that some of us need to concentrate on consuming foods that supply more of certain vitamins, minerals, and fiber. *Healthy People 2020* is a national initiative that includes Nutrition and Weight Status objectives related to eating a healthful diet and maintaining a healthy body weight. A healthful diet includes consuming a variety of nutrient-dense foods within and across the food groups, especially whole grains, fruits, vegetables, low-fat or fat-free milk or milk products, and lean meats and other protein sources; limiting intake of solid fats, cholesterol, added sugars, sodium (salt), and alcohol; and limiting intake of calories to meet energy needs.

1.6 A basic plan for health promotion and disease prevention includes eating a varied diet, performing regular physical activity, not smoking, not abusing nutrient supplements (if used), consuming adequate water and other fluids, getting enough sleep, limiting alcohol intake (if consumed), and limiting or appropriately coping with stress. The primary focus of nutrition planning should be on food, not on dietary supplements. The focus on foods to supply nutrient needs avoids the possibility of severe nutrient imbalances.

1.7 Studies show that the diets and other health habits of college students are not optimal. Students fall short of recommendations for servings of grains, vegetables, fruits, milk, and meat, opting instead for fats, sweets, and alcohol. This information is disturbing from a public health standpoint, because young adulthood is the time when many health behaviors are formed and will likely persist throughout life. Issues of particular importance on college campuses are weight control, making healthy meal choices, alcohol and binge drinking, and eating disorders.

Check Your Knowledge (Answers to the following multiple choice questions are below.)

1. Our primary psychological drive to eat that is affected by many external food-choice mechanisms is called
   a. hunger.
   b. appetite.
   c. satiety.
   d. feeding.

2. Energy-yielding nutrients include
   a. vitamins, minerals, and water.
   b. carbohydrates, proteins, and fats.
   c. trace minerals and fat-soluble vitamins.
   d. iron, vitamin C, and potassium.

3. The *essential* nutrients
   a. must be consumed at every meal.
   b. are required for infants but not adults.
   c. can be made in the body when they are needed.
   d. cannot be made by the body and therefore must be consumed to maintain health.

4. Sugars, starches, and dietary fibers are examples of
   a. proteins.
   b. vitamins.
   c. carbohydrates.
   d. minerals.

5. Which nutrient classes are most important in the regulation of body processes?
   a. vitamins
   b. carbohydrates
   c. minerals
   d. lipids
   e. Both a and c.

6. A kcal is a
   a. measure of heat energy.
   b. measure of fat in food.
   c. heating device.
   d. term used to describe the amount of sugar and fat in foods.

7. A food that contains 10 grams of fat would yield _____ kcal.
   a. 40
   b. 70
   c. 90
   d. 120

8. If you consume 300 grams of carbohydrate in a day that you consume 2400 kcal, the carbohydrates will provide _____% of your total energy intake.
   a. 12.5
   b. 30
   c. 50
   d. 60

9. Which of the following is true about the North American diet?
   a. Most of our protein comes from plant sources.
   b. About half of the carbohydrates come from simple sugars.
   c. Most of our fats come from plant sources.
   d. Most of our carbohydrates come from starches.

10. The _____ is a term used to describe the amount of weight college students gain during the first year of college.
    a. varsity 8
    b. stadium 7
    c. dormitory 12
    d. freshman 15

Answer Key: 1. b (LO 1.1), 2. b (LO 1.3), 3. d (LO 1.3), 4. c (LO 1.3), 5. e (LO 1.3), 6. a (LO 1.4), 7. c (LO 1.4), 8. c (LO 1.4), 9. b (LO 1.5), 10. d (LO 1.7)

Study Questions (Numbers refer to Learning Outcomes)

1. Describe the process that controls hunger and satiety in the body. List other factors that influence our food choices. **(LO 1.1)**

2. Describe how your food preferences have been shaped by the following factors:
   a. Exposure to foods at an early age
   b. Advertising (what is the newest food you have tried?)
   c. Eating out
   d. Peer pressure
   e. Economic factors **(LO 1.1)**

3. What products in your supermarket reflect the consumer demand for healthier foods? For convenience? **(LO 1.1)**

4. Name one chronic disease associated with poor nutrition habits. Now list a few corresponding risk factors. **(LO 1.2)**

5. Describe two sources of fat and explain why the differences are important in terms of overall health. **(LO 1.3)**

6. Identify three ways that water is used in the body. **(LO 1.3)**

7. Explain the concept of calories as it relates to foods. What are the values used to calculate kcals from grams of carbohydrate, fat, protein, and alcohol? **(LO 1.4)**

8. Wendy's Big Bacon Classic contains 44 grams carbohydrate, 36 grams fat, and 37 grams protein. Calculate the percentage of calories derived from fat. **(LO 1.4)**

9. According to national nutrition surveys, which nutrients tend to be underconsumed by many North Americans? Why do you think this is the case? **(LO 1.5)**

10. List four *Healthy People 2020* objectives for the United States. How would you rate yourself in each area? Why? **(LO 1.5 & 1.6)**

11. List five strategies to avoid weight gain during college. **(LO 1.7)**

What Would You Choose Recommendations

Even bleary-eyed procrastinators can fuel their bodies for a new day of higher education! *Skipping breakfast is not a smart plan.* After a period of fasting (i.e., overnight), the body and the brain need fuel to operate at peak efficiency. In addition, many research studies demonstrate that eating a sensible breakfast is a good way to control weight. Compared to those who eat breakfast, people who skip breakfast tend to crave higher-calorie foods, snack more throughout the day, and eat more at subsequent meals. Consider eating breakfast each day as part of your plan to fend off the freshman fifteen.

Grab-and-go food options, such as those available in vending machines or from fast-food establishments, are often high in calories but low in nutrients. For example, a low-fat granola bar has only 100 kcal and 3 grams of fat but offers little else in terms of nutrition. Also, a granola bar is not likely to stave off hunger for very long.

On the other hand, a fast-food breakfast sandwich will probably promote satiety but its calorie, fat, and sodium contents are too high. This type of sandwich provides 550 kcal, 23 grams of fat (38% of a day's total kcal in the sandwich and 35% of the

whole day's limit for fat), and 1490 mg sodium (just under the 1500 mg Adequate Intake for this nutrient). A fast-food breakfast sandwich can fit into an otherwise healthy diet on occasion but should not be part of your normal routine.

Keeping nutritious but convenient breakfast options accessible is a good strategy for any time-pressed college student. Whole-grain, fortified, ready-to-eat breakfast cereal with fat-free milk is a great choice: it is quick, provides a wide variety of vitamins and minerals, and boosts fiber intake. Adding a source of protein will help to support body processes and make you feel full for a longer time. Hard-boiled eggs or a handful of dry-roasted nuts provide protein in ready-to-eat form. A cup of low-fat yogurt offers protein with the added benefit of calcium. Fresh and dried fruit are portable and nutritious options for breakfast. Many fruit choices are loaded with potassium and vitamin C, plus they provide fiber. A 1.5-ounce box of raisins, which can be stored for months without a refrigerator, provides about 130 kcal, no fat or cholesterol, very little sodium, 2 grams of fiber, and 320 mg potassium.

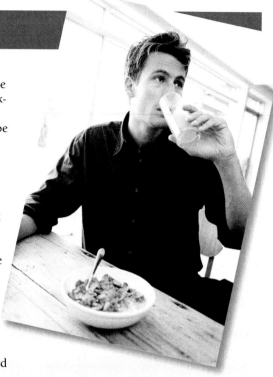

▲ With a little bit of planning, breakfast can be both quick and healthy.

So, the bowl of Wheaties with a banana and low-fat milk along with a yogurt, all from your dorm room "pantry," would be the healthiest choice for most.

Further Readings

1. Brown LB and others: College students can benefit by participating in a prepaid meal plan. *Journal of the American Dietetic Association* 105:445, 2005.

   Participation in a prepaid campus meal plan resulted in modest nutritional benefits to students through an increase in servings of foods from fruit, vegetable, and meat groups.

2. Center for Science in the Public Interest: *Guidelines for Responsible Food Marketing to Children.* Washington, DC, 2005. *www. cspinet.org/marketingguidelines.pdf.*

   These guidelines are written for all companies or organizations who manufacture, sell, market, advertise, or promote food to children. Criteria are provided for marketing food to children in a manner that does not undermine children's diets or harm their health. The guidelines address not only how food is marketed but also which foods are marketed to children.

3. Chiuve SE and others: Adherence to a low-risk, healthy lifestyle and risk of sudden cardiac death among women. *Journal of the American Medical Association* 306: 62, 2011.

   Sudden cardiac death causes more than half of all heart-related deaths and usually occurs as the first sign of heart disease, especially in women. Adherence to a healthy lifestyle and the risk of sudden cardiac death was studied in women from the Nurses' Health Study. Risk of sudden cardiac death dropped by 92% with a combination of the four healthy lifestyles (not smoking, not overweight, exercising 30 minutes/day or longer, and following the Mediterranean Diet). Women who ate a high proportion of vegetables, fruits, nuts, omega-3 fats, and fish, along with moderate amounts of alcohol and small amounts of red meat, had a 40% less risk than women whose diets least resembled this diet. Therefore, a healthy diet along with other healthy lifestyle factors appears to protect women from sudden cardiac death.

4. Choinière CJ, Lando A: *2008 Health and Diet Survey,* Food and Drug Administration, March 2010. *www.fda.gov/Food/Science-Research/ResearchAreas/ConsumerResearch/ucm193895.htm.*

   This report is a snapshot of the nations dietary habits based on the FDA 2008 telephone survey of more than 2500 adults in every state and the District of Columbia. One of the key findings was that more than half of consumers in the United States often read the food label when buying a product for the first time, and they are increasingly aware of the link between diet and heart disease..

5. Edmonds MJ and others: Body weight and percent body fat increase during the transition from high school to university in females. *Journal of the American Dietetic Association* 108:1033, 2008.

   The notion that weight gain occurs during the first year of university was studied in Canadian females making the transition from high school to university. There was a significant increase in body weight of 2.4 kg (5.28 pounds) during the first 6 to 7 months of university. Percent body fat also increased from 23.8% to 25.6%. Although dietary energy (calorie) intake did not increase, a decrease in moderate physical activity was an important predictor of weight. Body weight, therefore, may be modified by lifestyle factors during this formative period.

6. Federal Trade Commission: Marketing food to children and adolescents: A review of industry expenditures, activities, and self-regulation, a report to Congress. July 2008. *http://www.ftc.gov/opa/2008/07/foodmkting .shtm.*

This study by the Federal Trade Commission found that 44 major food and beverage marketers spent $1.6 billion to promote their products to children under 12 and adolescents ages 12 to 17 in the United States in 2006. The report states that food advertising to youth is dominated by advertising campaigns that combine traditional media, such as television, with previously unmeasured forms of marketing, such as packaging, in-store advertising, sweepstakes, and Internet. This advertising often involves cross-promotion with a new movie or popular television program. The report calls for all food companies "to adopt and adhere to meaningful, nutrition-based standards for marketing their products to children under 12."

7. Goris JM and others: Television food advertising and the prevalence of childhood overweight and obesity: A multicountry comparison. *Public Health Nutrition* 13:1003, 2010.

The higher prevalence of childhood obesity in the United States compared to other countries could be explained by greater exposure to TV food advertising. In a study of children ages 6 to 11 years in six countries, the contribution of TV food ads to the occurrence of childhood obesity was greatest for the United States at 16% to 40% and lowest in Great Britain, Sweden, and the Netherlands at 4% to 18%. Children in the United States were exposed to 11.5 minutes/day of TV food ads compared to only 1.8 minutes/day in the Netherlands. The authors conclude that the contribution of TV food ads to the prevalence of childhood obesity is significant in some countries and greatest in the United States.

8. Hoffman DY and others: Changes in body weight and fat mass of men and women in the first year of college: A study of the "freshman 15." *Journal of American College of Health* 55:41, 2006.

It is commonly thought that there is a high risk of gaining 15 pounds of weight during freshman year of college. In this study, changes in body weight and percentage of body fat were measured in first-year college students. Body weight increased by an average of almost 3 pounds (1.3 kilograms) and body fat increased an average of 0.7%. This study, therefore, found that weight and fat gain may occur during the first year of college.

9. Kochanek KD and others: *National Vital Statistics Reports,* Deaths: Preliminary Data for 2009: 59, 2011.

Preliminary U.S. data on deaths, death rates, life expectancy, leading causes of death, and infant mortality for 2009 are presented. Death rates decreased significantly from 2008 to 2009 for 10 of the 15 leading causes of death: heart diseases, cancer, chronic lower respiratory diseases, cerebrovascular diseases, accidents (unintentional injuries), Alzheimer's disease, diabetes mellitus, influenza and pneumonia, septicemia, and assault (homicide).

10. Litt, AS: *The College Student's Guide to Eating Well on Campus.* Tulip Hill Press, Glen Echo, MD, 2005.

This book provides important information on how to survive and eat well during your college years and covers how to avoid and spot eating disorders.

11. Oz D: *The Dorm Room Diet: The 10-Step Program for Creating a Healthy Lifestyle Plan That Really Works.* Newmarket Press, 2010.

This book is written to help students stay fit while at college. The 10-step program shows students how to stop eating out of emotional need; navigate the most common danger zones at school for unhealthy eating; get the exercise you need, even in your small dorm room; choose vitamins and supplements wisely; and relax and rejuvenate amid the stress of college life.

12. Rutledge PC and others: 21st birthday drinking: Extremely extreme. *Journal of Consulting and Clinical Psychology* 76:511, 2008.

A new level of extreme drinking goes beyond the four or five drinks in one sitting defined as "bingeing." At the University of Missouri, a study of 2518 students found 34% of men and 24% of women who imbibed on their 21st birthdays drank 21 alcoholic drinks or more. The authors conclude that interventions shown to be effective with general risky drinking may prove effective in reducing 21st birthday excess.

13. Shields DH and others: Gourmet coffee beverage consumption among college women. *Journal of the American Dietetic Association* 104:650, 2004.

A significant percentage of college women were shown to consume gourmet coffee beverages, which contributed additional calories and fat to their daily dietary intake.

14. Woolf K and others: Physical activity is associated with risk factors for chronic disease across adult women's life cycle. *Journal of the American Dietetic Association* 108:948, 2008.

The results of this study confirm that younger age and greater physical activity across the adult women's life cycle are associated with more favorable serum lipid levels; less inflammation; lower concentrations of insulin, glucose, and leptin in serum; and more favorable body composition. These factors are associated with reduced risk for several chronic diseases including cardiovascular disease, type 2 diabetes, and obesity.

15. U.S. Department of Health and Human Services. 2008 Physical Activity Guidelines for Americans. *www.health.gov/paguidelines.*

Inactivity remains relatively high among American children, adolescents, and adults. These science-based guidelines are designed to help Americans aged six and older use appropriate physical activity to improve their health. The guidelines include information about the health benefits of physical activity; how to do physical activity in a manner that meets the guidelines; how to reduce the risks of activity-related injury; and how to assist others in participating regularly in physical activity.

16. Vital Signs: State-Specific Obesity Prevalence Among Adults—United States, 2009. *Morbidity and Mortality Weekly Report* 59(30), 2010.

Each year state health departments collect obesity data through a series of telephone interviews with U.S. adults. Obesity is defined as body mass index (BMI) of 30 or higher. Prevalence of obesity has increased significantly since 1985. In 2009, nine of these states (Alabama, Arkansas, Kentucky, Louisiana, Mississippi, Missouri, Oklahoma, Tennessee, and West Virginia) had a prevalence of obesity equal to or greater than 30%; 33 states had a prevalence equal to or greater than 25%; only Colorado and the District of Columbia had a prevalence of obesity less than 20%.

17. Yanover T, Sacco WP: Eating beyond satiety and body mass index. *Eating and Weight Disorders* 13:119, 2008.

Eating beyond satiety (EBS), snacking, night eating, and hunger were examined in undergraduate females. EBS was the strongest predictor of body mass and therefore may be a variable to target in interventions to prevent and treat overweight and obesity.

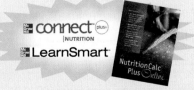

RATE YOUR PLATE

I. Examine Your Eating Habits More Closely

Choose one day of the week that is typical of your eating pattern. Using the first table found in Appendix E, list all foods and drinks you consumed for 24 hours. In addition, write down the approximate amounts of food you ate in units, such as cups, ounces, teaspoons, and tablespoons. After you record the amount of each food and drink consumed, indicate in the table why you chose to consume the item. Place the corresponding abbreviation in the space provided to indicate why you picked that food or drink.

FLVR	Flavor/texture	ADV	Advertisement	PEER	Peers
CONV	Convenience	WTCL	Weight control	NUTR	Nutritive value
EMO	Emotions	HUNG	Hunger	$	Cost
AVA	Availability	FAM	Family/cultural	HLTH	Health

There can be more than one reason for choosing a particular food or drink.

Application

Ask yourself what your most frequent reason is for eating or drinking. To what degree is health or nutritive value a reason for your food choices? Should you make these higher priorities?

II. Observe the Supermarket Explosion

Today's supermarkets carry up to 60,000 items, compared to 20,000 items 10 years ago. Think about your last grocery shopping trip and the items you purchased to eat. Following is a list of 20 newer food products added to supermarket shelves. Check the items that you have tried. Then use the key from Part I of the Rate Your Plate exercise to identify why you might have chosen these products.

_____ Prepackaged salad greens (variety packs other than iceberg lettuce) _____

_____ Gourmet or sprayable salad oils (e.g., walnut, almond, olive, or sesame oil) _____

_____ Gourmet vinegars (e.g., balsamic or rice) _____

_____ Prepackaged lunch products (e.g., nacho, pizza, taco, and tortilla Lunchables) _____

_____ Precooked frozen turkey patties, precooked bacon _____

_____ Bean soup mixes (e.g., lentil, black bean, combination bean soups) _____

_____ Microwavable sandwiches (e.g., Hotpockets, frozen sandwiches) _____

_____ Microwavable meals in a bowl (e.g., mac and cheese, soup) _____

_____ Refrigerated, precooked pasta (e.g., tortellini, fettucini) and accompanying sauces (e.g., pesto, tomato basil) _____
_____

_____ Imported grain products (e.g., risotto, farfalline, gnocchi, fusilli) _____

_____ Whole-grain pasta or rice _____

_____ Frozen dinners (list your favorite of any of the wide variety) _____

_____ Imported sauces for food preparation (e.g., hoisin or brown bean sauce; mandarin marinade, sesame, curry, or fire oils)
_____

_____ Bottled waters (flavored or unflavored) _____

_____ Trendy juices (e.g., draft apple cider, acai, pomegranate) _____

_____ Roasted and/or flavored coffees (e.g., beans, ground, instant, or k-cups) _____

_____ Gourmet jelly beans and candies (e.g., gummi coca-colas or imported chocolates) _____

_____ Instant hot cereal in a bowl (add water and go!) _____

_____ "Fast-shake" pancake mix (add water, shake, and ready to cook) _____

_____ Breakfast bars or cookies (e.g., granola or fruit-flavored bars) _____

_____ Meal replacement/fitness products (e.g., "energy" bars, high-protein bars, sports drinks) _____

_____ Low-carbohydrate meat and pasta dishes _____

_____ Low-calorie muffin tops, bagel thins _____

_____ Packaged yogurt smoothies _____

_____ Milk substitutes (e.g., rice milk, soy milk) _____

Finally, identify three new food products not on this list that you have seen in the past year. Discuss the appeal of these products to the North American consumer.

Chapter 2 Guidelines for Designing a Healthy Diet

Student Learning Outcomes

Chapter 2 is designed to allow you to:

2.1 Develop a healthy eating plan.

2.2 Outline the measurements used (ABCDEs) in nutrition assessment: **A**nthropometric, **B**iochemical, **C**linical, **D**ietary, and **E**nvironmental status.

2.3 Understand the basis of the scientific method as it is used in developing hypotheses and theories in the field of nutrition, including the determination of nutrient needs.

2.4 Describe what the Recommended Dietary Allowances (RDAs) and other dietary standards represent.

2.5 List the purpose and key recommendations of the Dietary Guidelines and the 2008 Physical Activity Guidelines for Americans.

2.6 Exemplify a meal that conforms to MyPlate recommendations.

2.7 Describe the components of the Nutrition Facts panel and the various health claims and label descriptors that are allowed.

2.8 Identify reliable sources of nutrition information.

What Would You Choose?

Living and learning in close quarters make it easy to share germs when flu season rolls around. You have heard that vitamin C supports the immune system, helping your body to fight infections. Many varieties of fruit juice and other beverages contain 100% of the Daily Value of vitamin C. In terms of nutrient density, is it better to get your vitamin C from a glass of orange juice or by eating a whole orange? How do oranges compare to orange juice in terms of energy density?

 Think about your choice as you read Chapter 2, then see our recommendations at the end of the chapter. To learn more about nutrient density and energy density, check out the Connect site: www.mcgrawhillconnect.com

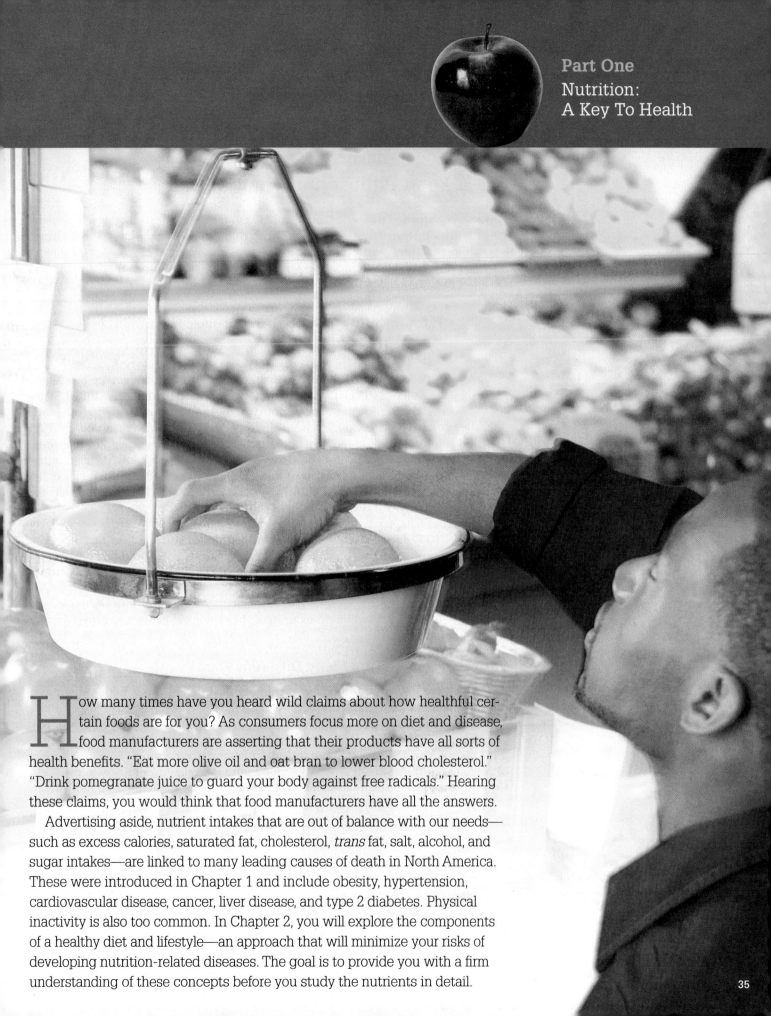

How many times have you heard wild claims about how healthful certain foods are for you? As consumers focus more on diet and disease, food manufacturers are asserting that their products have all sorts of health benefits. "Eat more olive oil and oat bran to lower blood cholesterol." "Drink pomegranate juice to guard your body against free radicals." Hearing these claims, you would think that food manufacturers have all the answers.

Advertising aside, nutrient intakes that are out of balance with our needs—such as excess calories, saturated fat, cholesterol, *trans* fat, salt, alcohol, and sugar intakes—are linked to many leading causes of death in North America. These were introduced in Chapter 1 and include obesity, hypertension, cardiovascular disease, cancer, liver disease, and type 2 diabetes. Physical inactivity is also too common. In Chapter 2, you will explore the components of a healthy diet and lifestyle—an approach that will minimize your risks of developing nutrition-related diseases. The goal is to provide you with a firm understanding of these concepts before you study the nutrients in detail.

Refresh Your Memory

As you begin your study of diet planning in Chapter 2, you may want to review:

- The terms in the margin in Chapter 1 and Table 1-1.

2.1 A Food Philosophy That Works

You may be surprised that what you should eat to minimize the risk of developing the nutrition-related diseases seen in North America is exactly what you have heard many times before: *Consume a variety of foods balanced by a moderate intake of each food.* Health professionals have recommended the same basic diet and health plan for the past 50 years:

- Control *how much* you eat.
- Pay attention to *what* you eat—choose whole grains, fruits, and vegetables.
- Stay physically active.

It is disappointing, however, that according to a recent survey conducted by the American Dietetic Association, two of five people in the United States believe that following a healthful diet means completely giving up foods they enjoy. To the contrary, a healthful diet does not have to mean deprivation and misery; it simply requires some basic nutrition know-how and planning. Besides, eliminating favorite foods typically does not work for "dieters" in the long run. The best plan consists of learning the basics of a healthful diet: variety, balance, and moderation. Monitoring total calorie intake is also important for many of us, especially if unwanted weight gain is taking place.

As noted in Chapter 1, many nutrition experts agree that there are no exclusively "good" or "bad" foods. Even so, many North Americans have diets that miss the mark when it comes to the foundations of healthy eating. Diets overloaded with fatty meats, fried foods, sugared soft drinks, and refined starches can result in substantial risk for nutrition-related chronic diseases.

Let's now define *variety*, *balance*, and *moderation*. We will also introduce two very important concepts that will help us to make healthy food choices: nutrient density and energy density.

Variety Means Eating Many Different Foods

Variety in your diet means choosing a number of different foods within any given food group rather than eating the "same old thing" day after day. Variety makes meals more interesting and helps ensure that a diet contains sufficient nutrients. A variety of foods is best because no one food meets all your nutrient needs. For example, meat provides protein and iron but little calcium and no vitamin C. Eggs are a source of protein, but they provide little calcium because the calcium is mostly in the shell. Cow's milk contains calcium but very little iron. None of these foods contains fiber.

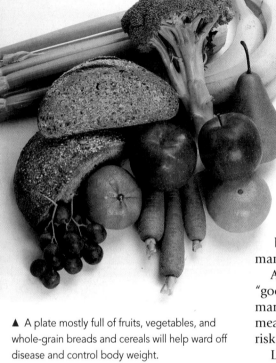

▲ A plate mostly full of fruits, vegetables, and whole-grain breads and cereals will help ward off disease and control body weight.

What do nutrition experts recommend for a healthy diet? Why are whole grains, fruits, and vegetables so important? How many servings do we need from each food group? How big is a serving? Are North Americans generally following the advice of the Dietary Guidelines? Chapter 2 provides some answers.

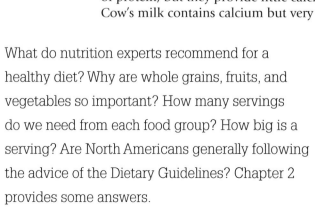
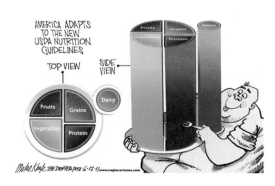

Carrots—a source of fiber and a pigment that forms vitamin A—may be your favorite vegetable. However, if you choose carrots every day as your only vegetable source, you may miss out on the vitamin folate. Other vegetables, such as broccoli and asparagus, are rich sources of this nutrient. Hopefully, you're beginning to get a sense of how different foods and food groups vary in the nutrients they contain. You'll learn much more about this in Chapters 8–12. For now, just recognize that you need a variety of foods in your diet because the required nutrients are scattered among many foods.

An added bonus of variety in the diet, especially within the fruit and vegetable groups, is the inclusion of a rich supply of **phytochemicals.** Recall from Chapter 1 that phytochemicals were discussed along with the nutrient classes. Many of these substances provide significant health benefits. Considerable research attention is focused on various phytochemicals in reducing the risk for certain diseases (e.g., cancer). You can't just buy a bottle of phytochemicals—they are generally available only within whole foods. Current multivitamin and mineral supplements contain few or none of these beneficial plant chemicals.

Numerous population studies show reduced cancer risk among people who regularly consume fruits and vegetables (see Further Readings 3 and 9). Researchers suspect that some phytochemicals present in the fruits and vegetables block the cancer process. Links between cancer and nutrition are described more thoroughly in the Nutrition and Your Health section in Chapter 16. Some phytochemicals also have been linked to a reduced risk of cardiovascular disease (see Further Reading 5). Could it be that, because humans evolved eating a wide variety of plant-based foods, the body developed with a need for these phytochemicals, along with the various nutrients present, to maintain optimal health?

Foods rich in phytochemicals are now part of a family of foods referred to as **functional foods.** A functional food provides health benefits beyond those supplied by the traditional nutrients it contains. For example, a tomato contains the phytochemical lycopene, so it can be called a functional food. You may hear this term more from the food industry in the future.

It will likely take many years for scientists to unravel all of the important effects of the myriad of phytochemicals in foods, and it is unlikely that all will ever be available or effective in supplement form. For this reason, leading nutrition and medical experts suggest that a diet rich in fruits, vegetables, and whole-grain breads and cereals is the most reliable way to obtain the potential benefits of phytochemicals.

A note of caution: Some research suggests that increasing dietary variety can lead to overeating. Thus, as one incorporates a wide variety of foods in a diet, attention to total calorie intake is also important to consider. Table 2-1 provides a number of suggestions for including more phytochemicals in your diet, as do the websites www.fruitsandveggiesmorematters.org and www.fruitsandveggiesmatter.gov.

functional foods Foods that provide health benefits beyond those supplied by the traditional nutrients they contain. For example, a tomato contains the phytochemical lycopene, so it can be called a functional food.

Balance Means Consuming Food from Each Group

One way to balance your diet as you consume a variety of foods is to select foods from each of these five major food groups every day:

- Grains
- Vegetables
- Fruits
- Dairy
- Protein

MyPlate, a food guide plan discussed later in this chapter, offers a visual reminder and advice to help you make smart choices from each of these food groups. A dinner consisting of a bean burrito, lettuce and tomato salad with oil-and-vinegar dressing, a glass of milk, and an apple covers all groups.

Balance also refers to matching your energy intake (how many total calories you consume) with energy expenditure (calories burned by metabolism and physical activity) over time. As you will see in Chapter 7, a prolonged imbalance between energy intake and energy expenditure leads to fluctuations in body weight.

CRITICAL THINKING

Andy would benefit from more variety in his diet. What are some practical tips he can use to increase his fruit and vegetable intake?

TABLE 2-1 Tips for Boosting the Phytochemical Content of a Diet

- Include vegetables in main and side dishes. Add these to rice, omelets, potato salad, and pastas. Try broccoli or cauliflower florets, mushrooms, peas, carrots, corn, or peppers.

- Look for quick-to-fix grain side dishes in the supermarket. Pilafs, couscous, rice mixes, and tabbouleh are just a few that you'll find.

- Choose fruit-filled cookies, such as fig bars, instead of sugar-rich cookies. Use fresh or canned fruit as a topping for pudding, hot or cold cereal, pancakes, and frozen desserts.

- Put raisins, grapes, apple chunks, pineapples, grated carrots, zucchini, or cucumber into coleslaw, chicken salad, or tuna salad.

- Be creative at the salad bar: Try fresh spinach, leaf lettuce, red cabbage, zucchini, yellow squash, cauliflower, peas, mushrooms, or red or yellow peppers.

- Pack fresh or dried fruit for snacks away from home instead of grabbing a candy bar or going hungry.

- Add slices of cucumber, zucchini, spinach, or carrot slivers to the lettuce and tomato on your sandwiches.

- Each week try one or two vegetarian meals, such as beans and rice or pasta; vegetable stir fry; or spaghetti and tomato sauce.

- If your daily protein intake exceeds the recommended amounts, reduce the meat, fish, or poultry in casseroles, stews, and soups by one-third to one-half and add more vegetables and legumes.

- Keep a container of fresh vegetables in the refrigerator for snacks.

- Choose fruit or vegetable juices (preferably 100% juice varieties) instead of soft drinks.

- Substitute tea for coffee or soft drinks on a regular basis.

- Have a bowl of fresh fruit on hand.

- Switch from crisp head lettuce to leaf lettuce, such as romaine.

- Use salsa as a dip for chips in place of creamy dips.

- Choose whole-grain breakfast cereals, breads, and crackers.

- Add flavor to your plate with ginger, rosemary, basil, thyme, garlic, onions, parsley, and chives in place of salt.

- Incorporate soy products, such as tofu, soy milk, soy protein isolate, and roasted soybeans into your meals (see Chapter 6).

Moderation Refers Mostly to Portion Size

Eating in moderation requires paying attention to portion sizes and planning your day's diet so that you do not overconsume any nutrients. This is especially important for fat, salt, and sugar because Americans typically consume too much of these food components—and too many calories overall. For example, if you plan to eat a bacon cheeseburger (relatively high in fat, salt, and calories) at lunch, you should eat foods such as fruits and salad greens (less concentrated sources of these nutrients) at other meals that same day. If you prefer whole milk to low-fat or fat-free milk, reduce the fat elsewhere in your meals. Try low-fat salad dressings, or use jam rather than butter or margarine on toast. Overall, it is more feasible to consume moderate portions of foods that supply lots of fat, salt, and sugar than to try to eliminate these foods altogether.

Let's be clear that moderation is important for all food components, not just fat, salt, and sugar. For example, many North Americans do not consume enough

nutrient density The ratio derived by dividing a food's nutrient content by its calorie content. When the food's contribution to our nutrient need for that nutrient exceeds its contribution to our calorie need, the food is considered to have a favorable nutrient density.

vitamin E, which is found in plant oils, nuts, and some fruits and vegetables. However, taking large doses of vitamin E (e.g., from supplements) can lead to excessive bleeding because of its effects on blood clotting. You *can* get too much of a good thing!

Nutrient Density Focuses on Nutrient Content

The **nutrient density** of a food is a characteristic used to determine its nutritional quality. Nutrient density of a food is determined by comparing its protein, vitamin, or mineral content with the amount of calories it provides. A food is deemed nutrient dense if it provides a large amount of a nutrient for a relatively small amount of calories when compared with other food sources. The higher a food's nutrient density, the better it is as a nutrient source. Comparing the nutrient density of different foods is an easy way to estimate their relative nutritional quality.

Generally, nutrient density is determined with respect to individual nutrients (see Further Reading 7). For example, many fruits and vegetables have a high content of vitamin C compared with their modest calorie content; that is, they are nutrient-dense foods for vitamin C. Figure 2-1 shows that fat-free milk is much more nutrient dense than sugared soft drinks for many nutrients, especially protein, vitamin A, riboflavin, and calcium.

As noted previously, menu planning should focus mainly on the total diet—not on the selection of one critical food as the key to an adequate diet. Nutrient-dense foods—such as fat-free and low-fat milk, lean meats, legumes (beans), oranges, carrots, broccoli, whole-wheat bread, and whole-grain breakfast cereals—do help balance less nutrient-dense foods—such as cookies and potato chips, which many people like to eat. The latter are often called empty-calorie foods because they tend to be high in sugar and/or fat but provide few other nutrients.

Eating nutrient-dense foods is especially important for people who consume diets relatively low in calories. This includes some older people and those following weight-loss diets (see Further Reading 4). This is because nutrient needs remain high even though calorie needs may be diminished.

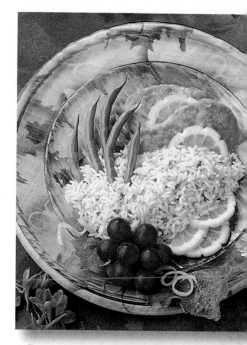

▲ Focus on nutrient-rich foods as you strive to meet your nutrient needs. The more colorful the food on your plate, the greater the content of nutrients and phytochemicals.

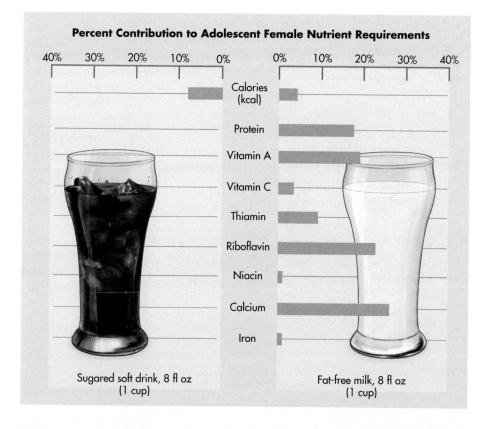

Sugared soft drink, 8 fl oz (1 cup)

Fat-free milk, 8 fl oz (1 cup)

FIGURE 2-1 ▶ Comparison of the nutrient contributions of a sugared soft drink with that of fat-free (i.e., nonfat or skim) milk. Choosing a glass of fat-free milk makes a significantly greater contribution to nutrient intake than does a sugared soft drink. An easy way to determine nutrient density from this chart is to compare the lengths of the bars indicating vitamin or mineral contribution with the bar that represents calorie contribution. For the soft drink, no nutrient surpasses calorie content. Fat-free milk, in contrast, has longer nutrient bars for protein, vitamin A, the vitamins thiamin and riboflavin, and the mineral calcium than it does for calories. Including many nutrient-dense foods in your diet is a good way to meet nutrient needs without exceeding calorie needs.

energy density A comparison of the calorie (kcal) content of a food with the weight of the food. An energy-dense food is high in calories but weighs very little (e.g., potato chips), whereas a food low in energy density has few calories but weighs a lot, such as an orange.

Energy (kcal) Density Affects Calorie Intake

Energy density is a measurement that best describes the calorie content of a food. Energy density of a food is determined by comparing the calorie (kcal) content with the weight of food. A food that is rich in calories but weighs relatively little is considered energy dense. Examples include nuts; cookies; fried foods in general; and even fat-free snacks, such as fat-free pretzels. Foods with low energy density include fruits, vegetables, and any food that incorporates lots of water during cooking, such as oatmeal (Table 2-2).

Researchers have shown that eating a meal with many foods of low energy density promotes satiety without contributing many calories (see Further Reading 11). This is probably because we typically consume a constant weight of food at a meal rather than a constant number of calories. How this constant weight of food is regulated is not known, but careful laboratory studies show that people consume fewer calories in a meal if most of the food choices are low in energy density, compared with foods high in energy density. Eating a diet low in energy density can aid in losing (or maintaining) weight.

Overall, foods with lots of water and fiber (i.e., low-energy-density foods) contribute few calories even though they help one feel full. Alternatively, foods with high energy density must be eaten in greater amounts to promote fullness. This is one more reason to eat a diet rich in fruits, vegetables, and whole-grain breads and cereals, a pattern that is typical of many ethnic diets throughout rural areas of the world.

Still, favorite foods, even if they are high in energy density, can have a place in your dietary pattern, but you will have to plan for them. For example, chocolate is a very energy-dense food, but a small portion at the end of a meal can supply a satisfying finale. In addition, foods with high energy density can help people with poor appetites, such as some older people, to maintain or gain weight.

The following sections of Chapter 2 describe various states of nutritional health and provide tools and nutrient guidelines for planning healthy diets to support overall health.

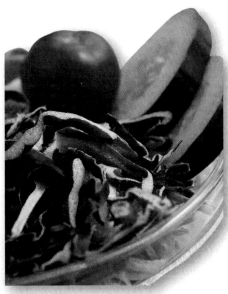

▲ Salads are low in energy density if we limit additional calories from salad dressing, bacon bits, cheese crumbles or cubes, and croutons.

TABLE 2-2 Energy Density of Common Foods (Listed in Relative Order)

Very Low Energy Density (less than 0.6 kcal per gram)	Low Energy Density (0.6 to 1.5 kcal per gram)	Medium Energy Density (1.5 to 4 kcal per gram)	High Energy Density (greater than 4 kcal per gram)
Lettuce	Whole milk	Eggs	Graham crackers
Tomatoes	Oatmeal	Ham	Fat-free sandwich cookies
Strawberries	Cottage cheese	Pumpkin pie	Chocolate
Broccoli	Beans	Whole-wheat bread	Chocolate chip cookies
Salsa	Bananas	Bagels	Tortilla chips
Grapefruit	Broiled fish	White bread	Bacon
Fat-free milk	Fat-free yogurt	Raisins	Potato chips
Carrots	Ready-to-eat breakfast cereals with 1% low-fat milk	Cream cheese	Peanuts
Vegetable soup		Cake with frosting	Peanut butter
		Pretzels	Mayonnaise
	Plain baked potato	Rice cakes	Butter or margarine
	Cooked rice		Vegetable oils
	Spaghetti noodles		

Data adapted from Rolls B, *The Volumetrics Eating Plan.* New York: HarperCollins, 2005.

CONCEPT CHECK

Healthy diet planning requires variety, balance, and moderation. Variety involves choosing different foods within each food group. Balance refers to consuming foods from each of the five food groups, as well as balancing calorie intake with calorie expenditure. Moderation implies limiting portion sizes with each food choice, so that the diet is not excessive in calories or any particular nutrient. Nutrient-dense foods, such as fat-free milk, fruits, vegetables, and whole-grain breads and cereals, supply many nutrients without contributing excessive calories. Consuming foods of low energy density, such as fruits and vegetables, may also help in weight control, because they promote satiety with relatively few calories.

MAKING DECISIONS

Some people frequently choose French fries as their vegetable. What is the nutrient content of French fries? Check the food composition supplement for the vitamin C content of French fries. How many servings would you need to eat to meet vitamin C needs (75 to 95 milligrams)?

(Answer: 4 to 5 servings)

2.2 States of Nutritional Health

The body's nutritional health is determined by considering the **nutritional state** of each needed nutrient. Three general categories of nutritional status are recognized: desirable nutrition, undernutrition, and overnutrition. The common term **malnutrition** can refer to either **overnutrition** or **undernutrition.** Neither state is conducive to good health. Furthermore, it is possible to be both overnourished (e.g., consume excess calories) and undernourished (e.g., consume too few essential vitamins and minerals) at the same time.

The amount of each nutrient needed to maintain a state of desirable nutrition is the basis for published dietary intake recommendations. Diet plans to meet those needs are discussed later in this chapter.

Desirable Nutrition

The **nutritional state** for a particular nutrient is desirable when body tissues have enough of the nutrient to support normal metabolic functions as well as surplus stores that can be used in times of increased need. A desirable nutritional state can be achieved by obtaining essential nutrients from a variety of foods.

Undernutrition

Undernutrition occurs when nutrient intake does not meet nutrient needs. At first, any surpluses are put to use; then, as stores are exhausted, health begins to decline. Many nutrients are in high demand due to constant cell loss and regeneration in the body, such as in the gastrointestinal tract. For this reason, the stores of certain nutrients, including many of the B vitamins, are exhausted rapidly and therefore require a regular intake. In addition, some women in North America do not consume sufficient iron to meet monthly losses and eventually deplete their iron stores (Fig. 2-2).

Once availability of a nutrient falls sufficiently low, biochemical evidence indicates that the body's metabolic processes have slowed or stopped. At this state of deficiency, there are no outward **symptoms;** thus, it is termed a **subclinical** deficiency. A subclinical deficiency can go on for some time before clinicians are able to detect its effects.

Eventually, clinical symptoms will develop. Clinical evidence of a nutritional deficiency—perhaps in the skin, hair, nails, tongue, or eyes—can occur within months but may take years to develop. Often, clinicians do not detect a problem until a deficiency produces outward symptoms, such as small areas of bruising on the skin from a vitamin C deficiency.

Overnutrition

Prolonged consumption of more nutrients than the body needs can lead to overnutrition. In the short run (e.g., 1 to 2 weeks), overnutrition may cause only a few symptoms, such as stomach distress from excess iron intake. If an excess intake continues, however, some nutrients may accumulate to toxic amounts, which can lead to serious disease. For example, too much vitamin A during pregnancy can cause birth defects.

nutritional state The nutritional health of a person as determined by anthropometric measurements (height, weight, circumferences, and so on), biochemical measurements of nutrients or their by-products in blood and urine, a clinical (physical) examination, a dietary analysis, and economic evaluation; also called nutritional status.

malnutrition Failing health that results from long-standing dietary practices that do not coincide with nutritional needs.

overnutrition A state in which nutritional intake greatly exceeds the body's needs.

undernutrition Failing health that results from a long-standing dietary intake that is not enough to meet nutritional needs.

symptom A change in health status noted by the person with the problem, such as stomach pain.

subclinical Stage of a disease or disorder not severe enough to produce symptoms that can be detected or diagnosed.

FIGURE 2-2 ▶ The general scheme of nutritional status. Green reflects good status, yellow marginal status, and red poor status (undernutrition or overnutrition). This general concept can be applied to all nutrients. Iron was chosen as an example because iron deficiency is the most common nutrient deficiency worldwide.

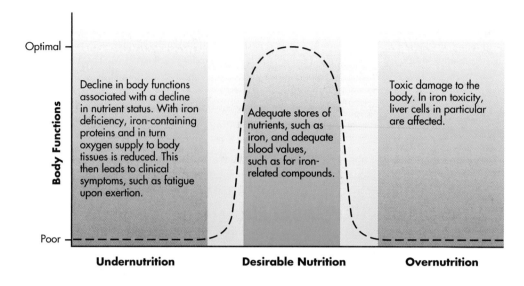

Decline in body functions associated with a decline in nutrient status. With iron deficiency, iron-containing proteins and in turn oxygen supply to body tissues is reduced. This then leads to clinical symptoms, such as fatigue upon exertion.

Adequate stores of nutrients, such as iron, and adequate blood values, such as for iron-related compounds.

Toxic damage to the body. In iron toxicity, liver cells in particular are affected.

Undernutrition   **Desirable Nutrition**   **Overnutrition**

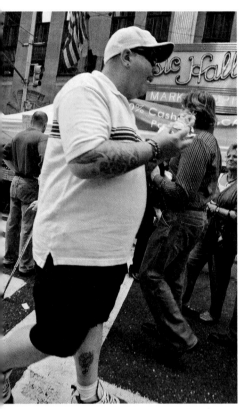

▲ The most common type of overnutrition in North America is the excess intake of calories, which often leads to obesity.

anthropometric assessment Measurement of body weight and the lengths, circumferences, and thicknesses of parts of the body.

biochemical assessment Measurement of biochemical functions (e.g., concentrations of nutrient by-products or enzyme activities in the blood or urine) related to a nutrient's function.

The most common form of overnutrition in developed nations is an excess intake of calories that leads to obesity. In the long run, outcomes of obesity include other serious diseases, such as type 2 diabetes and certain forms of cancer. Use the website www.shapeup.org to learn more about the importance of lifelong weight control.

For most vitamins and minerals, the gap between desirable intake and overnutrition is wide. Therefore, even if people take a typical balanced multivitamin and mineral supplement daily, they probably will not receive a harmful dose of any nutrient. The gap between desirable intake and overnutrition is smallest for vitamin A and the minerals calcium, iron, and copper. Thus, if you take nutrient supplements, keep a close eye on your total vitamin and mineral intake from both food and supplements to avoid toxicity (see Chapter 10 for further advice on use of nutrient supplements).

2.3 How Can Your Nutritional State Be Measured?

To find out how nutritionally fit *you* are, a nutritional assessment—either whole or in part—needs to be performed (Table 2-3). Generally, this is performed by a physician, often with the aid of a registered dietitian.

Analyzing Background Factors

Because family health history plays an important role in determining nutritional and health status, it must be carefully recorded and critically analyzed as part of a nutritional assessment. Other related background information includes: (1) a medical history, especially for any disease states or treatments that could decrease nutrient absorption or ultimate use; (2) a list of medications taken; (3) a social history (e.g., marital status, living conditions); (4) level of education to determine the degree of complexity that can be used in written materials and oral discussions; and (5) economic status to determine the ability to purchase, transport, and cook food.

Assessing Nutritional Status Using the ABCDEs

In addition to background factors, four nutritional-assessment categories complete the picture of nutritional status. **Anthropometric** measurements of height, weight (and weight changes), skinfold thicknesses, and body circumferences provide information about the current state of nutrition. Most measures of body composition are easy to obtain and are generally reliable. However, an in-depth examination of nutritional health is impossible without the more expensive process of **biochemical assessment.** This involves the measurement of the concentrations of nutrients and nutrient by-products in the blood, urine, and feces and of specific blood enzyme activities.

TABLE 2-3 Conducting an Evaluation of Nutritional Health

Parameters	Example
Background	Medical history (e.g., current diseases, past surgeries, current weight, weight history, and current medications)
	Social history (marital status, living conditions)
	Family health history
	Education level
	Economic status
Nutritional	Anthropometric assessment: height, weight, skinfold thickness, arm muscle circumference, and other parameters
	Biochemical (laboratory) assessment of blood and urine: enzyme activities, concentrations of nutrients or their by-products
	Clinical assessment (physical examination): general appearance of skin, eyes, and tongue; rapid hair loss; sense of touch; ability to walk
	Dietary assessment: usual intake or record of previous days' meals

A **clinical assessment** would follow, during which a health professional would search for any physical evidence (e.g., high blood pressure) of diet-related diseases or deficiencies. Then, a close look at the person's diet (**dietary assessment**), including a record of at least the previous few days' food intake, would help to determine any possible problem areas.

Finally, adding the **environmental assessment** (from the background analysis) provides further details about the living conditions, education level, and ability to purchase and prepare foods needed to maintain health. Now the true nutritional state of a person emerges. Taken together, these five assessments form the ABCDEs of nutritional assessment: anthropometric, biochemical, clinical, dietary, and environmental (Fig. 2-3).

MAKING DECISIONS

Nutritional Assessment

A practical example using the ABCDEs for evaluating nutritional status can be illustrated in a person who chronically abuses alcohol. Upon evaluation, the physician notes:

(A) Low weight for height, recent 10-pound weight loss, muscle wasting in the upper body
(B) Low amounts of the vitamins thiamin and folate in the blood
(C) Psychological confusion, facial sores, and uncoordinated movement
(D) Dietary intake of little more than wine and hamburgers for the last week
(E) Currently residing in a homeless shelter; $35.00 in wallet; unemployed

Evaluation: This person needs medical attention, including nutrient repletion.

Recognizing the Limitations of Nutritional Assessment

A long time may elapse between the initial development of poor nutritional health and the first clinical evidence of a problem. A diet high in saturated (typically solid) fat often increases blood cholesterol but without producing any clinical evidence for years. However, when the blood vessels become sufficiently blocked by cholesterol and other materials, chest pain during physical activity or a **heart attack** may occur. An active area of nutrition research is the development of better methods for early detection of nutrition-related problems such as heart attack risk.

clinical assessment Examination of general appearance of skin, eyes, and tongue; evidence of rapid hair loss; sense of touch; and ability to cough and walk.

dietary assessment Estimation of typical food choices relying mostly on the recounting of one's usual intake or a record of one's previous days' intake.

environmental assessment Includes details about living conditions, education level, and the ability of the person to purchase, transport, and cook food. The person's weekly budget for food purchases is also a key factor to consider.

heart attack Rapid fall in heart function caused by reduced blood flow through the heart's blood vessels. Often part of the heart dies in the process. Technically called a myocardial infarction.

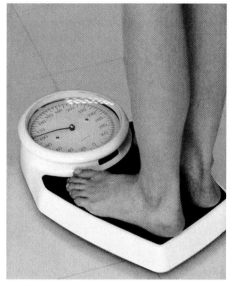

Anthropometric

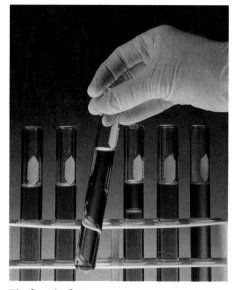

Biochemical

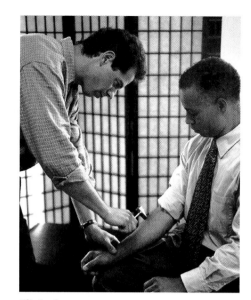

Clinical

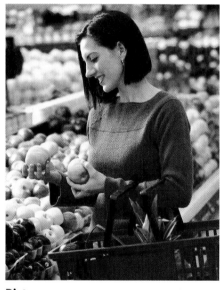

Dietary

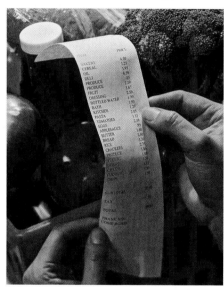

Environmental

FIGURE 2-3 ▶ A complete nutritional assessment includes anthropometric, biochemical, clinical, and dietary information. Environmental status adds further information, rounding out the ABCDEs of nutritional assessment.

Another example of a serious health condition with delayed symptoms is low bone density resulting from a calcium deficiency—a particularly relevant issue for adolescent and young adult females. Many young women do not consume the needed amount of calcium but suffer no obvious effects in their younger years. However, the bone structures of these women with low calcium intakes do not reach full potential during the years of growth, making osteoporosis more likely later in life.

Furthermore, clinical symptoms of some nutritional deficiencies (e.g., diarrhea, inability to walk normally, and facial sores) are not very specific. These may have causes other than poor nutrition. The long time it takes for symptoms to develop and their potential to be vague often make it difficult to establish a link between an individual's current diet and nutritional state.

Concern About the State of Your Nutritional Health Is Important

Table 1-7 in Chapter 1 portrayed the close relationship between nutrition and health. The good news is that people who focus on maintaining nutritional health are apt to enjoy a long, vigorous life. For example, a recent study found that women with a healthy lifestyle had a decreased risk for heart attacks (80% reduction) compared to women without such healthy practices. The healthy habits included:

- Consumed a healthy diet
  - Varied
  - Rich in fiber
  - Included some fish
  - Low in animal fat and *trans* fat
- Maintained a healthy weight
- Occasionally consumed alcohol in small amounts
- Exercised for at least 30 minutes daily
- Avoided use of tobacco

Should all adults follow this example (with optional use of alcohol)?

CONCEPT CHECK

A desirable nutritional state results when the body has enough nutrients to function fully and contains stores to use in times of increased needs. When nutrient intake fails to meet body needs, undernutrition develops. Symptoms of such an inadequate nutrient intake can take months or years to develop. Overloading the body with nutrients, leading to overnutrition, is another potential problem to avoid. Nutritional state can be assessed by using anthropometric, biochemical, clinical, dietary, and economic assessments (ABCDEs).

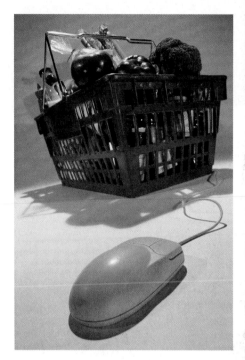

▲ Is there an app for that? Yes, there is! Health-conscious consumers can tap into a growing number of smartphone applications to help them stay on track with a healthy lifestyle. From calorie counters to pedometers to gentle reminders to get up and stretch, smartphone users have access to a virtual arsenal against diet-related disease. Log onto the Connect site to find links to apps from reputable sources.

2.4 Using the Scientific Method to Determine Nutrient Needs

How do we know what we know about nutrient needs? In a word, research. Like other sciences, the research that sets the foundation for nutrition knowledge has developed through the use of the *scientific method*, a testing procedure designed to detect and eliminate error.

MAKING DECISIONS

Research on Stomach Ulcers

Overall, the scientific method requires a skeptical attitude. A recent example of this need for skepticism involves stomach **ulcers.** Not so many years ago, everyone "knew" that stomach ulcers were caused by a stressful lifestyle and a poor diet. Then, in 1983, an Australian physician, Dr. Barry Marshall, reported in a respected medical journal that ulcers are usually caused by a common **microorganism** called *Helicobacter pylori*. Furthermore, he stated that a cure is possible using antibiotics. At first, other physicians were skeptical about this finding and continued to prescribe medications such as antacids that reduce stomach acid. But, as more studies were published demonstrating that patients using antibiotics were cured of ulcers, the medical profession eventually accepted the findings. Today, ulcers are managed for the most part by medications that destroy the microorganism. (We will discuss the treatment of stomach ulcers in more detail in Chapter 3.) Sound scientific discoveries will always be subject to challenge and change.

ulcer Erosion of the tissue lining, usually in the stomach (gastric ulcer) or the upper small intestine (duodenal ulcer). As a group these are generally referred to as peptic ulcers.

microorganism Bacterium virus, or other organism invisible to the naked eye, some of which cause diseases. Also called *microbe*.

hypotheses Tentative explanations by a scientist to explain a phenomenon.

scurvy The deficiency disease that results after a few weeks to months of consuming a diet that lacks vitamin C; pinpoint sites of bleeding on the skin are an early sign.

epidemiology The study of how disease rates vary among different population groups.

The first step of the scientific method is the observation of a natural phenomenon. Scientists then suggest possible explanations, called **hypotheses,** about its cause. At times, historical events can provide clues to important relationships in nutrition science, such as the link between vitamin C and **scurvy** (see Chapter 10). In a related approach, scientists may study diet and disease patterns among various populations, a research method called **epidemiology**.

theory An explanation for a phenomenon that has numerous lines of evidence to support it.

control group Participants in an experiment who are not given the treatment being tested.

placebo Generally a fake medicine or treatment used to disguise the treatments given to the participants in an experiment.

Historical and epidemiological findings can *suggest* hypotheses about the role of diet in various health problems. *Proving* the role of particular dietary components, however, requires controlled experiments. The data gathered from experiments may either support or refute each hypothesis. If the results of many experiments support a hypothesis, scientists accept the hypothesis as a **theory** (such as the theory of gravity). Often, the results from one experiment suggest a new set of questions (Fig. 2-4).

The most rigorous type of controlled experiment follows a randomized, double-blind, placebo-controlled study design. In this type of study, a group of participants—the experimental group—follows a specific protocol (e.g., consuming a certain food or nutrient), and participants in a corresponding **control group** follow their normal habits or consume a **placebo**. People are randomly assigned to each group, such as by the flip of a coin. Scientists then observe the experimental group over time to see if there is any effect not found in the control group.

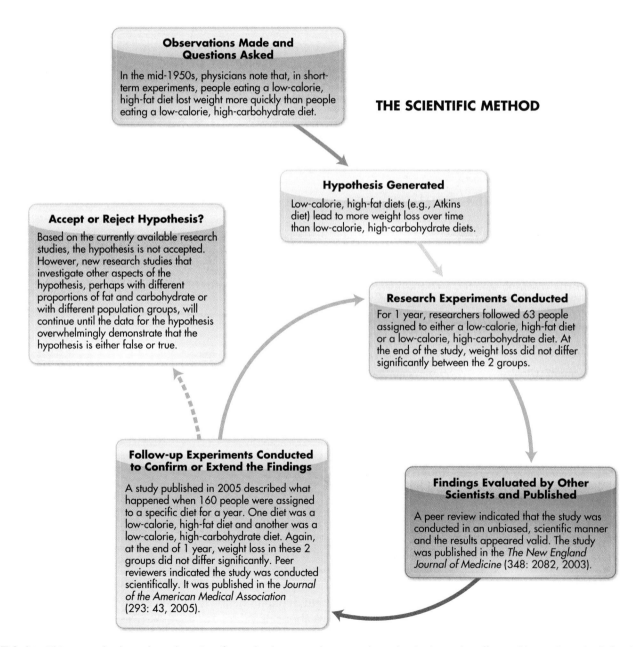

THE SCIENTIFIC METHOD

Observations Made and Questions Asked

In the mid-1950s, physicians note that, in short-term experiments, people eating a low-calorie, high-fat diet lost weight more quickly than people eating a low-calorie, high-carbohydrate diet.

Hypothesis Generated

Low-calorie, high-fat diets (e.g., Atkins diet) lead to more weight loss over time than low-calorie, high-carbohydrate diets.

Accept or Reject Hypothesis?

Based on the currently available research studies, the hypothesis is not accepted. However, new research studies that investigate other aspects of the hypothesis, perhaps with different proportions of fat and carbohydrate or with different population groups, will continue until the data for the hypothesis overwhelmingly demonstrate that the hypothesis is either false or true.

Research Experiments Conducted

For 1 year, researchers followed 63 people assigned to either a low-calorie, high-fat diet or a low-calorie, high-carbohydrate diet. At the end of the study, weight loss did not differ significantly between the 2 groups.

Follow-up Experiments Conducted to Confirm or Extend the Findings

A study published in 2005 described what happened when 160 people were assigned to a specific diet for a year. One diet was a low-calorie, high-fat diet and another was a low-calorie, high-carbohydrate diet. Again, at the end of 1 year, weight loss in these 2 groups did not differ significantly. Peer reviewers indicated the study was conducted scientifically. It was published in the *Journal of the American Medical Association* (293: 43, 2005).

Findings Evaluated by Other Scientists and Published

A peer review indicated that the study was conducted in an unbiased, scientific manner and the results appeared valid. The study was published in the *The New England Journal of Medicine* (348: 2082, 2003).

FIGURE 2-4 ▶ This example shows how the scientific method was used to test a hypothesis about the effects of low-calorie, high-fat diets on weight loss. Scientists consistently follow these steps when testing all types of hypotheses. Scientists do not accept a nutrition or another scientific hypothesis until it has been thoroughly tested using the scientific method.

Human experiments provide the most convincing evidence about relationships between nutrients and health, but they are often not practical or ethical. Thus, much of what we know about human nutritional needs and functions has been gleaned from animal experiments. The use of animal experiments to study the role of nutrition in certain human diseases depends on the availability of an **animal model**—a disease in laboratory animals that closely mimics a particular human disease. Often, however, if no animal model is available and human experiments are ruled out, scientific knowledge cannot advance beyond what can be learned from epidemiological studies.

Once an experiment is complete, scientists summarize the findings and seek to publish the results in scientific journals. Generally, before articles are published in scientific journals, they are critically reviewed by other scientists familiar with the subject, which helps to ensure that only high-quality, objective research findings are published.

Keep in mind, one experiment is never enough to prove a particular hypothesis or provide a basis for nutritional recommendations. Rather, through follow-up studies, the results obtained in one laboratory must be confirmed by experiments conducted in other laboratories and, possibly, under varying circumstances. Only then can we really trust and use the results. The more lines of evidence available to support an idea, the more likely it is to be true (Fig. 2-5).

Epidemiological studies may suggest hypotheses, but controlled experiments are needed to rigorously test hypotheses before nutrition recommendations can be made. For example, epidemiologists found that smokers who regularly consumed fruits and vegetables had a lower risk for lung cancer than smokers who ate few fruits and vegetables. Some scientists proposed that beta-carotene, a pigment present in many fruits and vegetables, may be responsible for reducing the damage that tobacco smoke creates in the lungs. However, in **double-blind studies** involving heavy smokers, the risk of lung cancer was found to be *higher* for those who took beta-carotene supplements than for those who did not (this is not true for the small amount of beta-carotene found naturally in foods). Soon after these results were reported, the U.S. federal agency supporting two other large ongoing studies that employed beta-carotene supplements called a halt to the research, stating that these supplements are ineffective in preventing both lung cancer and cardiovascular disease.

animal model Use of animals to study disease to understand more about human disease.

case-control study A study in which individuals who have a disease or condition, such as lung cancer, are compared with individuals who do not have the condition.

double-blind study An experimental design in which neither the participants nor the researchers are aware of each participant's assignment (test or placebo) or the outcome of the study until it is completed. An independent third party holds the code and the data until the study has been completed.

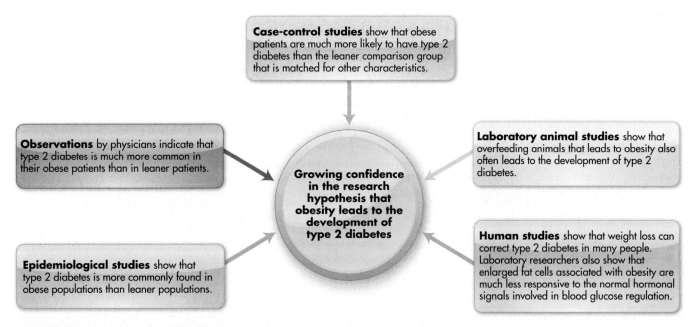

Case-control studies show that obese patients are much more likely to have type 2 diabetes than the leaner comparison group that is matched for other characteristics.

Observations by physicians indicate that type 2 diabetes is much more common in their obese patients than in leaner patients.

Laboratory animal studies show that overfeeding animals that leads to obesity also often leads to the development of type 2 diabetes.

Growing confidence in the research hypothesis that obesity leads to the development of type 2 diabetes

Epidemiological studies show that type 2 diabetes is more commonly found in obese populations than leaner populations.

Human studies show that weight loss can correct type 2 diabetes in many people. Laboratory researchers also show that enlarged fat cells associated with obesity are much less responsive to the normal hormonal signals involved in blood glucose regulation.

FIGURE 2-5 ▶ Data from a variety of sources can come together to support a research hypothesis. This diagram shows how various types of research data support the hypothesis that obesity leads to the development of type 2 diabetes (see Chapter 4).

2.5 Specific Nutrient Standards and Recommendations

The overarching goal of any healthy diet plan is to meet nutrient needs. To begin, we must determine what amount of each essential nutrient is necessary to maintain health. Most of the terms that describe nutrient needs fall under one umbrella term— **Dietary Reference Intakes (DRIs)**. The development of DRIs is an ongoing, collaborative effort between the Food and Nutrition Board of the Institute of Medicine in the United States and Health Canada (see Further Reading 2). Included under the DRI umbrella are **Recommended Dietary Allowances (RDAs)**, **Adequate Intakes (AIs)**, **Estimated Energy Requirements (EERs)**, and **Tolerable Upper Intake Levels (Upper Levels or ULs)**.

As you begin your study of nutrition, all these acronyms can seem like an alphabet soup of abbreviations! However, you can more easily sift through these nutrient standards if you have some basic knowledge about their development and use (summarized in Table 2-4).

Recommended Dietary Allowance

Dietary Reference Intakes (DRIs) Term used to encompass nutrient recommendations made by the Food and Nutrition Board of the National Academy of Sciences. These include RDAs, EARs, AIs, EERs, and ULs.

Recommended Dietary Allowance (RDA) Nutrient intake amount sufficient to meet the needs of 97% to 98% of the individuals in a specific life stage.

Adequate Intake (AI) Nutrient intake amount set for any nutrient for which insufficient research is available to establish an RDA. AIs are based on estimates of intakes that appear to maintain a defined nutritional state in a specific life stage.

Estimated Energy Requirement (EER) Estimate of the energy (kcal) intake needed to match the energy use of an average person in a specific life stage.

Tolerable Upper Intake Level (UL) Maximum chronic daily intake level of a nutrient that is unlikely to cause adverse health effects in almost all people in a specific life stage.

A Recommended Dietary Allowance (RDA) is the amount of a nutrient that will meet the needs of nearly all individuals (about 97%) in a particular age and gender group. A person can compare his or her individual intake of specific nutrients to the RDA. Although an intake slightly above or below the RDA for a particular nutrient is no reason for concern, a significant deviation below (about 70%) or above (about three times or more for some nutrients) the RDA for an extended time can eventually result in a deficiency or toxicity of that nutrient, respectively.

Adequate Intake

An RDA can be set for a nutrient only if there is sufficient information on the human needs for that particular nutrient. Today, there is not enough information on some nutrients, such as calcium, to set such a precise standard as an RDA. For this and other nutrients, the DRIs include a category called an Adequate Intake (AI). This standard is based on the dietary intakes of people that appear to be maintaining nutritional health. That amount of intake is assumed to be adequate, as no evidence of a nutritional deficiency is apparent.

TABLE 2-4 Recommendations within the Dietary Reference Intakes

RDA	Recommended Dietary Allowance. Use to evaluate your current intake for a specific nutrient. The further you stray above or below this value, the greater your chances of developing nutritional problems.
AI	Adequate Intake. Use to evaluate your current intake of nutrients, but realize that an AI designation implies that further research is required before scientists can establish a more definitive recommendation.
EER	Estimated Energy Requirement. Use to estimate calorie needs of the average person within a specific height, weight, gender, age, and physical activity pattern.
UL	Upper Level. Use to evaluate the highest amount of daily nutrient intake unlikely to cause adverse health effects in the long run in almost all people (97% to 98%) in a population. This number applies to chronic use and is set to protect even very susceptible people in the healthy general population. As intake increases above the Upper Level, the potential for adverse effects generally increases.
DV	Daily Value. Use as a rough guide for comparing the nutrient content of a food to approximate human needs. Typically, the Daily Value used on food labels refers to ages 4 years through adulthood. It is based on a 2000 kcal diet. Some Daily Values also increase slightly with higher calorie intakes (see Fig. 2-16 in the section on food labeling).

Estimated Energy Requirement

For calorie needs, we use the Estimated Energy Requirement (EER) instead of an RDA or AI. As described, the RDAs are set somewhat higher than the average needs for nutrients. This is fine for nutrients other than calories because a slight excess of vitamins and minerals is not harmful. However, a long-term excess of even a small amount of calories will lead to weight gain. Therefore, the calculation of EER needs to be more specific, taking into account age, gender, height, weight, and physical activity (e.g., sedentary or moderately active). In some cases, the additional calorie needs for growth and lactation are also included (see Chapters 7, 14, and 15 for the specific formulas used). Note that the EER is based on the "average" person. Thus, it can only serve as a starting point for estimating calorie needs.

Tolerable Upper Intake Level

A Tolerable Upper Intake Level (Upper Level or UL) has been set for some vitamins and minerals (see the inside cover). The UL is the highest amount of a nutrient unlikely to cause adverse health effects in the long run. As intake exceeds the UL, the risk of ill effects increases. These amounts generally should not be exceeded day after day, as toxicity could develop. For people eating a varied diet and/or using a balanced multivitamin and mineral supplement, exceeding the UL is unusual. Problems are more likely to arise with diets that promote excessive intakes of a limited variety of foods, with the use of many fortified foods, or with excessive doses of individual vitamins or minerals.

Daily Value

A nutrition standard more relevant to everyday life is the Daily Value (DV). This is a generic standard used on food labels. It is applicable to both genders from 4 years of age through adulthood, and is based on consuming a 2000 kcal diet. DVs are mostly set at or close to the highest RDA value or related nutrient standard seen in the various age and gender categories for a specific nutrient (see Appendix B). DVs have been set for vitamins, minerals, protein, and other dietary components. For fat and cholesterol, the DVs represent a maximum level, not a goal one should strive to reach. DVs allow consumers to compare their intake from a specific food to desirable (or maximum) intakes.

How Should These Nutrient Standards Be Used?

To sum up the acronyms described so far, the type of standard set for nutrients depends on the quality of available evidence. A nutrient recommendation backed by lots of experimental research will have an RDA. For a nutrient that still requires more research, only an AI is presented. We use the EER as a starting point for determining calorie needs. Some nutrients also have a UL if information on toxicity or adverse health effects is available. Periodically, new DRIs become available as expert committees review and interpret the available research.

RDAs and related standards are intended mainly for diet planning. Specifically, a diet plan should aim to meet the RDA or AI as appropriate and not to exceed the UL over the long term (Fig. 2-6). Specific RDA, AI, EER, and UL standards are printed on the inside cover of this book. To learn more about these nutrient standards, visit the link for Food and Nutrition on the Institute of Medicine's website (www.iom.edu).

CONCEPT CHECK

Standards for nutrient intake are included in the broad category of Dietary Reference Intakes (DRIs). The Recommended Dietary Allowances (RDAs) are the amounts of each nutrient that will meet the needs of healthy individuals within specific gender and age categories. If not enough information is available to set an RDA, an Adequate Intake (AI) value is used. Tolerable Upper Intake Levels (ULs) are the highest amounts of a nutrient unlikely to cause adverse health effects. ULs have been set for some vitamins and minerals.

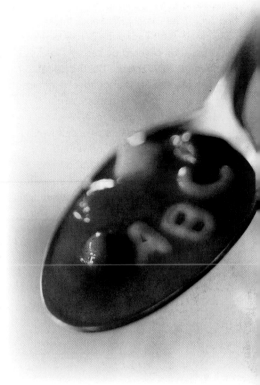

▲ With a little bit of study, you can master the alphabet soup of nutrition recommendations.

MAKING DECISIONS

Using Nutrient Recommendations

As nutrient intake increases, the Recommended Dietary Allowance (RDA) for the nutrient, if set, is eventually met and a deficient state is no longer present. An individual's needs most likely will be met since RDAs are set high to include almost all people. Related to the RDA concept of meeting an individual's needs are the standards of Adequate Intake (AI) and the Estimated Energy Requirement (EER). These can be used to estimate an individual's needs for some nutrients and calories, respectively. Still, keep in mind that these standards do not share the same degree of accuracy as the RDA. For example, EER may have to be adjusted upward if the individual is very physically active. Finally, as nutrient intake increases above the Upper Level (UL), poor nutritional health is again likely. However, this poor health is due now to the toxic effects of a nutrient, rather than those of a deficiency.

FIGURE 2-6 ▶ This figure shows the relationship of the Dietary Reference Intakes (DRIs) to each other and the percentage of the population covered by each. At intakes between the RDA and the UL, the risk of either an inadequate diet or adverse effects from the nutrient in question is close to 0. The UL is then the highest level of nutrient intake likely to pose no risks of adverse health effects to almost all individuals in the general population. At intakes above the UL, the margin of safety to protect against adverse effects is reduced. The AI is set for some nutrients instead of an RDA. The Food and Nutrition Board states that there is no established benefit for healthy individuals if they consume nutrient intakes above the RDA or AI.

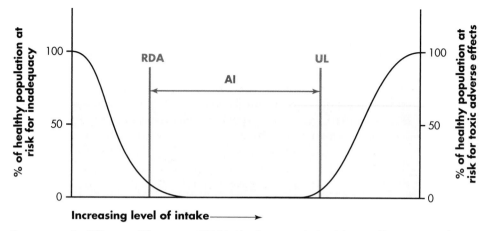

Recommended Dietary Allowance (RDA): The dietary intake level that is sufficient to meet the nutrient requirement of nearly all (97% to 98%) healthy individuals in a particular life stage and gender group. When set for a nutrient, aim for this intake.

Adequate Intake (AI): A recommended intake value based on observed or experimentally determined approximations or estimates of nutrient intake by a group (or groups) of healthy people that is assumed to be adequate—used when an RDA cannot be determined. When set for a nutrient, aim for this intake.

Tolerable Upper Intake Level (Upper Level or UL): The highest level of nutrient intake that is likely to pose no risk of adverse health effects for almost all individuals in the general population. As intake increases above the Upper Level, the risk of adverse effects increases.

2.6 Recommendations for Healthy Living

Since the early twentieth century, researchers have worked to translate the science of nutrition into practical terms so that people with no special training could estimate whether their nutritional needs were being met. Early food guidance systems aimed to reduce risk for nutrient deficiencies, but severe deficiency diseases are no longer common. Marginal deficiencies of calcium, iron, folate and other B vitamins, vitamin C, vitamin D, vitamin E, potassium, magnesium, and fiber are still a problem; but for many North Americans, major health problems stem from overconsumption of one or more of the following: calories, saturated fat, cholesterol, *trans* fat, alcohol, and sodium (see Further Reading 18).

The following sections of Chapter 2 will describe guidelines and tools for planning healthy lifestyles. You will notice how those core concepts of variety, balance, and moderation keep showing up throughout our discussions of the Dietary Guidelines, MyPlate, and the Physical Activity Guidelines.

Dietary Guidelines—The Basis for Menu Planning

The 2010 **Dietary Guidelines for Americans** provide nutrition and physical activity advice based on the latest and strongest scientific information to improve the health of all Americans age 2 and older (see Further Readings 17 and 20). The USDA and U.S. Department of Health and Human Services (DHHS) have published Dietary Guidelines since 1980 to aid diet planning. In light of the current epidemic of overweight and obesity—pressing health issues that now affect two-thirds of adults and one-third of children and adolescents—the message of calorie balance is woven throughout this seventh edition of the Dietary Guidelines.

The most important changes from the 2005 edition of the Dietary Guidelines include powerful emphases on reduction of total calories, sugar-sweetened beverages, saturated fat, and sodium. In addition, the report calls for a much-needed increase in physical activity among all population groups. Previous editions of the Dietary Guidelines have targeted healthy Americans, but these latest recommendations also include those at risk of developing chronic diseases. The health of children is highlighted. The new recommendations are also more culturally sensitive to reflect the

Dietary Guidelines for Americans General goals for nutrient intakes and diet composition set by the USDA and the U.S. Department of Health and Human Services.

Losing weight is a challenge that takes time and continual awareness of calorie balance. We live in an *obesogenic* environment. With around-the-clock access to an increasing variety of super-sized, energy-dense foods, the typical American consumes about 600 more kilocalories per day than in 1970. Furthermore, out of convenience or necessity, our work, school, and home lives are dominated by sedentary activities.

growing diversity and varied health concerns of the American population. Finally, the new Dietary Guidelines recognize the prevalence of food insecurity (see Chapter 12), aiming to help populations with limited access to food optimize the nutritional content of meals within their resource constraints.

The Dietary Guidelines give direction for the development of educational materials, aid policy makers, and serve as the basis for consumer nutrition messages (see Further Reading 12). Overall, Americans should use this information along with related tools, such as MyPlate and the Physical Activity Guidelines for Americans, to form lifestyle patterns that optimize health.

The report identifies 29 key recommendations (outlined in Figure 2-7) to support three major goals:

- Balance calories with physical activity to manage weight.
- Consume more of certain foods and nutrients, such as fruits, vegetables, whole grains, fat-free and low-fat dairy products, and seafood.
- Consume fewer foods with sodium (salt), saturated fats, *trans* fats, cholesterol, added sugars, and refined grains.

Appendix C contains nutrient guidelines for Canadians.

CRITICAL THINKING

Shannon has grown up eating the typical American diet. Having recently read and heard many media reports about the relationship between nutrition and health, she is beginning to look critically at her diet and is considering making changes. However, she doesn't know where to begin. What advice would you give her?

FIGURE 2-7 ▶ Key Recommendations from the 2010 Dietary Guidelines for Americans

BALANCING CALORIES TO MANAGE WEIGHT

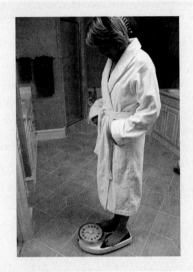

- Prevent and/or reduce overweight and obesity through improved eating and physical activity behaviors.
- Control total calorie intake to manage body weight. For people who are overweight or obese, this will mean consuming fewer calories from foods and beverages.
- Increase physical activity and reduce time spent in sedentary behaviors.
- Maintain appropriate calorie balance during each stage of life—childhood, adolescence, adulthood, pregnancy and breastfeeding, and older age.

Key Recommendations for Specific Population Groups

- Women of childbearing age: Achieve and maintain a healthy weight before becoming pregnant.
- *Pregnant women*: Gain weight within the 2009 Institute of Medicine gestational weight-gain guidelines.
- Adults ages 65 years and older: If overweight, avoid additional weight gain. For those with cardiovascular disease risk factors, lose weight to improve quality of life and reduce risk of chronic diseases and associated disabilities.

FOODS AND FOOD COMPONENTS TO REDUCE

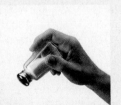

- Reduce daily sodium intake to less than 2300 mg and further reduce intake to 1500 mg among persons who are 51 and older and those of any age who are African-American or have hypertension, diabetes, or chronic kidney disease. The 1500-mg recommendation applies to about half of the U.S. population, including children, and the majority of adults.
- Consume less than 10% of calories from saturated fatty acids by replacing them with monounsaturated and polyunsaturated fatty acids.
- Consume less than 300 mg per day of dietary cholesterol.
- Keep *trans* fatty acid consumption as low as possible by limiting foods that contain synthetic sources of *trans* fats, such as partially hydrogenated oils, and by limiting other solid fats.
- Reduce the intake of calories from solid fats and added sugars.
- Limit the consumption of foods that contain refined grains, especially refined grain foods that contain solid fats, added sugars, and sodium.
- If alcohol is consumed, it should be consumed in moderation—up to one drink per day for women and two drinks per day for men—and only by adults of legal drinking age.

continued on next page

FIGURE 2-7 ▶ continued

FOODS AND NUTRIENTS TO INCREASE

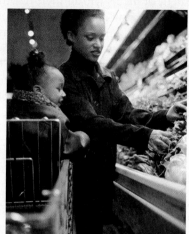

- Increase vegetable and fruit intake.

- Eat a variety of vegetables, especially dark-green and red and orange vegetables and beans and peas.

- Consume at least half of all grains as whole gains. Increase whole-grain intake by replacing refined grains with whole grains.

- Increase intake of fat-free or low-fat milk and milk products, such as milk, yogurt, cheese, or fortified soy beverages.

- Choose a variety of protein foods, which include seafood, lean meat and poultry, eggs, beans and peas, soy products, and unsalted nuts and seeds.

- Increase the amount and variety of seafood consumed by choosing seafood in place of some meat and poultry.

- Replace protein foods that are higher in solid fats with choices that are lower in solid fat and calories and/or sources of oils.

- Use oils to replace solid fats where possible.

- Choose foods that provide more potassium, dietary fiber, calcium, and vitamin D, which are nutrients of concern in American diets. These foods include vegetables, fruits, whole grains, and milk and milk products.

For women capable of becoming pregnant:

- Choose foods that supply heme iron (e.g., lean red meat), which is more readily absorbed by the body, additional iron sources, and enhancers of iron absorption, such as vitamin C-rich foods.

- Consume 400 micrograms per day of synthetic folic acid (from fortified foods and/or supplements) in addition to food forms of folate from a varied diet.

For women who are pregnant or breastfeeding:

- Consume 8 to 12 ounces of seafood per week from a variety of seafood types.

- Due to their high methyl mercury content, limit white (albacore) tuna to 6 ounces per week and do not eat the following four types of fish: tilefish, shark, swordfish, and king mackerel.

- If pregnant, take an iron supplement, as recommended by an obstetrician or other health care provider.

For individuals ages 50 years and older:

- Consume foods fortified with vitamin B-12, such as fortified cereals, or dietary supplements.

	Calorie Range (kcal)		
Children	Sedentary	⟶	Active
2–3 years	1000	⟶	1400
Females			
4–8 years	1200	⟶	1800
9–13	1400	⟶	2200
14–18	1800	⟶	2400
19–30	1800	⟶	2400
31–50	1800	⟶	2200
51+	1600	⟶	2200
Males			
4–8 years	1200	⟶	2000
9–13	1600	⟶	2600
14–18	2000	⟶	3200
19–30	2400	⟶	3000
31–50	2200	⟶	3000
51+	2000	⟶	2800

FIGURE 2-8 ▶ Estimates of calorie needs (kcals).

The full report contains background on the development of the Dietary Guidelines, many informative tables and charts to support the recommendations, and a comprehensive list of consumer behaviors and key strategies for achieving each recommendation. This information is available at www.health .gov/dietaryguidelines.

Balancing Calories to Manage Weight. As you will see in Chapter 7, the balance between calories consumed (from foods and beverages) and calories expended (through physical activity and metabolic processes) determines body weight. Consuming too many calories without increasing physical activity will inevitably lead to weight gain, which exacts an enormous toll on individuals and communities. Many chronic diseases, especially cardiovascular disease, type 2 diabetes, and osteoporosis, could be alleviated by meeting nutrient needs within calorie limits.

The Dietary Guidelines encourage all Americans to achieve and maintain a healthy body weight. Knowing how many calories you need each day is a good place to start (Fig. 2-8). You can calculate your EER on your own (see Chapter 7) or use an online calculator such as the one at www.ChooseMyPlate.gov. Once calorie needs are known, the next step is to become familiar with the calorie content of foods and beverages. Chapters 4, 5, and 6 will cover sources of calories in the diet. Finally, monitoring weight over time will allow you to see how your food and physical activity choices are balancing out.

Foods and Food Components to Reduce. Typical American diets contain too much sodium (salt), **solid fats** (e.g., butter), **added sugars,** and refined grains. Diets predominated by these food components especially increase risk for obesity, type 2 diabetes, hypertension, cardiovascular disease, and cancer.

Moderate alcohol consumption is associated with reduced risk of cardiovascular disease, deaths, and cognitive decline. However, those who do not drink should not begin drinking to attain these health benefits, because there are risks associated with even moderate alcohol consumption, including increased risk of breast cancer, violence, drowning, and injuries from falls and motor vehicle crashes. Heavy drinking is inherently risky and should be avoided altogether. More information about alcohol is presented in Chapter 16.

Foods and Nutrients to Increase. The Dietary Guidelines urge Americans to replace the problem foods we have discussed with nutrient-dense foods. Emphasize vegetables, fruits, whole grains, fat-free or low-fat milk and milk products, seafood, lean meats and poultry, eggs, beans and peas, and nuts and seeds. Instead of solid fats, choose foods made with vegetable oils.

These recommendations reflect the nutrient inadequacies of greatest public health concern: potassium, dietary fiber, calcium, and vitamin D. Individuals should strive to meet these goals without exceeding their calorie needs. Focusing on vegetables, fruits, whole grains, lean sources of protein, and low-fat or fat-free dairy products will not only contribute to nutrient adequacy but will also lower intake of problem nutrients, improve gastrointestinal function, aid in weight management, and decrease risk for a variety of chronic diseases.

A basic premise of the Dietary Guidelines is that nutrient needs should be met primarily through consuming foods. Foods provide an array of nutrients and other compounds that may benefit health. In certain cases, fortified foods and dietary supplements may be useful sources of one or more nutrients that otherwise might be consumed in less than recommended amounts. These are especially important for people whose typical food choices lead to a diet that cannot meet one or more nutrient recommendations, such as for vitamin D, vitamin E, or calcium. However, dietary supplements cannot and should not replace a healthy diet.

Building Healthy Eating Patterns. The Dietary Guidelines steer clear of a rigid prescription and, instead, promote an array of healthful options that can accommodate cultural, ethnic, traditional, and personal preferences, as well as food cost and availability factors. Well-studied examples of **eating patterns** consistent with the Dietary Guidelines include Dietary Approaches to Stop Hypertension (DASH), the USDA Food Patterns that accompanied MyPyramid (now MyPlate), vegetarian eating patterns, and Mediterranean-style eating patterns (see Further Reading 10). Common among these patterns are an abundance of vegetables and fruits, emphasis on whole grains, moderate amounts and varied sources of protein-rich foods, limited added sugars and solid fats, a high proportion of unsaturated fats compared to saturated fats, high potassium, and lower sodium.

The Dietary Guidelines and You. When applying the Dietary Guidelines, you need to consider your own state of health. Make specific changes and see whether they are effective for you. Note that results do not occur overnight and may not meet your expectations. Even when carefully following a diet low in saturated fat, some people continue to have high blood cholesterol. Other people can eat greater amounts of saturated fats and keep their blood cholesterol under control. Differences in genetic background are a key reason for these different responses, as you will learn in Chapter 3. Each of us must take into consideration our individual nutritional needs and

solid fats Fats that are solid at room temperature, such as butter and margarine. Foods containing solid fats tend to be high in saturated fatty acids or *trans* fatty acids.

added sugars Sugars or syrups that are added to foods during processing or preparation.

eating pattern A combination of foods and beverages that constitute an individual's complete dietary intake over time.

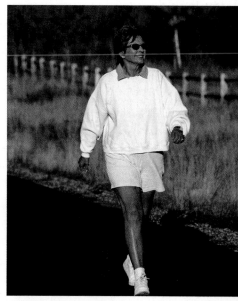

▲ Active means a lifestyle that includes physical activity equivalent to walking more than 3 miles per day at 3 to 4 miles per hour, in addition to the light physical activity associated with typical day-to-day life.

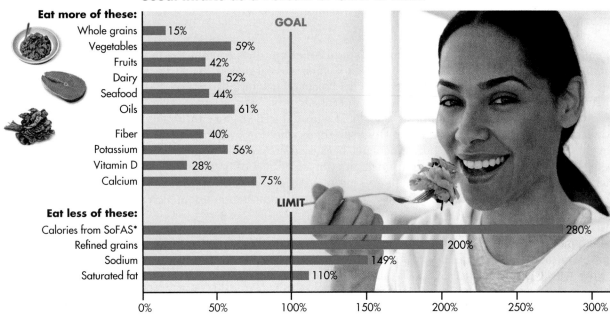

Usual Intake as a Percent of Goal or Limit

Eat more of these:

Whole grains	15%
Vegetables	59%
Fruits	42%
Dairy	52%
Seafood	44%
Oils	61%
Fiber	40%
Potassium	56%
Vitamin D	28%
Calcium	75%

GOAL

Eat less of these:

Calories from SoFAS*	280%
Refined grains	200%
Sodium	149%
Saturated fat	110%

LIMIT

0%   50%   100%   150%   200%   250%   300%

Percent of goal or limit

FIGURE 2-9 ▶

Comparing American Dietary habits to the Dietary Guidelines.

Source: Based on data from: U.S. Department of Agriculture, Agricultural Research Service and U.S. Department of Health and Human Services, Centers for Disease Control and Prevention. What We Eat in America, NHANES 2001–2004 or 2005–2006.

*SoFAS = solid fats and added sugars.
Note: Bars show average intakes for all individuals (ages 1 or 2 years or older, depending on the data source) as a percent of the recommended intake level or limit. Recommended intakes for food groups and limits for refined grains and solid fats and added sugars are based on amounts in the USDA 2000-calorie food pattern. Recommended intakes for fiber, potassium, vitamin D, and calcium are based on the highest AI or RDA for age 14 to 70 years. Limits for sodium are based on the UL and for saturated fat on 10% of calories. The protein foods group is not shown here because, on average, intake is close to recommended levels.

our risks of developing certain diseases (see Further Reading 6). Plan your diet with your specific needs in mind, taking into account your current health status and family history.

Whereas the Dietary Guidelines are not able to tailor a unique nutrition program for every North American citizen, they do provide adults with simple nutritional advice, which can be implemented by anyone willing to take a step toward good health. Table 2-5 provides examples of recommended diet changes based on the Dietary Guidelines. Although the cost of healthy eating is on the rise, you can make good choices and stay within your budget—canned or frozen fruits and vegetables and non-fat dry milk are a few of the available lower-cost foods.

Diet recommendations for adults have been issued by other scientific groups, such as the American Heart Association, U.S. Surgeon General, National Academy of Sciences, American Cancer Society, Canadian Ministries of Health (see Appendix C), and World Health Organization. All are consistent with the spirit of the Dietary Guidelines. These groups encourage people to modify their eating behaviors in ways that are both healthful and pleasurable.

MyPlate—A Menu-Planning Tool

The titles, food groupings, and shapes of food guides have evolved since the first edition published by the U.S. Department of Agriculture (USDA) nearly a century ago. The most recent food-guidance systems have incorporated physical activity and provided a means for individualization of dietary advice via interactive technology available on the Internet.

To keep pace with updated nutrition advice presented by the 2010 Dietary Guidelines for Americans and *Healthy People 2020* (see Chapter 1), MyPlate was released in 2011 as the leading depiction of healthy eating for Americans (Fig. 2-10). MyPlate,

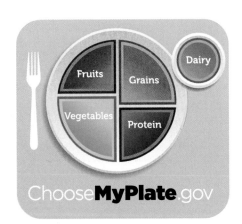

FIGURE 2-10 ▶ MyPlate is a visual representation of the advice contained in the 2010 Dietary Guidelines for Americans.

TABLE 2-5 Recommended Diet Changes Based on the Dietary Guidelines

If You Usually Eat This,	Try This Instead	Benefit
White bread	Whole-wheat bread	• Higher nutrient density, due to less processing • More fiber
Sugary breakfast cereal	Low-sugar, high-fiber cereal with fresh fruit	• Higher nutrient density • More fiber • More phytochemicals
Cheeseburger with French fries	Hamburger and baked beans	• Less saturated fat and *trans* fat • Less cholesterol • More fiber • More phytochemicals
Potato salad	Three-bean salad	• More fiber • More phytochemicals
Doughnuts	Bran muffin/bagel with light cream cheese	• More fiber • Less fat
Regular soft drinks	Diet soft drinks	• Fewer calories
Boiled vegetables	Steamed vegetables	• Higher nutrient density, due to reduced loss of water-soluble vitamins
Canned vegetables	Fresh or frozen vegetables	• Higher nutrient density, due to reduced loss of heat-sensitive vitamins • Lower in sodium
Fried meats	Broiled meats	• Less saturated fat
Fatty meats, such as ribs or bacon	Lean meats, such as ground round, chicken, or fish	• Less saturated fat
Whole milk	Low-fat or fat-free milk	• Less saturated fat • Fewer calories • More calcium
Ice cream	Sherbet or frozen yogurt	• Less saturated fat • Fewer calories
Mayonnaise or sour cream salad dressing	Oil-and-vinegar dressings or light creamy dressings	• Less saturated fat • Less cholesterol • Fewer calories
Cookies	Popcorn (air popped with minimal margarine or butter)	• Fewer calories and *trans* fat
Heavily salted foods	Foods flavored primarily with herbs, spices, lemon juice	• Lower in sodium
Chips	Pretzels	• Less fat

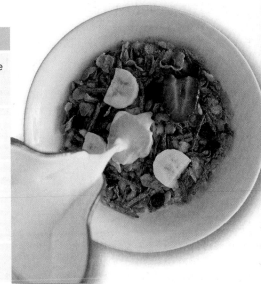

▲ Choose low-sugar, high-fiber cereal with fresh fruit instead of sugary breakfast cereal.

which replaces the familiar MyPyramid, shapes the key recommendations from the Dietary Guidelines into an easily recognizable and universally applicable visual: a place setting.

empty calories Calories from solid fats and/or added sugars. Foods with empty calories supply energy but few or no other nutrients.

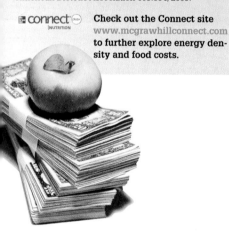

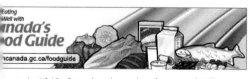

▲ In 1942, Canada released its first set of Official Food Rules. Since then, food guidance has evolved based on nutrition research and the changing needs of the population. Now, Health Canada publishes *Canada's Food Guide to Healthy Eating*, available in Appendix C.

Dishing Up MyPlate. Although it is not intended to stand alone as a source of dietary advice, MyPlate serves as a reminder of how to build a healthy plate at mealtimes (see Further Reading 19). It emphasizes important areas of the American diet that are in need of improvement. Recall from the discussion of the Dietary Guidelines that Americans need to increase the relative proportions of fruits, vegetables, whole grains, and fat-free or low-fat dairy products while simultaneously decreasing consumption of refined grains and high-fat meats.

The new MyPlate icon emphasizes five food groups:

- **Fruits** and **vegetables** cover half of the plate. These foods are dense sources of nutrients and health-promoting phytochemicals despite their low calorie contents.
- **Grains** occupy slightly more than one-fourth of the plate. The message to make half your grains whole is stressed throughout accompanying consumer-education materials.
- The remaining space on the plate is reserved for sources of **protein**. Specifically, the Dietary Guidelines recommend lean meats and poultry, plant sources of protein, and inclusion of fish twice a week.
- A cup of **dairy** appears next to the plate. Depending on personalized calorie recommendations, users should have 2 to 3 cups per day of low-fat or fat-free dairy products or other rich sources of calcium.

Unlike MyPyramid, MyPlate does not display a separate group for fats and oils, as they are mostly incorporated into other foods. Consumer messages tied to the MyPlate campaign reinforce recommendations to limit solid fats and focus instead on plant oils, which are sources of essential fatty acids and vitamin E.

Actionable Health Messages. Consumer research points to the need for simple, actionable health messages to capture the attention of the public and achieve successful behavior change. Accordingly, ChooseMyPlate.gov provides a series of succinct imperatives to help Americans make healthier food choices. Consumer messages include:

Balancing Calories

- Enjoy your food, but eat less.
- Avoid oversized portions.

Foods to Increase

- Make half your plate fruits and vegetables.
- Make at least half your grains whole.
- Switch to skim or 1% milk.

Foods to Reduce

- Compare sodium in foods like soup, bread, and frozen meals—and choose the foods with lower numbers.
- Drink water instead of sugary drinks.

Daily Food Plan. The Daily Food Plan is an interactive tool that estimates your calorie needs and suggests a food pattern based on your age, gender, height, and weight (Table 2-6). The Daily Food Plan provides useful information for each food group, including recommended daily amounts in common household measures, suggested oil intake, limits for **empty calories** and sodium, as well as advice for physical activity.

The recommended numbers of servings are given in cups for vegetables, fruits, and dairy foods. Grains and protein foods are listed in ounces. See Figure 2-11 for a description of what counts as a MyPlate serving. Pay close attention to the stated serving size for each choice when following your Daily Food Plan to help control calorie intake. Figure 2-12 provides a convenient guide to estimating common serving size measurements.

Modified daily food plans are also available for preschoolers, pregnant or breast-feeding mothers, and those interested in losing weight. Be sure to visit www.ChooseMyPlate.gov to generate your own Daily Food Plan.

TABLE 2-6 MyPlate Food-Intake Patterns Based on Calorie Needs

Daily Amount of Food from Each Group

Calorie Level	1000	1200	1400	1600	1800	2000	2200	2400	2600	2800	3000	3200
Fruits	1 cup	1 cup	1.5 cups	1.5 cups	1.5 cups	2 cups	2 cups	2 cups	2 cups	2.5 cups	2.5 cups	2.5 cups
Vegetables[1,2]	1 cup	1.5 cups	1.5 cups	2 cups	2.5 cups	2.5 cups	3 cups	3 cups	3.5 cups	3.5 cups	4 cups	4 cups
Grains[3]	3 oz-eq	4 oz-eq	5 oz-eq	5 oz-eq	6 oz-eq	6 oz-eq	7 oz-eq	8 oz-eq	9 oz-eq	10 oz-eq	10 oz-eq	10 oz-eq
Protein Foods	2 oz-eq	3 oz-eq	4 oz-eq	5 oz-eq	5 oz-eq	5.5 oz-eq	6 oz-eq	6.5 oz-eq	6.5 oz-eq	7 oz-eq	7 oz-eq	7 oz-eq
Dairy[4]	2 cups	2 cups	2 cups	3 cups	3 cups	3 cups	3 cups	3 cups	3 cups	3 cups	3 cups	3 cups
Oils[5]	3 tsp	4 tsp	4 tsp	5 tsp	5 tsp	6 tsp	6 tsp	7 tsp	8 tsp	8 tsp	10 tsp	11 tsp
Empty Calorie Limit[6]	140	120	120	120	160	260	270	330	360	400	460	600

oz-eq stands for ounce equivalent; tsp stands for teaspoon.

[1]Vegetables are divided into five subgroups (dark green, orange, legumes, starchy, and other). Over a week's time, a variety of vegetables should be eaten, especially green and orange vegetables.

[2]Dry beans and peas can be counted *either* as vegetables (dry beans and peas subgroup), *or* in the protein foods group. Generally, individuals who regularly eat meat, poultry, and fish would count dry beans and peas in the vegetable group. Individuals who seldom eat meat, poultry, or fish (vegetarians) would consume more dry beans and peas and count some of them in the protein foods group until enough servings from that group are chosen for the day.

[3]At least half of the grain servings should be whole-grain varieties.

[4]Most of the dairy servings should be fat-free or low-fat.

[5]Limit solid fats such as butter, stick margarine, shortening, and meat fat, as well as foods that contain these.

[6]Empty calories refers to added sugars and/or solid fats.

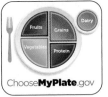

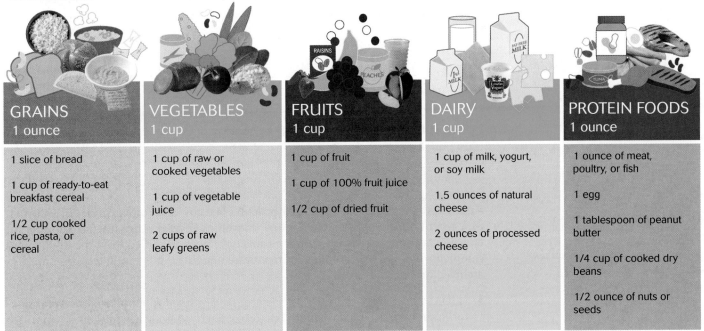

FIGURE 2-11 ▶ MyPlate: What counts as a serving?

Portion sizes

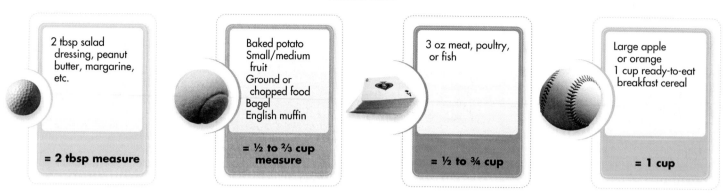

FIGURE 2-12 ▶ A golf ball, tennis ball, deck of cards, and baseball are standard-size objects that make convenient guides for judging serving sizes. Your hand provides an additional handy guide (for the greatest accuracy, compare your fist with a baseball, and adjust the following guides accordingly).

Fist = 1 cup

Thumb = 1 oz of cheese

Thumb tip to first joint = 1 tsp

Palm of hand = 3 oz

Handful = 1 or 2 oz of a snack food

MAKING DECISIONS

Measuring Your Portion Size

How familiar are you with serving size measurements? Common household units are listed in Appendix I with their metric equivalents. Ounces and fluid ounces differ. Ounces are a measure of weight, while fluid ounces are a measure of volume. Fluid ounces are based on the corresponding volume of water as the standard; 1 ounce of water by weight equals 1 fluid ounce. Any fluid more or less dense than water will yield a different number of fluid ounces per ounce of material.

MAKING DECISIONS

Empty Calories

MyPlate sets limits for empty calories, which come from solid fats and/or added sugars (Fig. 2-13). Solid fats and added sugars add calories to the diet but contribute few nutrients. Solid fats are solid at room temperature and include butter, beef fat, and shortening. Some solid fats, such as the marbling in a cut of ribeye steak, are naturally present in foods. Others, such as the shortening used to make a flaky croissant, are added during food processing or preparation. Added sugars include sugars and syrups that are added to foods during processing or preparation. Examples of foods that are major contributors of empty calories in the American diet are cakes, cookies, pastries, soft drinks, energy drinks, cheese, pizza, ice cream, and processed meats. The Daily Food Plans available on www.ChooseMyPlate.gov allow for 120 to 600 empty calories per day, depending on total energy needs:

Calorie Intake (kcal)	Empty Calories (kcal)	Calorie Intake (kcal)	Empty Calories (kcal)
1000*	140	2200	270
1200*	120	2400	330
1400*	120	2600	360
1600	120	2800	400
1800	160	3000	460
2000	260	3200	600

*Calorie intakes below 1600 kcal per day are generally intended for children 2 to 8 years of age. Unless under the guidance of a physician or registered dietitian, adults should consume at least 1600 kcal per day.

The International Food Information Council, available online at www.ific.org, is another great resource for current nutrition information.

Additional MyPlate Resources. ChooseMyPlate.gov also offers in-depth information regarding the Dietary Guidelines, as well as several other interactive tools for consumers. Many of these interactive tools have been modified from the MyPyramid campaign, but updates and improvements are ongoing. MyPyramid resources are also archived on the website.

- USDA's consumer brochure, *Let's Eat for the Health of It*, emphasizes several tips for improving Americans' diets (Fig. 2-14). Each tip is clearly broken down into specific actions the consumer can take. For example, one key recommendation

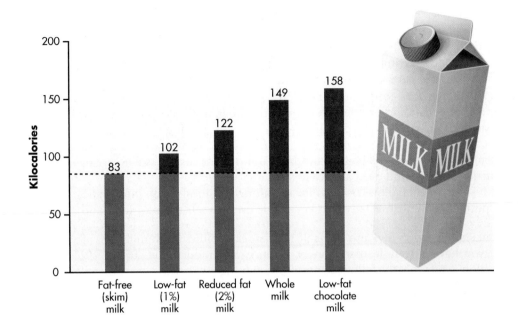

FIGURE 2-13 ▶ Empty calories come from solid fats and/or added sugars. This bar graph compares the amounts of empty calories in various types of milk.

Grains	Vegetables	Fruits	Dairy	Protein
Make half your grains whole grains	Vary your veggies	Focus on fruits	Get your calcium-rich foods	Go lean with protein
Use whole grains in mixed dishes, such as barley in vegetable soup or stews and bulgur wheat in casseroles or stir-fries. Add whole-grain flour or oatmeal when making cookies or other baked treats. Use the Nutrition Facts label and choose whole-grain products with a higher % Daily Value (%DV) for fiber. Many, but not all, whole-grain products are good or excellent sources of fiber.	Buy fresh vegetables in season. They cost less and are likely to be at their peak flavor. Include chopped vegetables in pasta sauce or lasagna. Allow children to pick a new vegetable to try while shopping.	Make most of your choices whole or cut-up fruit rather than fruit juice, for the benefits dietary fiber provides. Select fruits with more potassium often, such as bananas, prunes and prune juice, dried peaches and apricots, and orange juice. Add fruits like pineapple or peaches to kabobs as part of a barbeque meal.	Include milk or calcium-fortified soymilk as a beverage at meals. Choose fat-free or low-fat milk. If you avoid milk because of lactose intolerance, the most reliable way to get the health benefits of dairy products is to choose lactose-free alternatives within the Dairy Group, such as cheese, yogurt, lactose-free milk, or calcium-fortified soy milk or to consume the enzyme lactase before consuming milk.	The leanest beef cuts include round steaks and roasts (eye of round, top round, bottom round, round tip), top loin, sirloin, and chuck shoulder and arm roasts. Trim away all of the visible fat from meats and poultry before cooking. Choose beans, peas, or soy products as a main dish or part of a meal often.

Physical Activity

Find your balance between food and physical activity

- Do stretches, exercises, or pedal a stationary bike while watching television.
- Replace a coffee break with a brisk 10-minute walk. Ask a friend to go with you.
- Get the whole family involved—enjoy an afternoon bike ride with your kids.

Food Safety

Keep food safe to eat

- Wash your hands with warm water and soap for at least 20 seconds before and after handling food and after using the bathroom or changing diapers.
- Separate raw meat, poultry, seafood, and eggs from other foods in your grocery shopping cart, grocery bags, and in your refrigerator.
- Use a food thermometer, which measures the internal temperature of cooked meat, poultry, and egg dishes, to make sure that the food is cooked to a safe internal temperature.

FIGURE 2-14 ▶ These consumer tips have been developed by the USDA to help you build healthy meals with MyPlate. Many more tips are available at www.ChooseMyPlate.gov.

is "Cut back on foods high in solid fats, added sugars, and salt." One way a consumer can put this message into practice is to choose foods and drinks with little or no added sugars. Specific techniques associated with this recommendation include "Drink water instead of sugary drinks," "Select fruit for dessert," and "Choose 100% fruit juice instead of fruit-flavored drinks."

- USDA's Ten Tips Nutrition Education series provides access to one-page hand-outs for consumers and health educators. The materials cover a variety of topics, such as "Kid-friendly veggies and fruits," "Healthy eating for vegetarians," and "Got your dairy today?"
- Sample menus and recipes are available online for consumers who are ready to make a change and need a place to start.
- MyFood-a-Pedia allows users to locate calorie and food group information for specific food entries. Daily trackers enable users to self-monitor food and activity.

Menu Planning with MyPlate. Overall, MyPlate exemplifies the foundations of a healthy diet you have already learned: variety, balance, and moderation. To achieve optimal nutrition, remember the following points when using MyPlate to plan your daily menus:

- The guide does not apply to infants or children under 2 years of age. Daily Food Plans for children from ages 2 to 8 are based on average height and weight for age and gender.
- Variety is key to successful implementation of MyPlate. There is no single, perfect food that is absolutely essential to good nutrition. Each food is rich in some nutrients but deficient in at least one essential nutrient. Likewise, no food group is more important than another; each food group makes an important, distinctive contribution to nutritional intake (Table 2-7). Choose foods from each food group and also choose different foods within each food group. For a sample meal plan, see Table 2-8.
- The foods within a group may vary widely with respect to nutrients and calories. For example, the calorie content of 3 ounces of baked potato is 98 kcal, whereas that of 3 ounces of potato chips is 470 kcal. With respect to vitamin C, an orange has 70 mg and an apple has 10 mg.

Solid fats contribute almost 20% of total calories in typical American diets, but they have little to offer in terms of essential nutrients and dietary fiber. Instead of solid fats, choose foods containing plant oils.

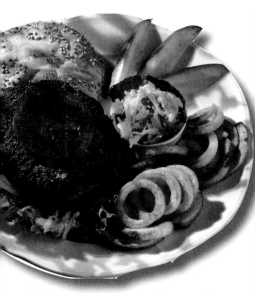

▲ Typical restaurant meals contain oversized portions that do not align with MyPlate.

TABLE 2-7 Nutrient Contributions of MyPlate Food Groups

Food Category	Major Nutrient Contributions
Grains	Carbohydrate Vitamins such as thiamin Minerals such as iron Fiber*
Vegetables	Carbohydrate Vitamins such as plant pigments that form vitamin A Minerals such as magnesium Fiber
Fruits	Carbohydrate Vitamins such as folate and vitamin C Minerals such as potassium Fiber
Dairy	Carbohydrate Protein Vitamins such as vitamin D Minerals such as calcium and phosphorus
Protein Foods	Protein Vitamins such as vitamin B-6 Minerals such as iron and zinc

*Whole-grain varieties

TABLE 2-8 Putting MyPlate into Practice.

Meal	Food Group
Breakfast	
1 small orange	Fruits
¾ cup Healthy Choice Low-fat Granola	Grains
with ½ cup fat-free milk	Dairy
½ toasted, small raisin bagel	Grains
with 1 tsp soft margarine	Oils
Optional: coffee or tea	
Lunch	
Turkey sandwich	
2 slices whole-wheat bread	Grains
2 oz turkey	Protein Foods
2 tsp mustard	
1 small apple	Fruits
2 oatmeal-raisin cookies (small)	Empty Calories
Optional: diet soft drink	
3 P.M. Study Break	
6 whole-wheat crackers	Grains
1 tbsp peanut butter	Protein Foods
½ cup fat-free milk	Dairy
Dinner	
Tossed salad	
1 cup romaine lettuce	Vegetables
½ cup sliced tomatoes	Vegetables
1½ tbsp Italian dressing	Oils
½ carrot, grated	Vegetables
3 oz broiled salmon	Protein Foods
½ cup rice	Grains
½ cup green beans	Vegetables
with 1 tsp soft margarine	Oils
Optional: coffee or tea	
Late-Night Snack	
1 cup "light" fruit yogurt	Dairy
Nutrient Breakdown	
1800 kcal	
Carbohydrate	56% of kcal
Protein	18% of kcal
Fat	26% of kcal

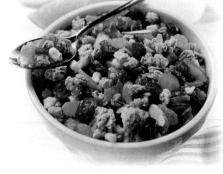
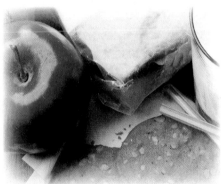
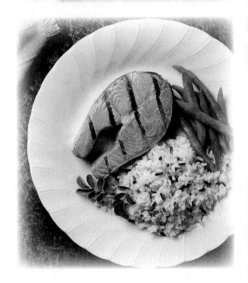

This menu meets nutrient needs for all vitamins and minerals for an average adult who needs 1800 kcal. For adolescents, teenagers, and older adults, add one additional serving of milk or other calcium-rich sources.

- Choose primarily low-fat and fat-free items from the dairy group. By reducing calorie intake in this way, you can select more items from other food groups. If milk causes intestinal gas and bloating, emphasize yogurt and cheese (see Chapter 4 for details on the problem of lactose maldigestion and lactose intolerance).

Check out CONNECT for links to alternative menu planning tools, such as the Healthy Eating Plate from Harvard School of Public Health. ⊞connect DRUG+ NUTRITION

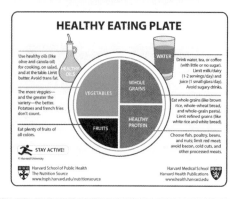

The **Exchange System** is an alternative menu-planning tool. This tool organizes foods based on calorie, protein, carbohydrate, and fat content. The result is a manageable framework for designing diets, especially for treatment of diabetes. For more information on the Exchange System, see Appendix D.

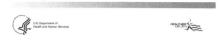

2008 Physical Activity Guidelines for Americans

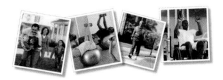

Be Active, Healthy, and Happy!

www.health.gov/paguidelines

▲ http://www.health.gov/PAGuidelines/.

- Include plant foods that are good sources of proteins, such as beans and nuts, at least several times a week because many are rich in vitamins (such as vitamin E), minerals (such as magnesium), and fiber.
- For vegetables and fruits, try to include a dark-green or orange vegetable for vitamin A and a vitamin-C rich fruit, such as an orange, every day. Do not focus primarily on potatoes (e.g., French fries) for your vegetable choices. Surveys show that fewer than 5% of adults eat a full serving of a dark-green vegetable on any given day. Increased consumption of these foods is important because they contribute vitamins, minerals, fiber, and phytochemicals.
- Choose whole-grain varieties of breads, cereals, rice, and pasta because they contribute vitamin E and fiber. A daily serving of a whole-grain, ready-to-eat breakfast cereal is an excellent choice because the vitamins (such as vitamin B-6) and minerals (such as zinc) typically added to it, along with fiber, help fill in common nutritional gaps.
- Include some plant oils on a daily basis, such as those in salad dressing, and eat fish at least twice a week. This supplies you with health-promoting essential fatty acids.

Reviews of MyPlate. Although MyPlate will promote important changes in American diets, it does have some limitations. Some critics say that the new icon is too simple. For example, it does not immediately provide information about overall calories, serving sizes, or number of servings to choose from each food group (recall the comic at the beginning of this chapter). However, many of these details will vary by person. Users will need to access the accompanying materials available on www.ChooseMyPlate.gov to obtain a personally tailored Daily Food Plan.

Food *quality* is just as important as food *quantity* when it comes to good nutrition. Consider the difference in calorie contents of the following two meals, both of which fit the proportions suggested by MyPlate:

Fried chicken fillet sandwich with mayonnaise on a white sandwich roll, 1 each	Skinless grilled chicken breast, 3 ounces
French fries, 1 medium order	Brown rice, prepared with reduced-fat tub margarine, 1 cup
Apple-filled pastry, 1 each	Steamed green beans, 1 cup
Whole milk, 1 cup	Cubed watermelon, 1 cup
1293 kcal	Skim milk, 1 cup
	513 kcal

The MyPlate icon does not address the types of foods to choose within each food group. Making appropriate food choices for weight management and prevention of diet-related chronic diseases requires consumers to have some nutrition knowledge. Fortunately, public health messages and online content related to MyPlate are available to educate Americans.

MyPlate shows how to build a healthy plate at mealtimes, but it does not adequately address the total diet, which, in reality, includes many snacks between meals. Consumer messages about healthy snacking will be a part of the consumer communications initiative over the next few years.

As with any public health campaign, it is possible that the people who need it most will overlook the MyPlate message. Educated consumers with access to interactive MyPlate tools likely already comply with many of the Dietary Guidelines. Populations with poor diets may be unlikely or unable to click through to find a personalized Daily Food Plan. The USDA's best response is to rely on the coordinated partnership of the National Communicator's Network to spread those actionable MyPlate messages, such as "Switch to fat-free or low-fat (1%) milk."

Overall, the new MyPlate icon is an attractive and relevant tool that immediately shows us how to build a healthy plate at meals. The strength of MyPlate lies in its simplicity. It conveys the major messages that are needed when shopping, cooking, and eating and can be enhanced with the details provided on www.ChooseMyPlate.gov and in forthcoming materials.

MAKING DECISIONS

The Mediterranean Diet Pyramid

Recently updated in 2009, the Mediterranean Diet Pyramid (Fig. 2-15) is a useful alternative to MyPlate. It is based on the dietary patterns of the southern Mediterranean region, which has enjoyed the lowest recorded rates of chronic diseases and the highest adult life expectancy. An abundance of research supports the health benefits of following the Mediterranean Diet (see Further Reading 14). Characteristics include:

- Foods from plant sources form the foundation of every meal.
- A variety of minimally processed and, wherever possible, seasonally fresh and locally grown foods are emphasized.
- Olive oil is the principal fat.
- Total fat ranges from less than 25% to over 35% of energy, with saturated fat no more than 7% to 8% of calories.
- Fish and seafood are consumed at least twice weekly.
- Lean or low-fat sources of protein, such as cheese, yogurt, poultry, and eggs, should be consumed in moderation.
- Red meats and sweet desserts are consumed less often.
- Regular physical activity is performed at a level that promotes a healthy weight, fitness, and well-being.
- Moderate wine drinking has health benefits.
- Water is the beverage of choice.

Oldways—a respected, international, nonprofit culinary think tank—also publishes the Latin-American Diet Pyramid and was the force behind development of the Whole Grain stamp seen on food packages.

Source: Oldways Food Issues Think Tank, 266 Beacon St., Boston, MA 02116, www.oldwayspt.org.

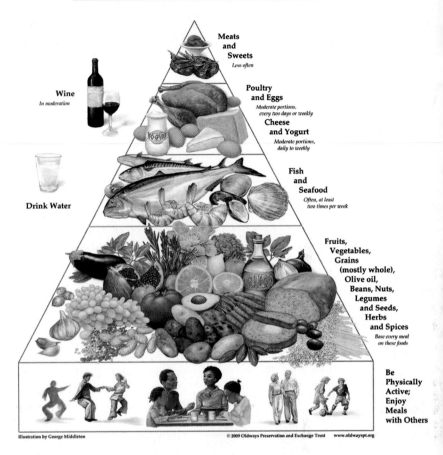

FIGURE 2-15 ▶ The Mediterranean Diet Pyramid is based on dietary patterns from the Mediterranean region, which has low rates of chronic diseases and high life expectancy.

How Does Your Plate Rate? Regularly comparing your daily food intake with your personalized Daily Food Plan recommendations is a relatively simple way to evaluate the quality of your overall diet. Identify the nutrients that are low in your diet based on the nutrients found in each food group (review Table 2-7). For example, if you do not consume enough servings from the milk group, your calcium intake is most likely too low. Look for foods that you enjoy that supply calcium, such as calcium-fortified orange juice.

For a more detailed analysis of your current diet, use the Food Tracker tool on www.ChooseMyPlate.gov. Your NutritionCalc software also helps you compare your food choices to MyPlate. With a detailed dietary analysis, you can compare your intakes of individual nutrients to the DRI standards and clearly see the areas that need improvement. Even small diet and exercise changes can have positive results.

Physical Activity Guidelines for Americans

In line with its goal for all Americans to live healthier, more prosperous, and more productive lives, the U.S. Department of Health and Human Services issued its first Physical Activity Guidelines for Americans in 2008 as a complement to the Dietary Guidelines (see Further Reading 16). The overarching idea is that regular physical activity—for people of all ages, races, ethnicities, and physical abilities—produces long-term health benefits. The guidelines are truly meant to inform the work of health professionals and policy makers, but consumer materials are available. *Be Active Your Way: A Guide for Adults*, available at www.health.gov, translates the guidelines into consumer-friendly, practical advice.

The key guidelines, listed in Table 2-9, provide measurable physical activity standards for Americans age 6 and older. Specific recommendations (not listed in Table 2-9) also apply to special population groups, including pregnant women, adults with disabilities, and people with chronic medical conditions. For adults, the guidelines emphasize that health benefits occur with at least 150 minutes per week of moderate-intensity physical activity. Adults may accumulate activity throughout the week in a variety of ways—extended sessions (e.g., 50 minutes on 3 days a week) or in short bursts throughout the week that amount to at least 150 minutes. Children and adolescents should strive to include 60 minutes of physical activity per day. For optimum benefits, include both aerobic and muscle-strengthening activities. Overall, physical activity should be enjoyable and safe for each individual.

A Coordinated Effort

The MyPlate icon fits together with a variety of educational tools as part of a multi-year Dietary Guidelines for Americans consumer communications initiative. USDA's Center for Nutrition Policy and Promotion heads up a National Communicator's Network to coordinate the efforts of public and private organizations, including the Department of Health and Human Services (sponsors of the 2008 Physical Activity Guidelines) as well as city governments, educational institutions, health networks, fitness centers, grocery chains, and a growing list of other organizations throughout the nation.

The Partnership program promotes a series of nutrition messages, starting with "Make half your plate fruits and vegetables." The campaign also incorporates the physical activity theme, "Be Active Your Way." The Dietary Guidelines Communications Message Calendar is available at http://www.choosemyplate.gov/downloads/MyPlate/DGCommunicationsMessageCalendar.pdf. Through a multifaceted media approach, this coordinated effort will help to expand the reach of the Dietary Guidelines, MyPlate, and Physical Activity Guidelines to individuals who, despite needing health improvements, may not be likely to access these tools.

▲ Americans of all ages should limit screen time—hours spent watching TV, at the computer, or playing video games.

CONCEPT CHECK

The 2010 Dietary Guidelines for Americans aim to improve the health of all Americans, ages 2 and older. Three major goals include: (1) balancing calories with physical activity to manage weight; (2) increasing intake of fruits, vegetables, whole grains, fat-free and low-fat dairy products, and seafood; and (3) reducing intake of foods with sodium, saturated fats, *trans* fats, cholesterol, added sugars, and refined grains. MyPlate and associated tools found at www.ChooseMyPlate.gov embody the Dietary Guidelines with a plate icon that serves as a reminder for healthy eating. Grains, fruits, vegetables, protein, and dairy are the five major food groups represented on MyPlate. The 2008 Physical Activity Guidelines for Americans advise a minimum of 150 minutes per week of moderate-intensity physical activity for adults or at least 60 minutes daily for children and adolescents.

TABLE 2-9 Selected Recommendations of the 2008 Physical Activity Guidelines for Americans*

Key Guidelines for Children and Adolescents

- Children and adolescents should do 60 minutes or more of physical activity daily.

  - Aerobic: Most of the 60 or more minutes a day should be either moderate- or vigorous-intensity aerobic physical activity and should include vigorous-intensity activity at least 3 days a week.

  - Muscle-strengthening: As part of their 60 or more minutes of daily physical activity, children and adolescents should include muscle-strengthening physical activity on at least 3 days of the week.

  - Bone-strengthening: As part of their 60 or more minutes of daily physical activity, children and adolescents should include bone-strengthening physical activity on at least 3 days of the week.

- It is important to encourage young people to participate in physical activities that are appropriate for their age, that are enjoyable, and that offer variety.

Key Guidelines for Adults

- All adults should avoid inactivity. Some physical activity is better than none, and adults who participate in any amount of physical activity gain some health benefits.

- For substantial health benefits, adults should do at least 150 minutes a week of moderate-intensity, or 75 minutes a week of vigorous-intensity aerobic physical activity, or an equivalent combination of moderate- and vigorous-intensity aerobic activity. Aerobic activity should be performed in episodes of at least 10 minutes, and preferably, it should be spread throughout the week.

- For additional and more extensive health benefits, adults should increase their aerobic physical activity to 300 minutes a week of moderate-intensity, or 150 minutes a week of vigorous-intensity aerobic physical activity, or an equivalent combination of moderate- and vigorous-intensity activity. Additional health benefits are gained by engaging in physical activity beyond this amount.

- Adults should also do muscle-strengthening activities that are moderate or high intensity and involve all major muscle groups on 2 or more days a week, as these activities provide additional health benefits.

Key Guidelines for Older Adults

- When older adults cannot do 150 minutes of moderate-intensity aerobic activity a week because of chronic conditions, they should be as physically active as their abilities and conditions allow.

- Older adults should do exercises that maintain or improve balance if they are at risk of falling.

- Older adults should determine their level of effort for physical activity relative to their level of fitness.

- Older adults with chronic conditions should understand whether and how their conditions affect their ability to do regular physical activity safely.

Key Guidelines for Safe Physical Activity

To do physical activity safely and reduce the risk of injuries and other adverse events, people should:

- Understand the risks and yet be confident that physical activity is safe for almost everyone.

- Choose to do types of physical activity that are appropriate for their current fitness level and health goals, because some activities are safer than others.

- Increase physical activity gradually over time whenever more activity is necessary to meet guidelines or health goals. Inactive people should "start low and go slow" by gradually increasing how often and how long activities are done.

- Protect themselves by using appropriate gear and sports equipment; looking for safe environments; following rules and policies; and making sensible choices about when, where, and how to be active.

- Be under the care of a health care provider if they have chronic conditions or symptoms. People with chronic conditions and symptoms should consult their health care provider about the types and amounts of activity appropriate for them.

*The 2008 Physical Activity Guidelines for Americans also include recommendations for pregnant women, adults with disabilities, and people with chronic medical conditions. These are available at www.health.gov.

2.7 Food Labels and Diet Planning

Today, nearly all foods sold in stores must be in a package that has a label containing the following information: the product name, name and address of the manufacturer, amount of product in the package, and ingredients listed in descending order by weight. This food and beverage labeling is monitored in North America by government agencies such as the Food and Drug Administration (FDA) in the United States (see Further Reading 15). The listing of certain food constituents also is required—specifically, on a Nutrition Facts panel (Fig. 2-16). Use the information in the Nutrition Facts panel to learn more about what you eat. The following components must be listed: total calories (kcal), calories from fat, total fat, saturated fat, *trans* fat, cholesterol, sodium, total carbohydrate, fiber, sugars, protein, vitamin A, vitamin C, calcium, and iron. In addition to these required components, manufacturers can choose to list polyunsaturated and monounsaturated fat, potassium, and others. Listing these components becomes *required* if the food is fortified with that nutrient or if a claim is made about the health benefits of the specific nutrient (see the upcoming section in Chapter 2 entitled "Health Claims on Food Labels").

Remember that the Daily Value is a generic standard used on the food label. The percentage of the Daily Value (% Daily Value or % DV) is usually given for each nutrient per serving. These percentages are based on a 2000 kcal diet. In other words, they are not as applicable to people who require considerably more or less than 2000 kcal per day with respect to fat and carbohydrate intake. DVs are mostly set at or close to the highest RDA value or related nutrient standard seen in the various age and gender categories for a specific nutrient.

Serving sizes on the Nutrition Facts panel must be consistent among similar foods. This means that all brands of ice cream, for example, must use the same serving size on their label. (These serving sizes may differ from those of MyPlate because those on food labels are based on typical serving sizes.) In addition, food claims made on packages must follow legal definitions (Table 2-10). For example, if a product claims to be "low sodium," it must have 140 milligrams of sodium or less per serving.

Many manufacturers list the Daily Values set for dietary components such as fat, cholesterol, and carbohydrate on the Nutrition Facts panel. This can be useful as a reference point. As noted, they are based on 2000 kcal; if the label is large enough, amounts based on 2500 kcal are listed as well for total fat, saturated fat, carbohydrate, and other components. As mentioned, DVs allow consumers to compare their intake from a specific food to desirable (or maximum) intakes.

Exceptions to Food Labeling

Foods such as fresh fruits and vegetables and fish currently are not required to have Nutrition Facts labels. However, many grocers have voluntarily chosen to provide their customers with information about these products. The next time you are at the grocery store, ask where you might find information on the fresh products that do not have a Nutrition Facts panel. You will likely find a poster or pamphlet near the product; often, these pamphlets contain recipes that use your favorite fruit, vegetable, or fish fillet. They may even assist you in your endeavor to improve your diet.

Protein deficiency is not a public health concern in the United States, so declaration of the % Daily Value for protein is not mandatory on foods for people over 4 years of age. If the % Daily Value for protein is given on a label, FDA requires that the product be analyzed for protein quality. This procedure is expensive and time-consuming, so many companies opt not to list a % Daily Value for protein. However, labels on food for infants and children under 4 years of age must

The Nutrition Facts label uses the term "calorie" to express energy content in some cases, but kilocalorie (kcal) values are actually listed.

Nutrient and herbal supplement labels have a different layout with a "Supplement Facts" heading. The Nutrition and Your Health section at the end of this chapter and Chapter 10 show examples of these labels.

▼ Use the Nutrition Facts label to learn more about the nutrient content of the foods you eat. Nutrient content is expressed as a percent of Daily Value. Canadian food laws and related food labels have a slightly different format (review Appendix C).

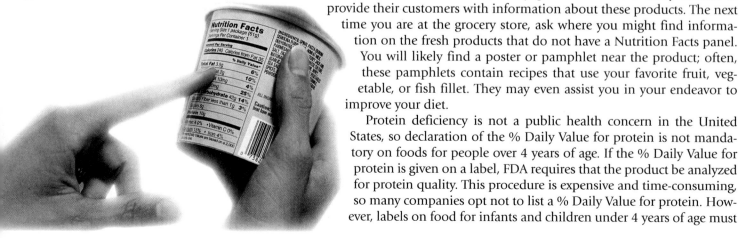

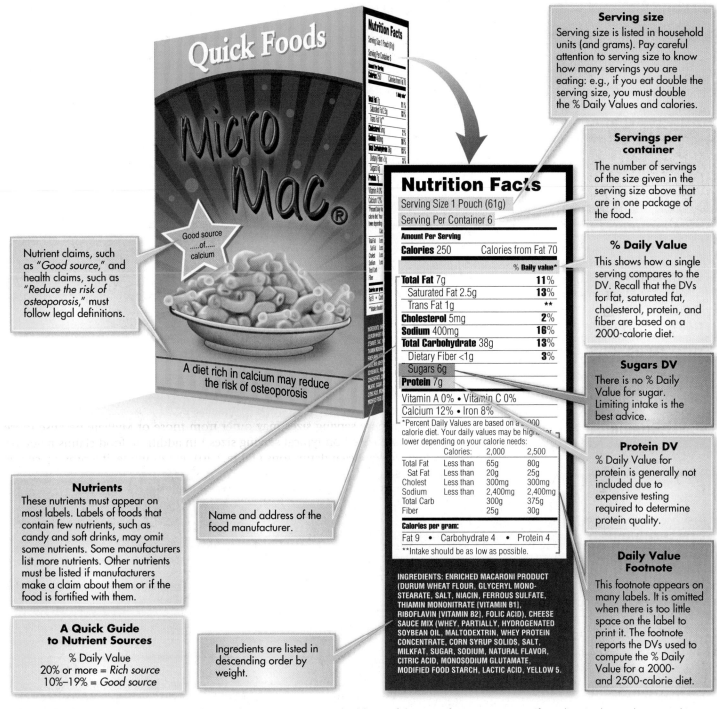

Serving size

Serving size is listed in household units (and grams). Pay careful attention to serving size to know how many servings you are eating: e.g., if you eat double the serving size, you must double the % Daily Values and calories.

Servings per container

The number of servings of the size given in the serving size above that are in one package of the food.

% Daily Value

This shows how a single serving compares to the DV. Recall that the DVs for fat, saturated fat, cholesterol, protein, and fiber are based on a 2000-calorie diet.

Sugars DV

There is no % Daily Value for sugar. Limiting intake is the best advice.

Protein DV

% Daily Value for protein is generally not included due to expensive testing required to determine protein quality.

Daily Value Footnote

This footnote appears on many labels. It is omitted when there is too little space on the label to print it. The footnote reports the DVs used to compute the % Daily Value for a 2000- and 2500-calorie diet.

Nutrient claims, such as "*Good source,*" and health claims, such as "*Reduce the risk of osteoporosis,*" must follow legal definitions.

Nutrients

These nutrients must appear on most labels. Labels of foods that contain few nutrients, such as candy and soft drinks, may omit some nutrients. Some manufacturers list more nutrients. Other nutrients must be listed if manufacturers make a claim about them or if the food is fortified with them.

A Quick Guide to Nutrient Sources

% Daily Value
20% or more = *Rich source*
10%–19% = *Good source*

Name and address of the food manufacturer.

Ingredients are listed in descending order by weight.

Nutrition Facts

Serving Size 1 Pouch (61g)
Serving Per Container 6

Amount Per Serving

Calories 250   Calories from Fat 70

	% Daily value*
Total Fat 7g	**11**%
Saturated Fat 2.5g	**13**%
Trans Fat 1g	**
Cholesterol 5mg	**2**%
Sodium 400mg	**16**%
Total Carbohydrate 38g	**13**%
Dietary Fiber <1g	**3**%
Sugars 6g	
Protein 7g	

Vitamin A 0% • Vitamin C 0%
Calcium 12% • Iron 8%

*Percent Daily Values are based on a 2,000 calorie diet. Your daily values may be higher or lower depending on your calorie needs:

	Calories:	2,000	2,500
Total Fat	Less than	65g	80g
Sat Fat	Less than	20g	25g
Cholest	Less than	300mg	300mg
Sodium	Less than	2,400mg	2,400mg
Total Carb		300g	375g
Fiber		25g	30g

Calories per gram:
Fat 9 • Carbohydrate 4 • Protein 4

**Intake should be as low as possible.

INGREDIENTS: ENRICHED MACARONI PRODUCT (DURUM WHEAT FLOUR, GLYCERYL MONO-STEARATE, SALT, NIACIN, FERROUS SULFATE, THIAMIN MONONITRATE (VITAMIN B1), RIBOFLAVIN (VITAMIN B2), FOLIC ACID), CHEESE SAUCE MIX (WHEY, PARTIALLY, HYDROGENATED SOYBEAN OIL, MALTODEXTRIN, WHEY PROTEIN CONCENTRATE, CORN SYRUP SOLIDS, SALT, MILKFAT, SUGAR, SODIUM, NATURAL FLAVOR, CITRIC ACID, MONOSODIUM GLUTAMATE, MODIFIED FOOD STARCH, LACTIC ACID, YELLOW 5.

FIGURE 2-16 ▶ Food packages must list product name, name and address of the manufacturer, amount of product in the package, and ingredients. The Nutrition Facts panel is required on virtually all packaged food products. The % Daily Value listed on the label is the percent of the amount of a nutrient needed daily that is provided by a single serving of the product. Canadian food labels use a slightly different group of health claims and label descriptors (see Appendix C).

include the % Daily Value for protein, as must the labels on any food carrying a claim about protein content (see Chapter 15).

Health Claims on Food Labels

As a marketing tool directed toward the health-conscious consumer, food manufacturers like to claim that their products have all sorts of health benefits. The FDA has

TABLE 2-10 Definitions for Nutrient Claims Allowed on Food Labels

Sugar

- **Sugar free**: less than 0.5 grams (g) per serving.

- **No added sugar; without added sugar; no sugar added:**

  - No sugars were added during processing or packing, including ingredients that contain sugars (for example, fruit juices, applesauce, or jam).

  - Processing does not increase the sugar content above the amount naturally present in the ingredients. (A functionally insignificant increase in sugars is acceptable for processes used for purposes other than increasing sugar content.)

  - The food that it resembles and for which it substitutes normally contains added sugars.

  - If the food doesn't meet the requirements for a low- or reduced-calorie food, the product bears a statement that the food is not low calorie or calorie reduced and directs consumers' attention to the Nutrition Facts panel for further information on sugars and calorie content.

- **Reduced sugar**: at least 25% less sugar per serving than reference food

Calories

- **Calorie free**: fewer than 5 kcal per serving

- **Low calorie**: 40 kcal or less per serving and, if the serving is 30 g or less or 2 tablespoons or less, per 50 g of the food

- **Reduced or fewer calories**: at least 25% fewer kcal per serving than reference food

Fiber

- **High fiber**: 5 g or more per serving. (Foods making high-fiber claims must meet the definition for low fat, or the level of total fat must appear next to the high-fiber claim.)

- **Good source of fiber**: 2.5 to 4.9 g per serving

- **More or added fiber**: at least 2.5 g more per serving than reference food

Fat

- **Fat free**: less than 0.5 g of fat per serving

- **Saturated fat free**: less than 0.5 g per serving, and the level of *trans* fatty acids does not exceed 0.5 g per serving

- **Low fat**: 3 g or less per serving and, if the serving is 30 g or less or 2 tablespoons or less, per 50 g of the food. 2% milk can no longer be labeled low fat, as it exceeds 3 g per serving. *Reduced fat* will be the term used instead.

- **Low saturated fat**: 1 g or less per serving and not more than 15% of kcal from saturated fatty acids

- **Reduced or less fat**: at least 25% less per serving than reference food

- **Reduced or less saturated fat**: at least 25% less per serving than reference food

Cholesterol

- **Cholesterol free**: less than 2 milligrams (mg) of cholesterol and 2 g or less of saturated fat per serving

- **Low cholesterol**: 20 mg or less of cholesterol and 2 g or less of saturated fat per serving or, if the serving is 30 g or less or 2 tablespoons or less, per 50 g of the food

- **Reduced or less cholesterol**: at least 25% less cholesterol than reference food and 2 g or less of saturated fat per serving

Sodium

- **Sodium free**: less than 5 mg per serving

- **Very low sodium**: 35 mg or less per serving and, if the serving is 30 g or less or 2 tablespoons or less, per 50 g of the food

- **Low sodium**: 140 mg or less per serving or, if the serving is 30 g or less or 2 tablespoons or less, per 50 g of the food

- **Light in sodium**: at least 50% less per serving than reference food

- **Reduced or less sodium**: at least 25% less per serving than reference food

Other Terms

- **Fortified or enriched**: Vitamins and/or minerals have been added to the product in amounts in excess of at least 10% of that normally present in the usual product. Enriched generally refers to replacing nutrients lost in processing, whereas fortified refers to adding nutrients not originally present in the specific food.

- **Healthy**: An individual food that is low fat and low saturated fat and has no more than 360 to 480 mg of sodium or 60 mg of cholesterol per serving can be labeled "healthy" if it provides at least 10% of the Daily Value for vitamin A, vitamin C, protein, calcium, iron, or fiber.

- **Light or lite**: The descriptor *light* or *lite* can mean two things: first, that a nutritionally altered product contains one-third fewer kcal or half the fat of reference food (if the food derives 50% or more of its kcal from fat, the reduction must be 50% of the fat) and, second, that the sodium content of a low-calorie, low-fat food has been reduced by 50%. In addition, "light in sodium" may be used for foods in which the sodium content has been reduced by at least 50%. The term *light* may still be used to describe such properties as texture and color, as long as the label explains the intent—for example, "light brown sugar" and "light and fluffy."

Diet: A food may be labeled with terms such as *diet, dietetic, artificially sweetened,* or *sweetened with nonnutritive sweetener* only if the claim is not false or misleading. The food can also be labeled *low calorie* or *reduced calorie.*

Good source: *Good source* means that a serving of the food contains 10% to 19% of the Daily Value for a particular nutrient. If 5% or less, it is a *low source.*

High: *High* means that a serving of the food contains 20% or more of the Daily Value for a particular nutrient.

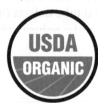

Organic: Federal standards for organic foods allow claims when much of the ingredients do not use chemical fertilizers or pesticides, genetic engineering, sewage sludge, antibiotics, or irradiation in their production. At least 95% of ingredients (by weight) must meet these guidelines to be labeled "organic" on the front of the package. If the front label instead says "made with organic ingredients," only 70% of the ingredients must be organic. For animal products, the animals must graze outdoors, be fed organic feed, and cannot be exposed to large amounts of antibiotics or growth hormones.

Natural: The food must be free of food colors, synthetic flavors, or any other synthetic substance.

The following terms apply only to meat and poultry products regulated by USDA.

Extra lean: less than 5 g of fat, 2 g of saturated fat, and 95 mg of cholesterol per serving (or 100 g of an individual food)

Lean: less than 10 g of fat, 4.5 g of saturated fat, and 95 mg of cholesterol per serving (or 100 g of an individual food)

Many definitions are from FDA's *Dictionary of Terms,* as established in conjunction with the 1990 Nutrition Labeling and Education Act (NLEA).
g = grams; mg = milligrams

legal oversight over most food products and permits some health claims with certain restrictions.

Overall, claims on foods fall into one of four categories:

- Health claims—closely regulated by FDA
- Preliminary health claims—regulated by FDA but evidence may be scant for the claim
- Nutrient claims—closely regulated by FDA (review Table 2-10)
- Structure/function claims—as discussed in the Nutrition and Your Health section at the end of this chapter, these are not FDA-approved or necessarily valid

Table 2-10 lists the definitions for nutrient claims on food labels. Currently, FDA limits the use of health messages to specific instances in which there is significant scientific agreement that a relationship exists between a nutrient, food, or food constituent and the disease. The claims allowed at this time may show a link between the following:

- A diet with enough calcium and vitamin D and a reduced risk of osteoporosis
- A diet low in total fat and a reduced risk of some cancers
- A diet low in saturated fat and cholesterol and a reduced risk of cardiovascular disease (typically referred to as heart disease on the label)
- A diet rich in fiber—containing grain products, fruits, and vegetables—and a reduced risk of some cancers
- A diet low in sodium and high in potassium and a reduced risk of hypertension and stroke
- A diet rich in fruits and vegetables and a reduced risk of some cancers
- A diet adequate in the synthetic form of the vitamin folate (called folic acid) and a reduced risk of neural tube defects (a type of birth defect) (see Chapter 12)
- Use of sugarless gum and a reduced risk of tooth decay, especially when compared with foods high in sugars and starches
- A diet rich in fruits, vegetables, and grain products that contain fiber and a reduced risk of cardiovascular disease. Oats (oatmeal, oat bran, and oat flour) and psyllium are two fiber-rich ingredients that can be singled out in reducing the risk of cardiovascular disease, as long as the statement also says the diet should also be low in saturated fat and cholesterol.
- A diet rich in whole-grain foods and other plant foods, as well as low in total fat, saturated fat, and cholesterol, and a reduced risk of cardiovascular disease and certain cancers
- A diet low in saturated fat and cholesterol that also includes 25 grams of soy protein and a reduced risk of cardiovascular disease. The statement "one serving of the (name of food) provides _____ grams of soy protein" must also appear as part of the health claim.
- Fatty acids from oils present in fish and a reduced risk of cardiovascular disease
- Margarines containing plant stanols and sterols and a reduced risk of cardiovascular disease (see Chapter 5 for more details on plant stanols and sterols)

A "may" or "might" qualifier must be used in the statement.

In addition, before a health claim can be made for a food product, it must meet two general requirements. First, the food must be a "good source" (before any fortification) of fiber, protein, vitamin A, vitamin C, calcium, or iron. The legal definition of "good source" appears in Table 2-10. Second, a single serving of the food product cannot contain more than 13 grams of fat, 4 grams of saturated fat, 60 milligrams of cholesterol, or 480 milligrams of sodium. If a food exceeds any one of these requirements, no health claim can be made for it, despite its other nutritional qualities. For example, even though whole milk is high in calcium, its label can't make the health

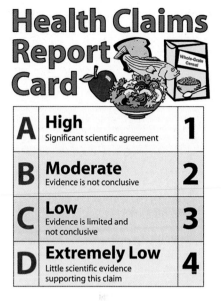

▲ In 2003, FDA unveiled a new process, including the Health Claims Report card, to provide more science-based, FDA-regulated health information on food product labels. This process is used to rank the claim based on the amount of scientific evidence and agreement. Only the first three classes are allowed.

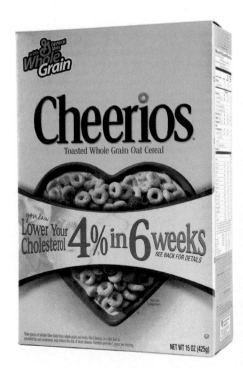

▲ Specific health claims can be made on food labels for whole-grain cereals.

claim about calcium and osteoporosis because whole milk contains 5 grams of saturated fat per serving. In another example, a health claim regarding fat and cancer can be made only if the product contains 3 grams or less of fat per serving, the standard for low-fat foods.

MAKING DECISIONS

Health Claims

FDA allows the three preliminary classes of health claims shown in the preceding section as long as the label qualifies the food with a disclaimer such as "this evidence is not conclusive." These preliminary health claims haven't shown up on many foods at this time (nuts, such as walnuts, and fish have been some of the first examples). These claims also cannot be used on foods considered unhealthy (review Table 2-10 for the definition of healthy with regard to a food).

CONCEPT CHECK

The Nutrition Facts panel on a food label provides key information for helping track one's food intake. Nutrient quantities are compared with the Daily Values and expressed on a percentage basis (% Daily Value). This information can be used to either increase or reduce intake of specific nutrients. Health and nutrient claims on food labels are closely regulated by FDA. Fruits, vegetables, whole-grain breads and cereals, soy, and good sources of calcium are prominent among the foods that can make specific health claims.

2.8 Epilogue

The tools discussed in Chapter 2 greatly aid in menu planning. Menu planning can start with MyPlate. The totality of choices made within the groups can then be evaluated using the Dietary Guidelines. Individual foods that make up a diet can be examined more closely using the Daily Values listed on the Nutrition Facts panel of the product. For the most part, these Daily Values are in line with the Recommended Dietary Allowances and related nutrient standards. The Nutrition Facts panel is especially useful in identifying nutrient-dense foods—foods high in a specific nutrient, such as the vitamin folate, but low in the relative amount of calories provided—and the energy-dense foods—foods that fill you up without providing a lot of calories. Generally speaking, the more you learn about and use these tools, the more they will benefit your diet.

Evaluating Nutrition Claims and Dietary Supplements

The following suggestions should help you make healthful and logical nutrition decisions:

1. Apply the basic principles of nutrition as outlined in this chapter (along with the 2010 Dietary Guidelines for Americans and related resources in Chapter 2) to any nutrition claim including those on websites. Do you note any inconsistencies? Do reliable references support the claims? Beware of the following:
   - Testimonials about personal experience
   - Disreputable publication sources
   - Promises of dramatic results (rarely true)
   - Lack of evidence from other scientific studies

2. Examine the background and scientific credentials of the individual, organizations, or publication making the nutritional claim. Usually, a reputable author is one whose educational background or present affiliation is with a nationally recognized university or medical center that offers programs or courses in the field of nutrition, medicine, or a closely allied specialty.

3. Be wary if the answer is "Yes" to any of the following questions about a health-related nutrition claim:
   - Are only advantages discussed and possible disadvantages ignored?
   - Are claims made about "curing" disease? Do they sound too good to be true?
   - Is extreme bias against the medical community or traditional medical treatments evident? Physicians as a group strive to cure diseases in their patients, using what proven techniques are available. They do not ignore reliable cures.
   - Is the claim touted as a new or secret scientific breakthrough?

4. Note the size and duration of any study cited in support of a nutrition claim. The larger it is and the longer it went on, the more dependable its findings. Also consider the type of study: epidemiology versus case-control versus double-blind. Check out the group studied; a study of men or women in Sweden may be less relevant than one of men or women of Southern European, African, or Hispanic descent, for example. Keep in mind that "contributes to," "is linked to," or "is associated with" does not mean "causes."

5. Beware of press conferences and other hype regarding the latest findings. Much of this will not survive more detailed scientific evaluation.

6. When you meet with a nutrition professional, you should expect that he or she will do the following:
   - Ask questions about your medical history, lifestyle, and current eating habits.
   - Formulate a diet plan tailored to your needs, as opposed to simply tearing a form from a tablet that could apply to almost anyone.
   - Schedule follow-up visits to track your progress, answer any questions, and help keep you motivated.
   - Involve family members in the diet plan, when appropriate.
   - Consult directly with your physician and readily refer you back to your physician for those health problems a nutrition professional is not trained to treat.

7. Avoid practitioners who prescribe **megadoses** of vitamin and mineral supplements for everyone.

8. Examine product labels carefully. Be skeptical of any promotional information about a product that is not clearly stated on the label. A product is not likely to do something not specifically claimed on its label or package insert (legally part of the label).

Dietary Supplements

A cautious approach to nutrition-related advice and products is even more important today because of broad changes in U.S. federal law passed in 1994.

The Dietary Supplement Health and Education Act (DSHEA) of 1994 classified vitamins, minerals, amino acids, and herbal remedies as "foods," which restrains the U.S. Food and Drug Administration (FDA) from regulating them as tightly as drugs and food additives. According to this act, rather than the manufacturer having to prove a dietary supplement is safe, FDA must prove it is unsafe before preventing its sale. In contrast, the safety of food additives and drugs must be demonstrated to FDA's satisfaction before they are marketed.

megadose Large intake of a nutrient beyond estimates of needs or what would be found in a balanced diet; 2 to 10 times human needs is a starting point.

▶ Recently, major nutrition organizations put together 10 red flags that they consider signals for poor nutrition advice:

1. Recommendations that promise a quick fix
2. Dire warnings of dangers from a single product or regimen
3. Claims that sound too good to be true
4. Simplistic conclusions drawn from a complex study
5. Recommendations based on a single study
6. Dramatic statements refuted by reputable scientific organizations
7. Lists of "good" and "bad" foods
8. Recommendations made to help sell a product
9. Recommendations based on studies published without peer review
10. Recommendations from studies that ignore differences among individuals or groups

▶ The FDA can act if evidence accumulates showing that a product is harmful. This has been true for some herbal remedies marketed as dietary supplements, such as ephedra.

Currently, a dietary supplement (or herbal product) can be marketed in the United States without FDA approval if (1) there is a history of its use or other evidence that it is expected to be reasonably safe when used under the conditions recommended or suggested in its labeling, and (2) the product is labeled as a dietary supplement. The Supplement Facts panel resembles the Nutrition Facts panel on foods and is required on all dietary supplements. It is permissible for the labels on such products to claim a benefit related to a classic nutrient-deficiency disease, describe how a nutrient affects human body structure or function (called structure/function claims), and claim that general well-being results from consumption of the ingredient(s). Examples could be "maintains bone health" or "improves blood circulation." However, the label of products bearing such claims also must prominently display in boldface type the following disclaimer: "This statement has not been evaluated by the Food and Drug Administration. This product is not intended to diagnose, treat, cure, or prevent disease" (Fig. 2-17). Despite this warning, when consumers find these products on the shelves of supermarkets,

health-food stores, and pharmacies, they may mistakenly assume FDA has carefully evaluated the products.

Many of us are willing to try untested nutrition products and believe in their miraculous actions. Popular products claim to increase muscle growth, enhance sexuality, boost energy, reduce body fat, increase strength, supply missing nutrients, increase longevity, and even improve brain function. Clearly, many nutritional products commonly found in stores are not strictly regulated in terms of effectiveness and safety (see Further Reading 13). The amount and potency of dietary supplements have also been in question. In June 2007, FDA issued long-awaited standards that require supplement manufacturers to test the purity, strength, and composition of all their products. The usefulness of supplements is discussed further in the Nutrition and Your Health section in Chapter 10, "Dietary Supplements—Who Needs Them?"

If you embark on a self-cure by means of such products, you will probably waste money and possibly risk ill health. A better approach is to consult a physician or **registered dietitian** first (see Further Reading 1). You can find a registered dietitian in North America by consulting the Yellow Pages in the telephone directory, contacting the local dietetic association, calling the dietary department of a local hospital, or visiting www.eatright.org/ or www.dietitians.ca. Make sure the person has the credentials "R.D." after his/her name ("R.D.N." is also used in Canada). This indicates the person has completed rigorous classroom and clinical training in nutrition and participates in continuing education. Appendix H also lists many reputable sources of nutrition advice for your use. Finally, the following websites can help you evaluate ongoing nutrition and health claims:

Supplement Facts

Serving Size 1 Softgel	
Each Softgel Contains	**% DV**
Ginseng Extract *(Panax ginseng)* (root) 100 mg (Standardized to 4% Ginsenosides)	*

*Daily Value (DV) not established.

INGREDIENTS: Gelatin, Soybean Oil, Panax Ginseng Extract, Vegetable Oil, Lecithin, Palm Oil, Glycerin, Sorbitol, Yellow Beeswax, Hydrogenated Coconut Oil, Titanium Dioxide, Yellow 5, Blue 1, Red 40, Green 3, Chlorophyll.

**DIST. BY NUTRA ASSOC., INC.
4411 WHITE POINT RD., SPRING CITY, IL 12345**

Suggested use: Adults- 1 to 2 capsules daily taken with a full glass of water, or as a tea, add one to two capsules to a cup of hot water.

When you need to perform your best, take ginseng.

This statement has not been evaluated by the Food and Drug Administration. This product is not intended to diagnose, treat, cure, or prevent disease.

- Suggested serving size
- Product and amount
- Name and address of manufacturer
- Suggested use
- Structure/function claim
- Standard FDA disclaimer

FIGURE 2-17 ▶ Supplement Facts label on an herbal product. Note the structure/function claim and the FDA disclaimer. Any nutrients or other food constituents would also be listed if contained in the product.

registered dietitian (R.D.) A person who has completed a baccalaureate degree program approved by the American Dietetic Association, performed at least 1200 hours of supervised professional practice, passed a registration examination, and complies with continuing education requirements.

www.acsh.org/
American Council on Science and Health

www.quackwatch.org/
Quackwatch: Your Guide to Quackery,
Health Fraud, and Intelligent Decisions

www.ncahf.org/
National Council Against Health Fraud

http://dietary-supplements.info.nih.gov/
National Institutes of Health, Office
of Dietary Supplements

www.fda.gov/
U.S. Food and Drug Administration

Overall, nutrition is a rapidly advancing
field and there are always new findings.

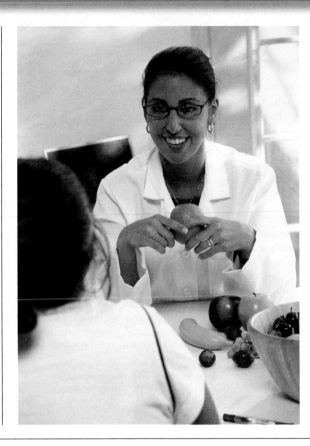

◀ Registered dietitians are a reliable source of nutrition advice.

Case Study Dietary Supplements

While Whitney was driving to campus last week, she heard an advertisement for a supplement containing a plant substance recently imported from China. It supposedly gives people more energy and helps one cope with the stress of daily life. This advertisement caught Whitney's attention because she has been feeling run-down lately. She is taking a full-course load and has been working 30 hours a week at a local restaurant to try to make ends meet. Whitney doesn't have a lot of extra money. Still, she likes to try new things and this recent breakthrough from China sounded almost too good to be true. After searching for more information about this supplement on the Internet, she discovered that the recommended dose would cost $60 per month. Because Whitney is looking for some help with her low energy level, she decides to order a 1-month supply.

Answer the following questions, and check your response in Appendix A.

1. Is the advertised supplement regulated by the FDA or other government agency?
2. What type of label claim is the phrase "increases energy," and does it require government approval?
3. Can Whitney feel confident that the supplement is safe and effective?
4. Is the amount of active ingredients in supplements tightly controlled?
5. Does it make sense for Whitney to spend the extra $60 per month for this supplement?
6. What advice would you give Whitney about the fact that she has been feeling run-down lately?

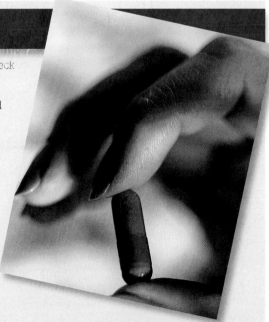

▲ Do you agree with Whitney's decision to try this supplement?

Summary (Numbers refer to numbered sections in the chapter.)

2.1 A healthy eating plan is based on consuming a *variety* of foods *balanced* by a moderate intake of each food and will minimize the risk of developing nutrition-related diseases.

Nutrient density reflects the nutrient content of a food in relation to its calorie content. Nutrient-dense foods are relatively rich in nutrients, in comparison with calorie content.

Energy density of a food is determined by comparing calorie content with the weight of food. A food rich in calories but weighing relatively very little, such as nuts, cookies, fried foods in general, and most snack foods (including fat-free brands), is considered energy dense. Foods with low energy density include fruits, vegetables, and any food that incorporates lots of water during cooking, such as oatmeal.

2.2 A person's nutritional state can be categorized as *desirable nutrition,* in which the body has adequate stores for times of increased needs; *undernutrition,* which may be present with or without clinical symptoms; and *overnutrition,* which can lead to vitamin and mineral toxicities and various chronic diseases.

2.3 Evaluation of nutritional state involves analyzing background factors, as well as anthropometric, biochemical, clinical, dietary, and environmental assessments. It is not always possible to detect nutritional inadequacies via nutrition assessment because symptoms of deficien-

cies are often nonspecific and may not appear for many years.

2.4 The scientific method is the procedure for testing the validity of possible explanations of a phenomenon, called hypotheses. Experiments are conducted to either support or refute a specific hypothesis. Once we have enough experimental information to support a specific hypothesis, it then can be called a theory. All of us need to be skeptical of new ideas in the nutrition field, waiting until many lines of experimental evidence support a concept before adopting any suggested dietary practice.

2.5 Recommended Dietary Allowances (RDAs) are set for many nutrients. These amounts yield enough of each nutrient to meet the needs of healthy individuals within specific gender and age categories. Adequate Intake (AI) is the standard used when not enough information is available to set a more specific RDA. Estimated Energy Requirements (EERs) set calorie needs for both genders at various ages and physical activity patterns. Tolerable Upper Intake Levels (Upper Levels or ULs) for nutrient intake have been set for some vitamins and minerals.

All of the many dietary standards fall under the term *Dietary Reference Intakes (DRIs).* Daily Values are used as a basis for expressing the nutrient content of foods on the Nutrition Facts panel and are based for the most part on the RDAs.

2.6 Dietary Guidelines for Americans have been issued to help improve the health of all Americans ages 2 and older. The guidelines emphasize balancing calories to manange weight; performing regular physical activity; moderating consumption of fat, *trans* fat, cholesterol, sugar, salt, and alcohol; eating plenty of whole-grain products, fruits, and vegetables; and safely preparing and storing foods, especially perishable foods.

MyPlate and accompanying online tools are designed to translate nutrient recommendations into a food plan that exhibits variety, balance, and moderation. The best results are obtained by using low-fat or fat-free dairy products; incorporating some vegetable proteins in the diet in addition to animal-protein foods; including citrus fruits and dark-green vegetables; and emphasizing whole-grain breads and cereals.

2.7 Food labels, especially the Nutrition Facts panels, are a useful tool to track your nutrient intake and learn more about the nutritional characteristics of the foods you eat. Any health claims listed must follow criteria set by FDA.

N&YH Apply the basic principles of nutrition to evaluate any nutrition claim. Dietary supplements can be marketed in the United States without FDA approval. Certain health claims can be made on supplement labels, although few have been thoroughly evaluated by reputable scientists.

Check Your Knowledge (Answers to the following questions are below.)

1. Anthropometric measurements include
   a. height, weight, skinfolds, and body circumferences.
   b. blood concentrations of nutrients.
   c. a diet history of the previous days' intake.
   d. blood levels of enzyme activities.

2. Foods with *high* nutrient density offer the _____ nutrients for the _____ calories.
   a. least, lowest
   b. least, most
   c. most, lowest
   d. most, most

3. A meal of a bean burrito, tossed salad, and glass of milk represents foods from all MyPlate food groups except
   a. dairy.   c. vegetables.
   b. protein.   d. fruits.

4. The Dietary Guidelines for Americans were recently revised in
   a. 2000   c. 2008
   b. 2005   d. 2010

5. The term Daily Value is used on
   a. restaurant menus.
   b. food labels.
   c. medical charts.
   d. None of the above.

6. The Tolerable Upper Intake Level, or UL, is used to
   a. estimate calorie needs of the average person.
   b. evaluate the highest amount of daily nutrient intake unlikely to cause adverse health effects.
   c. evaluate your current intake for a specific nutrient.
   d. compare the nutrient content of a food to approximate human needs.

7. The current food label must list
   a. a picture of the product.
   b. a uniform and realistic serving size.

c. the RDA for each age group.

d. ingredients alphabetically.

8. Dietary supplements are tightly regulated by the
   a. FDA.
   b. USDA.
   c. FTC.
   d. None of the above.

9. The scientific method begins with
   a. a hypothesis.
   b. research experiments.
   c. publication of research findings.
   d. observations made and questions asked.

10. The most common type of undernutrition in industrialized nations, such as the United States, is
    a. anorexia.
    b. protein deficiency.
    c. obesity.
    d. iron deficiency.

Study Questions (Numbers refer to Learning Outcomes)

1. Among your classmates, you observe that students who consume coffee get better grades. Provide an example of how you could use the scientific method to examine the effects of coffee consumption on academic performance **(LO 2.3)**.

2. How would you explain the concepts of nutrient density and energy density to a fourth-grade class **(LO 2.1)**?

3. Trace the progression, in terms of physical results, of a person who went from an overnourished to an undernourished state **(LO 2.2)**.

4. How could the nutritional state of the person at each state in question 3 be evaluated **(LO 2.2)**?

5. Describe the philosophy underlying the creation of MyPlate. What dietary changes would you need to make to comply with the healthy eating guidelines exemplified by MyPlate on a regular basis **(LO 2.6)**?

6. Describe the intent of the Dietary Guidelines for Americans. Point out one criticism for their general application to all North American adults **(LO 2.5)**.

7. Based on the discussion of the Dietary Guidelines for Americans, suggest two key dietary changes the typical North American adult should consider making **(LO 2.5)**.

8. How do RDAs and AIs differ from Daily Values in intention and application **(LO 2.4)**?

9. Dietitians encourage all people to read labels on food packages to learn more about what they eat. What four nutrients could easily be tracked in your diet if you read the Nutrition Facts panels regularly on food products **(LO 2.7)**?

10. What would you list as the top five sources of reliable nutrition information? What makes these sources reliable **(LO 2.8)**?

What Would You Choose Recommendations

An 8-ounce glass of orange juice provides 114 kcal, 24 grams of sugar, 0 grams of fiber, and 72 mg of vitamin C. The weight of this serving of orange juice is about 250 grams, or almost 9 ounces (there are about 28 grams in 1 ounce). To estimate energy density, compare the calorie content of this food to its weight: 114 kcal/250 grams = 0.456 kcal/gram. To find nutrient density for vitamin C, calculate a ratio of vitamin C content to the calorie content of the food: 72 milligrams of vitamin C/114 kcal = 0.63 mg vitamin C/kcal.

A whole, fresh, medium orange has about 60 kcal, 12 grams of sugar, 3 grams of fiber, and 70 mg of vitamin C. The weight of an orange is about 130 grams. Comparing calorie content to weight of the food results in 60 kcal/130 grams = 0.462 kcal/gram for energy density. Nutrient density for vitamin C is calculated as 70 milligrams of vitamin C/60 kcal = 1.17 mg vitamin C/kcal.

Oranges and orange juice have about the same energy density, but the nutrient density for vitamin C is almost twice as high as that for orange juice. Oranges and 100% orange juice are both good choices in terms of energy density, and both are rich sources of vitamin C. The RDA for vitamin C is 75 mg/day for women and 90 mg/day for men. A person who is trying to restrict calorie intake while still consuming adequate nutrients should choose the whole, fresh orange instead of the orange juice as a source of vitamin C because it has higher nutrient density—it provides excellent nutrition in fewer calories than the serving of orange juice. Whole fruits also provide more fiber and phytochemicals than juice. Be assured that 100% fruit juice is still a healthy choice. When choosing your servings of fruit, choose whole fruits more often than fruit juice to get the best nutrition in the fewest calories.

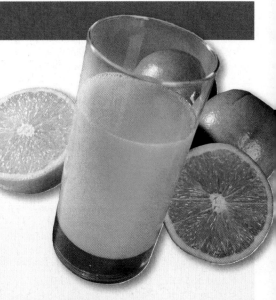

▲ The nutrient density of whole oranges surpasses that of orange juice.

Further Readings

1. ADA Reports: Position of the American Dietetic Association: Food and nutrition misinformation. *Journal of the American Dietetic Association* 106:601, 2006.

   Much food and nutrition misinformation pervades North American society. Individuals should carefully consider the training of those who give advice and be assured that registered dietitians are credible and reliable resources.

2. Barr SI: Introduction to dietary reference intakes. *Applied Physiology, Nutrition, and Metabolism* 31:61, 2006.

   The development of the Dietary Reference Intakes (DRIs) was a joint initiative by the United States and Canada to update and replace the former Recommended Nutrient Intakes for Canadians and the Recommended Dietary Allowances for Americans. The new DRIs are described.

3. Kennedy ET: Evidence for nutritional benefits in prolonging wellness. *American Journal of Clinical Nutrition* 83:410S, 2006.

   The interaction between genes; the environment; and lifestyle factors, especially diet and physical activity, are involved in healthy aging. The need to consider all the lifestyle and environmental factors contributing to suboptimal eating and lifestyle patterns is discussed.

4. Mobley AR and others: Putting the nutrient-rich foods index into practice. *Journal of the American College of Nutrition* 28:427S, 2009.

   In response to a need for a standardized definition of nutrient density as well as a growing interest among consumers and food manufacturers in front-of-pack labeling to convey nutrient information in a glance, the Nutrient Rich Foods Coalition formulated a Nutrient-Rich Foods educational tool and a symbol, called My5, which conveys nutrient content of a food within the context of a healthy diet.

5. Reedy J, Krebs-Smith SM: A comparison of food-based recommendations and nutrient values of three food guides: USDA's MyPyramid, NHLBI's dietary approaches to stop hypertension eating plan, and Harvard's healthy eating pyramid. *Journal of the American Dietetic Association* 108: 522, 2008.

   The three food guides share consistent messages to eat more fruits, vegetables, legumes, and whole grains; eat less added sugar and saturated fat; and emphasize plant oils.

6. Rolls B: *The volumetric eating plan: Techniques and recipes for feeling full on fewer calories.* Harper, New York, 2005.

   Energy density of food choices strongly affects total calories consumed at a meal and throughout the day. The volumetric eating plan includes techniques and recipes that decrease energy density of the diet—incorporating more fiber and water—which helps people lower their calories without feeling deprived.

7. Rowe S and others: Translating the Dietary Guidelines for Americans 2010 to bring about real behavior change. *Journal of the American Dietetic Association* 111:28, 2011.

   Nutition experts devised a set of recommendations to assist health professionals, government authorities, and food manufacturers in implementing the Dietary Guidelines for Americans, 2010. The coordination of efforts of educators, health care providers, policy makers, and industry leaders is needed to reach the public. Nutrition messages should be simple and targeted. Along with efforts to encourage people to want to change their habits, food manufacturers should make gradual changes in food composition to better align products with the goals of the Dietary Guidelines. Education efforts should begin at an early age and should be sensitive to differences in culure and ethnic background.

8. Sheth A and others: Potential liver damage associated with over-the-counter vitamin supplements. *Journal of the American Dietetic Association* 108:1536, 2008.

   This case report provides an example of the potential for liver damage associated with long-term intakes of megadose dietary supplements. In this case, a patient developed liver cirrhosis after long-term (2 years) daily ingestion of over-the-counter dietary supplements containing 13,000 micrograms of vitamin A. Such adverse effects indicate the need for medical supervision of use of these products.

9. Sofi F and others: Adherence to Mediterranean Diet and health status: Meta-analysis. *British Medical Journal* 337:a1344, 2008.

   A systematic review found that greater adherence to a Mediterranean Diet is associated with a significant reduction in overall mortality (9%), mortality from cardiovascular diseases (9%), incidence of mortality from cancer (6%), and incidence of Parkinson's disease and Alzheimer's disease (13%). These results indicate that a Mediterranean-like dietary pattern should be encouraged for primary prevention of major chronic diseases.

10. Taylor CL, Wilkening VL: How the nutrition food label was developed, Part 1: The nutrition facts panel. Part 2: The purpose and promise of nutrition claims. *The Journal of the American Dietetic Association* 108: 437, 618, 2008.

    These articles offer insight into the development of the nutrition label and discuss its role in improving the diet and health of Americans. The issues discussed highlight the fact that the nutrition label is a "work in progress."

11. U.S. Department of Health and Human Services. *2008 Physical Activity Guidelines for Americans.* 2008. www.health.gov/ PAGuidelines/.

    Inactivity remains high among American children, adolescents, and adults, putting Americans at unnecessary risk of disease. The Guidelines provide science-based guidance to help Americans aged six and older improve their health through appropriate physical activity.

12. U.S. Department of Health and Human Services. *Dietary Guidelines for Americans, 2010.* 2011. www.health.gov/ dietaryguidelines/2010.

    The most recent Dietary Guidelines have three overarching goals. 1.) balance calories with physical activity to manage weight; 2.) consume more fruits, vegetables, whole grains, fat-free and low-fat dairy products, and seafoods; and 3.) consume fewer foods with sodium, saturated fats, trans fats, cholesterol, added sugars, and refined grains.

13. United States Department of Agriculture. *USDA's MyPlate.* 2011. www.choosemyplate .gov.

    MyPlate replaces MyPyramid as the icon depicting healthy eating for Americans. In addition to the graphic representations of MyPlate, www. ChooseMyPlate.gov. provides Daily Food Plans specific to individual energy needs, several interactive tools for consumers, and resources for health educators. Building a healthy meal with balanced proportions of fruits, vegetables, grains, protein, and dairy will help Americans reach the goals set forth by the Dietary Guidelines.

14. Watts ML and others: The art of translating nutritional science into dietary guidance: History and evolution of the Dietary Guidelines for Americans. *Nutrition Reviews* 69:404, 2011.

    The U.S. government has issued dietary guidance for more than 100 years. Over time, the guidelines have become more firmly rooted in scientific evidence and more specific to the target audience. There is widespread recognition that successful implementation of dietary guidance requires the coordination of stakeholders at all levels—policy makers, health care providers, educators, industry, and consumers.

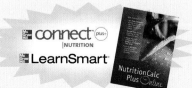

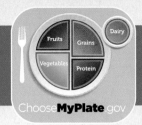
I. Does your Diet Compare to MyPlate?

Using your food-intake record from Chapter 1, place each food item in the appropriate group of the accompanying MyPlate chart. That is, for each food item, indicate how many servings it contributes to each group based on the amount you ate (see Food Composition Table Supplement for serving sizes). Many of your food choices may contribute to more than one group. For example, spaghetti with meat sauce contributes to three categories; grains, vegetables, and protein. After entering all the values, add the number of servings consumed in each group. Finally, compare your total in each food group with the recommended number of servings shown in Table 2-6 or obtained from the www.ChooseMyPlate.gov website. Enter a minus sign (−) if your total falls below the recommendation or a plus sign (+) if it equals or exceeds the recommendation.

Indicate the number of servings from MyPlate that each food yields:

Food or Beverage	Amount Eaten	Grains	Vegetables	Fruits	Dairy	Protein	Oils
Group totals							
Recommended servings							
Shortages/overages in numbers of servings							

II. Are You Putting Health Advice into Practice?

The broad range of diet and physical activity advice provided by the 2010 Dietary Guidelines for Americans, 2008 Physical Activity Guidelines for Americans, and MyPlate can seem overwhelming. Fill out the following inventory to see how well you comply with the basic intent of these consumer health guidelines and identify areas in which you need improvement.

Build a Healthy Plate

Y	N	Do fruits and vegetables cover at least half of your plate at meal times?
Y	N	Do you use fruits, vegetables, or unsalted nuts as snacks?
Y	N	Do you use either skim or 1% milk?
Y	N	Do you consume at least three servings of whole grains per day?
Y	N	Do you include seafood as your source of protein at least twice per week?
Y	N	Do you include beans as your source of protein at least once per week?
Y	N	Do you consume alcohol in moderation (≤1 drink/day for women; ≤2 drinks/day for men)?
Y	N	Do you use a meat thermometer to determine if your foods are thoroughly cooked?
Y	N	Do you clean hands, food contact surfaces, and fruits and vegetables before preparation?

Cut Back on Foods High in Solid Fats, Added Sugars, and Salt

Y	N	Do you choose water or other calorie-free beverages to drink most of the time?
Y	N	When you drink juice, do you choose 100% fruit juice?
Y	N	Do you use the Nutrition Facts panel to select foods low in sodium?
Y	N	Do you use spices and herbs instead of salt to season your food?
Y	N	Do you use vegetable oils rather than butter, lard, or shortening when preparing foods?
Y	N	Do you select foods that are reduced-fat, low-fat, or fat-free?

Eat the Right Amount of Calories for You

Y	N	Is your weight within a healthy range?
Y	N	Do you know how many calories you need per day?
Y	N	Do you limit your portions to one serving (i.e., as listed on food labels) of most foods?
Y	N	Do you stop eating when you are satisfied rather than uncomfortably full?
Y	N	Do you prepare most of your own foods?
Y	N	When eating out, do you seek out nutrition information on menu items?
Y	N	Do you take home leftovers or share meals with a friend when dining out?

Be Physically Active Your Way

Y	N	Do you exercise at least 150 minutes per week?
Y	N	Do you include aerobic and muscle-strengthening activities into your exercise routine?
Y	N	Do you protect yourself from injury when participating in physical activity?
Y	N	Does your exercise routine match your current level of fitness, ability, and health?

III. Applying the Nutrition Facts Label to Your Daily Food Choices

Imagine that you are at the supermarket looking for a quick meal before a busy evening. In the frozen food section, you find two brands of frozen cheese manicotti (see labels a and b). Which of the two brands would you choose? What information on the Nutrition Facts label in the figure contributed to this decision?

_____

_____

_____

_____

(a)

Nutrition Facts

Serving Size 1 Package (260g)
Servings Per Container 1

Amount Per Serving

Calories 390   Calories from Fat 160

	% Daily Value*
Total Fat 18g	**27**%
Saturated Fat 9g	**45**%
Trans Fat 2g	**
Cholesterol 45mg	**14**%
Sodium 880mg	**36**%
Total Carbohydrate 38g	**13**%
Dietary Fiber 4g	**15**%
Sugars 12g	
Protein 17g	

Vitamin A 10% • Vitamin C 4%

Calcium 40% • Iron 8%

*Percent Daily Values are based on a 2,000 calorie diet. Your daily values may be higher or lower depending on your calorie needs:

		Calories:	2,000	2,500
Total Fat	Less than		65g	80g
Sat Fat	Less than		20g	25g
Cholesterol	Less than		300mg	300mg
Sodium	Less than		2,400mg	2,400mg
Total Carbohydrate			300g	375g
Dietary Fiber			25g	30g

Calories per gram:
Fat 9 • Carbohydrate 4 • Protein 4

**Intake of _trans_ fat should be as low as possible.

(b)

Nutrition Facts

Serving Size 1 Package (260g)
Servings Per Container 1

Amount Per Serving

Calories 230   Calories from Fat 35

	% Daily Value*
Total Fat 4g	**6**%
Saturated Fat 2g	**10**%
Trans Fat 1g	**
Cholesterol 15mg	**4**%
Sodium 590mg	**24**%
Total Carbohydrate 28g	**9**%
Dietary Fiber 3g	**12**%
Sugars 10g	
Protein 19g	

Vitamin A 10% • Vitamin C 10%

Calcium 35% • Iron 4%

*Percent Daily Values are based on a 2,000 calorie diet. Your daily values may be higher or lower depending on your calorie needs:

		Calories:	2,000	2,500
Total Fat	Less than		65g	80g
Sat Fat	Less than		20g	25g
Cholesterol	Less than		300mg	300mg
Sodium	Less than		2,400mg	2,400mg
Potassium			3,500mg	3,500mg
Total Carbohydrate			300g	375g
Dietary Fiber			25g	30g

Calories per gram:
Fat 9 • Carbohydrate 4 • Protein 4

**Intake of _trans_ fat should be as low as possible.

Chapter 3 The Human Body: A Nutrition Perspective

Student Learning Outcomes

Chapter 3 is designed to allow you to:

3.1   Understand some basic roles of nutrients in human physiology.

3.2   Identify the functions of the common cellular components.

3.3   Define tissue, organ, and organ system.

3.4   Identify the role of the cardiovascular and lymphatic systems in nutrition.

3.5   List basic characteristics of the nervous system and its role in nutrition.

3.6   List basic characteristics of the endocrine system, especially the pancreas, and its role in nutrition.

3.7   List basic characteristics of the immune system and its role in nutrition.

3.8   Outline the overall processes of digestion and absorption in the mouth, stomach, small intestine, and large intestine, as well as the roles played by the liver, gallbladder, and pancreas.

3.9   List basic characteristics of the urinary system and and its role in nutrition.

3.10 Understand the importance of the body storage areas for nutrients.

3.11 Understand the emerging field of nutrigenomics.

3.12 Identify the major nutrition-related gastrointestinal health problems and approaches to treatment.

What Would You Choose?

For spring break, you are volunteering to help build a house with Habitat for Humanity. You are carpooling with some friends and staying in a retreat house. Unfortunately, the travel, budget, living accommodations, and your building schedule won't allow for home-cooked meals this week. Being out of your normal routine and relying on fast-food sandwiches and pizza have left you feeling constipated. This reminds you that you will need to make smarter choices at fast-food establishments. To decrease your constipation which menu combination would you choose from a pizza buffet?

a 2 slices of pepperoni pizza, 2 cups of tossed salad

b 2 slices of veggie pizza, 1 cup of bean and pasta soup

c 2 slices of ham and pineapple pizza, 1 cup of pasta with Alfredo sauce

d 2 slices of cheese pizza, 1 garlic breadstick with marinara sauce

Think about your choices as you read Chapter 3, then see our recommendations at the end of the chapter. To learn more about the connection between our diets and our bodies, check out the Connect site: www.mcgrawhillconnect.com

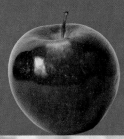

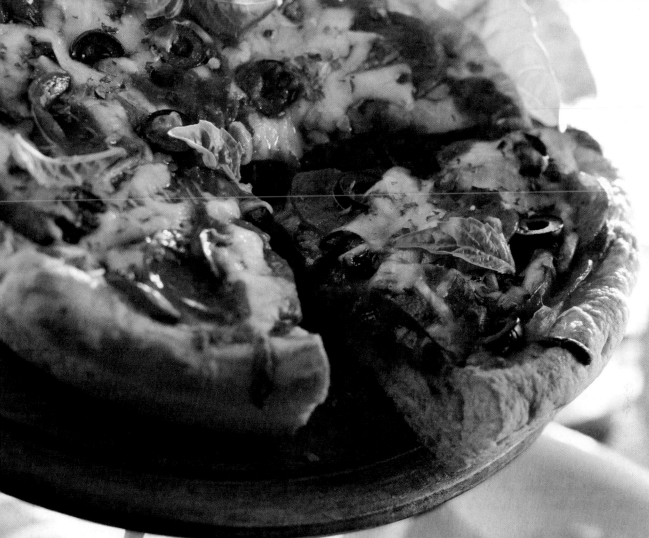

erely eating food won't nourish you. You must first digest the food by breaking it down into usable forms of the essential nutrients that can be absorbed into the bloodstream. Once nutrients are taken up by the bloodstream, they can be distributed to and used by body cells.

We rarely think about, let alone control, digesting and absorbing foods. Except for a few voluntary responses—such as deciding what and when to eat, how well to chew food, and when to eliminate the remains—most digestion and absorption processes control themselves. As suggested in the comic in this chapter, we don't consciously decide when the pancreas will secrete digestive substances into the small intestine or how quickly foodstuffs will be propelled down the intestinal tract. Various hormones and the nervous system mostly control these functions. Your only awareness of these involuntary responses may be a hunger pang right before lunch or a "full" feeling after eating that last slice of pizza.

Let's examine digestion and absorption as well as other aspects of human physiology that support nutritional health. In the process you will become acquainted with the basic anatomy (structure) and physiology (function) of the circulatory system, nervous system, endocrine system, immune system, digestive system, urinary system, and storage capabilities of the human body.

Refresh Your Memory

As you begin your study of human physiology in Chapter 3, you may want to review:

- Cell structure and function from previous coursework in university-level biology courses
- Each of the body's organ systems from any previous biology training

3.1 Nutrition's Role in Human Physiology

Overall, the human body is a coordinated unit of many highly structured organ systems (Fig. 3-1). Together, these system are composed of trillions of cells. Each cell is a self-contained, living entity. Cells of the same type normally join together, using intercellular substances to form **tissues,** such as muscle tissue. One, two, or more tissues then combine in a particular way to form more complex structures, called **organs.** All organs contribute to nutritional health, and a person's overall nutritional state determines how well each organ functions. At a still higher level of coordination, several organs can cooperate for a common purpose to form an **organ system,** such as the digestive system.

Chemical processes (reactions) occur constantly in every living cell: The production of new substances is balanced by the breaking down of older ones. An example is the constant formation and degradation of bone. For this turnover of substances to occur, cells require a continuous supply of energy in the form of dietary carbohydrate, protein, and/or fat. Cells also need water; building supplies, especially protein and minerals; and chemical regulators, such as the vitamins. Almost all cells also need a steady supply of oxygen. These substances enable the tissues, made from individual cells, to function properly.

Getting an adequate supply of all nutrients to the body's cells begins with a healthy diet. To assure optimal use of nutrients, the body's cells, tissues, organs, and organ systems also must work efficiently.

tissues Collections of cells adapted to perform a specific function.

organ A group of tissues designed to perform a specific function—for example, the heart, which contains muscle tissue, nerve tissue, and so on.

organ system A collection of organs that work together to perform an overall function.

FRANK & ERNEST® by Bob Thaves

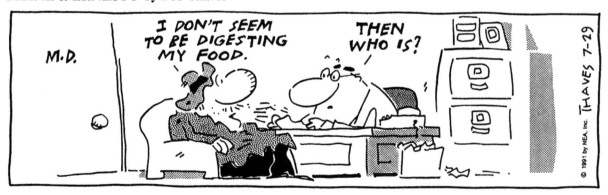

Some popular (fad) diets suggest not combining meat and potatoes to improve digestion and that fruit should only be eaten before noon. These diets might also claim that foods get stuck in the body and in turn putrefy and create toxins. Are there any scientific reasons to suggest that the timing of our food intake should optimize digestion? Do certain food practices improve digestion and subsequent absorption? This chapter provides some answers.

FRANK AND ERNEST reprinted by permission of Newspaper Enterprise Association, Inc.

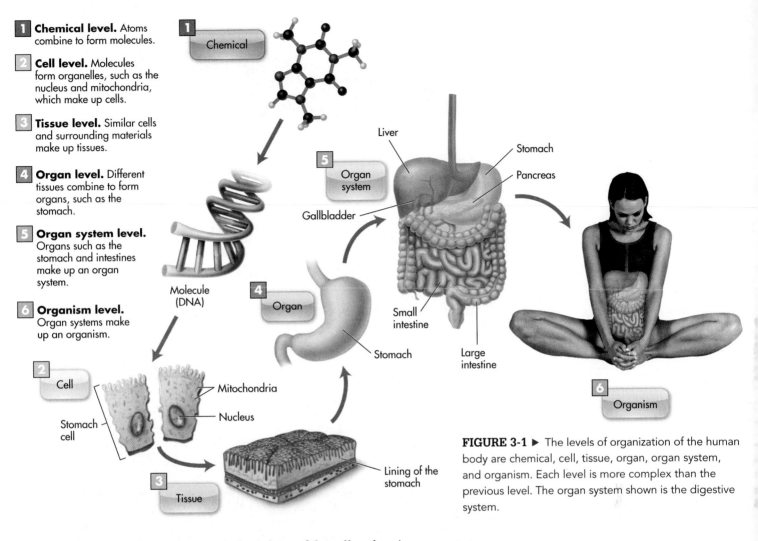

1 Chemical level. Atoms combine to form molecules.

2 Cell level. Molecules form organelles, such as the nucleus and mitochondria, which make up cells.

3 Tissue level. Similar cells and surrounding materials make up tissues.

4 Organ level. Different tissues combine to form organs, such as the stomach.

5 Organ system level. Organs such as the stomach and intestines make up an organ system.

6 Organism level. Organ systems make up an organism.

FIGURE 3-1 ▶ The levels of organization of the human body are chemical, cell, tissue, organ, organ system, and organism. Each level is more complex than the previous level. The organ system shown is the digestive system.

Chapter 3 covers the anatomy and physiology of the cell and major organ systems, especially as they relate to human nutrition. The information you are about to study is limited to the components of the various organ systems specifically influenced by the more than 45 essential nutrients discussed in this text.

3.2 The Cell: Structure, Function, and Metabolism

The cell is the basic structural and functional component of life. Living organisms are made of many different kinds of cells specialized to perform particular functions, and all cells are derived from preexisting cells. In the human body, all cells have certain common features. These cells have compartments and specialized structures that perform particular functions; these components are called **organelles** (Fig. 3-2). There are at least 15 different organelles. Eight of the most important organelles will be discussed. The numbers following the names of the cell structures correspond to the structures illustrated in Figure 3-2. Metabolism, the chemical processes that take place in body cells, will also be discussed.

organelles Compartments, particles, or filaments that perform specialized functions within a cell.

Cell (Plasma) Membrane 1

There is an outside and inside to every cell, separated by the cell (plasma) membrane. This membrane holds the cellular contents together and regulates the direction and flow of substances into and out of the cell. Cell-to-cell communication also occurs by way of this membrane.

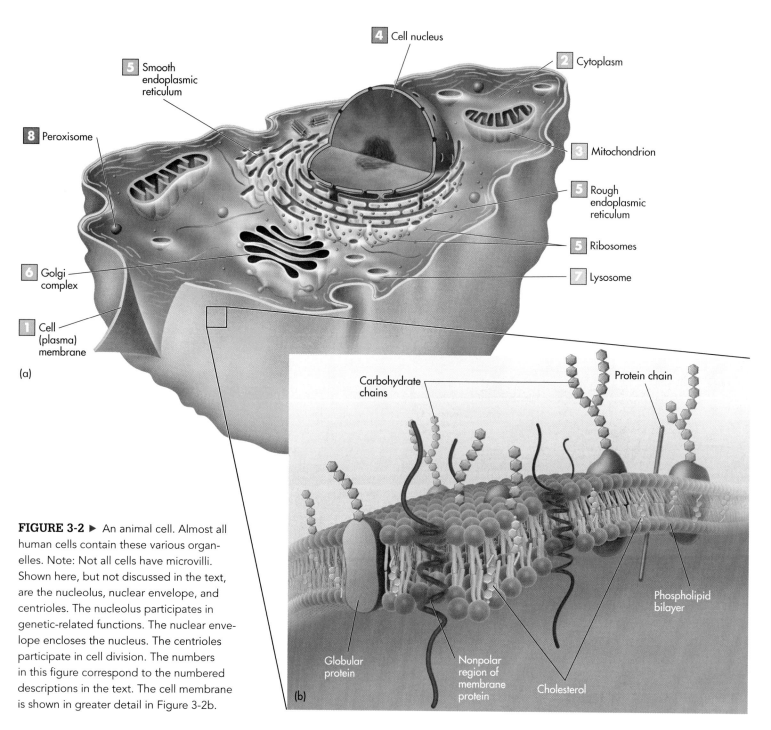

FIGURE 3-2 ▶ An animal cell. Almost all human cells contain these various organelles. Note: Not all cells have microvilli. Shown here, but not discussed in the text, are the nucleolus, nuclear envelope, and centrioles. The nucleolus participates in genetic-related functions. The nuclear envelope encloses the nucleus. The centrioles participate in cell division. The numbers in this figure correspond to the numbered descriptions in the text. The cell membrane is shown in greater detail in Figure 3-2b.

phospholipid Any of a class of fat-related substances that contain phosphorus, fatty acids, and a nitrogen-containing component. Phospholipids are an essential part of every cell.

enzyme A compound that speeds the rate of a chemical process but is not altered by that process. Almost all enzymes are proteins.

The cell membrane, illustrated in Figure 3-2(b), is a lipid bilayer (or double membrane) of **phospholipids** with their water-soluble heads facing both the interior of the cell and the exterior of the cell. Their water-insoluble tails are tucked into the center portion of the cell membrane.

Cholesterol is another component of the cell membrane. It is fat soluble, so it is embedded within the bilayer. This cholesterol provides rigidity and thus stability to the membrane.

There are also various proteins embedded in the cell membrane. Proteins provide structural support, act as transport vehicles, and function as **enzymes** that affect chemical processes within the membrane (see the later section on digestion for more about enzymes). Some proteins form open channels that allow water-soluble substances to pass into and out of the cell. Proteins on the outside surface of the membrane act as receptors, snagging essential substances that the cell needs and drawing them into the cell. Other proteins act as gates that open and close to control the flow of various particles into and out of the cell.

In addition to the lipid and protein, the membrane also contains carbohydrates that mark the exterior of the cell. These carbohydrates are combined either with protein or fat, and they help send messages to the cell's organelles and act as identification markers for the cell. In addition, they detect invaders and initiate defensive actions. In sum, these carbohydrates provide tags that are important to cellular identity and interaction.

Cytoplasm 2

The **cytoplasm** is the combination of fluid material and organelles within the cell, not including the nucleus. A small amount of energy for use by the cell can be produced by chemical processes that occur in the cytoplasm. This contributes to the survival of all cells and is the sole source of energy production in red blood cells. This energy production is called **anaerobic** metabolism because it doesn't require oxygen.

Organelles. Included within the cytoplasm are organelles. As described in the next two pages, they carry out vital roles in cell functions.

Mitochondria 3

Mitochondria are sometimes called the "power plants," or the powerhouse of the cell. These organelles are capable of converting the food energy in energy-yielding nutrients (carbohydrate, protein, and fat) to a form of energy that cells can use. This is an **aerobic** process that uses the oxygen we inhale, as well as water, enzymes, and other compounds (see Chapter 10 for details). With the exception of red blood cells, all cells contain mitochondria; only the size, shape, and quantity vary.

Cell Nucleus 4

With the exception of the red blood cell, all cells have one or more nuclei. The **cell nucleus** is bounded by its own double membrane. The nucleus contains the genetic material responsible for controlling actions that occur in the cell. The genetic material consists of **genes** on **chromosomes** made up of **deoxyribonucleic acid (DNA)**. DNA is the "code book" that contains directions for making substances, specifically proteins, the cell needs. This code book remains in the nucleus of the cell, but sends its information to other cell organelles by way of a similar "messenger" molecule called **ribonucleic acid (RNA)**. The information on the DNA is copied onto the RNA through the process of **transcription** and then moves out to the cytoplasm through pores in the nuclear membrane. The RNA carries the transcribed DNA code to protein-synthesizing sites called **ribosomes.** There, the RNA code is used in the process of **translation** to make a specific protein (see Chapter 6 for details on protein synthesis). This process is also known as **gene expression.**

All of the DNA in a cell is copied during cell replication. DNA is a double-stranded molecule, and when the cell begins to divide, each strand is separated and an identical copy of each is made. Thus, each new DNA contains one new strand of DNA and one strand from the original DNA. In this way, the genetic code is preserved from one cell generation to the next. (The mitochondria contain their own DNA, so they reproduce themselves within a cell independent of action in the cell's nucleus.)

cytoplasm The fluid and organelles (except the nucleus) in a cell.

anaerobic Not requiring oxygen.

mitochondria The main sites of energy production in a cell. They contain the pathway for oxidizing fat for fuel, among other metabolic pathways.

aerobic Requiring oxygen.

cell nucleus An organelle bound by its own double membrane and containing chromosomes, the genetic information for cell protein synthesis and cell replication.

gene A specific segment on a chromosome. Genes provide the blueprint for the production of cell proteins.

chromosome A single, large DNA molecule and its associated proteins; contains many genes to store and transmit genetic information.

deoxyribonucleic acid (DNA) The site of hereditary information in cells; DNA directs the synthesis of cell proteins.

ribonucleic acid (RNA) The single-stranded nucleic acid involved in the transcription of genetic information and translation of that information into protein structure.

transcription Information on DNA needed to make a protein is copied onto RNA.

ribosomes Cytoplasmic particles that mediate the linking together of amino acids to form proteins; may exist freely in the cytoplasm or attached to endoplasmic reticulum.

translation The information contained in RNA is used to determine the amino acids in a protein.

gene expression Use of DNA information on a gene to produce a protein. Thought to be a major determination of cell development.

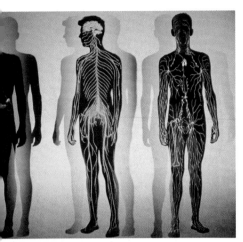

▲ The body is made up of numerous organ systems including the endocrine, nervous, and circulatory systems shown here.

endoplasmic reticulum (ER) An organelle in the cytoplasm composed of a network of canals running through the cytoplasm. Part of the endoplasmic reticulum contains ribosomes.

Golgi complex The cell organelle near the nucleus that processes newly synthesized protein for secretion or distribution to other organelles.

secretory vesicles Membrane-bound vesicles produced by the Golgi apparatus; contain protein and other compounds to be secreted by the cell.

lysosome A cellular organelle that contains digestive enzymes for use inside the cell for turnover of cell parts.

peroxisome A cell organelle that destroys toxic products within the cell.

adenosine triphosphate (ATP) The main energy currency for cells. ATP energy is used to promote ion pumping, enzyme activity, and muscular contraction.

Endoplasmic Reticulum (ER) 5

The outer membrane of the cell nucleus is continuous with a network of tubes called the **endoplasmic reticulum (ER)**. Part of the endoplasmic reticulum (termed the rough [as opposed to smooth] endoplasmic reticulum) contains the ribosomes, where the RNA code is translated into proteins during protein synthesis. Many of these proteins play a central role in human nutrition. Parts of the endoplasmic reticulum also are involved in lipid synthesis, detoxification of toxic substances, and calcium storage and release in the cell.

Golgi Complex 6

The **Golgi complex** is a packaging site for proteins used in the cytoplasm or exported from the cell. It consists of sacs within the cytoplasm in which proteins are "packaged" as **secretory vesicles** for secretion by the cell.

Lysosomes 7

Lysosomes are the cell's digestive system. They are sacs that contain enzymes for the digestion of foreign material. Sometimes known as "suicide bags," they are responsible for digesting worn-out or damaged cell components. Certain cells associated with immune functions contain many lysosomes (see the later section on the immune system).

Peroxisomes 8

Peroxisomes contain enzymes that detoxify harmful chemicals. Peroxisomes get their name from the fact that hydrogen peroxide (H_2O_2) is formed as a result of such enzyme action. Peroxisomes also contain a protective enzyme called *catalase*, which prevents excessive accumulation of hydrogen peroxide in the cell, which would be very damaging. Peroxisomes also play a minor role in metabolizing one possible source of energy for cells—alcohol.

Cell Metabolism

Metabolism refers to the entire network of chemical processes involved in maintaining life. It encompasses all the sequences of chemical reactions that occur in the body's cells. These biochemical reactions take place in the cell cytoplasm and organelles that we have just discussed. They enable us to release and use energy from foods, synthesize one substance from another, and prepare waste products for excretion.

The reactions of metabolism that take place within your body can be categorized into one of two types. One type of reaction, anabolic, puts different molecules together and, therefore, requires energy. The other type of reaction, catabolic, takes molecules apart and, therefore, releases energy. The metabolism of the nutrients, carbohydrates, proteins, and fats are interrelated and yield energy. The other nutrients, vitamins and minerals, contribute to the enzyme activity that supports metabolic reactions in the cell.

The metabolism of energy production begins in the cytoplasm with the initial anaerobic breakdown of glucose. The remaining aerobic steps of energy production take place in the mitochondria. Ultimately, the cells of the body use these interconnected processes to convert the energy found in food to energy stored in the high-energy compound, **adenosine triphosphate (ATP)**. You will learn more about the metabolism of energy sources in Chapter 10, "Nutrition: Fitness and Sports."

<u>CONCEPT CHECK</u>

In Chapter 1, you learned that fat (lipids), protein, and carbohydrate function as fuels. Now you recognize that these nutrients also serve as structural materials in the cell membrane. This is typical of many nutrients; they can carry out multiple functions. The cell receives nutrients and other substances through the cell membrane by using various transport systems.

The basic structural unit in the body is the cell. Within the cell are a variety of organelles with unique functions to perform. Although there is no typical cell, virtually all cells have the same organelles, each performing the same essential task.

3.3 Body Systems

As noted earlier, when groups of similar cells work together to accomplish a specialized task, the arrangement is referred to as a tissue. Humans are composed of four primary types of tissue: **epithelial, connective, muscle,** and **nervous.** Epithelial tissue is composed of cells that cover surfaces both inside and outside the body. For example, the lining of the respiratory tract is made up of epithelial cells. These cells of epithelial tissue secrete important substances, absorb nutrients, and excrete waste. Connective tissue supports and protects the body, stores fat, and produces blood cells. Muscle tissue is designed for movement. Nervous tissue found in the brain and spinal cord is designed for communication. These four types of tissues then go on to form various organs, and ultimately, organ systems (Table 3-1).

We will focus primarily on the digestive system in Chapter 3. The nutrients we consume in food are unavailable until such time as they have been processed by the digestive system. This employs chemical and mechanical means to alter food so that the nutrients can be released and absorbed into the body for distribution to body tissues.

Sometimes organs within a system can serve another system. For example, the basic function of the digestive system is to convert the food we eat into absorbable nutrients. At the same time, the digestive system serves the immune system by preventing dangerous pathogens from invading the body and causing illness. As you study nutrition, you will note the multiple roles played by many organs (Fig. 3-3).

The overriding theme of human nutrition is to understand the actions of nutrients as they affect different cells, tissues, organs, and organ systems. Each type of organ system is impacted by nutrient intake and simultaneously determines how each nutrient is used.

Our task now is to explore the key systems in the body as they specifically relate to the study of human nutrition: circulatory (cardiovascular and lymphatic), nervous, endocrine, immune, digestive, and urinary systems. This part of Chapter 3 will set the stage for a more detailed look at these and other organ systems in later chapters covering various aspects of human nutrition.

Also in this chapter, we will introduce the emerging area of genetics and nutrition. Throughout this book, discussions will point out how you can personalize nutrition advice based on your genetic background. In this way, you can identify and avoid the "controllable" risk factors that would contribute to development of genetically linked diseases present in your family.

epithelial tissue The surface cells that line the outside of the body and all external passages within it.

connective tissue Protein tissue that holds different structures in the body together. Some body structures are made up of connective tissue—notably, tendons and cartilage. Connective tissue also forms part of bone and the nonmuscular structures of arteries and veins.

muscle tissue A type of tissue adapted to contract to cause movement.

nervous tissue Tissue composed of highly branched, elongated cells, which transport nerve impulses from one part of the body to another.

cardiovascular system The body system consisting of the heart, blood vessels, and blood. This system transports nutrients, waste products, gases, and hormones throughout the body and plays an important role in immune responses and regulation of body temperature.

lymphatic system A system of vessels and lymph that accepts fluid surrounding cells and large particles, such as products of fat absorption. Lymph eventually passes into the bloodstream from the lymphatic system.

3.4 Cardiovascular System and Lymphatic System

The body has two separate organ systems that circulate fluids in the body: the **cardiovascular system** and the **lymphatic system.** The cardiovascular system consists of the heart and blood vessels. The lymphatic system consists of lymphatic vessels and

TABLE 3-1 Organ Systems of the Body

System	Major Components	Functions Related to Nutrition
Cardiovascular	Heart, blood vessels, and blood	Transports nutrients, waste products, gases, and hormones throughout the body and plays a role in the immune response and the regulation of body temperature
Lymphatic	Lymph vessels, lymph nodes, and other lymph organs	Removes foreign substances from the blood and lymph, combats disease, maintains tissue fluid balance, and aids in fat absorption
Nervous	Brain, spinal cord, nerves, and sensory receptors	A major regulatory system: detects sensation, controls movements, and controls physiological and intellectual functions
Endocrine	Endocrine glands, such as the pituitary, thyroid, and adrenal glands	A major regulatory system: participates in the regulation of metabolism, reproduction, and many other functions through the action of hormones
Immune	White blood cells, lymph vessels and nodes, spleen, thymus gland, and other lymph tissues	Provides defense against foreign invaders; formation of white blood cells
Digestive	Mouth, esophagus, stomach, intestines, and accessory structures (liver, gallbladder, and pancreas)	Performs the mechanical and chemical processes of digestion, absorption of nutrients, and elimination of wastes
Urinary	Kidneys, urinary bladder, and the ducts that carry urine	Removes waste products from the circulatory system and regulates the acidity, chemical composition, and water content of the blood
Integumentary	Skin, hair, nails, and sweat glands	Protects the body, regulates temperature, prevents water loss, and produces a substance that converts to vitamin D upon sun exposure
Skeletal	Bones, associated cartilage, and joints	Supports the body, and allows for body movement, produces blood cells, and stores minerals
Muscular	Smooth, cardiac, and skeletal muscle	Produces body movement, maintains posture, and produces body heat
Respiratory	Lungs and respiratory passages	Exchanges gases (oxygen and carbon dioxide) between the blood and the atmosphere and regulates blood acid-base (pH) balance
Reproductive	Gonads, accessory structures, and genitals of males and females	Performs the processes of reproduction and influences sexual functions and behaviors

lymph A clear fluid that flows through lymph vessels; carries most forms of fat after their absorption by the small intestine.

plasma The fluid, extracellular portion of the circulating blood. This includes the blood serum plus all blood-clotting factors. In contrast, serum is the fluid that remains after clotting factors have been removed from plasma.

a number of lymph tissues. Blood flows through the cardiovascular system, while **lymph** flows through the lymphatic system.

Cardiovascular System

The heart is a muscular pump that normally contracts and relaxes 50 to 90 times per minute when the body is at rest. This continual pumping, measured by taking your pulse, keeps blood moving through the blood vessels. The blood that flows through the cardiovascular system is composed of **plasma**, red blood cells, white blood cells, platelets, and many other substances. It travels two basic routes. In the first route, blood circulates from the right side of the heart, through the lungs, and then back to the heart. In the lungs, blood picks up oxygen and releases carbon dioxide. After this exchange of gases has taken place, blood is said to be *oxygenated* and returns to the left side of your heart. In the second route, the oxygenated blood circulates from the left side of the heart to all other body cells, eventually returning back to the right side of the heart (Fig. 3-4). After blood has circulated throughout the body, it is *deoxygenated*. (As you review the cardiovascular system, recall from your previous studies of biology that *left* and *right* designations of the heart refer to the left and right sides of your body, not of the page in your textbook.)

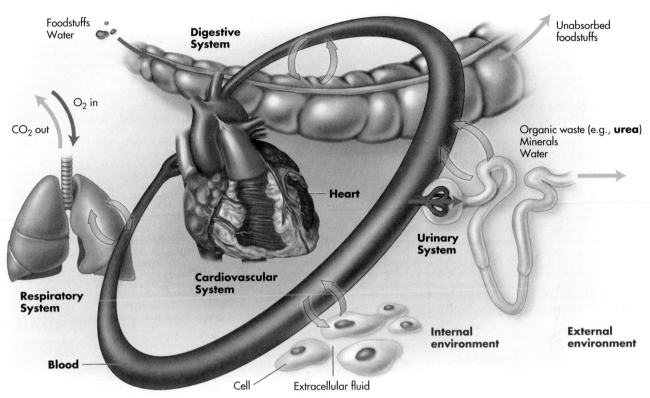

FIGURE 3-3 ▶ Exchanges of nutrients occur between our external environment and the internal environment of the circulatory system via the digestive, respiratory, and urinary systems. Overall, the human body is a combination of 12 systems working together to support cell needs.

In the cardiovascular system, blood leaves the heart via **arteries,** which branch into **capillaries,** a network of tiny blood vessels. Exchange of nutrients, oxygen, and waste products between the blood and cells occurs through the minute, web-like pores of the capillaries (Fig. 3-5). Capillaries service every region of the body via individual capillary beds only one cell layer thick. The blood then returns to the heart via the **veins.**

The cardiovascular system distributes nutrients absorbed from food and oxygen from the air to all body cells (review Fig. 3-3). Other functions include delivery of hormones to their target cells, maintenance of a constant body temperature, and distribution of white blood cells throughout the body to protect against pathogens as part of the immune system (see the later section, "Immune System").

Portal Circulation in the Gastrointestinal Tract. Water and nutrients are transferred to the circulatory system through capillary beds. Once absorbed through the stomach or intestinal wall, nutrients reach one of two destinations. Some nutrients are taken up by cells in the intestines and portions of the stomach to nourish those organs. Most of the nutrients from recently eaten foods, however, are transferred into **portal circulation.** To enter portal circulation, the nutrients pass from the intestinal capillaries into veins that eventually merge into a very large vein called a **portal vein.** Unlike most veins in the body—which carry blood back to the heart—this portal vein leads directly to the liver. This enables the liver to process absorbed nutrients before they enter the general circulation of the bloodstream. Overall, portal circulation represents a special form of circulation in the cardiovascular system.

Lymphatic System

The **lymphatic system** is also a circulatory system. It consists of a network of lymphatic vessels and the fluid (lymph) that moves through them. Lymph is similar to

artery A blood vessel that carries blood away from the heart.

capillary A microscopic blood vessel that connects the smallest arteries and veins; site of nutrient, oxygen, and waste exchange between body cells and the blood.

vein A blood vessel that carries blood to the heart.

portal circulation The portion of the circulatory system that uses a large vein (portal vein) to carry nutrient-rich blood from capillaries in the intestines and portions of the stomach to the liver.

urea Nitrogenous waste product of protein metabolism; major source of nitrogen in the urine.

portal vein Large vein leaving the intestine and stomach and connecting to the liver.

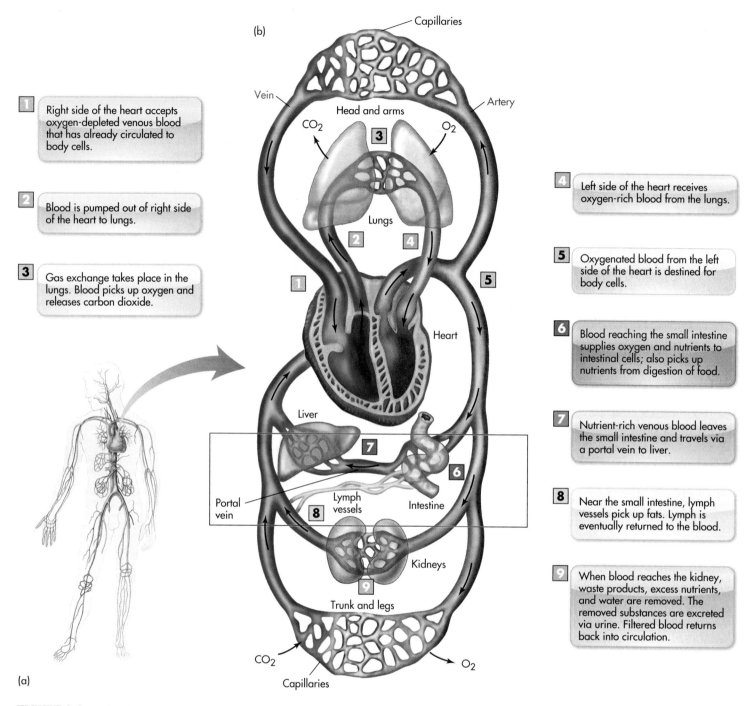

1 Right side of the heart accepts oxygen-depleted venous blood that has already circulated to body cells.

2 Blood is pumped out of right side of the heart to lungs.

3 Gas exchange takes place in the lungs. Blood picks up oxygen and releases carbon dioxide.

4 Left side of the heart receives oxygen-rich blood from the lungs.

5 Oxygenated blood from the left side of the heart is destined for body cells.

6 Blood reaching the small intestine supplies oxygen and nutrients to intestinal cells; also picks up nutrients from digestion of food.

7 Nutrient-rich venous blood leaves the small intestine and travels via a portal vein to liver.

8 Near the small intestine, lymph vessels pick up fats. Lymph is eventually returned to the blood.

9 When blood reaches the kidney, waste products, excess nutrients, and water are removed. The removed substances are excreted via urine. Filtered blood returns back into circulation.

FIGURE 3-4 ▶ Blood circulation through the body. Figure (a) shows the heart and some examples of the major arteries and veins of the cardiovascular system. Figure (b) shows the paths that blood takes from the heart to the lungs (1–3), back to the heart (4), and through the rest of the body (5–9). The red color indicates blood richer in oxygen; blue is for blood carrying more carbon dioxide. Keep in mind that arteries and veins go to all parts of the body.

blood, consisting largely of blood plasma that has found its way out of capillaries and into the spaces between cells. It contains a full array of the various white blood cells that play an important role in the immune system. However, neither red blood cells nor platelets are present. Lymph is collected in tiny lymph vessels all over the body and moves through even larger vessels until it eventually enters the cardiovascular system through major veins near the heart. This flow is driven by muscle contractions arising from normal body movements.

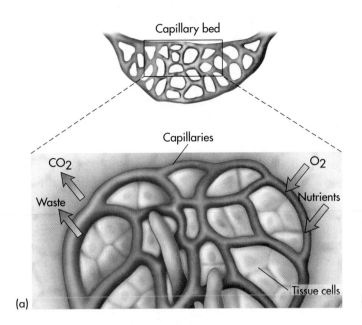

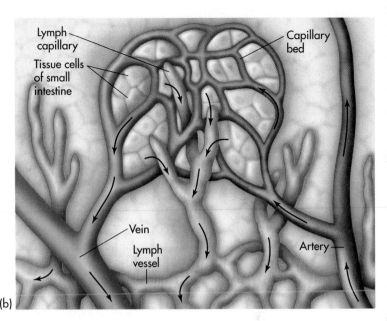

FIGURE 3-5 ▶ Capillary and lymph vessels. (a) Exchange of oxygen (O_2) and nutrients for carbon dioxide (CO_2) and waste products occurs between the capillaries and the surrounding tissue cells. (b) Lymph vessels are also present in capillary beds, such as in the small intestine. Lymph vessels in the small intestine are also called lacteals. The lymph vessels have closed ends and are important for fat absorption.

Lymphatic Circulation in the Gastrointestinal Tract. Besides contributing to the defense of the body against invading pathogens, lymphatic vessels that serve the small intestine play an important role in nutrition. These vessels pick up and transport the majority of products of fat digestion and fat absorption. These fat-related products are too large to enter the bloodstream directly and therefore are generally emptied into the bloodstream only after passing through the lymphatic system. The lymph vessels also take up excess fluid that collects between cells and returns it to the bloodstream.

CONCEPT CHECK

Blood is transported from the right side of the heart to the capillaries in the lungs. Carbon dioxide is removed and oxygen is taken up by red blood cells. The oxygenated blood returns to the left side of the heart. Here it is pumped into general circulation. In the capillaries, oxygen is released from the red blood cells and delivered through pores in the capillaries to the surrounding cells. Nutrients also are distributed from the bloodstream to body cells via the capillaries. Carbon dioxide released from cells travels through the capillary pores to the blood.

The lymph system serves several purposes: the transport of absorbed dietary fats, the uptake and return to the bloodstream of excess fluid that collects between cells, and the defense of the body against invading pathogens.

3.5 Nervous System

The **nervous system** is a regulatory system that centrally controls most body functions. The nervous system can detect changes occurring in various organs and the external environment and initiate corrective action when needed to maintain a constant internal body environment. The nervous system also regulates activities that change almost instantly, such as muscle contractions and perception of danger. The body has many receptors that receive information about what is happening within the body and in the outside environment. For the most part these receptors are found in our

nervous system The body system consisting of the brain, spinal cord, nerves, and sensory receptors. This system detects sensations, directs movements, and controls physiological and intellectual functions.

neuron The structural and functional unit of the nervous system. Consists of a cell body, dendrites, and an axon.

synapse The space between one neuron and another neuron (or cell).

neurotransmitter A compound made by a nerve cell that allows for communication between it and other cells.

eyes, ears, skin, nose, and stomach. We act on information from these receptors via the nervous system.

The basic structural and functional unit of the nervous system is the **neuron.** These are elongated, highly branched cells. The body contains about 100 billion neurons. Neurons respond to electrical and chemical signals, conduct electrical impulses, and release chemical regulators. Overall, neurons allow us to perceive what is occurring in our environment, engage in learning, store vital information in memory, and control the body's voluntary (and involuntary) actions.

The brain stores information, reacts to incoming information, solves problems, and generates thoughts. In addition, the brain plans a course of action based on the other sensory inputs. Responses to the stimuli are carried out mostly through the rest of the nervous system.

Simply put, the nervous system receives information through stimulation of various receptors, processes this information, and sends out signals through its various branches for an action that needs to be taken. Actual transmission of the signal occurs through a change in the concentration of two nutrients, sodium and potassium, in the neuron. There is an influx of sodium into the neuron and a loss of potassium as the message is sent. Concentrations of these minerals are then restored to normal amounts in the neuron after the signal passes, making it ready to conduct another message.

When the signal must bridge a gap **(synapse)** between the branches of different neurons, the message is generally converted to a chemical signal called a **neurotransmitter.** The neurotransmitter is then released into the gap, and its target may be another neuron or another type of cell, such as a muscle cell (Fig. 3-6). If the signal is sent to another neuron, this allows it to continue on to its final destination. The neurotransmitters

FIGURE 3-6 ▶ Transmission of a message from one neuron to another neuron or to another type of cell that relies on neurotransmitters. Vesicles containing neurotransmitters, formed within the neuron, fuse with the membrane of the neuron and the neurotransmitter is released into the synapse. The neurotransmitter then binds to the receptors on the nearby neuron (or cell). In this way, the message is transmitted from one neuron to another or to the cell that ultimately performs the action directed by the message.

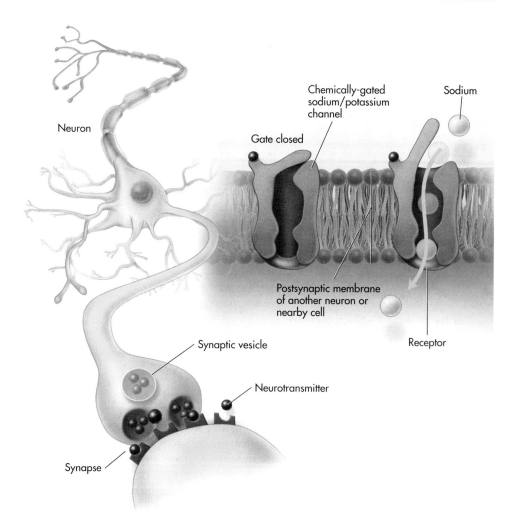

used in this process are often made from common nutrients found in foods, such as amino acids. The amino acid tryptophan is converted to the neurotransmitter serotonin, and the amino acid tyrosine is converted to the neurotransmitters **norepinephrine** and **epinephrine** (also called adrenaline).

Other nutrients also play a role in the nervous system. Calcium is needed for the release of neurotransmitters from neurons. Vitamin B-12 plays a role in the formation of the **myelin sheath,** which provides insulation around specific parts of most neurons. Finally, a regular supply of carbohydrate in the form of glucose is important for supplying fuel for the brain. The brain can use other calorie sources, but generally relies on glucose.

3.6 Endocrine System

The **endocrine system** plays a major role in the regulation of metabolism, reproduction, water balance, and many other functions by producing hormones in the **endocrine glands** of the body and subsequently releasing them into the blood (Table 3-2). The term *hormone* comes from the Greek word for "to stir or excite." A true hormone is a regulatory compound that has a specific site of synthesis from which it then enters the bloodstream to reach target cells. Hormones are the messengers of the body. They can be permissive (turn on), antagonistic (turn off), or synergistic (work in cooperation with another hormone) in performing a task. Some compounds must undergo chemical changes before they can function as hormones. For example, vitamin D, synthesized in the skin or obtained from food, is converted into an active hormone by chemical changes made in the liver and kidneys.

The hormone **insulin,** synthesized in and released from the pancreas, helps control the amount of glucose in the blood (Fig. 3-7). Insulin is mostly produced when glucose in the blood rises to a certain level, usually after a meal. At this point, insulin is released and it travels to the muscle, adipose, and liver cells of the body. Among its many functions, insulin allows for the movement of glucose from the blood into muscle and adipose cells. In the liver cells, insulin causes an increase in stored glycogen by stimulating the synthesis of glycogen from glucose. Once a sufficient amount of glucose has been cleared from the blood, the production of insulin lessens. The hormones epinephrine, norepinephrine, glucagon, and growth hormone have just the opposite effect on blood glucose. They all cause an increase in blood glucose through a variety of actions (Table 3-2). **Thyroid hormones,** synthesized in and released from the thyroid gland

norepinephrine A neurotransmitter from nerve endings and a hormone from the adrenal gland. It is released in times of stress and is involved in hunger regulation, blood glucose regulation, and other body processes.

epinephrine A hormone also known as *adrenaline;* it is released by the adrenal glands (located on each kidney) at times of stress. It acts to increase glycogen breakdown in the liver, among other functions.

myelin sheath A lipid and protein combination (lipoprotein) that covers nerve fibers.

endocrine system The body system consisting of the various glands and the hormones these glands secrete. This system has major regulatory functions in the body, such as reproduction and cell metabolism.

endocrine gland A hormone-producing gland.

thyroid hormones Hormones produced by the thyroid gland that among their functions increase the rate of overall metabolism in the body.

TABLE 3-2 Some Hormones of the Endocrine System with Nutritional Significance

Hormone	Gland/Organ	Target	Effect	Role in Nutrition
Insulin	Pancreas	Adipose (fat) and muscle cells	Decreased blood glucose	Uptake and storage of glucose, fat, and amino acids by cells
Glucagon	Pancreas	Liver	Increased blood glucose	Release of glucose from liver stores, release of fat from adipose tissue
Epinephrine, Norepinephrine	Adrenal glands	Heart, blood vessels, brain, lungs	Increased body metabolism and blood glucose	Release of glucose and fat into the blood
Growth hormone	Pituitary gland	Most cells	Promotion of amino acid uptake by cells, increased blood glucose	Promotion of protein synthesis and growth, increased fat use for energy
Thyroid hormones	Thyroid gland	Most organs	Increased oxygen consumption, overall growth, brain development of the nervous system	Protein synthesis, increased body metabolism

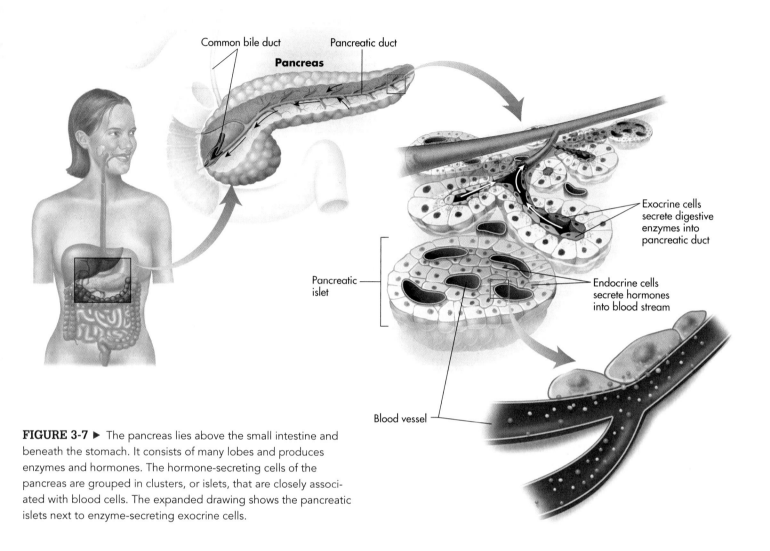

FIGURE 3-7 ▶ The pancreas lies above the small intestine and beneath the stomach. It consists of many lobes and produces enzymes and hormones. The hormone-secreting cells of the pancreas are grouped in clusters, or islets, that are closely associated with blood cells. The expanded drawing shows the pancreatic islets next to enzyme-secreting exocrine cells.

receptor A site in a cell at which compounds (such as hormones) bind. Cells that contain receptors for a specific compound are partially controlled by that compound.

help to control the body's rate of metabolism. Other hormones are especially important in regulating digestive processes (see the later section, "Digestive System").

Hormones are not taken up by all cells in the body, but only those with the correct **receptor** protein. These binding sites are highly specific for a certain hormone. They are generally found on the cell membrane. The hormone attaches to its receptor on the cell membrane. This binding activates additional compounds called second messengers within the cell to carry out the assigned task. This is true of insulin. A few hormones can penetrate the cell membrane and eventually bind to receptors on the DNA in the nucleus (e.g., thyroid hormone and estrogen).

CONCEPT CHECK

The functional unit of the nervous system is the neuron. Communication between neurons themselves, and other types of cells, is via neurotransmitters released into the synapse between the cells.

In the endocrine system, hormones are produced by glands in response to a change in the internal or external environment of the body. The gland secretes the hormone into the blood, and the blood delivers it to target cells. The hormone either attaches to receptors in the cell membrane and, through the action of second messengers, causes changes within the cell, or enters the cell and binds to the DNA in the cell to cause changes within the cell.

3.7 Immune System

Many types of body cells and body components work in cooperation as part of the **immune system** to maintain a defense against infection (Fig. 3-8). The components that work as part of the immune system include the skin, intestinal cells, and white blood cells. Several nutrients, including protein; minerals iron, copper, and zinc; and vitamins A, B-6, B-12, C, and folate have important roles in the immune system. These nutrients are key factors in the synthesis, growth, development, and activity of immune cells and additional factors that kill pathogens. It is easy to demonstrate the importance of nutritional health for immune function. Early humans were plagued by famine and thus, malnutrition; this contributed to infections, often leading to death. Today, largely because of better nutrition, most of the world avoids that cycle.

We are born with most aspects of immune function; these are termed **non-specific** (or innate) because the targets are a variety of microorganisms. In contrast, white blood cells produce **immunoglobulins,** also called **antibodies,** that target specific organisms or foreign proteins called **antigens.** These immunoglobulins constitute **specific** (or adaptive) immune function. Once exposed, a memory is created such that a second exposure to the substance will produce a more vigorous and rapid attack.

Skin

The skin is a large component of the immune system, forming an almost continuous barrier surrounding the body. Invading microorganisms have difficulty penetrating the skin. However, if the skin is split by lesions, bacteria can easily penetrate this barrier. Skin health is poor during deficiencies of such nutrients as essential fatty acids, vitamin A, niacin, and zinc. Vitamin A deficiency also decreases gland secretions in the skin that contain the enzyme **lysozyme,** capable of killing bacteria. Bacterial eye infections are common in developing countries, often as a result of a vitamin A deficiency.

Intestinal Cells

The cells of the intestines form an important barrier to invading microorganisms. The cells are packed closely together, producing a physical barrier to microorganisms. In addition, specialized cells that produce immune factors—such as immunoglobulins—are scattered throughout the intestinal tract. These immune factors bind to the invading microorganisms, preventing them from entering the bloodstream. These factors are part of the mucosal membrane aspect of immunity.

Nutrient deficiencies can cause the intestinal cells to break down weakening the mucosal membrane so that microorganisms more easily enter the body and cause infections. Thus, two common results of undernutrition related to an impaired immune system are diarrhea and bacterial infections of the bloodstream. To protect the health of the intestinal tract, an adequate nutrient intake is necessary—especially of protein, vitamin A, vitamin B-6, vitamin B-12, vitamin C, folate, and zinc.

MAKING DECISIONS

Immune Status

Although many studies show that a healthy nutritional state is associated with good immune status, other studies show that an overabundance of certain nutrients can harm the immune system. For example, taking too much zinc may decrease immune function (see Chapter 12).

FIGURE 3-8 ▶ Just as the roof and other external structures of a house protect the inside environment from outside elements, host protective factors (shown on the bricks) of the immune system "shelter" humans from threats such as diseases and toxins (shown in the rain).

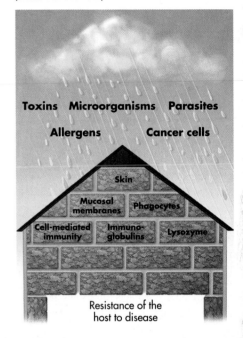

immune system The body system consisting of white blood cells, lymph glands and vessels, and various other body tissues. The immune system provides defense against foreign invaders, primarily due to the action of various types of white blood cells.

non-specific immunity Defenses that stop the invasion of pathogens; requires no previous encounter with a pathogen.

immunoglobulins Proteins found in the blood that bind to specific antigens; also called antibodies. The five major classes of immunoglobulins play different roles in antibody-mediated immunity.

antigen Any substance that induces a state of sensitivity and/or resistance to microorganisms or toxic substances after a lag period; foreign substance that stimulates a specific aspect of the immune system.

antibody Blood protein (immunoglobulin) that binds foreign proteins found in the body. This helps to prevent and control infections.

specific immunity Function of lymphocytes directed at specific antigens.

lysozyme An enzyme produced by a variety of cells; it can destroy bacteria by rupturing their cell membranes.

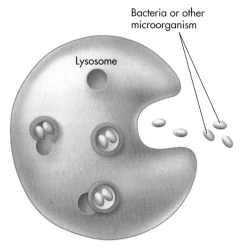

Phagocyte

FIGURE 3-9 ▶ One class of white blood cell, phagocytes, can ingest bacteria, fungi, viruses, and other foreign particles in the process of phagocytosis. An indentation is formed and the particle is engulfed by the cell. The foreign material is eventually digested by lysosomes in the cell.

white blood cells One of the formed elements of the circulating blood system; also called *leukocytes*. White blood cells are able to squeeze through intracellular spaces and migrate. They phagocytize bacteria, fungi, and viruses, as well as detoxify proteins that may result from allergic reactions, cellular injury, and other immune system cells.

phagocytes Cells that engulf substances; include neutrophils and macrophages.

phagocytosis Process in which a cell forms an indentation, and particles or fluids enter the indentation and are engulfed by the cell.

cell-mediated immunity A process in which certain white blood cells come in contact with the invading cells to destroy them.

digestive system System consisting of the gastrointestinal tract and accessory structures (liver, gallbladder, and pancreas). This system performs the mechanical and chemical processes of digestion, absorption of nutrients, and elimination of wastes.

digestion Process by which large ingested molecules are mechanically and chemically broken down to produce basic nutrients that can be absorbed across the wall of the GI tract.

absorption The process by which substances are taken up from the GI tract and enter the bloodstream or the lymph.

White Blood Cells

Once a microorganism enters the bloodstream, **white blood cells** move in to attack it. Several types of white blood cells participate in this response and function in unique ways. For example, a class called **phagocytes** circulates throughout the circulatory system and ingests and sometimes digests microorganisms and foreign particles (via lysosomes present in the cells) in a process called **phagocytosis** (Fig. 3-9). Other white blood cells participate in **cell-mediated immunity**, achieved when certain immune cells recognize foreign cells or proteins and directly attack and destroy them. Immunoglobulins, also known as antibodies and made by these cells, elicit an antibody-antigen response that binds microorganisms and proteins that are foreign to the body and destroys them, and then creates a template (memory) that allows future recognition of the microorganism or foreign protein. Recognition allows more rapid attacks in the future.

Some white blood cells live only a few days. Their constant resynthesis requires steady nutrient intake. The immune system needs the following nutrients: (1) iron to produce an important killing factor; (2) copper for synthesis of a specific type of white blood cell; and (3) protein, vitamin B-6, vitamin B-12, vitamin C, and folate for general cell synthesis and, later, cell activity. Zinc and vitamin A are also needed for the overall growth and development of immune cells.

CONCEPT CHECK

Many types of body cells and body components work in cooperation as part of the immune system to maintain a defense against infection. The skin forms an almost continuous barrier surrounding the body. Cell secretions contain the enzyme lysozyme. Specialized cells in the intestines and certain white blood cells secrete antibodies (immunoglobulins). Phagocytes roam throughout the circulatory system and ingest and sometimes digest microorganisms and foreign particles. Other white blood cells participate in cell-mediated immunity. This occurs when certain immune cells recognize foreign cells and directly attack them. Many nutrients, including protein, iron, copper, zinc, vitamin B-6, B-12, C, and folate, are needed for the overall growth and development of immune cells.

3.8 Digestive System

The foods and beverages we consume, for the most part, must undergo extensive alteration by the **digestive system** to provide us with usable nutrients. The processes of **digestion** and **absorption** take place in a long tube that is open at both ends and extends from the mouth to the anus. This tube is called the **gastrointestinal (GI) tract** (Fig. 3-10). Nutrients from the food we eat must pass through the walls of the GI tract—from the inside to the outside—to be absorbed into the bloodstream. The organs that make up the GI tract, as well as some additional accessory organs located nearby, are collectively known as the digestive system.

In the digestive system, food is broken down mechanically and chemically. Mechanical digestion takes place as soon as you begin chewing your food and continues as muscular contractions simultaneously mix and move food through the length of the GI tract (as part of a process known as **motility**). Chemical digestion refers to the chemical breakdown of foods by substances secreted into the GI tract. Finally, the digestive system eliminates wastes. In addition to nutrients that arise from digestion of food, the bacteria that live in the large intestine produce vitamin K and the vitamin biotin, some of which we can absorb and use.

Most of the processes of digestion and absorption are under autonomic control; that is, they are involuntary. Almost all of the functions involved in digestion and absorption are controlled by signals from the nervous system, hormones from the

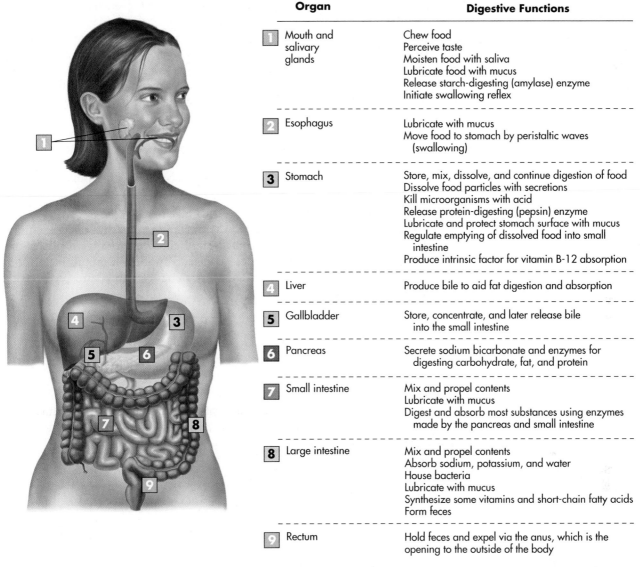

Organ	Digestive Functions
1 Mouth and salivary glands	Chew food Perceive taste Moisten food with saliva Lubricate food with mucus Release starch-digesting (amylase) enzyme Initiate swallowing reflex
2 Esophagus	Lubricate with mucus Move food to stomach by peristaltic waves (swallowing)
3 Stomach	Store, mix, dissolve, and continue digestion of food Dissolve food particles with secretions Kill microorganisms with acid Release protein-digesting (pepsin) enzyme Lubricate and protect stomach surface with mucus Regulate emptying of dissolved food into small intestine Produce intrinsic factor for vitamin B-12 absorption
4 Liver	Produce bile to aid fat digestion and absorption
5 Gallbladder	Store, concentrate, and later release bile into the small intestine
6 Pancreas	Secrete sodium bicarbonate and enzymes for digesting carbohydrate, fat, and protein
7 Small intestine	Mix and propel contents Lubricate with mucus Digest and absorb most substances using enzymes made by the pancreas and small intestine
8 Large intestine	Mix and propel contents Absorb sodium, potassium, and water House bacteria Lubricate with mucus Synthesize some vitamins and short-chain fatty acids Form feces
9 Rectum	Hold feces and expel via the anus, which is the opening to the outside of the body

FIGURE 3-10 ▶ Physiology of the GI tract. Many organs cooperate in a regulated fashion to allow the digestion and absorption of nutrients in foods.

endocrine system, and hormone-like compounds. Many common ailments arise from problems with the digestive system. Several of these digestive problems are discussed in the "Nutrition and Your Health" section at the end of this chapter.

The digestive system is composed of six separate organs; each organ performs one, or more, specific job(s). Let's look briefly at the role of each organ. These organs are listed in Figure 3-10 and in the flowchart on the next page. More detailed descriptions of digestive processes will be explained in later chapters as each nutrient is introduced.

Mouth

The mouth performs many functions in the digestion of food. Besides chewing food to reduce it to smaller particles, the mouth also senses the taste of the foods we consume. The tongue, through the use of its taste buds, identifies foods on the basis of their specific flavor(s). Sweet, sour, salty, bitter, and **umami** comprise the primary taste sensations we experience. Surprisingly, the nose and our sense of smell greatly contribute to our ability to sense the taste of food. When we chew a food, chemicals are released that stimulate the nasal passages. Thus, it makes perfect sense that when

gastrointestinal (GI) tract The main sites in the body used for digestion and absorption of nutrients. It consists of the mouth, esophagus, stomach, small intestine, large intestine, rectum, and anus. Also called the *digestive tract*.

motility Generally, the ability to move spontaneously. It also refers to movement of food through the GI tract.

umami A brothy, meaty, savory flavor in some foods. Monosodium glutamate enhances this flavor when added to foods.

GI Tract Components and Flow

Mouth

↓

Esophagus (10 inches long)

↓

Stomach—4-cup (1-liter) capacity. Food remains about 2 to 3 hours, or longer for large meals.

↓

Small intestine—duodenum (10 in long), jejunum (4 ft long), ileum (5 ft long)—about 10 ft (3.1 meters) in total length. Food remains about 3 to 10 hours.

↓

Large intestine (colon)—cecum, ascending colon, transverse colon, descending colon, sigmoid colon—3½ ft (1.1 meters) in total length. Food can remain up to 72 hours.

↓

Rectum

↓

Anus

saliva Watery fluid, produced by the salivary glands in the mouth, that contains lubricants, enzymes, and other substances.

salivary amylase A starch-digesting enzyme produced by salivary glands.

we have a cold and our noses are stuffed up and congested, even our most favorite foods will not taste as good as they normally do.

The taste of food, or the anticipation of it, signals the rest of the GI tract to prepare for the digestion of food. Once in the mouth, mechanical and chemical digestion begins. Salivary glands produce **saliva,** which functions as a solvent so that food particles can be further separated and tasted. In addition, saliva contains a starch-digesting enzyme, **salivary amylase** (see Chapter 4 for more on starch-digesting enzymes).

Enzymes are a key part of digestion. Each enzyme is specific to one type of chemical process. For example, enzymes that recognize and digest table sugar (sucrose) ignore milk sugar (lactose). Besides working on only specific types of chemicals, enzymes are sensitive to acidic and alkaline conditions, temperature, and the types of vitamins and minerals they require. Digestive enzymes that work in the acidic environment of the stomach do not work well in the alkaline environment of the small intestine. Overall, enzymes work to hasten certain events that take place in the body (Fig. 3-11).

The pancreas and the small intestine produce most of the digestive enzymes; however, the mouth and the stomach also contribute their own enzymes to digestion. **Mucus,** another component of saliva, makes it easy to swallow a mouthful of food. The food then travels to the esophagus. The important secretions and products of digestion are listed in Table 3-3.

MAKING DECISIONS

Enzymes and Digestion

The authors of some popular (fad) diet books contend that eating certain combinations of foods, such as meats and fruits together, hinders the digestive process. However, does this make sense in light of our newly gained knowledge about GI tract physiology? The body is able to increase the production of certain digestive enzymes in response to the type of diet consumed. The GI tract can respond to the nutritional makeup and amount of food consumed because of this fine-tuning. Once consumed, foods are attacked by multiple enzymes to release nutrients and other compounds for absorption.

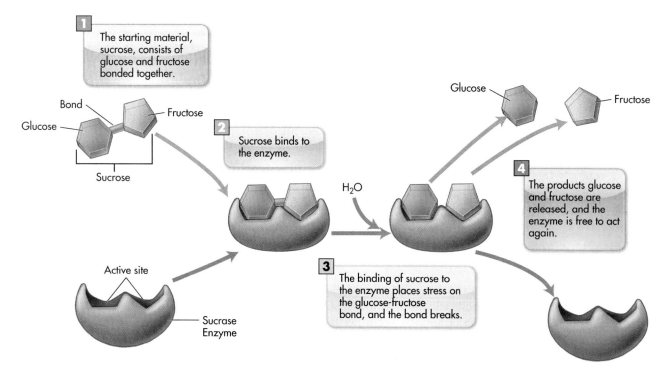

FIGURE 3-11 ▶ A model of enzyme action. The enzyme sucrase splits the sugar sucrose into two simpler sugars; glucose and fructose. [Note that sometimes energy input is needed to make reactions occur.]

TABLE 3-3 Important Secretions and Products of the Digestive Tract

Secretion	Site of Production	Purpose
Saliva	Mouth	Partial starch digestion using **salivary amylase,** lubrication of food for swallowing
Mucus	Mouth, stomach, small intestine, large intestine	Protects GI tract cells, lubricates food as it travels through the GI tract
Enzymes	Mouth, stomach, small intestine, pancreas	Promote digestion of carbohydrates, fats, and proteins into forms small enough for absorption (Examples: **amylases, lipases, proteases)**
Acid	Stomach	Promotes digestion of protein among other functions
Bile	Liver (stored in gallbladder)	Aids fat digestion in the small intestine by suspending fat in water using **bile acids, cholesterol,** and **lecithin**
Bicarbonate	Pancreas, small intestine	Neutralizes stomach acid when it reaches the small intestine
Hormones	Stomach, small intestine, pancreas	Stimulate production and/or release of acid, enzymes, bile, and bicarbonate; help regulate peristalsis and overall GI tract flow (Examples: gastrin, secretin, insulin, cholecystokinin, glucagon)

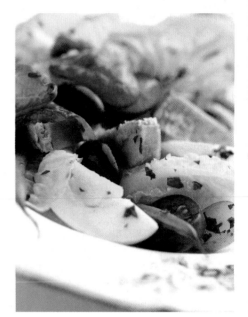

▲ The body digests the foods as they are presented—the order in which foods are eaten plays no role in digestion.

Esophagus

The **esophagus** is a long tube that connects the **pharynx** with the stomach. Near the pharynx is a flap of tissue (called the **epiglottis**) that prevents the **bolus** of swallowed food from entering the trachea (wind pipe) (Fig. 3-12). During swallowing, food lands on the epiglottis, folding it down to cover the opening of the trachea. Breathing also stops automatically. These responses ensure that swallowed food will only travel down the esophagus. If food instead travels down the trachea, choking may occur (the victim will not be able to speak or breathe). A group of techniques to treat such a person are called the Heimlich maneuver (see www.heimlichinstitute.org for details).

At the top of the esophagus, nerve fibers release signals to tell the GI tract that food has been consumed. This results in an increase in gastrointestinal muscle action, called **peristalsis.** These continual waves of muscle contractions, followed by muscle relaxation, force the food down the digestive tract from the esophagus onward (Fig. 3-13).

At the end of the esophagus is the **lower esophageal sphincter,** a muscle that constricts (closes) after food enters the stomach. The main function of sphincters is to prevent the backflow of GI tract contents. Sphincters respond to various stimuli, such as signals from the nervous system, hormones, acidic versus alkaline conditions, and pressure that builds up around the sphincter. The primary function of the lower esophageal sphincter is to prevent the acidic contents of the stomach from flowing back up into the esophagus—which can cause some of the health problems we will discuss in the "Nutrition and Your Health" section at the end of Chapter 3.

Stomach

The stomach is a large sac that can hold up to 4 cups (or 1 quart) of food for several hours until all of the food is able to enter the small intestine. Stomach size varies individually and can be reduced surgically as a radical treatment for obesity (more on this in Chapter 7). While in the stomach, the food is mixed with gastric juice,

mucus A thick fluid secreted by many cells throughout the body. It contains a compound that has both carbohydrate and protein parts. It acts as a lubricant and means of protection for cells.

amylase Starch-digesting enzyme produced by the salivary glands and pancreas.

lipase Fat-digesting enzyme produced by the salivary glands, stomach, and pancreas.

protease Protein-digesting enzyme produced by the stomach, small intestine, and pancreas.

esophagus A tube in the GI tract that connects the pharynx with the stomach.

pharynx The organ of the digestive tract and respiratory tract located at the back of the oral and nasal cavities, commonly known as the throat.

epiglottis The flap that folds down over the trachea during swallowing.

bolus A moistened mass of food swallowed from the oral cavity into the pharynx.

peristalsis A coordinated muscular contraction used to propel food down the gastrointestinal tract.

lower esophageal sphincter A circular muscle that constricts the opening of the esophagus to the stomach. Also called the *gastroesophageal sphincter.*

FIGURE 3-12 ▶ The process of swallowing. (a) During swallowing, food does not normally enter the trachea because the epiglottis closes over the larynx. (b) The closed epiglottis allows food to proceed down the esophagus. When a person chokes, food becomes lodged in the trachea, blocking air flow to the lungs. (c) The food should move down the esophagus.

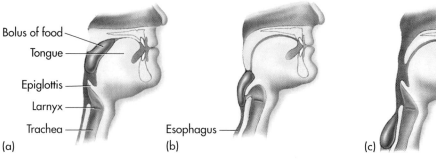

Bolus of food
Tongue
Epiglottis
Larnyx
Trachea
(a)

Esophagus
(b)

(c)

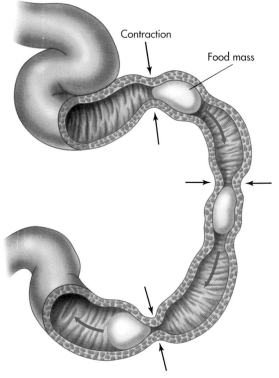

Contraction

Food mass

FIGURE 3-13 ▶ Peristalsis. Peristalsis is a progressive type of movement, propelling material from point to point along the GI tract. To begin this, a ring of contraction occurs where the GI wall is stretched, passing the food mass forward. The moving food mass triggers a ring of contraction in the next region, which pushes the food mass even farther along. The result is a ring of contraction that moves like a wave along the GI tract, pushing the food mass down the tract.

chyme A mixture of stomach secretions and partially digested food.

pyloric sphincter Ring of smooth muscle between stomach and small intestine.

intrinsic factor A proteinlike compound produced by the stomach that enhances vitamin B-12 absorption.

villi (singular, **villus**) The fingerlike protrusions into the small intestine that participate in digestion and absorption of food.

which contains water, a very strong acid, and enzymes. (Gastric is a term pertaining to the stomach.) The acid in the gastric juice maintains the acidity of the stomach contents and, thereby destroys the biological activity of proteins, converts inactive digestive enzymes to their active form, partially digests food protein, and makes dietary minerals soluble so that they can be absorbed. The mixing that takes place in the stomach produces a watery food mixture, called **chyme,** which slowly leaves the stomach a teaspoon (5 milliliters) at a time and enters the small intestine. Following a meal, the stomach contents are emptied into the small intestine over the course of 1 to 4 hours. The **pyloric sphincter,** located at the base of the stomach, controls the rate at which the chyme is released into the small intestine (Fig. 3-14). There is very little absorption of nutrients from the stomach, except for some alcohol.

You might wonder how the stomach prevents itself from being digested by the acid and enzymes it produces. First, the stomach has a thick layer of mucus that lines and protects it. The production of acid and enzymes also requires the release of a specific hormone (gastrin). This release happens primarily when we are eating or thinking about eating. Last, as the concentration of acid in the stomach increases, hormonal control causes acid production to taper off.

One other important function of the stomach is the production of a substance called **intrinsic factor.** This vital proteinlike compound is essential for the absorption of vitamin B-12.

Small Intestine

The small intestine is about 10 feet (3 meters) long, beginning at the stomach and ending at the large intestine (colon) (Fig. 3-15). The small intestine is considered "small" because of its narrow (1 inch [2.5 centimeters]) diameter. Most of the digestion and absorption of food occurs in the small intestine. The chyme secreted from the stomach is moved through the small intestine by peristaltic contractions so that it can be well mixed with the digestive juices of the small intestine (review Fig. 3-13). These juices contain many enzymes that function in the breakdown of carbohydrates, protein, and fat, as well as in the preparation of vitamins and minerals for absorption.

The physical structure of the small intestine is very important to the body's ability to digest and absorb the nutrients it needs. The lining of the small intestine is called the mucosa and is folded many times; within these folds are fingerlike projections called **villi.** These "fingers" are constantly moving, which helps them trap food to enhance absorption. Each individual villus (singular) is made up of many **absorptive cells,** and each of these cells has a highly folded cap. The combined folds, villi, and caps in the small intestine increase its surface area 600 times beyond that of a simple tube (Fig. 3-16).

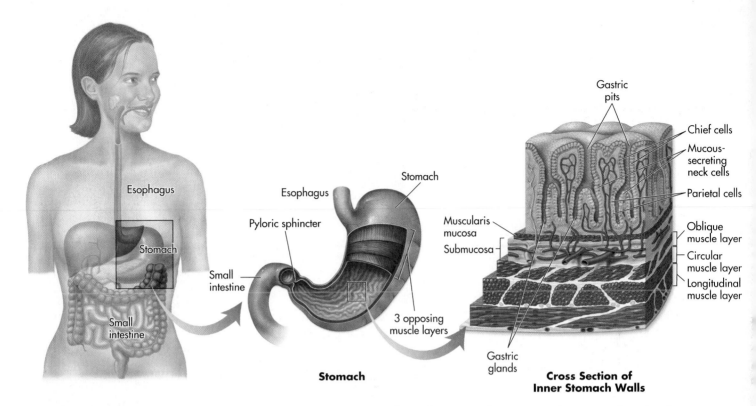

FIGURE 3-14 ▶ Physiology of the stomach. The interior surface mucous cells produce mucus for protection from stomach acid and enzymes. Parietal cells produce the hydrochloric acid (HCL), and chief cells produce the enzymes. Mucous neck cells, scattered among the cells in the gastric pits, also produce mucus. The exterior surface is made up of three types of muscle layers.

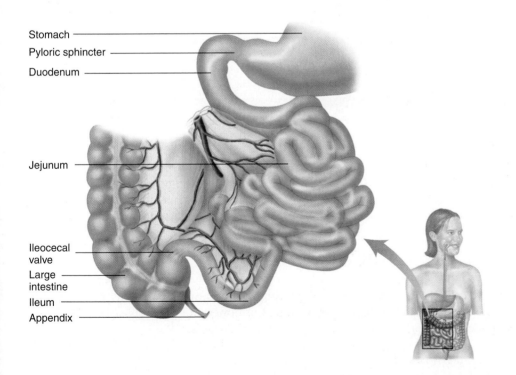

FIGURE 3-15 ▶ The small intestine and beginning of the large intestine. The three parts of the small intestine are the duodenum, jejunum, and ileum. Notice the smaller diameter of the small intestine, compared with the large intestine.

The absorptive cells have a short life. New intestinal absorptive cells are constantly produced in the crypts of the small intestine (Fig. 3-16) and appear daily along the surface of each villus "finger." This is probably because absorptive cells are subjected to a harsh environment, so renewal of the intestinal cell lining is necessary. This rapid cell turnover leads to high nutrient needs for the small intestine. Fortunately, many of

absorptive cells Intestinal cells that line the villi; and participate in nutrient absorption.

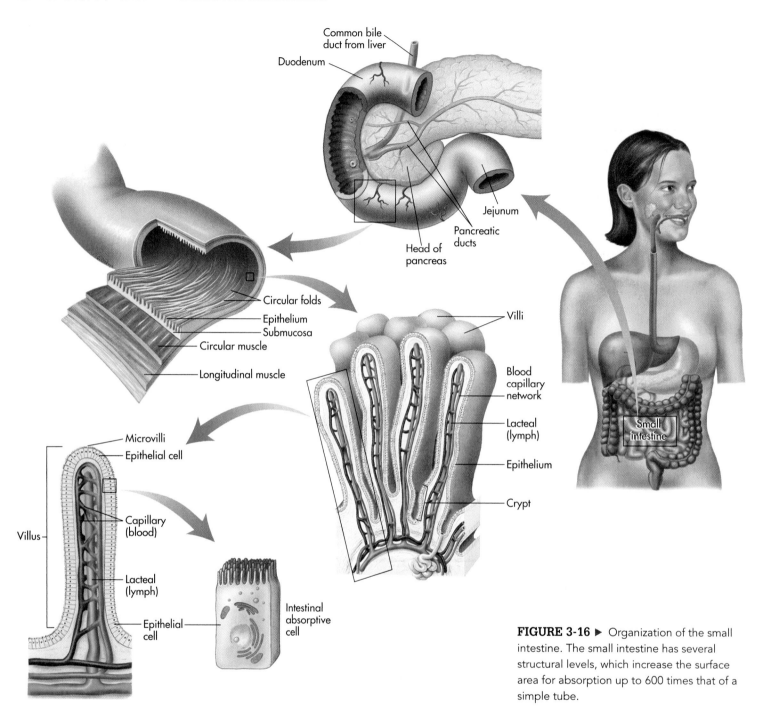

FIGURE 3-16 ▶ Organization of the small intestine. The small intestine has several structural levels, which increase the surface area for absorption up to 600 times that of a simple tube.

the old cells can be broken down and have their component parts reused. The health of the cells is further enhanced by various hormones and other substances that participate in or are produced as part of the digestive process.

The small intestine absorbs nutrients through the intestinal wall through various means and processes, as illustrated in Figure 3-17:

- **Passive diffusion:** When the nutrient concentration is higher in the cavity (lumen) of the small intestine than in the absorptive cells, the difference in nutrient concentration drives the nutrient into the absorptive cells by diffusion. Fats, water, and some minerals are absorbed by passive diffusion.

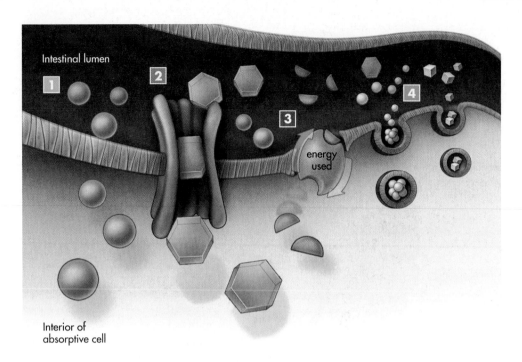

Intestinal lumen

energy used

Interior of absorptive cell

FIGURE 3-17 ▶ Nutrient absorption relies on four major absorptive processes. **1** Passive diffusion (in blue) is diffusion of nutrients across the absorptive cell membranes. **2** Facilitated diffusion (in green) uses a carrier protein to move nutrients down a concentration gradient. **3** Active absorption (in purple) involves a carrier protein as well as energy to move nutrients (against a concentration gradient) into absorptive cells. **4** Phagocytosis and pinocytosis (in green and brown) are forms of active transport in which the absorptive cell membrane forms an indentation that engulfs a nutrient to bring it into the cell.

- **Facilitated diffusion:** Some compounds require a carrier protein to drive them into absorptive cells. This type of absorption is called faciliated diffusion. Fructose is one example of a compound that makes use of such a carrier to allow for facilitated diffusion.
- **Active absorption:** In addition to the need for a carrier protein, some nutrients also require energy input to move from the lumen of the small intestine into the absorptive cells. This mechanism makes it possible for cells to take up nutrients even when they are consumed in low concentrations. Some sugars, such as glucose, are actively absorbed, as are amino acids.
- **Phagocytosis** and **pinocytosis:** In a further means of active absorption, absorptive cells literally engulf compounds (phagocytosis) or liquids (pinocytosis). As described earlier, a cell membrane can form an indentation of itself so that when particles or fluids move into the indentation, the cell membrane surrounds and engulfs them. This process is used when an infant absorbs immune substances from human milk (see Chapter 14).

Once absorbed, water-soluble compounds such as glucose and amino acids go to the capillaries and then on to the portal vein. Recall that the liver is the end of this process. Most fats eventually go into the lymph vessels. In doing so, they can eventually enter the bloodstream (see the earlier section on the circulatory system for details; and review Figs. 3-4 and 3-5).

Undigested food cannot be absorbed into cells of the small intestine. Any undigested food that reaches the end of the small intestine must pass through the **ileocecal sphincter** on the way to the large intestine (Fig. 3-18). This sphincter prevents the contents of the large intestine from reentering the small intestine.

ileocecal sphincter The ring of smooth muscle between the end of the small intestine and the large intestine.

Large Intestine

When the contents of the small intestine enter the large intestine, the material left bears little resemblance to the food originally eaten. Under normal circumstances, only a minor amount (5%) of carbohydrate, protein, and fat escape absorption to reach the large intestine (Table 3-4).

FIGURE 3-18 ▶ The parts of the colon: cecum ascending colon, transverse colon, descending colon, and sigmoid colon.

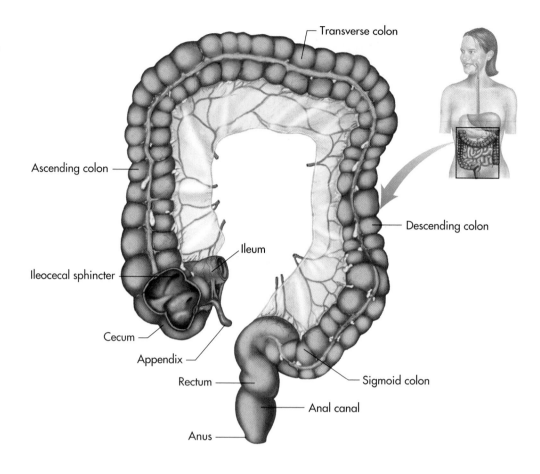

Transverse colon

Ascending colon

Descending colon

Ileum

Ileocecal sphincter

Cecum

Appendix

Rectum

Sigmoid colon

Anal canal

Anus

Physiologically, the large intestine differs from the small intestine in that there are no villi or digestive enzymes. The absence of villi means that little absorption takes place in the large intestine in comparison to the small intestine. Nutrients absorbed from the large intestine include water, some vitamins, some fatty acids, and the minerals sodium and potassium. Unlike the small intestine, the large intestine has a number of mucus-producing cells. The mucus secreted by these cells functions to hold the feces together and to protect the large intestine from the bacterial activity within it. The large intestine is home to a large population of bacteria (over 500 different species). Whereas the stomach and small intestine have some bacterial activity, the large intestine is the organ most heavily colonized with bacteria. Starting at infancy, the diet plays a major part in determining the type of bacteria in our digestive tracts. The number and type of bacteria in the human colon recently has become of great interest. Research has shown that intestinal bacteria play a significant role in the maintenance of health, especially health of the colon. It is speculated that higher levels of beneficial organisms can reduce the activity of disease-causing bacteria. This is another illustration of the intestinal tract working as an important immune organ. The strains *bifidobacteria* and *lactobacilli* are typically associated with health, whereas *clostridia* are considered problematic. These bacteria are able to break down some of the remaining food products that enter the large intestine, such as the milk sugar lactose (in lactose intolerant people), and some components of fiber. The products of bacterial metabolism in the large intestine, which include various acids, can then be absorbed.

Foods containing certain live microorganisms such as lactobacilli have been linked to some health benefits, such as improving intestinal tract health. These microorganisms are called **probiotics** because once consumed, they take up residence in the large

probiotic Product that contains specific types of bacteria. Use is intended to colonize the large intestine with the specific bacteria in the product. An example is yogurt.

TABLE 3-4 Major Sites of Absorption Along the GI Tract

Organ	Primary Nutrients Absorbed
Stomach	Alcohol (20% of total)
	Water (minor amount)
Small intestine	Calcium, magnesium, iron, and other minerals
	Glucose
	Amino acids
	Fats
	Vitamins
	Water (70% to 90% of total)
	Alcohol (80% of total)
	Bile acids
Large intestine	Sodium
	Potassium
	Some fatty acids
	Gases
	Water (10% to 30% of total)

intestine and confer a health benefit. You can find these probiotic microorganisms in certain forms of fluid milk, fermented milk, yogurt, and in pill form (see Further Reading 13). A related term is **prebiotic.** These are substances that increase growth of probiotic microorganisms. One example is fructooligosaccharides (see Table 1-5 in Chapter 1 for dietary sources). The beneficial organisms of the large intestine and their use as probiotics are highlighted in "Newsworthy Nutrition" and will be discussed further in Chapter 4 when we explore their use as probiotics.

Some water remains in the material that enters the large intestine because the small intestine absorbs only 70% to 90% of the fluid it receives, which includes large amounts of GI-tract secretions produced during digestion. The remnants of a meal also contain some minerals and some fiber. Because water is removed from the large intestine, its contents become semisolid by the time they have passed through the first two-thirds of it. What remains in the **feces,** besides water and undigested fiber, is tough connective tissues (from animal foods); bacteria from the large intestine; and some body wastes, such as parts of dead intestinal cells.

Rectum

The feces or stool remains in the last portion of the large intestine, the **rectum,** until muscular movements push it into the **anus** to be eliminated. The presence of feces in the rectum stimulates elimination. The anus contains two **anal sphincters** (internal and external), one of which is under voluntary control (external sphincter). Relaxation of this sphincter allows for elimination.

prebiotic Substance that stimulates bacterial growth in the large intestines.

rectum Terminal portion of the large intestine.

anus Last portion of the GI tract; serves as an outlet for that organ.

anal sphincters A group of two sphincters (inner and outer) that help control expulsion of feces from the body.

gallbladder An organ attached to the underside of the liver; site of bile storage, concentration, and eventual secretion.

bile A liver secretion stored in the gallbladder and released through the common bile duct into the first segment of the small intestine. It is essential for the digestion and absorption of fat.

See Nutrition and Your Health: Common Problems with Digestion at the end of Chapter 3.

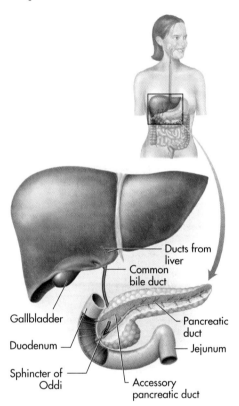

FIGURE 3-19 ▶ The liver, gallbladder, and pancreas are accessory organs that work with the GI tract. The liver produces bile, stored in the gallbladder and released into the duodenum portion of the small intestine, via the common bile duct, to help digest fat. The pancreas secretes pancreatic juice containing water, bicarbonate, and digestive enzymes into the duodenum via the common bile duct. The common bile duct from the liver and gallbladder and the pancreatic duct join together at the sphincter of Oddi to deliver bile, pancreatic enzymes, and bicarbonate to the duodenum.

Accessory Organs

The liver, **gallbladder,** and pancreas work with the GI tract and are considered accessory organs to the process of digestion (review Fig. 3-10). These accessory organs are not part of the GI tract through which food passes, but they play necessary roles in the process of digestion. These organs secrete digestive fluids into the GI tract and enable the process of converting food into absorbable nutrients.

The liver produces a substance called **bile.** The bile is stored and concentrated in the gallbladder until the gallbladder receives a hormonal signal to release the bile. This signal is induced by the presence of fat in the small intestine. Bile is released and delivered to the small intestine via a tube called the bile duct (Fig. 3-19).

In action, bile is like soap. Components of the bile enable large portions of fat to break into smaller bits so that they can be suspended in water (Chapter 5 will cover this process in detail). Interestingly, some of the bile constituents can be "recycled" in a process known as **enterohepatic circulation.** These components of bile are reabsorbed from the small intestine, returned to the liver via the portal vein, and reused.

In addition to bile, the liver releases a number of other unwanted substances that travel with the bile to the gallbladder and end up in the small intestine and eventually in the large intestine for excretion. The liver functions in this manner to remove unwanted substances from the blood. (Other byproducts are excreted via the urine; see the next section, "Urinary System.")

The pancreas manufactures hormones and pancreatic juice. The hormones include glucagon and insulin, which as noted earlier function in glucose regulation (review Fig. 3-7). Pancreatic juice contains water, bicarbonate, and a variety of digestive enzymes capable of breaking apart carbohydrates, proteins, and fats into small fragments. Bicarbonate is a base that neutralizes the acidity of chyme as it moves from the stomach into the small intestine. In contrast to the stomach, the small intestine, does not have a protective layer of mucus, because mucus would impede nutrient absorption. Instead, the neutralizing capacity of bicarbonate from the pancreas protects the walls of the small intestine from erosion by acid, which would otherwise lead to formation of an ulcer (see the "Nutrition and Your Health" section at the end of Chapter 3).

CONCEPT CHECK

Digestion is a mechanical and chemical process mediated by enzymes and coordinated by hormones and nerves. Whereas swallowing and ultimate elimination of feces from the anus are voluntary, the majority of the digestive processes are involuntary. The stomach initiates the process of digestion by mixing food with gastric juice and converting this partially digested food into chyme. The products of digestion are molecules of the original food or beverage small enough to be absorbed into the villi of the small intestine and transferred to the blood or lymph. For the most part, nutrients are absorbed in the small intestine; only a few are absorbed in the large intestine. Any dietary component that escapes digestion by human or bacterial enzymes exits the body as feces.

3.9 Urinary System

The **urinary system** is composed of two kidneys, one on each side of the spinal column. Each kidney is connected to the bladder by a **ureter.** The bladder is emptied by way of the **urethra** (Fig. 3-20). The main function of the kidneys is to remove waste from the body. The kidneys are constantly filtering blood to control its composition. This results in the formation of urine, mostly water, along with dissolved waste products of metabolism such as urea, and excess and unneeded water-soluble vitamins and various minerals.

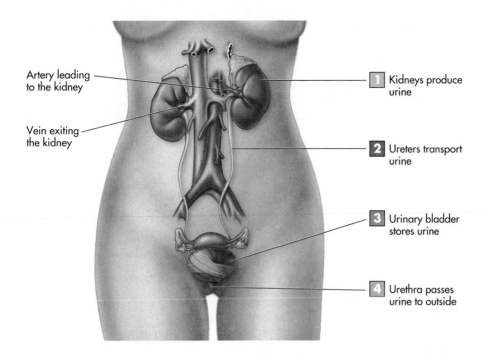

Artery leading to the kidney

Vein exiting the kidney

1 Kidneys produce urine

2 Ureters transport urine

3 Urinary bladder stores urine

4 Urethra passes urine to outside

FIGURE 3-20 ▶ Organs of the urinary system. The kidneys, **1** bean-shaped organs located on either side of the spinal column, filter waste from the blood and form urine, which is transported to the bladder by the ureters **2** and stored in the bladder **3** as urine. The urethra **4** transports the urine to outside the body. The urinary system of the female is shown. The male's urinary system is the same, except that the urethra extends through the penis.

enterohepatic circulation A continual recycling of compounds such as bile acid between the small intestine and the liver.

urinary system The body system consisting of the kidneys, urinary bladder, and the ducts that carry urine. This system removes waste products from the circulatory system and regulates blood acid-base balance, overall chemical balance, and water balance in the body.

ureter Tube that transports urine from the kidney to the urinary bladder.

urethra Tube that transports urine from the urinary bladder to the outside of the body.

pH A measure of relative acidity or alkalinity of a solution. The pH scale is 0 to 14. A pH of 7 is neutral; A pH below 7 is acidic; a pH above 7 is alkaline.

erythropoietin A hormone secreted mostly by the kidneys that enhances red blood cell synthesis and stimulates red blood cell release from bone marrow.

Together with the lungs, the kidneys also maintain the acid-base balance **(pH)** of the blood. The kidneys also convert a form of vitamin D into its active hormone form and produce a hormone that stimulates red blood cell synthesis (**erythropoietin;** see Chapter 12 for information on misuse of this hormone by some athletes). During times of fasting, the kidneys even produce glucose from certain amino acids. Thus, the kidneys perform many important functions related to nutrition and are a vital component of the body.

The proper function of the kidneys is closely tied to the strength of the cardiovascular system, particularly its ability to maintain adequate blood pressure, and the consumption of sufficient fluid. Uncontrolled diabetes, hypertension, and drug abuse are harmful to the kidneys.

3.10 Nutrient Storage Capabilities

The human body must maintain reserves of nutrients, otherwise we would need to eat continuously. Storage capacity varies for each different nutrient. Most fat is stored in adipose tissue, made up of cells designed specifically for this. Short-term storage of carbohydrate occurs in muscle and liver in the form of glycogen. The blood maintains a small reserve of glucose and amino acids. Many vitamins and minerals are stored in the liver, while other nutrient stores are found in other sites in the body.

When people do not meet certain nutrient needs, these nutrients are obtained by breaking down a tissue that contains high concentrations of the nutrient. For example, calcium is taken from bone and protein is taken from muscle. In cases of long-term deficiency, these nutrient losses weaken and harm these tissues.

Many people believe that if too much of a nutrient is obtained—for example, from a vitamin or mineral supplement—only what is needed is stored and the rest is excreted by the body. Though true for some nutrients, such as vitamin C, the large dosages of other nutrients frequently found in supplements, such as vitamin A and iron, can cause harmful side effects because they are not readily excreted. This is one reason why obtaining your nutrients primarily (or exclusively) from a balanced diet is the safest means to acquire the building blocks you need to maintain the good health of all organ systems.

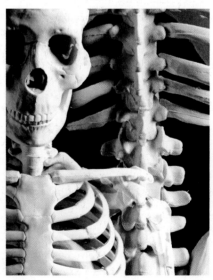

▲ The skeletal system provides a reserve of calcium for day-to-day needs when dietary intake is inadequate. Long-term use of this reserve, however, reduces bone strength.

CONCEPT CHECK

The urinary system removes the wastes produced by the body and many nutrients ingested in excess of storage capacity and need. The kidneys maintain the chemical composition and acidity of the blood. In addition, the kidneys help convert vitamin D to its active form and produce a hormone needed for red blood cell synthesis.

In well-nourished individuals, nutrients are constantly present in the blood for immediate use and are stored in the body tissues for later use when sufficient amounts are not consumed from food. However, when the body suffers a nutrient deficiency after an inadequate diet is consumed over a long period, vital tissues will be broken down for their nutrients, which can lead to ill health. Additionally, too much of any nutrient can be detrimental. It's best to focus primarily (or exclusively) on obtaining all essential nutrients from a balanced diet rather than mostly from dietary supplements.

3.11 Nutrition and Genetics

epigenome The way that the genome is marked and packaged inside the cell nucleus.

epigenetics Inherited changes in gene expression caused by mechanisms other than changes in the DNA sequence.

Once nutrients and other dietary components are taken up by cells, they may interact with our genes and have an effect on gene expression. The growth, development, and maintenance of cells, and ultimately of the entire organism, are directed by genes present in the cells. Each gene essentially represents a recipe, noting the ingredients (amino acids) and how those ingredients should be put together (to make proteins). The products (proteins) of all the recipes in the cookbook (the human genome) would then make up the human organism. The genome and the **epigenome**, the way the genome is marked and packaged inside a cell's nucleus, control the expression of individual traits, such as height, eye color, and susceptibility to many diseases. **Epigenetics** refers to inherited changes in gene expression caused by mechanisms other than changes in the underlying DNA sequence. While our genome contains the code for the proteins that can be made by our bodies, our epigenome is an extra layer of instructions that influences gene activity. In many cases it is the epigenome that can be repaired by treatments, or affected by diet, rather than the genetics.

The causes of chronic diseases are complex and include a significant genetic component. Fortunately, the science of genetics is moving swiftly such that medical breakthroughs are beginning to touch our lives. Genetic discoveries are leading to new drugs that disrupt disease processes at the molecular level and to tests that predict our risk for disease. In 2008, scientists discovered more than 100 genetic variations associated with many medical conditions associated with aging, including type 2 diabetes, Alzheimer's disease, osteoporosis, high blood pressure, and heart disease.

A genetic variation can directly affect the proteins encoded by our genes and result in different:

- nutrient requirements among individuals.
- susceptibilities to diseases.
- effects of environmental factors (such as our diet) on our genes and their proteins.

The Emerging Field of Nutrigenomics

nutrigenomics Study of how food impacts health through its interaction with our genes and its subsequent effect on gene expression.

In the near future, genetic information will enhance the ability of health professionals to help individuals manage diseases and optimize health. Nutritional genomics or **nutrigenomics** is the study of how food impacts health through its interaction with our genes and its subsequent effect on gene expression. Nutrigenomics also includes the study of how genes determine our nutritional requirements. Research in this area highlights the fallacy of a "one-size-fits-all" approach to nutrition interventions for disease prevention and management. It is becoming clear that the general nutrient requirements do not apply to certain genetic subgroups. Research is very active in identifying these subgroups and classifying the human genetic variation that may affect nutrient utilization and physiological function and therefore their unique nutrient requirements (see Further Readings 5, 14, and 15).

In addition to the direct effect of genes on disease risk, in many cases, genes influence the effect of diet and nutrition on disease development and progression. In some cases, a food component can cause a gene to be turned on or off, thus manipulating the production of proteins that can affect—positively or negatively—development or progression of diseases. With a better understanding of the interactions between genes and our diet, it will not be long before dietary recommendations may be personalized to help those with various genetically-linked diseases (see Further Reading 7).

Nutritional Diseases with a Genetic Link

Studies of families, including those with twins and adopted children, provide strong support for the effects of genetics in various disorders. In fact, family history is considered to be an important risk factor in the development of many nutrition-related diseases.

Cardiovascular Disease. There is strong evidence that cardiovascular disease is the result of gene-environment interactions. About 1 of every 500 people in North America has a defective gene that greatly delays cholesterol removal from the bloodstream. As discussed in Chapter 1, elevated blood cholesterol is one major risk factor for development of cardiovascular disease. The gene-diet interactions being discovered for cardiovascular disease, particularly the cases of high blood lipid levels, will likely be the first to lead to nutrition plans personalized to decrease cardiovascular disease risk. Another genetic variation can cause abnormally high levels of an amino acid called homocysteine, which increases cardiovascular disease risk. Diet changes can help these people, but medications and even surgery are needed to address these problems.

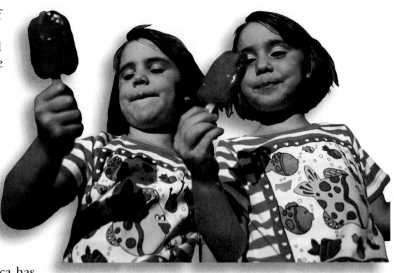

▲ Studies of twins have provided strong evidence for the interaction between genes and diet and their combined effects on disease risk.

Obesity. Most obese North Americans have at least one obese parent. This strongly suggests a genetic link. Findings from many human studies suggest that a variety of genes (likely 60 or more) are involved in the regulation of body weight. Little is known, however, about the specific nature of these genes in humans or how the actual changes in body metabolism (such as lower calorie-burning in general or fat use in particular) are produced.

Still, although some individuals may be genetically predisposed to store body fat, whether they do so depends on how many calories they consume relative to their needs. A common concept in nutrition is that *nurture*—how people live and the environmental factors that influence them—allows *nature*—each person's genetic potential—to be expressed. Although not every person with a genetic tendency toward obesity becomes obese, those genetically predisposed to weight gain have a higher lifetime risk than individuals without a genetic predisposition to obesity.

Diabetes. Both of the two common types of diabetes—type 1 and type 2—have genetic links. Evidence for these genetic links comes from studies of families, including twins, and from the high incidence of diabetes among certain population groups (e.g., South Asians or Pima Indians). Diabetes, in fact, is a complex disease with more than 200 genes identified as possible causes. Only sensitive and expensive testing can determine who is at risk. Type 2 diabetes is the most common form of diabetes (90% of all cases), and also has a strong link to obesity. Typically a genetic tendency for type 2 diabetes is expressed once a person becomes obese but often not before, again illustrating that nurture affects nature.

Cancer. A few types of cancer (e.g., some forms of colon [large intestine] and breast cancer) have a strong genetic link, and genetics may play a role in others, such as **prostate cancer.** Because obesity increases the risk of several forms of cancer, a long-standing excess calorie intake is also a risk factor. Although genes are an important determinant in the development of cancer, environmental and lifestyle factors, such as excessive sun exposure and a poor diet, also contribute significantly to the risk profile.

CRITICAL THINKING

Wesley notices that at family gatherings his parents, uncles, aunts, and older siblings typically drink excessive amounts of alcohol. His father has been arrested for driving while intoxicated, as has one of his aunts. Two of his uncles died before the age of 60 from alcohol abuse. As Wesley approaches the age of legal drinking, he wonders if he is destined to fall into the pattern of alcohol abuse. What advice would you give to Wesley concerning his future use of alcohol?

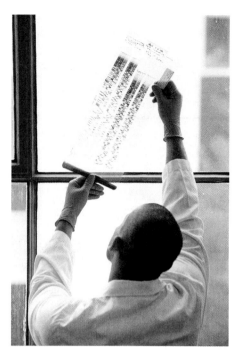

▲ Genetic testing for disease susceptibility will be more common in the future as the genes that increase the risk of developing various diseases are isolated and decoded.

The following weblinks will help you gather more information about genetic conditions and testing:

http://nutrigenomics.ucdavis.edu/
Center for Excellence for Nutritional Genomics. Website dedicated to promoting the new science of nutritional genomics

www.geneticalliance.org
Alliance of Genetic Support Groups

www.kumc.edu/gec/support
Information on genetic and rare conditions

www.cancer.gov/cancertopics/prevention-genetics-causes
Genetics information from the National Cancer Institute

http://www.genome.gov/
National Human Genome Research Institute (at the National Institutes of Health) website. Describes the latest research finding, discusses some ethical issues, and provides a talking glossary.

http://history.nih.gov/exhibits/genetics/
Revolution in Progress: Human Genetics and Medical Research

MAKING DECISIONS

Research is opening the way for "personalized nutrition" that uses the results of genetic testing to determine which diet will work most effectively with the person's genetic makeup. There are genetic tests available for at least 1500 diseases and conditions, but mechanisms are not in place to ensure that the tests are based on adequate evidence or that marketing claims are truthful. Many companies are already tailoring genetic testing services and products for certain genetic profiles even though there are insufficient data on which to base genotype-specific recommendations. Most of these offers are online. As we discussed in Chapter 2, caution is always needed when evaluating nutrition information and claims. Genetic testing is no exception. Some DNA-testing companies are responsible organizations, and some are not. Some are offering DNA tests to determine the best weight-loss diets or the best supplements. These marketing schemes belittle the science of genetics to consumers. Use the principles outlined in Chapter 2 to evaluate any genetic testing services or products.

Your Genetic Profile

From this discussion, you can see that your genes can greatly influence your risk of developing certain diseases. By recognizing your potential for developing a particular disease, you can avoid behavior that further raises your risk. How can you figure out your genetic profile? Genetic testing can be valuable if it confirms that you carry a gene for a disease that you can do something about in terms of protecting against it. Testing is also of interest when you do not know your family medical history or there are gaps in your family tree. About 1000 genetic tests have become available in recent years. It typically costs about $1000 to have your DNA read to reveal the diseases to which you are most susceptible. Many tests are covered by health insurance plans. The Genetic Information Nondiscrimination Act (GINA) became a law in May 2008, and prohibits health insurers from raising premiums or denying coverage based on genetic information and applies to people who have genes that carry the risk of disease. DNA testing includes providing a saliva sample from which your DNA will be separated. Certain areas of the genome are then read and measured in the process known as genotyping. After this 1-to 2-month process, you receive your DNA profile, which will supplement what you already know about your family history. You can also compare your DNA profile to future findings from DNA research.

Many of the genes involved in common diseases, such as diabetes, are still unknown. Although there are genetic tests available for some diseases, your family history of certain diseases is still a much better indicator of your genetic profile and risk of disease. Put together a family tree of illnesses and deaths by compiling a few key facts on your primary relatives: siblings, parents, aunts and uncles, and grandparents, as suggested in the "Rate Your Plate" section. In general, the greater number of your relatives who had a genetically transmitted disease and the closer they are related to you, the greater your risk. If there is a significant family history of a certain disease, lifestyle changes may be appropriate. For example, women with a family history of breast cancer should avoid becoming obese, should minimize alcohol use, and should obtain mammograms regularly.

Figure 3-22 shows an example of a family tree (also called a *genogram*). High-risk conditions include two or more first-degree relatives in a family with a specific disease (first-degree relatives include one's parents, siblings, and offspring). Another sign of risk of inherited disease is development of the disease in a first-degree relative before the age of 50 to 60 years. In the family depicted in Figure 3-21, prostate cancer killed the man's father. Knowing this, the man should be tested regularly for prostate cancer. His sisters should have frequent mammograms and other preventive practices because their mother died of breast cancer. Because heart attack and stroke are also common in the family, all the children should adopt a lifestyle that minimizes the risk of developing these conditions, such as avoiding excessive animal fat and salt intake. Colon cancer is also evident, so careful screening throughout life is important.

Information about our genetic makeup will increasingly influence our dietary and lifestyle choices. Throughout this book we will discuss "controllable" risk factors that could contribute to development of genetically linked diseases present in your family. This information will help you personalize nutrition advice based on your genetic background and identify and avoid the risk factors that could lead to the diseases present in your family.

This review of human anatomy, physiology, and genetics from a nutrition perspective sets the stage for developing a more detailed understanding of the nutrients. Chapters 4, 5, and 6 will build on this information.

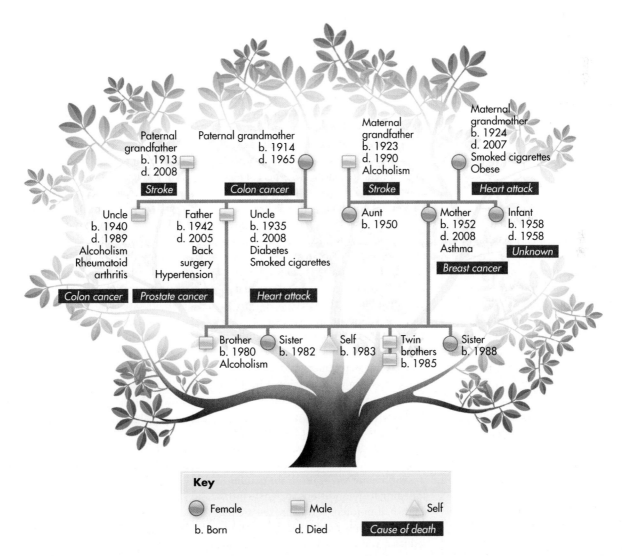

FIGURE 3-21 ▶ Example of a family tree for Justin, designated as "Self" at the trunk of the tree. The gender of each family member is identified by color (blue squares for males, orange circles for females). Dates of birth (b) and death (d) are listed below each family member. If deceased, the cause of death is highlighted using white text against a red background. Other medical conditions the family members experienced are noted beneath each name. Create your own family tree of frequent diseases using the diagram in "Rate Your Plate" and this figure as a guide. Then show your family tree to your physician to get a more complete picture of what the information means for your health.

Common Problems with Digestion

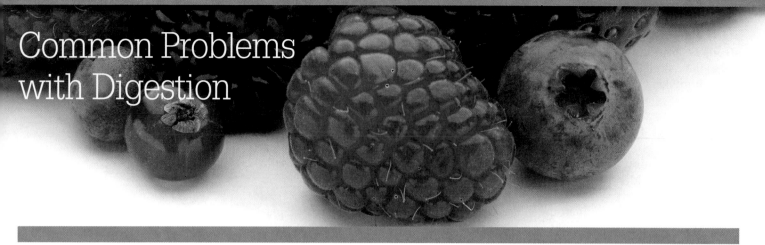

The fine-tuned organ system we call the digestive system can develop problems. Knowing about these common problems can help you avoid or lessen them. Two common GI tract-related problems are diverticulosis and lactose maldigestion and intolerance. These disorders will be discussed in Chapter 4 after you learn more about carbohydrates.

Ulcers

A peptic **ulcer** can occur when the lining of the esophagus, stomach, or small intestine is eroded by the acid secreted by the stomach cells (Fig. 3-22). As the stomach lining deteriorates in ulcer development, it loses its protective mucus layer, and the acid further erodes the stomach tissue. Acid can also erode the lining of the esophagus and the first part of the small intestine, the duodenum. In young people, most ulcers occur in the small intestine, wheras in older people they occur primarily in the stomach.

Millions of North Americans develop ulcers during their lifetimes. As a result, billions of healthcare dollars are spent annually on the treatment of peptic ulcers and their complications. Fortunately, our understanding of ulcer formation has increased, resulting in a variety of improved treatment options. The typical symptom of an ulcer is pain about 2 hours after eating. Stomach acid acting on a meal irritates the ulcer after most of the meal has moved from the site of the ulcer.

Not long ago, the major cause of ulcer disease was thought to be excess acid. Therefore, neutralizing and curtailing the secretion of stomach acid were the logical treatment choices. Although acid is still a significant player in ulcer formation, the principal causes of ulcer disease are currently thought to be infection of the stomach by the acid-resistant bacteria, *Helicobacter pylori (H. pylori)*; heavy use of nonsteroidal anti-inflammatory drugs **(NSAIDS),** such as aspirin; and disorders that cause excessive acid production in the stomach. Stress is regarded as a predisposing factor for ulcers, especially if the person is infected with *H. pylori* or has certain anxiety disorders. Cigarette smoking is also known to cause ulcers, increase ulcer complications such as bleeding, and lead to ulcer treatment failure.

The *H. pylori* bacteria is found in more than 80% of patients with stomach and duodenal ulcers. The bacteria is common but results in ulcer disease in only 10% to 15% of those infected. Although the mechanism of how *H. pylori* causes ulcers is not well understood, treatment of the infection with antibiotics heals the ulcers and prevents their recurrence. Two Australian physicians were awarded the Nobel Prize in 2005 "for their discovery of the bacterium *Helicobacter pylori* and its role in gastritis and peptic ulcer disease."

NSAIDs are medications for painful inflammatory conditions such as arthritis. Aspirin, ibuprofen, and naproxen are the most commonly used NSAIDs. NSAIDs reduce the mucus secreted by the stomach. Newer medications, called "Cox-2 inhibitors" (e.g., celecoxib [Celebrex]), have been used as a replacement for NSAIDs because they are less likely to cause stomach ulcers. They do offer some advantages over NSAIDs, but they may not be totally safe for some people, especially those with a history of cardiovascular disease or strokes.

The primary risk associated with an ulcer is the possibility that it will erode entirely through the stomach or intestinal wall. The GI contents could then spill into the body cavities, causing a massive infection. In addition, an ulcer may erode a blood vessel, leading to substantial blood loss. For these reasons, it is important not to ignore the early warning signs of ulcer development, including a persistent gnawing or burning near the stomach that may occur immediately following a meal or awaken you at night. In addition to the pain that may improve with food, other signs and symptoms of ulcers are weight loss, nausea, vomiting, loss of appetite, and abdominal bloating.

In the past, milk and cream therapy was used to help cure ulcers. Clinicians now know that milk and cream are two of the worst foods for an ulcer. The calcium in these foods stimulates stomach acid secretion and actually inhibits ulcer healing.

Today, a combination of approaches is used for ulcer therapy. People infected with *H. pylori* are given antibiotics as well as stomach acid-blocking medica-

ulcer Erosion of the tissue lining, usually in the stomach or the upper small intestine. As a group these are generally referred to as *peptic ulcers*.

NSAIDs Nonsteroidal anti-inflammatory drugs; includes aspirin, ibuprofen (Advil®), and naproxen (Aleve®).

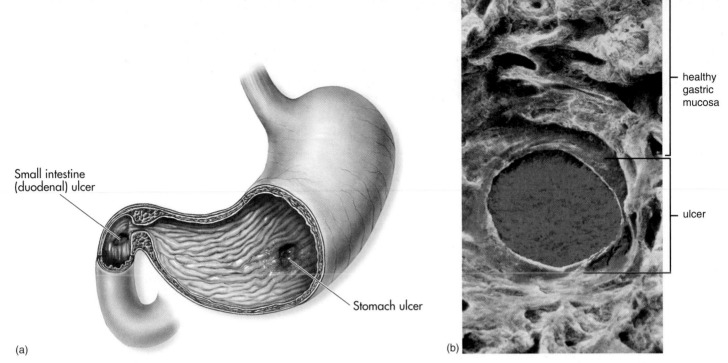

(a)   (b)

FIGURE 3-22 ▶ (a) A peptic ulcer in the stomach or small intestine. *H. pylori* bacteria and NSAIDs (e.g., aspirin) cause ulcers by impairing mucosal defense, especially in the stomach. In the same way, smoking, genetics, and stress can impair mucosal defense, as well as cause an increase in the release of pepsin and stomach acid. All of these factors can contribute to ulcers. (b) Close-up of a stomach ulcer. This needs to be treated or eventual perforation of the stomach is possible.

▶ When suffering from persistent heartburn or GERD, see a doctor if you have:

- Difficulty swallowing or pain when swallowing
- Heartburn that has persisted for more than 10 years
- Initial onset of heartburn after age 50
- Heartburn that resists treatment with medications
- Sudden, unexplained weight loss
- Chest pain
- Blood loss or anemia
- Blood in stool or vomit

tions called **proton** (proton is another name for the hydrogen ion that creates acidity) **pump inhibitors** (e.g., omeprazole [Prilosec], esomeprazole [Nexium], and lansoprazole [Prevacid]). In many cases, there is a 90% cure rate for *H. pylori* infections in the first week of this treatment. Recurrence is unlikely if the infection is cured, but an incomplete cure almost certainly leads to repeated ulcer formation (see Further Reading 2).

Antacid medications may also be part of ulcer care, as is a class of medicines called **H2 blockers**. These include cimetidine (Tagamet), ranitidine (Zantac), nizatidine (Axid), and famotidine (Pepcid), all of which prevent **histamine**-related acid secretion in the stomach. Medications that coat the ulcer, such as sucralfate (Carafate), are also commonly used.

People with ulcers should refrain from smoking and minimize the use of NSAIDs. These practices reduce the mucus secreted by the stomach. Overall, a combination of lifestyle therapy and medical treatment has so revolutionized ulcer

therapy that dietary changes are of minor importance today. Current diet-therapy approaches recommend avoiding foods that increase ulcer symptoms (Table 3-5).

proton pump inhibitor A medication that inhibits the ability of gastric cells to secrete hydrogen ions. Low doses of this class of medications are also available without prescription (e.g., omeprazole [Prilosec]).

H₂ blocker Medication, such as cimetidine (Tagamet®), that blocks the increase of stomach acid production caused by histamine.

histamine A breakdown product of the amino acid histidine that stimulates acid secretion by the stomach and has other effects on the body, such as contraction of smooth muscles, increased nasal secretions, relaxation of blood vessels, and changes in relaxation of airways.

TABLE 3-5 Recommendations to Prevent Ulcers and Heartburn from Occurring or Recurring

Ulcers

1. Stop smoking if you are now a smoker.

2. Avoid large doses of aspirin, ibuprofen, and other NSAID compounds unless a physician advises otherwise. For people who must use these medications, FDA has approved an NSAID combined with a medication to reduce gastric damage. The medication reduces gastric acid production and enhances mucus secretion.

3. Limit consumption of coffee, tea, and alcohol (especially wine), if this helps.

4. Limit consumption of pepper, chili powder, and other strong spices, if this helps.

5. Eat nutritious meals on a regular schedule; include enough fiber (see Chapter 4 for sources of fiber).

6. Chew foods well.

7. Lose weight if you are currently overweight.

Heartburn

1. Follow ulcer prevention recommendations.

2. Wait about 2 hours after a meal before lying down.

3. Don't overeat. Eat smaller meals that are low in fat.

4. Elevate the head of the bed at least 6 inches.

Heartburn

About half of North American adults experience occasional heartburn, also known as acid reflux (Fig. 3-23). This gnawing pain in the upper chest is caused by the movement of acid from the stomach into the esophagus. The recurrent and therefore more serious form of the problem is called **gastroesophageal reflux disease (GERD).** Unlike the stomach, the esophagus has very little mucus lining to protect it, so acid quickly erodes the lining of the esophagus, causing pain. Symptoms may also include nausea, gagging, cough, or hoarseness. GERD is characterized by the occurrence of such symptoms of acid reflux two or more times per week. People who have GERD experience occasional relaxation of the gastroesophageal sphincter. Typically it should be relaxed only during swallowing, but in individuals with GERD it is relaxed at other times as well.

The majority of heartburn sufferers say it significantly affects their quality of life, particularly their enjoyment of many favorite foods. On a more serious note, however, if left untreated, heartburn can, over time, damage the lining of the esophagus, leading to chronic esophageal inflammation and an increased risk of esophageal cancer (see Further Reading 8). Heartburn sufferers should follow the general recommendations given in Table 3-5. For occasional heartburn, quick relief can be found with over-the-counter (OTC) antacids. Taking antacids will reduce the acid in the stomach but will not stop the acid reflux. For more persistent (few days a week or everyday) heartburn or GERD, the H2 blockers or PPIs, discussed in the previous section on ulcers, may be needed. PPIs provide long-lasting relief by reducing stomach acid production and should be taken before the first meal of the day because they take longer to work. If the proper medications are not effective at controlling GERD, surgery may be

gastroesophageal reflux disease (GERD) Disease that results from stomach acid backing up into the esophagus. The acid irritates the lining of the esophagus, causing pain.

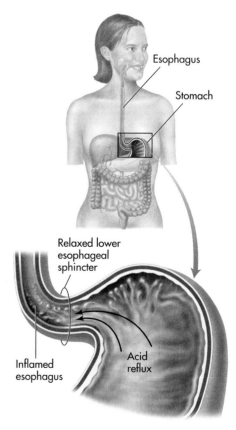

FIGURE 3-23 ▶ Heartburn results from stomach acid refluxing into the esophagus.

Esophagus

Stomach

Relaxed lower esophageal sphincter

Inflamed esophagus

Acid reflux

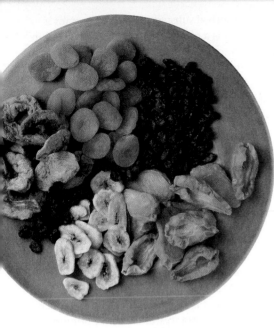

▲ Dried fruits are a natural source of fiber and can help prevent constipation when consumed with an adequate amount of fluid.

needed to strengthen the weakened esophageal sphincter (see Further Reading 3). A popular theory is that relaxation of the lower esophageal sphincter allows acid and stomach contents to flow back into the esophagus. This situation will be more of a problem when lying down.

Both pregnancy and obesity can lead to heartburn (see Further Reading 6). These conditions result in increased production of estrogen and progesterone, which relax the lower esophageal sphincter, making heartburn more likely. In obesity, adipose tissue turns certain circulating hormones into estrogen; thus, the more adipose tissue one has, the more estrogen produced.

Constipation and Laxatives

Constipation, difficult or infrequent evacuation of the bowels, is commonly reported by adults. Slow movement of fecal material through the large intestine causes constipation. As more fluid is absorbed during the extended time the feces stay in the large intestine, they become dry and hard.

Constipation can result when people regularly ignore their normal bowel reflexes for long periods. People may ignore normal urges when it is inconvenient to interrupt occupational or social activities. Muscle spasms of an irritated large intestine can also slow the movement of feces and contribute to constipation. Calcium, iron supplements, and medications such as antacids can also cause constipation.

Eating foods with plenty of fiber, such as whole-grain breads, cereals, and beans, along with drinking adequate fluid to avoid dehydration, is the best method for treating mild cases of constipation. Fiber stimulates peristalsis by drawing water into the large intestine and helping form a bulky, soft fecal output. Dried fruits are a good source of fiber and therefore can also help stimulate the bowel. Additional fluid should be consumed to facilitate fiber's action in the large intestine. In addition, people with constipation may need to develop more regular bowel habits; allowing the same time each day for a bowel move-

ment can help train the large intestine to respond routinely. Finally, relaxation facilitates regular bowel movements, as does regular physical activity.

Laxatives, as well as various other medications, can also lessen constipation. Some laxatives work by irritating the intestinal nerve junctions to stimulate the peristaltic muscles, while others that contain fiber draw water into the intestine to enlarge fecal output. The larger output stretches the peristaltic muscles, making them rebound and then constrict. Regular use of laxatives, however, should be supervised by a physician. Overall the bulk-forming fiber laxatives are the safest to use.

Hemorrhoids

Hemorrhoids, also called *piles,* are swollen veins of the rectum and anus. The blood vessels in this area are subject to intense pressure, especially during bowel movements. Added stress to the vessels from pregnancy, obesity, prolonged sitting, violent coughing or sneezing, or straining during bowel movements, particularly with constipation, can lead to a hemorrhoid. Hemorrhoids can develop unnoticed until a strained bowel movement precipitates symptoms, which may include pain, itching, and bleeding.

Itching, caused by moisture in the anal canal, swelling, or other irritation, is perhaps the most common symptom. Pain, if present, is usually aching and steady. Bleeding may result from a hemorrhoid and appear in the toilet as a bright red streak in the feces. The sensation of a mass in the anal canal after a bowel movement is symptomatic of an internal hemorrhoid that protrudes through the anus.

Anyone can develop a hemorrhoid, and about half of adults over age 50 do. Diet, lifestyle, and possibly heredity play

constipation A condition characterized by infrequent bowel movements.

laxative A medication or other substance that stimulates evacuation of the intestinal tract.

a role. For example, a low-fiber diet can lead to hemorrhoids as a result of straining during bowel movements. If you think you have a hemorrhoid, you should consult your physician. Rectal bleeding, although usually caused by hemorrhoids, may also indicate other problems, such as cancer.

A physician may suggest a variety of self-care measures for hemorrhoids. Pain can be lessened by applying warm, soft compresses or sitting in a tub of warm water for 15 to 20 minutes. Dietary recommendations are the same as those for treating constipation, emphasizing the need to consume adequate fiber and fluid. Over-the-counter remedies, such as Preparation H, can also offer relief of symptoms.

Irritable Bowel Syndrome

Many adults (25 million or more in the United States alone) have irritable bowel syndrome, noted as a combination of cramps, gassiness, bloating, and irregular bowel function (diarrhea, constipation, or alternating episodes of both). It is more common in younger women than in younger men. In older adults the ratio is closer to 50:50. The disease leads to about 3.5 million visits to physicians in the United States each year.

Symptoms associated with irritable bowel syndrome include visible abdominal distention, pain relief after a bowel movement, increased stool frequency, loose stools with pain onset, mucus in stool, and a feeling of incomplete elimination even after a bowel movement.

The cause is thought to be altered intestinal peristalsis coupled with a decreased pain threshold for abdominal distension—in other words, a minor amount of abdominal bloating causes pain that the average person would not sense. It is also noteworthy that up to 50% of sufferers report a history of verbal or sexual abuse.

Therapy is individualized and can include a trial of high-fiber foods (soluble fiber is more effective than insoluble fiber) or elimination diets that focus on avoiding dairy products and gas-forming foods, such as legumes, certain vegetables (cabbage, beans, and broccoli), and some fruits (grapes, raisins, cherries, and cantaloupe). Herbal formulations, certain probiotics, and cognitive behavioral therapy have been shown to decrease symptoms of irritable bowel syndrome and improve overall quality of life (see Further Reading 1). The patient should moderate or eliminate caffeine-containing foods/beverages altogether. Low-fat and more frequent, small meals may help because large meals can trigger contractions of the large intestine. Other strategies include a reduction in stress, psychological counseling, and certain antidepressant and other medications. Hypnosis has been shown to relieve symptoms in severe cases.

Referral to a registered dietitian can be beneficial, as many patients experience improvement with the elimination of specific problem foods. A good patient/physician relationship is also necessary for the treatment of irritable bowel syndrome; however, before any single treatment is applauded, note that response to placebos alone has been as high as 70% in this population. Although irritable bowel syndrome can be uncomfortable and upsetting, it is harmless as it carries no risk for cancer or other serious digestive problems. The website www.ibsgroup.org provides further information.

Diarrhea

Diarrhea, a GI tract disease that generally lasts only a few days, is defined as increased fluidity, frequency, or amount of bowel movements compared to a person's usual pattern. Most cases of diarrhea result from infections in the intestines, with bacteria and viruses the usual offending agents. They produce substances that cause the intestinal cells to secrete fluid rather than absorb fluid. Another form of diarrhea can be caused by consumption of substances not readily absorbed, such as the sugar alcohol sorbitol found in sugarless gum (see Chapter 4) or large amounts of a high-fiber source such as bran. When consumed in large amounts, the unabsorbed substance draws much water into the intestines, in turn leading to diarrhea. Treatment of diarrhea generally requires drinking lots of fluid during the affected stage; reduced intake of the poorly absorbed substance also is important if that is a cause. Prompt treatment—within 24 to 48 hours—is especially important for infants and older people, as they are more susceptible to the effects of dehydration associated with diarrhea (see Chapters 15 and 16). Diarrhea that lasts more than 7 days in adults should be investigated by a physician as it can be a symptom of more serious intestinal disease, especially if there is also blood in the stool.

Gallstones

Gallstones are a major cause of illness and surgery, affecting 10% to 20% of U.S. adults. Gallstones are pieces of solid material that develop in the gallbladder when substances in the bile—primarily cholesterol (80% of gallstones)—form crystal-like particles. They may be as small as a grain of sand or as large as a golf ball. These stones are caused by a combination of factors, with excess weight being the primary modifiable factor, especially in women 20 to 60 years old. Other factors include genetic background (e.g., Native Americans), advanced age (> 60 years for both women and men), reduced activity of the gallbladder (contracts less than normal), altered bile composition (e.g., too much cholesterol or not enough bile salts), diabetes, and diet (e.g., low-fiber diets). In addition, gallstones may develop during rapid weight loss or prolonged fasting (as the liver metabolizes more fat, it secretes more cholesterol into the bile).

Attacks due to gallstones include intermittent pain in the upper right abdomen, gas and bloating, nausea or vomiting, or other health problems. Surgical removal of the gallbladder is the most common method for treating gallstones (500,000 surgeries per year in the United States).

Prevention of gallstones revolves around avoiding becoming overweight, especially for women. Avoiding rapid weight loss (> 3 pounds per week), limiting animal protein and focusing more on plant protein intake (especially some nut intake), and following a high-fiber diet can help as well. Regular physical activity is also recommended, as is moderate to no caffeine and alcohol intake.

Less Common Digestive Disorders

In **cystic fibrosis**—an inherited disease of infants, children, and sometimes adults—the pancreas often develops thick mucus that blocks its ducts, and active cells then die. As a result, the pancreas is not able to effectively deliver its digestive enzymes into the small intestine. Digestion of carbohydrate, protein, and—most notably—fat then is impaired. Often the missing enzymes must be ingested in capsule form with meals to aid in digestion. Another intestinal problem gaining attention is **celiac disease.** People with this disease experience an allergic reaction to the protein gluten in certain cereals, such as wheat and rye. This reaction damages the absorptive cells, resulting in a much-reduced surface area due to flattening of the villi. Elimination of wheat, rye, and certain other grains from the diet typically cures the problem.

Summary

Overall, typical medical disorders of the GI tract arise from differences in anatomical features and lifestyle habits among individuals. Because of the importance of various nutrition and lifestyle habits, such as adequate fiber and fluid intake, as well as not smoking or abusing NSAID medications, nutrition and lifestyle therapy is often effective in helping treat GI tract disorders.

cystic fibrosis Inherited disease that can cause overproduction of mucus. Mucus can block the pancreatic duct, decreasing enzyme output.

celiac disease Immunological or allergic reaction to the protein gluten in certain grains, such as wheat and rye. The effect is to destroy the intestinal enterocytes, resulting in a much reduced surface area due to flattening of the villi. Elimination of wheat, rye, and certain other grains from the diet restores the intestinal surface.

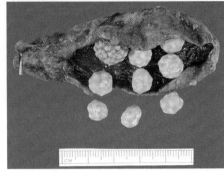

▲ Gallbladder and gallstones seen after surgical removal from the body. Size and composition of the stones vary from one case to another.

Case Study Gastroesophageal Reflux Disease

Caitlin is a 20-year-old college sophomore. Over the last few months, she has been experiencing regular bouts of heartburn. This usually happens after a large lunch or dinner. Occasionally she has even bent down after dinner to pick up something and had some stomach contents travel back up her esophagus and into her mouth. This especially frightened Caitlin, so she visited the University Health Center.

The nurse practitioner at the Center told Caitlin it was good that she came in for a checkup because she suspects Caitlin has a disease called gastroesophageal reflux disease (GERD). She tells Caitlin that this can lead to serious problems, such as a rare form of cancer if not controlled. She provides Caitlin with a pamphlet describing GERD and schedules an appointment with a physician for further evaluation.

Answer the following questions, and check your response in Appendix A.

1. What dietary and lifestyle habits likely contribute to Caitlin's symptoms of GERD?
2. What is the dietary and lifestyle management advice that will help Caitlin cope with this health problem?
3. What types of medications have been especially useful for treating this problem?
4. Overall, how will Caitlin cope with this health problem, and will it ever go away?
5. Why is management of GERD so important?

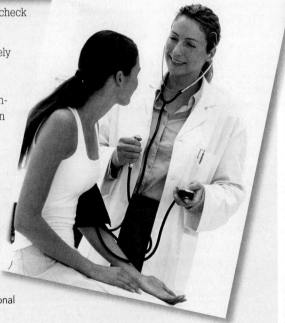

▶ Caitlin was wise to see a health professional about her persistent heartburn.

Summary (Numbers refer to numbered sections in the chapter.)

3.1 Cells join together to make up tissues, tissues unite to form organs, and organs work together as an organ system.

3.2 The basic structural unit of the human body is the cell. A most all cells contain the same organelles (nucleus, mitochondria, endoplasmic reticulum, lysosomes, peroxisomes, and cytoplasm), but cell structure varies according to the type of job they must perform.

3.3 Epithelial, connective, muscle, and nervous, are the four primary types of tissues in the human body. Each type of organ system is affected by nutrient intake.

3.4 Blood is pumped from the heart to the lungs, picking up oxygen. Blood delivers essential nutrients, oxygen, and water to all body cells. Nutrients and wastes are exchanged between blood and cells across the cell membrane. This exchange occurs in the capillaries. Water-soluble compounds absorbed by the small intestine cells enter the portal vein and travel to the liver. Fat-soluble compounds enter the lymphatic system, which eventually connects to the bloodstream.

3.5 The nervous system's neurons are the body's communication network. They control and manage all other organ systems of the body. Neurotransmitters are used to carry the message from one neuron to another (or to another cell).

3.6 The endocrine system produces hormones, which chemically regulate almost all other cells.

3.7 The immune system protects the body from invading pathogens. We activate immunity, such as production of antibodies (immunoglobulins), when we come in contact with a pathogen.

3.8 The gastrointestinal (GI) tract consists of the mouth, esophagus, stomach, small intestine, large intestine (colon), rectum, and anus.

Spaced along the GI tract are ring-like valves (sphincters) that regulate the flow of foodstuffs. Muscular contractions, called *peristalsis,* move the foodstuffs down the GI tract. A variety of nerves, hormones, and other substances control the activity of sphincters and peristaltic muscles.

Digestive enzymes are secreted by the mouth, stomach, wall of the small intestine, and pancreas. The presence of food in the small intestine stimulates the release of pancreatic enzymes.

The major absorptive sites consist of fingerlike projections called *villi,* located in the small intestine. Absorptive cells cover the villi. This intestinal lining is continually renewed. Absorptive cells can perform various forms of passive diffusion and active absorption.

Little digestion and absorption occur in the stomach or large intestine, but some protein is digested in the stomach. Some constituents of fiber and undigested starch are broken down by bacteria in the large intestine and some of the products are absorbed; any undigested fiber that remains is eliminated in the feces.

Final water and mineral absorption takes place in the large intestine. Products from bacterial breakdown of some fibers and other substances are also absorbed here. The presence of feces in the rectum provides the impetus for elimination.

The liver, gallbladder, and pancreas participate in digestion and absorption. Products from these organs, such as enzymes and bile, enter the small intestine help in digesting protein, fat, and carbohydrate.

3.9 The urinary system, including the kidneys, is responsible for filtering the blood, removing body wastes, and maintaining the chemical composition of the blood.

3.10 Limited stores of nutrients are present in the blood for immediate use and stored to a greater or lesser extent in body tissues for later use when sufficient food is unavailable. When the body suffers a nutrient deficiency caused by a poor diet, it breaks down vital tissues for their nutrients, which can lead to ill health. Additionally, too much of any nutrient can be detrimental.

3.11 Genetic background influences the risk for many health-related diseases. Examining one's family tree provides clues for an individual to such risks. Preventative measures are then import ant to implement, especially with respect to diet.

N&YH Common GI-tract diseases, such as heartburn, constipation, and irritable bowel syndrome, can be treated with diet changes. These can include increasing fiber intake and avoiding large meals high in fat. Medications are also very helpful in many cases.

Check Your Knowledge (Answers to the following questions are below.)

1. The stomach is protected from digesting itself by producing
   a. bicarbonate.
   b. a thick layer of mucus.
   c. hydroxyl ions to neutralize acid.
   d. antipepsin that destroys enzymes.

2. The lower esophageal sphincter is located between the
   a. stomach and esophagus.
   b. stomach and duodenum.
   c. ileum and the cecum.
   d. colon and the anus.

3. A muscular contraction that propels food down the GI tract is called
   a. a sphincter.
   b. enterohepatic circulation.
   c. gravitational pull.
   d. peristalsis.

4. Bicarbonate ions (HCO_3-) from the pancreas
   a. neutralize acid in the stomach.
   b. are synthesized in the pyloric sphincter.
   c. neutralize bile in the duodenum.
   d. neutralize the acid in the duodenum.

5. Most digestive processes occur in the
   a. mouth.
   b. stomach.
   c. small intestine.
   d. large intestine.
   e. colon.

6. Bile is formed in the _____ and stored in the _____.
   a. stomach, pancreas
   b. duodenum, kidney
   c. liver, gallbladder
   d. gallbladder, liver

7. Much of the digestion that occurs in the large intestine is caused by
   a. lipase.
   c. saliva.
   b. pepsin.
   d. bacteria.

8. Nexium ("the purple pill") acts as a(n)
   a. H₂ blocker.
   b. laxative.
   c. analgesic.
   d. proton pump inhibitor.

9. The study of how food impacts health through interaction with genes is
   a. nutrigenomics.
   b. epidemiology.
   c. immunology.
   d. genetics.

10. Energy production that takes place in the cytoplasm is anaerobic metabolism because it does not require
   a. water.
   b. oxygen.
   c. anabolic steroids.
   d. anaerobic bacteria.

Answer Keys: 1. b (LO 3.11), 2. a (LO 3.8), 3. d (LO 3.8), 4. d (LO 3.8), 5. c (LO 3.8), 6. c (LO 3.8), 7. d, 8. d (LO 3.12), 9. a, 10. b (LO 3.2)

Study Questions (Numbers refer to Learning Outcomes)

1. Identify at least one function of the 12 organ systems related to nutrition **(LO 3.3)**

2. Draw and label parts of the cell, and explain the function of each organelle as it relates to human nutrition. **(LO 3.2)**

3. Trace the flow of blood from the right side of the heart and back to the same site. How is blood routed through the small intestine? Which class of nutrients enters the body via the blood? Via the lymph? **(LO 3.4)**

4. Explain why the small intestine is better suited than the other GI tract organs to carry out the absorptive process. **(LO 3.8)**

5. Identify the four basic tastes. Give an example of one food that exemplifies each of these basic taste sensations. **(LO 3.8)**

6. What is one role of acid in the process of digestion? Where is it secreted? **(LO 3.8)**

7. Contrast the processes of active absorption and passive diffusion of nutrients. **(LO 3.8)**

8. Identify two accessory organs that empty their contents into the small intestine. How do the digestive substances secreted by these organs contribute to the digestion of food? **(LO 3.8)**

9. In which organ systems would the following substances be found?
   chym **(LO 3.8)**, plasma **(LO 3.4)**, lymph **(LO 3.4)**, urine **(LO 3.9)**

10. Describe the nutrition-related diseases for which genetics or family history is considered to be an important risk factor. **(LO 3.11)**

What Would You Choose Recommendations

Constipation results from slow movement of fecal material through the large intestine. Increasing fiber and water in your diet can often relieve constipation without the aid of an over-the-counter laxative. To boost your fiber intake, choose whole grains, fruits, vegetables, and legumes (beans). This can be a tough task when most of the menu options you will find in fast-food restaurants and convenience stores are low in fiber.

As you select your pizza, look for slices with extra vegetables or fruit. This will increase the fiber content by about 1 gram per slice. Pizza with whole-grain crust, would add another 1 gram of fiber per slice. These are small improvements, so you will probably still need to look for additional fiber sources.

What about your side dish? Unless they are made with whole grains, the pasta and breadsticks will not add much fiber to your meal. A breadstick and a cup of pasta with Alfredo sauce provide about 1 and 2 grams

of fiber, respectively. These carbohydrate-rich add-ons are supplying extra calories and would be better off skipped. The salad provides about 1 to 3 grams of fiber, depending on its size and ingredients. The core ingredients of tossed salad—lettuce, cucumbers, tomato—are mostly water and not particularly high in fiber. Toppings such as cheese, egg, or diced meat will not help relieve constipation. Instead, dried fruit (e.g., dried cranberries or raisins) and nuts supply some additional fiber.

An even better choice, however, is the soup! A cup of bean and pasta soup is just what the doctor ordered to help relieve constipation. It provides about 6 grams of fiber and some extra water, as well.

Lastly, be sure to drink plenty of water. Dehydration is an often overlooked cause of constipation. Water helps lubricate the digestive tract and adds bulk to the feces when absorbed by fiber in the large intestine.

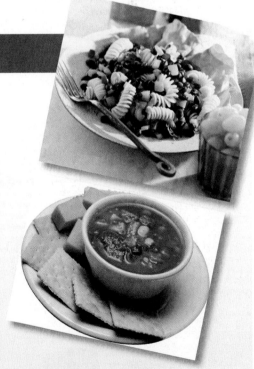

▶ Whole-grain pasta and beans used in salads and soups are good sources of fiber that can prevent intestinal issues such as constipation.

Further Readings

1. Camilleri M: Probiotics and irritable bowel syndrome: Rationale, putative mechanisms, and evidence of clinical efficacy. *Journal of Clinical Gastroenterology* 40:264, 2006.

   The evidence that Bifidobacteria or Lactobacilli species alone or in the specific probiotic combination of VSL#3 are beneficial for treatment of symptoms in IBS is discussed.

2. Consumers Union : Drugs to treat heartburn and stomach acid reflux: The proton pump inhibitors—comparing effectiveness, safety, and price ConsumerReportHealth.org/Best Buy Drugs, 16 pp. May 2010. www.consumer reports.org/health/resources/pdf/best-buy-drugs/PPIsUpdate-FINAL.pdf

   PPIs are the most widely prescribed medicines in the United States to treat heartburn and GERD in individuals who have symptoms that persist, are chronic or severe, or are unrelieved by antacids or H2 blockers. The seven available PPI medicines were found to be roughly equal in effectiveness and safety but differed in cost. The report recommended three of the less expensive drugs that are available without a prescription.

3. Galmiche J-P, Deshpande AR: Laparoscopic antireflux surgery versus esomeprazole treatment for chronic GERD: The LOTUS Randomized Clinical Trial. *Journal of the American Medical Association* 305(19): 1969, 2011.

   Study Taking daily medication (Nexium) or undergoing a minimally invasive surgery to treat acid reflux disease control the worst symptoms of the disease in many people. More than 500 persons were studied and after 5 years, 92% of people in the medication group and 85% in the surgery group reported having no GERD symptoms, or symptoms that were easy to live with.

4. Gosden RG, Feinberg AP: Genetics and epigenetics, Nature's pen-and-pencil set. *New England Journal of Medicine* 356:731; 2007.

   Epigenetics refers to inherited changes in gene expression caused by mechanisms other than changes in the underlying DNA sequence. Epigenetic information is like a code written in pencil in the margins around the DNA, which is written in indelible ink. In many cases it is the epigenome that can be repaired by treatments, or affected by diet.

5. Institute of Medicine: *Nutrigenomics and beyond: Informing the future.* Washington, DC: The National Academy Press, 2007.

   This report summarizes the state of nutritional genomics research and policy. It includes guidance for further development and translation of this knowledge into nutrition practice and policy.

6. Jacobson BC and others: Body mass index and symptoms of gastroesophageal reflux in women. *New England Journal of Medicine* 354:2340, 2006.

   BMI was associated with symptoms of GERD in 10,545 participants in the Nurses' Health Study. Even moderate weight gain caused or exacerbated symptoms of reflux.

7. Katsanis SH and others: A case study of personalized medicine. *Science* 320:53, 2008.

   Personalized medicine promises to revolutionize health care by tailoring treatments based on individual genetic information. The need for regulating personalized genomic medicine in a manner beneficial to public health is discussed. Currently, in most states companies are not required to demonstrate clinical validity before offering new genetic tests.

8. Layke JC, Lopez PP: Esophageal cancer. A review and update. *American Family Physician* 73:2187, 2006.

   Esophageal cancer is aggressive and is commonly diagnosed at an advanced stage with a poor prognosis. Associations among the development of esophageal cancer, Helicobacter pylori *infection and GERD are discussed. Despite increased use of proton pump inhibitors and eradication of H. pylori, the number of new cases of esophageal cancer continues to grow.*

9. Lynch A, Webb C: What are the most effective nonpharmacologic therapies for irritable bowel syndrome? *Journal of Family Practice* 57:57, 2008.

   Herbal formulations, certain probiotics, elimination diets based on immunoglobulin G antibodies, cognitive behavioral therapy, and self-help books are discussed because they have been shown to decrease global symptoms of irritable bowel syndrome (IBS) and improve overall quality of life. Soluble fiber is more effective than insoluble fiber at improving IBS symptoms.

10. Muller-Lisser and others: Myths and misconceptions about constipation. *American Journal of Gastroenterology* 100:232, 2005.

    Increasing fiber intake and avoiding dehydration help in mild cases of constipation. More difficult cases require physician evaluation and likely the use of laxatives and other medications.

11. Niewinski MM: Advances in celiac disease and gluten-free diet. *Journal of the American Dietetic Association* 108:661, 2008.

    Recognition of celiac disease as a disorder, is increasing. This review focuses on the gluten-free diet and the importance for all patients with celiac disease to receive expert dietary counseling. Recent advances in the gluten-free diet are discussed.

12. Omoruyi O, Holten KB: How should we manage GERD? *Journal of Family Practice* 55:410, 2006.

    Guidelines for the use of proton pump inhibitors, H2 blockers, and surgery for the treatment of GERD are presented.

13. Santosa S and others: Probiotics and their potential health claims. *Nutrition Reviews* 64:265, 2006.

    This paper provides strong evidence of the ability of different probiotic strains to prevent and treat diarrhea, and some forms of irritable bowel syndrome.

14. Stover PJ: Influence of human genetic variation on nutritional requirements. *American Journal of Clinical Nutrition* 83:436S, 2006.

    The complexity of the interaction between genes and diet is discussed as well as the reevaluation of criteria used to determine RDAs relative to the contribution of genetic variation to optimal nutrition for individuals.

15. Stover PJ, Caudill MA: Genetic and epigenetic contributions to human nutrition and health: Managing genome-diet interactions. *Journal of the American Dietetic Association* 108:1480, 2008.

    This article discusses ways that nutritional genomics will facilitate the establishment of genome-informed nutrient and food-based dietary guidelines for disease prevention and healthful aging, individualized medical nutrition therapy for disease management, and targeted public health nutrition interventions that maximize benefits and minimize adverse outcomes within genetically diverse human populations.

16. Wallace TC and others: Human gut microbiota and its relationship to health and disease. *Nutrition Review* 69 (7): 392, 2011.

    Evidence is available from over 700 research studies to support the growing interest in the benefits of probiotics and prebiotics and to aid the development of intervention strategies and practical guidelines for their use in the prevention and treatment of gastrointestinal tract disorders.

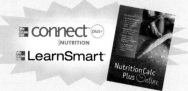

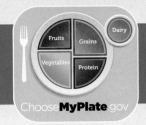

RATE YOUR PLATE

I. Are You Taking Care of Your Digestive Tract?

People need to think about the health of their digestive tracts. There are symptoms we need to notice, as well as habits we need to practice to protect it. The following assessment is designed to help you examine your habits and symptoms associated with the health of your digestive tract. Put a *Y* in the blank to the left of the question to indicate yes and an *N* to indicate no.

_____ 1. Are you currently experiencing greater than normal stress and tension?

_____ 2. Do you have a family history of digestive tract problems (e.g., ulcers, hemorrhoids, recurrent heartburn, constipation)?

_____ 3. Do you experience pain in your stomach region about 2 hours after you eat?

_____ 4. Do you smoke cigarettes?

_____ 5. Do you take aspirin frequently?

_____ 6. Do you have heartburn at least once per week?

_____ 7. Do you commonly lie down after eating a large meal?

_____ 8. Do you drink alcoholic beverages more than two or three times per day?

_____ 9. Do you experience abdominal pain, bloating, or gas 1½ to 2 hours after consuming milk products?

_____ 10. Do you often have to strain while having a bowel movement?

_____ 11. Do you consume less than 9 (women) or 13 (men) cups of a combination of water and other fluids per day?

_____ 12. Do you perform physical activity for less than 60 minutes or more on most or all days of the week (e.g., jog, swim, walk briskly, row, stair climb)?

_____ 13. Do you eat a diet relatively low in fiber (recall that significant fiber is found in whole fruits, vegetables, legumes, nuts and seeds, whole-grain breads, and whole-grain cereals)?

_____ 14. Do you frequently have diarrhea?

_____ 15. Do you frequently use laxatives or antacids?

Add up the number of yes answers and record the total. If your score is from 8 to 15, your habits and symptoms put you at risk for experiencing future digestive tract problems. Take particular note of the habits to which you answered yes. Consider trying to cooperate more with your digestive tract.

II. Create Your Family Tree for Health-Related Concerns

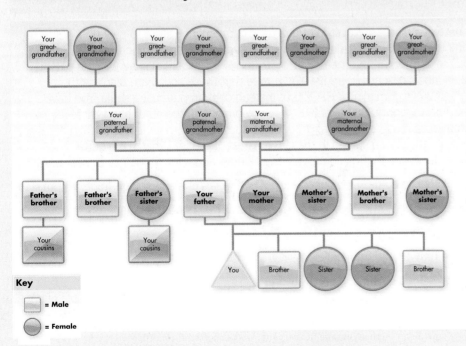

Adapt this diagram to your family tree. Under each heading, list year born, year died (if applicable), major diseases that developed during the person's lifetime, and cause of death (if applicable). Figure 3-21 provides one such example.

You are likely to be at risk for any diseases listed. Creating a plan for preventing such diseases when possible, especially those that developed in your family members before age 50 to 60 years, is advised. Speak with your physician about any concerns arising from this exercise.

Chapter 4 Carbohydrates

Student Learning Outcomes

Chapter 4 is designed to allow you to:

4.1 Identify the basic structures and food sources of the major carbohydrates—monosaccharides, disaccharides, polysaccharides (e.g., starches), and fiber.

4.2 Describe food sources of carbohydrate and list some alternative sweeteners.

4.3 Explain how carbohydrates are digested and absorbed, including the consequences of lactose maldigestion (and lactose intolerance).

4.4 List the functions of carbohydrate in the body and the problems that result from not eating enough carbohydrate.

4.5 Describe the regulation of blood glucose and discuss how other nutrients can be converted to blood glucose.

4.6 Outline the beneficial effects of fiber on the body.

4.7 State the RDA for carbohydrate and various guidelines for carbohydrate intake.

4.8 Identify the consequences of diabetes, and explain appropriate dietary measures that will reduce the adverse effects of this health problem.

What Would You Choose?

In between classes, you stop at a nearby convenience store to pick up a cold drink that will quench your thirst and fill your growling stomach. Immediately, you reach for your favorite cola but the Jones Soda Co.® display with its personalized labels catches your eye. You notice that these sodas are made with no high-fructose corn syrup (HFCS) but instead contain pure cane sugar. You have heard news reports that liken HFCS to poison, but on the other hand, there are commercials saying HFCS is just the same as sugar. Is there a nutritional difference between the added sugars in these two types of sodas? What is the better beverage choice that could provide the calories and energy of an afternoon snack?

a 20-ounce bottle of regular cola (e.g., Coca-Cola®) containing high-fructose corn syrup

b 20-ounce bottle of diet cola (e.g., Coke Zero®) containing aspartame

c 12-ounce bottle of Jones Soda Co.® Pure Cane Root Beer Soda

d ½ pint (8 fluid ounces) of low-fat (1%) chocolate milk

e 16-ounce bottle of water

 connect plus+ | NUTRITION

Think about your choice as you read Chapter 4, then see our recommendations at the end of the chapter. To learn more about various sweeteners, including how HFCS is made and arguments for and against use of HFCS, check out the Connect site: www.mcgrawhillconnect.com

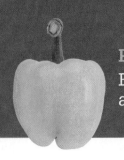

What did you eat to obtain the energy you are using right now? Chapters 4, 5, and 6 will examine this question by focusing on the main nutrients the human body uses for fuel. These nutrients are carbohydrates (on average, 4 kcal per gram) and fats and oils (on average, 9 kcal per gram). Although protein (on average, 4 kcal per gram) *can* be used for energy needs, the body typically reserves this nutrient for other processes.

It is likely that you have recently consumed fruits, vegetables, dairy products, cereal, breads, and pasta. These foods supply carbohydrates. Although

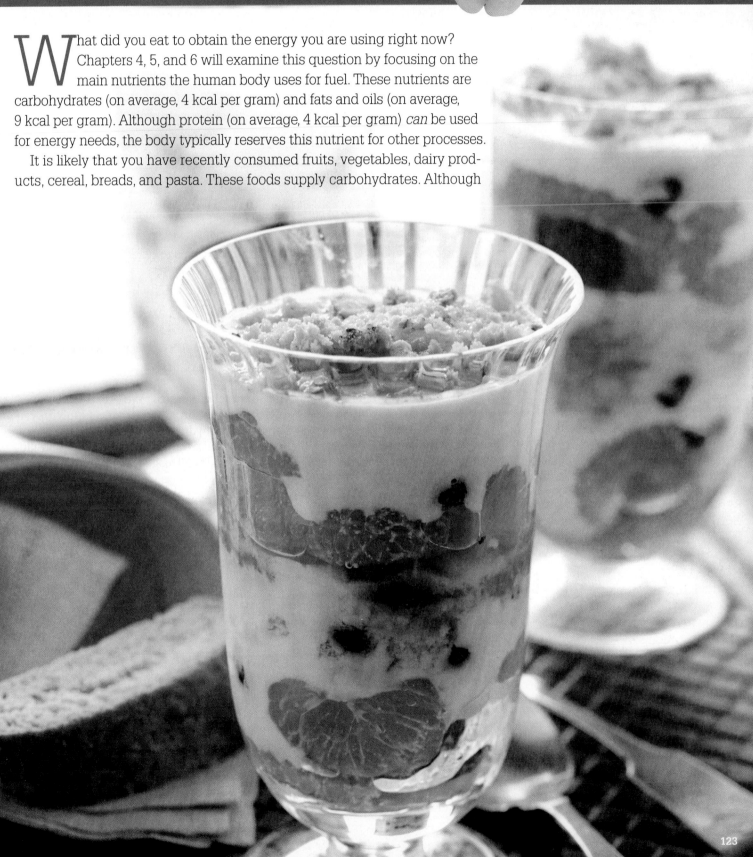

some carbohydrate sources are more beneficial than others (for example, whole-grain bread compared to white bread, as suggested in the Ziggy comic in this chapter), carbohydrates should be a major part of our diets. Many people think carbohydrate-rich foods cause weight gain but they do not any more so than fat or protein. In fact, pound for pound, carbohydrates are much less fattening than fats and oils. Furthermore, high-carbohydrate foods, especially fiber-rich foods such as fruits, vegetables, whole-grain breads and cereals, and legumes, provide many important health benefits in addition to the calories they contain. Almost all carbohydrate-rich foods, except pure sugars, provide several essential nutrients and should generally constitute 45% to 65% of our daily calorie intake. Let's take a closer look at carbohydrates.

Refresh Your Memory

As you begin your study of carbohydrates in Chapter 4, you may want to review:

- The concept of energy density and the health claims for various carbohydrates in Chapter 2
- The processes of digestion and absorption in Chapter 3
- The hormones that regulate blood glucose in Chapter 3

4.1 Carbohydrates—An Introduction

Carbohydrates are a main fuel source for some cells, especially those in the brain, nervous system, and red blood cells. Muscles also rely on a dependable supply of carbohydrates to fuel intense physical activity. Carbohydrates provide on average 4 kcal per gram and are a readily available fuel for all cells, both in the form of blood glucose and **glycogen** stored in the liver and muscles. The glycogen stored in the liver can be used to maintain blood glucose concentrations in times when you have not eaten for several hours or the diet does not supply enough carbohydrates. Regular intake of carbohydrates is important, because liver glycogen stores are depleted in about 18 hours if no carbohydrate is consumed. After that point, the body is forced to produce carbohydrates, largely from breakdown of proteins in the body. This eventually leads

glycogen A carbohydrate made of multiple units of glucose with a highly branched structure. It is the storage form of glucose in humans and is synthesized (and stored) in the liver and muscles.

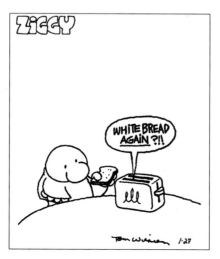

A class of carbohydrate that needs more attention in our diet is fiber. Why is this so? As Ziggy is reminded, white bread is a poor source of fiber. Which health problems typically result from a limited intake of fiber? Which foods are good sources of fiber? How much fiber is enough? Too much? Chapter 4 provides some answers.

to health problems including the loss of muscle tissue. To obtain adequate energy, the Food and Nutrition Board recommends that 45% to 65% of the calories we consume each day be from carbohydrates. (See the Acceptable Macronutrient Distribution Range table in the DRI charts in the back pages of this book.)

Despite their important role as a calorie source, some forms of carbohydrate promote health more than others. As you will see in this chapter, whole-grain breads and cereals have greater health benefits than refined and processed forms of carbohydrate. Choosing the healthiest carbohydrate sources most often, while moderating intake of less healthful sources, contributes to a healthy diet. It is difficult to eat so little carbohydrate that body fuel needs are not met, but it is easy to overconsume the simple carbohydrates that can contribute to health problems. Let's explore this concept further as we look at carbohydrates in detail.

Green plants create the carbohydrates in our foods. Leaves capture the sun's solar energy in their cells and transform it to chemical energy. This energy is then stored in the chemical bonds of the carbohydrate glucose as it is produced from carbon dioxide from the air and water from the soil. This complex process is called **photosynthesis** (Fig. 4-1).

$$\text{6 carbon dioxide} + \text{6 water (solar energy)} \rightarrow \text{glucose} + \text{6 oxygen}$$
$$(CO_2) \qquad\qquad (H_2O) \qquad (C_6H_{12}O_6) \quad (O_2)$$

Translated into English, this reads: 6 molecules of carbon dioxide combine with 6 molecules of water to form one molecule of **glucose**. Converting solar energy into chemical bonds in the sugar is a key part of the process. Six molecules of oxygen are then released into the air.

4.2 Simple Carbohydrates

As the name suggests, most carbohydrate molecules are composed of carbon, hydrogen, and oxygen atoms. Simple forms of carbohydrates are called **sugars**. Larger, more complex forms are primarily called either **starches** or **fibers**, depending on their digestibility by human GI tract enzymes. Starches are the digestible form. The Concept Map on page 127 summarizes the forms and characteristics of carbohydrates.

Monosaccharides and disaccharides are often referred to as *simple sugars* because they contain only one or two sugar units. Food labels lump all of these sugars under one category, listing them as "sugars."

▲ Fruits such as oranges and pears are an excellent source of carbohydrate, including sugar, starch, and fiber.

photosynthesis Process by which plants use energy from the sun to synthesize energy-yielding compounds, such as glucose.

glucose A six-carbon monosaccharide that usually exists in a ring form; found as such in blood, and in table sugar bonded to fructose; also known as *dextrose*.

sugar A simple carbohydrate with the chemical composition $(CH_2O)_n$. The basic unit of all sugars is glucose, a six-carbon ring structure. The primary sugar in the diet is sucrose, which is made up of glucose and fructose.

starch A carbohydrate made of multiple units of glucose attached together in a form the body can digest; also known as *complex carbohydrate*.

fiber Substances in plant foods not digested by the processes that take place in the stomach or small intestine. These add bulk to feces. Fibers naturally found in foods are also called dietary fiber.

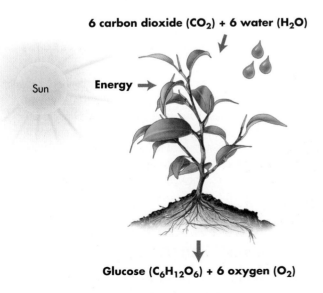

6 carbon dioxide (CO₂) + 6 water (H₂O)

Sun

Energy →

Glucose (C₆H₁₂O₆) + 6 oxygen (O₂)

FIGURE 4-1 ▶ A summary of photosynthesis. Plants use carbon dioxide, water, and energy to produce glucose. Glucose is then stored in the leaf but can also undergo further metabolism to form starch and fiber in the plant. With the addition of nitrogen from soil or air, glucose also can be transformed into protein.

Monosaccharides

FIGURE 4-2 ▶ Chemical forms of the important monosaccharides.

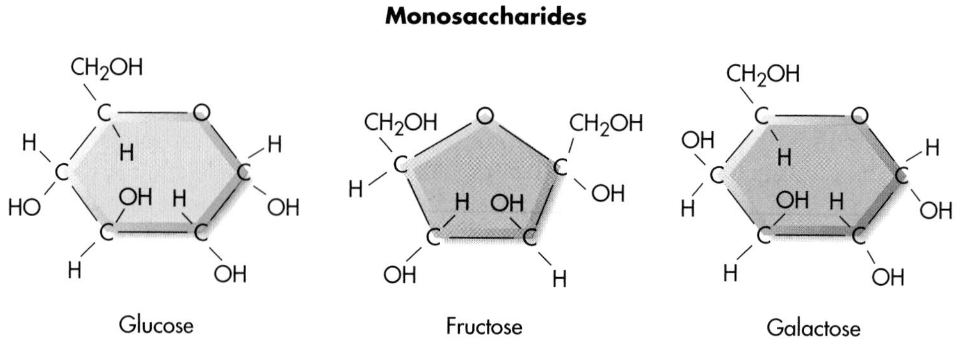

Glucose   Fructose   Galactose

Monosaccharides—Glucose, Fructose, and Galactose

monosaccharide Simple sugar, such as glucose, that is not broken down further during digestion.

simple sugar Monosaccharide or disaccharide in the diet.

sucrose Fructose bonded to glucose; table sugar.

fructose A six-carbon monosaccharide that usually exists in a ring form; found in fruits and honey; also known as *fruit sugar*.

high-fructose corn syrup Corn syrup that has been manufactured to contain 42 and 90% fructose.

galactose A six-carbon monosaccharide that usually exists in a ring form; closely related to glucose.

lactose Glucose bonded to galactose; also known as *milk sugar*.

disaccharide Class of sugars formed by the chemical bonding of two monosaccharides.

maltose Glucose bonded to glucose.

Monosaccharides are the **simple sugar** units (*mono* means one) that serve as the basic unit of all carbohydrate structures. The most common monosaccharides in foods are glucose, fructose, and galactose (Fig. 4-2).

Glucose is the major monosaccharide found in the body. Glucose is also known as *dextrose*, and glucose in the bloodstream may be called blood sugar. Glucose is an important source of energy for human cells, although foods contain very little carbohydrate as this single sugar. Most glucose comes from the digestion of starches and **sucrose** (common table sugar) from our food. The latter is made up of the monosaccharides glucose and fructose. For the most part, sugars and other carbohydrates in foods are eventually converted to glucose in the liver. This glucose then goes on to serve as a source of fuel for cells.

Fructose, also called *fruit sugar*, is another common monosaccharide. After it is consumed, fructose is absorbed by the small intestine and then transported to the liver, where it is quickly metabolized. Much is converted to glucose, but the rest goes on to form other compounds, such as fat, if fructose is consumed in very high amounts. Most of the free fructose in our diets comes from the use of **high-fructose corn syrup** in soft drinks, candies, jams, jellies, and many other fruit products and desserts (see the later discussion on nutritive sweeteners and in What Would You Choose?). Fructose also is found naturally in fruits and forms half of each sucrose molecule.

The sugar **galactose** has nearly the same structure as glucose. Large quantities of pure galactose do not exist in nature. Instead, galactose is usually found bonded to glucose in **lactose**, a sugar found in milk and other milk products. After lactose is digested and absorbed, galactose arrives in the liver. There it is either transformed into glucose or further metabolized into glycogen.

MAKING DECISIONS

Nutrient Metabolism

Now is a good time to begin emphasizing a key concept in nutrition: the difference between *intake* of a substance and the body's *use* of that substance. The body often does not use all nutrients in their original states. Some of these substances are broken down and later reassembled into the same or a different substance when and where they are needed. For example, much of the galactose in the diet is metabolized to glucose. When later required for the production of milk in the mammary gland of a lactating female, galactose is resynthesized from glucose to help form the milk sugar lactose. Knowing this, do you think it is necessary for a lactating women to drink milk to make milk?

Disaccharides—Sucrose, Lactose, and Maltose

Disaccharides are formed when two monosaccharides combine (*di* means two). The disaccharides in food are sucrose, lactose, and **maltose**. All contain glucose.

Disaccharides

Sucrose: glucose + fructose
Lactose: glucose + galactose
Maltose: glucose + glucose

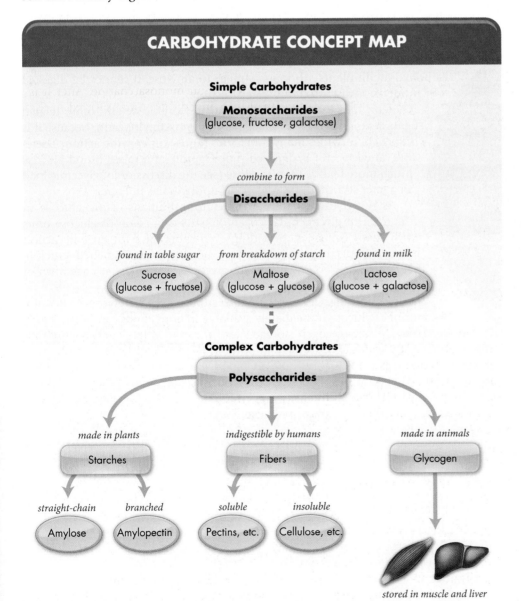

Sucrose

FIGURE 4-3 ▶ Chemical form of the disaccharide sucrose.

Sucrose forms when the two sugars glucose and fructose bond together (Fig. 4-3). Sucrose is found naturally in sugarcane, sugar beets, honey, and maple sugar. These products are processed to varying degrees to make brown, white, and powdered sugars. Animals do not produce sucrose or much of any carbohydrate except glycogen.

Lactose forms when glucose bonds with galactose during the synthesis of milk. Again, our major food source for lactose is milk products. A later section on lactose maldigestion and lactose intolerance discusses the problems that result when a person can't readily digest lactose.

◀ This Concept Map summarizes the various forms and characteristics of the simple and complex carbohydrates.

CARBOHYDRATE CONCEPT MAP

Simple Carbohydrates

Monosaccharides
(glucose, fructose, galactose)

combine to form

Disaccharides

found in table sugar
Sucrose
(glucose + fructose)

from breakdown of starch
Maltose
(glucose + glucose)

found in milk
Lactose
(glucose + galactose)

Complex Carbohydrates

Polysaccharides

made in plants
Starches

indigestible by humans
Fibers

made in animals
Glycogen

straight-chain
Amylose

branched
Amylopectin

soluble
Pectins, etc.

insoluble
Cellulose, etc.

stored in muscle and liver

Maltose results when starch is broken down to just two glucose molecules bonded together. Maltose plays an important role in the beer and liquor industry. In the production of alcoholic beverages, starches in various cereal grains are first converted to simpler carbohydrates by enzymes present in the grains. The products of this step—maltose, glucose, and other sugars—are then mixed with yeast cells in the absence of oxygen. The yeast cells convert most of the sugars to alcohol (ethanol) and carbon dioxide, a process called **fermentation**. Little maltose remains in the final product. Few other food products or beverages contain maltose. In fact, most maltose that we ultimately digest in the small intestine is produced during our own digestion of starch.

4.3 Complex Carbohydrates

In many foods, single-sugar units are bonded together to form a chain, known as a polysaccharide (*poly* means many). **Polysaccharides**, also called *complex carbohydrates* or *starch*, may contain 1000 or more glucose units and are found chiefly in grains, vegetables, and fruits. When food labels list "Other Carbohydrates," this primarily refers to starch content.

Plants store carbohydrate in two forms of starch digestible by humans: **amylose** and **amylopectin**. Amylose, a long, straight chain of glucose units, comprises about 20% of the digestible starch found in vegetables, beans, breads, pasta, and rice. Amylopectin is a highly branched chain and makes up the remaining 80% of digestible starches in the diet (Fig. 4-4). Cellulose (a fiber) is another complex carbohydrate in plants. Although similar to amylose, it cannot be digested by humans, as discussed in the next section.

The enzymes that break down starches to glucose and other related sugars act only at the end of a glucose chain. Amylopectin, because it is branched, provides many more sites (ends) for enzyme action. Therefore, amylopectin is digested more rapidly and raises blood glucose much more readily than amylose (see the discussion of glycemic load in a later section of Chapter 4, "Carbohydrates in Foods").

As noted earlier, animals—including humans—store glucose in the form of glycogen. Glycogen consists of a chain of glucose units with many branches, providing even more sites for enzyme action than amylopectin (review Fig. 4-4). Because of its branched structure that can be broken down quickly, glycogen is an ideal storage form of carbohydrate in the body.

The liver and muscles are the major storage sites for glycogen. Because the amount of glucose immediately available in body fluids can provide only about 120 kcal, these glycogen storage sites for carbohydrate energy—amounting to about 1800 kcal—are extremely important. Of this 1800 kcal, liver glycogen (about 400 kcal) can readily contribute to blood glucose. Muscle glycogen stores (about 1400 kcal) cannot raise blood glucose, but instead supply glucose for muscle use, especially during high-intensity and endurance exercise (see Chapter 10 for a detailed discussion of carbohydrate use in exercise).

fermentation The conversion of carbohydrates to alcohols, acids, and carbon dioxide without the use of oxygen.

polysaccharides Carbohydrates containing many glucose units, from 10 to 1000 or more.

amylose A digestible straight-chain type of starch composed of glucose units.

amylopectin A digestible branched-chain type of starch composed of glucose units.

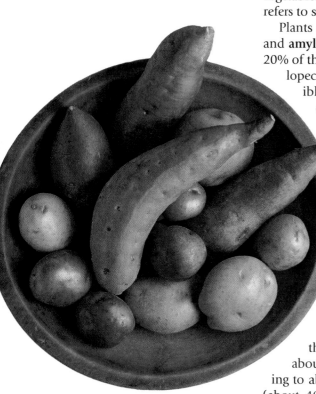

▲ Root vegetables such as potato, yams, and tapioca are high in amylopectin starch.

MAKING DECISIONS

Animal Sources of Carbohydrates

If animals store glycogen in their muscles, are meats, fish, and poultry a good source of carbohydrates? No—animal products are not good food sources of this (or any other) carbohydrate because glycogen stores quickly degrade after the animal dies.

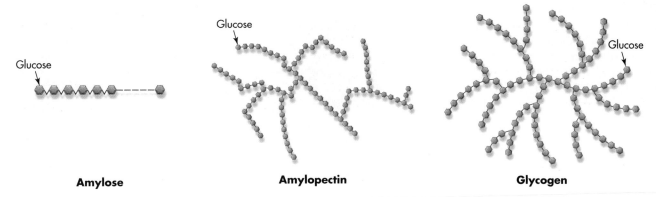

Glucose

Glucose

Glucose

Amylose

Amylopectin

Glycogen

FIGURE 4-4 ▶ Some common starches, amylose and amylopectin, and glycogen. We consume essentially no glycogen. All glycogen found in the body is made by our cells, primarily in the liver and muscles.

4.4 Fiber

Fiber as a class is mostly made up of polysaccharides, but they differ from starches insofar as the chemical links that join the individual sugar units cannot be digested by human enzymes in the GI tract. This prevents the small intestine from absorbing the sugars that make up the various fibers. Fiber is not a single substance but a group of substances with similar characteristics (Table 4-1). The group is comprised of the carbohydrates **cellulose**, **hemicelluloses**, **pectins**, **gums**, and **mucilages**, as well as the noncarbohydrate, **lignin**. In total, these constitute all the nonstarch polysaccharides in foods. Nutrition Facts labels generally do not list these individual forms of fiber, but instead lump them together under the term **dietary fiber**.

Cellulose, hemicelluloses, and lignin form the structural parts of plants. Bran fiber is rich in hemicelluloses and lignin. (The woody fibers in broccoli are partly lignin.) Bran layers form the outer covering of all grains, so **whole grains** (i.e., unrefined) are good sources of bran fiber (Fig. 4-5). Because the majority of these fibers neither readily dissolve in water nor are easily metabolized by intestinal bacteria, they are called **nonfermentable** or insoluble fibers.

Pectins, gums, and mucilages are contained around and inside plant cells. These fibers either dissolve or swell when put into water and are therefore called **viscous** or soluble fibers. They also are readily fermented by bacteria in the large intestine. These fibers are found in salad dressings, some frozen desserts, jams, and jellies as gum arabic, guar gum, locust bean gum, and various pectin forms. Some forms of hemicelluloses also fall into the soluble category.

Most foods contain mixtures of soluble and insoluble fibers. Food labels do not generally distinguish between the two types, but, manufacturers have the option to do so. Often, if food is listed as a good source of one type of fiber, it usually contains some

cellulose An undigestible nonfermentable straight-chain polysaccharide made of glucose molecules.

hemicellulose A nonfermentable fiber containing xylose, galactose, glucose, and other monosaccharides bonded together.

pectin A viscous fiber containing chains of galacturonic acid and other monosaccharides; characteristically found between plant cell walls.

mucilages A viscous fiber consisting of chains of galactose, mannose, and other monosaccharides; characteristically found in seaweed.

lignins A nonfermentable fiber made up of a multiringed alcohol (noncarbohydrate) structure.

dietary fiber Fiber found in food.

whole grains Grains containing the entire seed of the plant, including the bran, germ, and endosperm (starchy interior). Examples are whole wheat and brown rice.

nonfermentable fiber A fiber that is not easily metabolized by intestinal bacteria.

TABLE 4-1 Classification of Fibers

Type	Component(s)	Physiological Effects	Major Food Sources
Nonfermentable or Insoluble			
Noncarbohydrate form	Lignin	Increases fecal bulk	Whole grains, wheat bran
Carbohydrate form	Cellulose, hemicelluloses	Increases fecal bulk Decreases intestinal transit time	All plants, wheat products Wheat, rye, rice, vegetables
Viscous or Soluble			
Carbohydrate form	Pectins, gums, mucilages, some hemicelluloses	Delays stomach emptying; slows glucose absorption; can lower blood cholesterol	Citrus fruits, apples, bananas, oat products, carrots, barley, beans, thickeners added to foods

FIGURE 4-5 ▶ Viscous and nonfermentable fiber. (a) The skin of an apple consists of the nonfermentable fiber cellulose, which provides structure for the fruit. The viscous fiber pectin "glues" the fruit cells together. (b) The outside layer of a wheat kernel is made of layers of bran—primarily hemicellulose, a nonfermentable fiber—making this whole grain a good source of fiber. Overall, fruits, vegetables, whole-grain breads and cereals, and beans are rich in fiber.

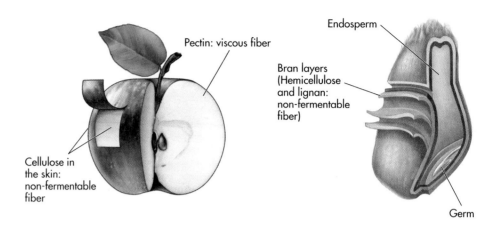

Pectin: viscous fiber

Endosperm

Bran layers (Hemicellulose and lignan: non-fermentable fiber)

Cellulose in the skin: non-fermentable fiber

Germ

viscous fiber A fiber that is readily fermented by bacteria in the large intestine.

functional fiber Fiber added to foods that has been shown to provide health benefits.

total fiber Combination of dietary fiber and functional fiber in a food. Also just called *fiber*.

of the other type of fiber as well. The definition of fiber has recently been expanded to include both the dietary fiber found naturally in foods and additional fiber that is added to foods. This second category is called **functional fiber;** a fiber of this type must show beneficial effects in humans to be included in the category. **Total fiber** (or just the term *fiber*) is then the combination of dietary fiber and functional fiber in the food product. Currently the Nutrition Facts label only includes the category dietary fiber; the label has yet to be updated to reflect the latest definition of fiber.

A newly studied category of functional fiber are the prebiotics. Prebiotics include a group of short-chain carbohydrates or oligosaccharides, resistant to digestion, but fermented by bacteria in the colon. They are thought to stimulate the growth or activity of beneficial bacteria in the large intestine and therefore promote the host's health.

CONCEPT CHECK

Important monosaccharides in nutrition are glucose, fructose, and galactose. Glucose is a primary energy source for body cells. Disaccharides form when two monosaccharides bond together. Important disaccharides in nutrition are sucrose (glucose + fructose), maltose (glucose + glucose), and lactose (glucose + galactose). Once digested into monosaccharides and absorbed, most carbohydrates are transformed into glucose by the liver.

Amylose, amylopectin, and glycogen are all polysaccharides, which function as storage forms of glucose. Amylose and amylopectin are the major digestible plant polysaccharides and contain multiple glucose units bonded together. Glycogen is a storage form of glucose in our liver and muscle cells.

Fiber is essentially the portion of plant food that remains undigested as it enters the large intestine. There are two general classes of fiber: nonfermentable and viscous. Nonfermentable (insoluble) fibers are mostly made up of cellulose, hemicelluloses, and lignins. Viscous (soluble) fibers are made up mostly of pectins, gums, and mucilages. Both nonfermentable and viscous fibers are resistant to human digestive enzymes, but bacteria in the large intestine can break down viscous fibers.

4.5 Carbohydrates in Foods

The food components that yield the highest percentage of calories from carbohydrates are table sugar, honey, jam, jelly, fruit, and plain baked potatoes (Fig. 4-6). Corn flakes, rice, bread, and noodles all contain at least 75% of calories as carbohydrates. Foods with moderate amounts of carbohydrate calories are peas, broccoli, oatmeal, dry beans and other legumes, cream pies, French fries, and fat-free milk. In these foods, the carbohydrate content is diluted either by protein, as in the case of fat-free milk, or by fat, as in the case of a cream pie. Foods with essentially no carbohydrates include beef, eggs, chicken, fish, vegetable oils, butter, and margarine.

Food Sources of Carbohydrate

FIGURE 4-6 ▶ Food sources of carbohydrates compared to the RDA of 130 grams for carbohydrate.

Food Item	Carbohydrate (grams)	% RDA
RDA	130	100%
Baked potato, 1 each	51	39%
Cola drink, 12 fluid oz	39	30%
Plain M&M's, ½ oz	30	23%
Banana, 1 each	28	22%
Cooked rice, ½ cup	22	17%
Cooked corn, ½ cup	21	16%
Light yogurt, 1 cup	19	15%
Kidney beans, ½ cup	19	15%
Spaghetti noodles, ½ cup	19	15%
Orange, 1 each	16	12%
Seven grain bread, 1 slice	12	9%
Fat-free milk, 1 cup	12	9%
Pineapple chunks, ½ cup	10	8%
Cooked carrots, ½ cup	8	6%
Peanuts, 1 ounce	6	5%

Key:
- ■ Grains
- ■ Vegetables
- ■ Fruits
- ■ Dairy
- ■ Protein
- ■ Empty calories
- ■ Oils

ChooseMyPlate.gov

The percentage of calories from carbohydrate is more important than the total amount of carbohydrate in a food when planning a healthy high-carbohydrate diet. Figure 4-7 shows that the grain, vegetable, fruit, and dairy groups contain the most nutrient-dense sources of carbohydrate. In planning a healthy high-carbohydrate diet, you need to emphasize whole grains, fruits, and vegetables, rather than potato chips and French fries, because these foods contain too much fat. Currently, the top five carbohydrate sources for U.S. adults are white bread, soft drinks, cookies and cakes (including doughnuts), sugars/syrups/jams, and potatoes. Clearly, many North Americans (teenagers included) should take a closer look at their main carbohydrate sources and strive to improve them from a nutritional standpoint by including more whole-grain versions of breads, pasta, rice, and cereals, as well as fruits and vegetables.

Starch

Starches contribute much of the carbohydrate in our diets. Recall that plants store glucose as polysaccharides in the form of starches. Thus, plant-based foods, such as beans, potatoes, and the grains (wheat, rye, corn, oats, barley, and rice) used to make breads, cereals, and pasta, are the best sources of starch. A diet rich in these starches provides ample carbohydrate, as well as many micronutrients.

Fiber

Fiber can be found in many of the same foods as starch, so a diet rich in grains, beans, and potatoes also can provide significant amounts of dietary fiber (especially insoluble cellulose, hemicellulose, and lignins). Because much of the fiber in whole grains

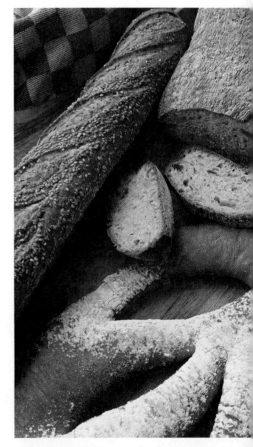

▲ Breads are a rich source of carbohydrate, especially starch and fiber.

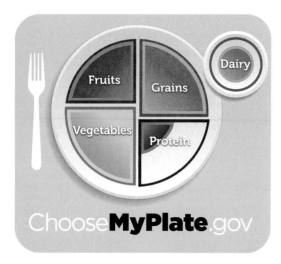

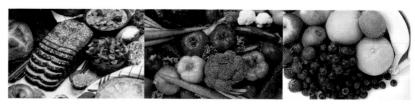

MyPlate:
Sources of Carbohydrates

Grains	Vegetables	Fruits	Dairy	Protein
• All varieties	• All varieties	• All varieties	• Milk • Yogurt	• Beans • Nuts
15 grams per serving	5 grams per serving	18 grams per serving	12 grams per serving	4-10 grams per serving

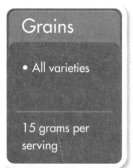 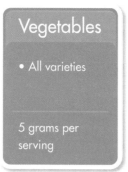 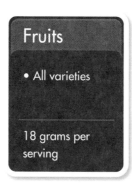 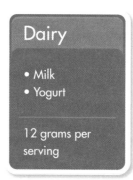 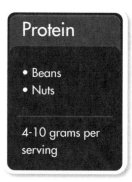

FIGURE 4-7 ▶ Sources of carbohydrates from MyPlate. The fill of the background color (none, 1/3, 2/3, or completely covered) within each group in the plate indicates the average nutrient density for carbohydrate in that group. Overall, the grain group, vegetable group, fruit group, and dairy group contain many foods that are nutrient-dense sources of carbohydrate. With regard to physical activity, carbohydrates are a key fuel in most endeavors.

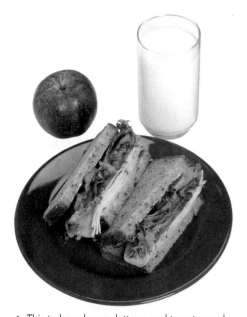

▲ This turkey, cheese, lettuce, and tomato sandwich on whole-grain bread with an apple and glass of low-fat milk fits on **MyPlate** in the right proportions and offers excellent carbohydrate sources of fruits, vegetables, whole grains, and low-fat dairy.

is found in the outer layers, which are removed in processing, highly processed grains are low in fiber. Soluble fibers (pectin, gums, mucilages) are found in the skins and flesh of many fruits and berries; as thickeners and stabilizers in jams, yogurts, sauces, and fillings; and in products that contain psyllium and seaweed.

For individuals who have difficulties consuming adequate dietary fiber, fiber is available as a supplement or as an additive to certain foods (functional fiber). In this way, individuals with relatively low dietary fiber intakes can still obtain the health benefits of fiber.

Nutritive Sweeteners

The various substances that impart sweetness to foods fall into two broad classes: nutritive sweeteners, which can provide calories for the body; and alternative sweeteners, which for the most part provide no calories. As shown in Table 4-2, the alternative sweeteners are much sweeter on a per-gram basis than the nutritive sweeteners. The taste and sweetness of sucrose make it the benchmark against which all other sweeteners are measured. Sucrose is obtained from sugar cane and sugar beet plants. Both sugars and sugar alcohols provide calories along with sweetness. Sugars are found in many different food products, whereas sugar alcohols have rather limited uses.

Sugars. All of the monosaccharides (glucose, fructose, and galactose) and disaccharides (sucrose, lactose, and maltose) discussed earlier are designated *nutritive sweeteners* (Table 4-3). Many forms of sugar are used in food products and result in an intake of about 82 grams or 16 teaspoons of sugar per day.

TABLE 4-2 The Sweetness of Sugars (Nutritive) and Alternative Sweeteners

Type of Sweetener	Relative Sweetness* (Sucrose = 1)	Typical Sources
Sugars		
Lactose	0.2	Dairy products
Maltose	0.4	Sprouted seeds
Glucose	0.7	Corn syrup
Sucrose	1.0	Table sugar, most sweets
Invert sugar[†]	1.3	Some candies, honey
Fructose	1.2–1.8	Fruit, honey, some soft drinks
Sugar Alcohols		
Sorbitol	0.6	Dietetic candies, sugarless gum
Mannitol	0.7	Dietetic candies
Xylitol	0.9	Sugarless gum
Maltitol	0.9	Baked goods, chocolate, candies
Alternative Sweeteners		
Tagatose (Naturlose™)	0.9	Ready-to-eat breakfast cereals, diet soft drinks, meal replacement bars, frozen desserts, candy, frosting
Cyclamate[‡]	30	Tabletop sweetener, medicines
Stevia (Truvia®)	100–300	Tabletop sweetener, food ingredient
Aspartame (Equal®)	180	Diet soft drinks, diet fruit drinks, sugarless gum, tabletop sweetener
Acesulfame-K (Sunette®)	200	Sugarless gum, diet drink mixes, tabletop sweetener, puddings, gelatin desserts
Saccharin (Sweet'N Low®)	300	Diet soft drinks, tabletop sweetener
Sucralose (Splenda®)	600	Diet soft drinks, tabletop sweetener, sugarless gums, jams, frozen desserts
Neotame	7000 to 13,000	Tabletop sweetener, baked goods, frozen desserts, jams

*On a per gram basis.

[†]Sucrose broken down into glucose and fructose.

[‡]Not available in the United States, but available in Canada.

From the *American Dietetic Association*, 2004, and other sources (see Further Reading 1).

High-fructose corn syrup (HFCS) is made by an enzymatic process that converts some of the glucose in cornstarch into fructose, which tastes sweeter than glucose. It is called "high-fructose" corn syrup because it contains 55% fructose, compared to sucrose, which contains only 50% fructose. In the United States, corn is abundant and inexpensive compared to sugar cane or sugar beets, much of which is imported. Food manufacturers prefer HFCS because it is easy to transport, has better shelf-stability, and improves food properties. Because of its low cost and broad range of food-processing applications, HFCS is now used in all kinds of foods, from soft drinks to barbecue sauce. An average American consumes about 60 pounds of HFCS each year. The dramatic rise in obesity has paralleled the increase in HFCS consumption over the past 40 years, and some researchers speculate that properties of the HFCS are to blame. Read more about this in the Newsworthy Nutrition column in the margin and in our recommendations for What Would You Choose?

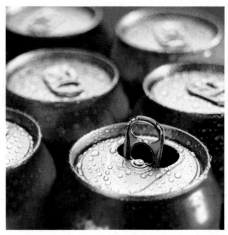

▲ Soft drinks are typical sources of either sugars or alternative sweeteners, depending on the type of soft drink chosen.

NEWSWORTHY NUTRITION

Link between high-fructose corn syrup and obesity

The intake of high-fructose corn syrup (HFCS) from 1967 to 2000 was studied and compared to the development of obesity. HFCS consumption increased >1000% between 1970 and 1990. It was estimated that Americans consume 132 to 316 kcal daily from HFCS. The increase in HFCS use has paralleled the increase in obesity. Differences in the digestion, absorption, and metabolism of fructose compared to glucose have been suggested as explanations for the relationship between HFCS and obesity. Studies of HFCS in humans, however, have been unable to separate the effects of the widely consumed sweetener from the impact of physical inactivity, large portion sizes, smoking cessation, increased consumption of foods prepared outside the home, and other environmental factors.

Source: Bray GA and others. Consumption of high-fructose corn syrup in beverages may play a role in the epidemic of obesity. *American Journal of Clinical Nutrition*, 79(4):537, 2004 (see Further Reading 4).

connect NUTRITION **Check out the Connect site** www.mcgrawhillconnect.com **to further explore HFCS and obesity.**

TABLE 4-3 Names of Sugars Used in Foods

Sugar	Invert sugar	Honey	Maple syrup
Sucrose	Glucose	Corn syrup or sweeteners	Dextrose
Brown sugar	Sorbitol		Fructose
		High-fructose corn syrup	
Confectioner's sugar (powdered sugar)	Levulose		Maltodextrins
	Polydextrose	Molasses	Caramel
Turbinado sugar	Lactose	Date sugar	Fruit sugar

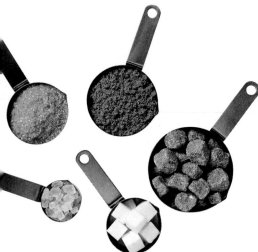

▲ There are many forms of sugar on the market. Used in many foods, together they contribute to our daily intake of approximately 82 grams (16 teaspoons) of sugars in our diets.

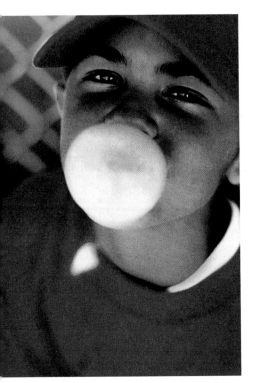

▲ Sugarless gum is typically sweetened with sugar alcohols.

sorbitol Alcohol derivative of glucose that yields about 3 kcal/g but is slowly absorbed from the small intestine; used in some sugarless gums and dietetic foods.

xylitol Alcohol derivative of the 5-carbon monosaccharide xylose.

In addition to sucrose and high-fructose corn syrup, brown sugar, turbinado sugar (sold as raw sugar), honey, maple syrup, and other sugars are also added to foods. Brown sugar is essentially sucrose containing some molasses that is not totally removed from the sucrose during processing or is added to the sucrose crystals. Turbinado sugar is a partially refined version of raw sucrose. Maple syrup is made by boiling down and concentrating the sap that runs during the late winter in sugar maple trees. Because pure maple syrup is expensive, most pancake syrup is primarily corn syrup and high-fructose corn syrup with maple flavor added.

Honey is a product of plant nectar that has been altered by bee enzymes. The enzymes break down much of the nectar's sucrose into fructose and glucose. Honey offers essentially the same nutritional value as other simple sugars—a source of energy and little else. However, honey is not safe to feed to infants because it can contain spores of the bacterium *Clostridium botulinum* that causes fatal food-borne illness. Unlike the acidic environment of an adult's stomach, which inhibits the growth of the bacteria, an infant's stomach does not produce much acid, making infants susceptible to the threat that this bacterium poses.

Sugar Alcohols. Food manufacturers and consumers have numerous options for obtaining sweetness while consuming less sugar and calories. Overall, sugar alcohols and alternative sweeteners enable people with diabetes to enjoy the flavor of sweetness while controlling sugars in their diets; they also provide noncaloric or very-low-calorie sugar substitutes for persons trying to lose (or control) body weight.

Sugar alcohols such as **sorbitol** and **xylitol** are used as nutritive sweeteners. Sugar alcohols contribute fewer calories (about 2.6 kcal per gram) than sugars. They also are absorbed and metabolized to glucose more slowly than are simple sugars. Because of this, they remain in the intestinal tract for a longer time and in large quantities can cause diarrhea. In fact, any products that may be consumed in amounts that may result in a daily ingestion of 50 grams of sugar alcohols, must bear this labeling statement: "Excess consumption may have a laxative effect."

Sugar alcohols are used in sugarless gum, breath mints, and candy. Unlike sucrose, sugar alcohols are not readily metabolized by bacteria to acids in the mouth and thus do not promote tooth decay (see the later section on problems linked to carbohydrate intake).

Sugar alcohols must be listed on labels. If only one sugar alcohol is used in a product, its name must be listed. However, if two or more are used in one product, they are grouped together under the heading "sugar alcohols." The caloric value of each sugar alcohol used in a food product is calculated so that when one reads the total amount of calories a product provides, it includes the sugar alcohols in the overall amount.

Alternative Sweeteners

Alternative sweeteners in increasing order of sweetness include **tagatose**, **cyclamate**, **stevia**, **aspartame**, **acesulfame-K**, **saccharin**, **sucralose**,and **neotame**. Unlike sugar alcohols, alternative sweeteners yield little or no calories when consumed in amounts typically used in food products. All except cyclamate are currently available in the United States. Cyclamate was banned for use in the United States in 1970, although it has never been conclusively proven to cause health problems when used appropriately. Cyclamate is used in Canada as a sweetener in medicines and as a tabletop sweetener.

The safety of sweeteners is determined by the FDA and is indicated by an **Acceptable Daily Intake (ADI)** guideline. The ADI is the amount of alternative sweetener considered safe for daily use over one's lifetime. ADIs are based on studies in laboratory animals and are set at a level 100 times less than the level at which no harmful effects were noted in animal studies. Alternative sweeteners can be used safely by adults and children. Although general use is considered safe during pregnancy, pregnant women may want to discuss this issue with their health-care providers.

Saccharin. The oldest alternative sweetener, saccharin, was first produced in 1879 and is currently approved for use in more than 90 countries. It represents about half of the alternative sweetener market in North America (typically packaged in pink packets, including Sweet 'N Low®). Based on laboratory animal studies, saccharin was once thought to increase the risk of bladder cancer but it is no longer listed as a potential cause of cancer.

Aspartame. Aspartame is in widespread use throughout the world (typically packaged in blue packets, including Equal®). It has been approved for use by more than 90 countries, and its use has been endorsed by the World Health Organization, the American Medical Association, the American Diabetes Association, and other groups.

The components of aspartame are the amino acids phenylalanine and aspartic acid, along with methanol. Recall that amino acids are the building blocks of proteins, so aspartame is more of a protein than a carbohydrate. Aspartame yields about 4 kcal per gram, but it is about 200 times sweeter than sucrose. Thus, only a small amount of aspartame is needed to obtain the desired sweetness, and the amount of calories added is insignificant unless the product is consumed in unusually high amounts. Aspartame is used in beverages, gelatin desserts, chewing gum, toppings and fillings in precooked bakery goods, and cookies. Aspartame does not cause tooth decay. Like other proteins, however, aspartame is damaged when heated for a long time and thus would lose its sweetness if used in products requiring cooking.

Some complaints have been filed with FDA by people claiming to have had adverse reactions to aspartame: headaches, dizziness, seizures, nausea, and other side effects. It is important for people who are sensitive to aspartame to avoid it, but the percentage of sensitive people is likely to be extremely small.

The acceptable daily intake of aspartame set by FDA is 50 milligrams per kilogram of body weight. This is equivalent to the aspartame in about 14 cans of diet soft drink for an adult or about 80 packets of Equal®. Aspartame appears to be safe for pregnant women and children, but some scientists suggest cautious use by these groups, especially young children, who need ample calories to grow.

Sucralose. Sucralose (Splenda®) is 600 times sweeter than sucrose. It is made by adding three chlorines to sucrose. Sucralose is approved for use as an additive to foods such as soft drinks, gum, baked goods, syrups, gelatins, frozen dairy desserts such as ice cream, jams, processed fruits and fruit juices, and for tabletop use. Sucralose doesn't break down under high heat conditions and can be used in cooking and baking. It is also excreted as such in the feces. The small amount absorbed is excreted in the urine.

Sugar alcohols as a class are also called polyols.

stevia Alternative sweetener derived from South American shrub; 100 to 300 times sweeter than sucrose.

aspartame Alternative sweetener made of 2 amino acids and methanol; about 200 times sweeter than sucrose.

sucralose Alternative sweetener that has chlorines in place of 3 hydroxyl (—OH) groups on sucrose; 600 times sweeter than sucrose.

acesulfame K Alternative sweetener that yields no energy to the body; 200 times sweeter than sucrose.

saccharin Alternative sweetener that yields no energy to the body; 300 times sweeter than sucrose.

neotame General-purpose, nonnutritive sweetener that is approximately 7000 to 13,000 times sweeter than table sugar. It has a chemical structure similar to aspartame's.

Persons with an uncommon disease called **phenylketonuria (PKU)**, which interferes with the metabolism of phenylalanine, should avoid aspartame because of its high phenylalanine content. A warning label is required on products containing aspartame, alerting people with PKU that a product with aspartame contains phenylalanine.

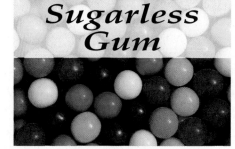

INGREDIENTS: SORBITOL, GUM BASE, MANNITOL, GLYCEROL, HYDROGENATED GLUCOSE SYRUP, XYLITOL, ARTIFICIAL AND NATURAL FLAVORS, ASPARTAME, RED 40, YELLOW 6 AND BHT (TO MAINTAIN FRESHNESS). PHENYLKETONURICS: CONTAINS PHENYLALANINE.

Sugarless Gum

▲ Sugar alcohols and the alternative sweetener aspartame are used to sweeten this product. Note the warning for people with phenylketonuria PKU that this product is made with aspartame and, thus, contains phenylalanine.

Acceptable Daily Intake (ADI) Estimate of the amount of a sweetener that an individual can safely consume daily over a lifetime. ADIs are given as mg per kg of body weight per day.

phenylketonuria (PKU) Disease caused by a defect in the liver's ability to metabolize the amino acid phenylalanine into the amino acid tyrosine; untreated, toxic by-products of phenylalanine build up in the body and lead to mental retardation.

Neotame. Neotame was recently approved by FDA for use as a general-purpose sweetener in a wide variety of food products, other than meat and poultry. Neotame is a nonnutritive, high-intensity sweetener that, depending on its food application, is approximately 7000 to 13,000 times sweeter than table sugar. It has a chemical structure similar to aspartame. Neotame is heat stable and can be used as a tabletop sweetener as well as in cooking applications. Examples of uses for which it has been approved include baked goods, nonalcoholic beverages (including soft drinks), chewing gum, confections and frostings, frozen desserts, gelatins and puddings, jams and jellies, processed fruits and fruit juices, toppings, and syrups. Neotame is safe for use by the general population, including children, pregnant and lactating women, and people with diabetes. In addition, no special labeling for people with phenylketonuria is needed because neotame is not broken down in the body to its amino acid components.

Acesulfame-K. The alternative sweetener acesulfame-K (the *K* stands for potassium; Sunette®) was approved by the FDA in July 1988. It is approved for use in more than 40 countries and has been in use in Europe since 1983. Acesulfame-K is 200 times sweeter than sucrose. It contributes no calories to the diet because it is not digested by the body, and it does not cause dental caries.

Unlike aspartame, acesulfame-K can be used in baking because it does not lose its sweetness when heated. In the United States, it is currently approved for use in chewing gum, powdered drink mixes, gelatins, puddings, baked goods, tabletop sweeteners, candy, throat lozenges, yogurt, and nondairy creamers; additional uses may soon be approved. One recent trend is to combine it with aspartame in soft drinks.

Tagatose. Tagatose, sold as Naturlose,® is a slightly altered form of the simple sugar fructose. It is approved for use in ready-to-eat breakfast cereals, diet soft drinks, meal replacement bars, frozen desserts, candy, frosting, and chewing gum. Tagatose is poorly absorbed, so it yields only 1.5 kcal per gram to the body. Use also does not raise the risk for dental caries, nor does it increase blood glucose. Eventual fermentation in the large intestine may even lead to a beneficial effect on that organ (i.e., a prebiotic effect, covered in Chapter 3).

Stevia. Stevia, sold as the dietary supplement Sweet Leaf®, is an alternative sweetener derived from a South American shrub. Stevia extracts are 100 to 300 times sweeter than sucrose but provide no energy. It has been used in teas and as a sweetener in Japan since the 1970s, and the FDA recently (December 2008) stated that stevia is considered generally recognized as safe (GRAS) for use in foods. Stevia can be purchased as a dietary supplement in natural and health food stores and as an alternative sweetener in grocery stores.

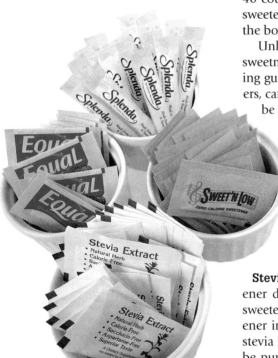

▲ A variety of alternative sweeteners are available.

CONCEPT CHECK

Table sugar, honey, jam, fruit, and plain baked potatoes contain the highest percentage of calories from carbohydrates. Foods such as cream pies, potato chips, whole milk, and oatmeal contain moderate amounts of carbohydrate. Common nutritive sweeteners added to foods include sucrose, maple sugar, honey, brown sugar, and high-fructose corn syrup. For people who want to limit calories from sugar intake, other sweeteners are available and include the sugar alcohols, saccharin, aspartame, sucralose, neotame, acesulfame-K, tagatose, and stevia. Of these, aspartame is the most common alternative sweetener in use.

4.6 Making Carbohydrates Available for Body Use

As discussed in Chapter 3, simply eating a food does not supply nutrients to body cells. Digestion and absorption must occur first.

Digestion

Food preparation can be viewed as the start of carbohydrate digestion because cooking softens tough connective structures in the fibrous parts of plants, such as broccoli stalks. When starches are heated, the starch granules swell as they soak up water, making them much easier to digest. All of these effects of cooking generally make carbohydrate-containing foods easier to chew, swallow, and break down during digestion.

The enzymatic digestion of starch begins in the mouth, when the saliva, which contains an enzyme called salivary **amylase**, mixes with the starchy products during the chewing of the food. This amylase breaks down starch into many smaller units, primarily disaccharides, such as maltose (Fig. 4-8). You can taste this conversion while chewing a saltine cracker. Prolonged chewing of the cracker causes it to taste sweeter as some starch breaks down into the sweeter disaccharides, such as maltose. Still, food is in the mouth for such a short amount of time that this phase of digestion is negligible. In addition, once the food moves down the esophagus and reaches the stomach, the acidic environment inactivates salivary amylase.

amylase Starch-digesting enzyme from the salivary glands or pancreas.

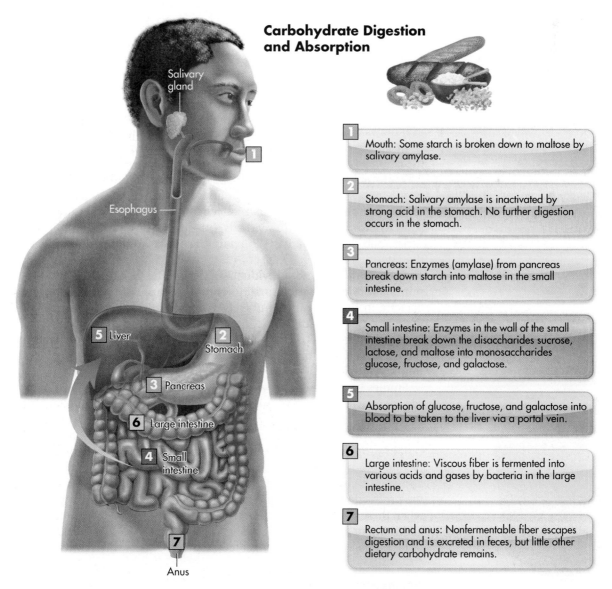

Carbohydrate Digestion and Absorption

1 Mouth: Some starch is broken down to maltose by salivary amylase.

2 Stomach: Salivary amylase is inactivated by strong acid in the stomach. No further digestion occurs in the stomach.

3 Pancreas: Enzymes (amylase) from pancreas break down starch into maltose in the small intestine.

4 Small intestine: Enzymes in the wall of the small intestine break down the disaccharides sucrose, lactose, and maltose into monosaccharides glucose, fructose, and galactose.

5 Absorption of glucose, fructose, and galactose into blood to be taken to the liver via a portal vein.

6 Large intestine: Viscous fiber is fermented into various acids and gases by bacteria in the large intestine.

7 Rectum and anus: Nonfermentable fiber escapes digestion and is excreted in feces, but little other dietary carbohydrate remains.

FIGURE 4-8 ▶ Carbohydrate digestion and absorption. Enzymes made by the mouth, pancreas, and small intestine participate in the process of digestion. Most carbohydrate digestion and absorption take place in the small intestine. Chapter 3 covered the physiology of digestion and absorption in detail.

maltase An enzyme made by absorptive cells of the small intestine; this enzyme digests maltose to two glucoses.

sucrase An enzyme made by absorptive cells of the small intestine; this enzyme digests sucrose to glucose and fructose.

lactase An enzyme made by absorptive cells of the small intestine; this enzyme digests lactose to glucose and galactose.

lactose maldigestion (primary and secondary) Primary lactose maldigestion occurs when production of the enzyme lactase declines for no apparent reason. Secondary lactose maldigestion occurs when a specific cause, such as long-standing diarrhea, results in a decline in lactase production. When significant symptoms develop after lactose intake, it is then called lactose intolerance.

lactose intolerance A condition in which symptoms such as abdominal gas and bloating appear as a result of severe lactose maldigestion.

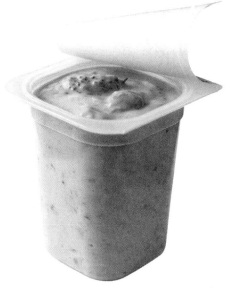

▲ Use of yogurt helps lactose maldigesters meet calcium needs.

When the carbohydrates reach the small intestine, the more alkaline environment of the intestine is better suited for further carbohydrate digestion. The pancreas releases enzymes, such as pancreatic amylase, to aid the last stage of starch digestion. After amylase action, the original carbohydrates in a food are now present in the small intestine as the monosaccharides glucose and fructose, originally present as such in food, and disaccharides (maltose from starch breakdown, lactose mainly from dairy products, and sucrose from food and that added at the table).

The disaccharides are digested to their monosaccharide units once they reach the wall of the small intestine, where the specialized enzymes on the absorptive cells digest each disaccharide into monosaccharides. The enzyme **maltase** acts on maltose to produce two glucose molecules. **Sucrase** acts on sucrose to produce glucose and fructose. **Lactase** acts on lactose to produce glucose and galactose.

Lactose Maldigestion and Lactose Intolerance. Lactose maldigestion is a normal pattern of physiology that often begins to develop after early childhood, at about ages 3 to 5 years. It can lead to symptoms of abdominal pain, gas, and diarrhea after consuming lactose, generally when eaten in large amounts. This *primary* form of lactose maldigestion is estimated to be present in about 75% of the world's population, although not all of these individuals experience symptoms. (When significant symptoms develop after lactose intake, it is then called **lactose intolerance**.) Another form of the problem, *secondary* lactose maldigestion, is a temporary condition in which lactase production is decreased in response to another condition, such as intestinal diarrhea. The symptoms of lactose intolerance include gas, abdominal bloating, cramps, and diarrhea. The bloating and gas are caused by bacterial fermentation of lactose in the large intestine. The diarrhea is caused by undigested lactose in the large intestine as it draws water from the circulatory system into the large intestine.

In North America, approximately 25% of adults show signs of decreased lactose digestion in the small intestine. Many lactose maldigesters are Asian Americans, African Americans, and Latino/Hispanic Americans, and the occurrence increases as people age. It is hypothesized that approximately 3000 to 5000 years ago, a genetic mutation occurred in regions that relied on milk and dairy foods as a main food source, allowing those individuals (mostly in northern Europe, pastoral tribes in Africa, and the Middle East) to retain the ability to maintain high lactase output for their entire lifetime.

Still, many of these individuals can consume moderate amounts of lactose with minimal or no gastrointestinal discomfort because of eventual lactose breakdown by bacteria in the large intestine (see Further Reading 12). Thus, it is unnecessary for these people to greatly restrict their intake of lactose-containing foods, such as milk and milk products. These calcium-rich food products are important for maintaining bone health. Obtaining enough calcium and vitamin D from the diet is much easier if milk and milk products are included in a diet.

Studies have shown that nearly all individuals with decreased lactase production can tolerate ½ to 1 cup of milk with meals, and that most individuals adapt to intestinal gas production resulting from the fermentation of lactose by bacteria in the large intestine. Combining lactose-containing foods with other foods also helps because certain properties of foods can have positive effects on rates of digestion. For example, fat in a meal slows digestion, leaving more time for lactase action. Hard cheese and yogurt also are more easily tolerated than milk. Much of the lactose is lost in the production of cheese, and the active bacteria cultures in yogurt digest the lactose when these bacteria are broken apart in the small intestine and release their lactase. In addition, an array of products, such as low-lactose milk (Lactaid®, Dairy Ease®) and lactase pills, is available to assist lactose maldigesters when needed.

Absorption

Monosaccharides found naturally in foods and those formed as by-products of starch and disaccharide digestion in the mouth and small intestine generally follow an active absorption process. Recall from Chapter 3 that this is a process that requires a specific carrier and energy input for the substance to be taken up by the absorptive cells in the small intestine. Glucose and its close relative, galactose, undergo active absorption. They are pumped into the absorptive cells along with sodium.

Fructose is taken up by the absorptive cells via facilitated diffusion. In this case, a carrier is used, but no energy input is needed. This absorptive process is thus slower than that seen with glucose or galactose. So, large doses of fructose are not readily absorbed and can contribute to diarrhea as the monosaccharide remains in the small intestine and attracts water.

Once glucose, galactose, and fructose enter the absorptive cells, some fructose is metabolized into glucose. The single sugars in the absorptive cells are then transferred to the portal vein that goes directly to the liver. The liver then metabolizes those sugars by transforming the monosaccharides galactose and fructose into glucose and:

- Releasing it directly into the bloodstream for transport to organs such as the brain, muscles, kidneys, and adipose tissues
- Producing glycogen for storage of carbohydrate
- Producing fat (minor amount, if any)

Of these three options, producing fat is the least likely, except when carbohydrates are consumed in high amounts and overall calorie needs are exceeded.

Unless an individual has a disease that causes malabsorption, or an intolerance to a carbohydrate such as lactose (or fructose), only a minor amount of some sugars (about 10%) escapes digestion. Any undigested carbohydrate travels to the large intestine and is fermented there by bacteria. The acids and gases produced by bacterial metabolism of the undigested carbohydrate are absorbed into the bloodstream. Scientists suspect that some of these products of bacterial metabolism promote the health of the large intestine by providing it with a source of calories.

MAKING DECISIONS

Fermentable Fiber

Bacteria in the large intestine ferment soluble fibers into such products as acids and gases. The acids, once absorbed, also provide calories for the body. In this way, soluble fibers provide about 1.5 to 2.5 kcal per gram. Although the intestinal gas (flatulence) produced by this bacterial fermentation is not harmful, it can be painful and sometimes embarrassing. Over time, however, the body tends to adapt to a high-fiber intake, eventually producing less gas.

Name some potentially gas-forming foods. Are these foods good sources of soluble fiber?

CONCEPT CHECK

Carbohydrate digestion is the process of breaking down larger carbohydrates into smaller units, and eventually to monosaccharide forms. The enzymatic digestion of starches in the body begins in the mouth with salivary amylase. Enzymes made by the pancreas and small intestine complete the digestion of carbohydrates to single sugars in the small intestine. Lactose maldigestion is a condition that results when cells of the intestine do not make sufficient lactase, the enzyme necessary to digest lactose, resulting in symptoms such as abdominal gas, pain, and diarrhea. Most people with lactose maldigestion can tolerate cheeses and yogurt, as well as moderate amounts of milk. When significant symptoms develop after lactose intake, it is called lactose intolerance. Following primarily an active absorption process, glucose and galactose (resulting from the digestive process or present in the meal) are taken up by absorptive cells in the intestine. Fructose undergoes facilitated absorption. All of the monosaccharides then enter the portal vein that goes directly to the liver. The liver finally exercises its metabolic options, producing glucose, glycogen, and even fat if carbohydrates are consumed in great excess and overall calorie needs are exceeded.

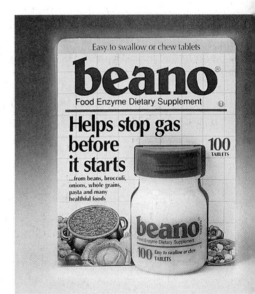

▲ Beano® is a dietary supplement that contains natural digestive enzymes. Such products can be used to reduce intestinal gas produced by bacterial metabolism of undigested sugars in beans and some vegetables in the large intestine.

4.7 Putting Simple Carbohydrates to Work in the Body

As just discussed, all of the digestible carbohydrate that we eat is eventually converted to glucose. Glucose then is the form of carbohydrate that goes on to function in body metabolism. The other sugars can generally be converted to glucose and the starches are broken down to yield glucose, so the functions described here apply to most carbohydrates. The functions of glucose in the body start with supplying calories to fuel the body.

Yielding Energy

The main function of glucose is to supply calories for use by the body. Certain tissues in the body, such as red blood cells, can use only glucose and other simple carbohydrate forms for fuel. Most parts of the brain and central nervous system also derive energy only from glucose, unless the diet contains almost none. In that case, much of the brain can use partial breakdown products of fat—called **ketone bodies**—for energy needs. Other body cells, including muscle cells, can use simple carbohydrates as fuel but many of these cells can also use fat or protein for energy needs.

Sparing Protein from Use as an Energy Source and Preventing Ketosis

A diet that supplies enough digestible carbohydrates to prevent breakdown of proteins for energy needs is considered *protein sparing*. Under normal circumstances, digestible carbohydrates in the diet mostly end up as blood glucose, and protein is reserved for functions such as building and maintaining muscles and vital organs. However, if you don't eat enough carbohydrates, your body is forced to make glucose from body proteins, draining the pool of amino acids available in cells for other critical functions. During long-term starvation, the continuous withdrawal of proteins from the muscles, heart, liver, kidneys, and other vital organs can result in weakness, poor function, and even failure of body systems.

In addition to the loss of protein, when you don't eat enough carbohydrates, the metabolism of fats is inefficient. In the absence of adequate carbohydrate, fats don't break down completely in metabolism and instead form ketone bodies. This condition, known as **ketosis**, should be avoided because it disturbs the body's normal acid-base balance and leads to other health problems. This is a good reason to question the long-term safety of the low-carbohydrate diets that have been popular.

MAKING DECISIONS

Carbohydrates and Protein Sparing

The wasting of protein that occurs during long-term fasting can be life threatening. This has prompted companies that make formulas for rapid weight loss to include sufficient carbohydrate in the products to decrease protein breakdown and thereby protect vital tissues and organs, including the heart. Most of these very low-calorie products are powders that can be mixed with different types of fluids and are consumed five or six times per day. When considering any weight-loss products, be sure that your total diet provides at least the RDA for carbohydrate.

Regulating Glucose

Under normal circumstances, a person's blood glucose concentration is regulated within a narrow range. Recall from Chapter 3 that when carbohydrates are digested

ketone bodies Partial breakdown products of fat that contain three or four carbons.

ketosis The condition of having a high concentration of ketone bodies and related breakdown products in the bloodstream and tissues.

▲ When following a weight-loss diet, be sure that your diet provides at least the RDA for carbohydrate.

and taken up by the absorptive cells of the small intestine, the resulting monosaccharides are transported directly to the liver. One of the liver's roles, then, is to guard against excess glucose entering the bloodstream after a meal. The liver works in concert with the pancreas to regulate blood glucose.

When the concentration of glucose in the blood is high, such as during and immediately after a meal, the pancreas releases the hormone **insulin** into the bloodstream. Insulin delivers two different messages to various body cells to cause the level of glucose in the blood to fall. First, insulin directs the liver to store the glucose as glycogen. Second, insulin directs muscle, adipose, and other cells to remove glucose from the bloodstream by taking it into those cells. By triggering both glycogen synthesis in the liver and glucose movement out of the bloodstream into certain cells, insulin keeps the concentration of glucose from rising too high in the blood (Fig. 4-9).

On the other hand, when a person has not eaten for a few hours and blood glucose begins to fall, the pancreas releases the hormone **glucagon**. This hormone has the opposite effect of insulin. It prompts the breakdown of liver glycogen into glucose, which is then released into the bloodstream. In this way, glucagon keeps blood glucose from falling too low.

A different mechanism increases blood glucose during times of stress. **Epinephrine** (adrenaline) is the hormone responsible for the "flight or fight" reaction. Epinephrine and a related compound are released in large amounts from the adrenal glands (located on each kidney) and various nerve endings in response to a perceived threat, such as a car approaching head-on. These hormones cause glycogen in the liver to be quickly broken down into glucose. The resulting rapid flood of glucose from the liver into the bloodstream helps promote quick mental and physical reactions.

In essence, the actions of insulin on blood glucose are balanced by the actions of glucagon, epinephrine, and other hormones. If hormonal balance is not maintained, such as during over- or underproduction of insulin or glucagon, major changes in blood glucose concentrations occur. The disease, type 1 diabetes, is an example of the underproduction of insulin. To maintain blood glucose within an acceptable range, the body relies on a complex regulatory system. This provides a safeguard against extremely high blood glucose (**hyperglycemia**) or low blood glucose (**hypoglycemia**). The failure of blood glucose regulation will be discussed in the Nutrition and Your Health section at the end of this chapter.

insulin A hormone produced by the pancreas. Among other processes, insulin increases the synthesis of glycogen in the liver and the movement of glucose from the bloodstream into body cells.

glucagon A hormone made by the pancreas that stimulates the breakdown of glycogen in the liver into glucose; this ends up increasing blood glucose. Glucagon also performs other functions.

epinephrine A hormone also known as *adrenaline*; it is released by the adrenal glands (located on each kidney) and various nerve endings in the body. It acts to increase glycogen breakdown in the liver, among other functions.

hyperglycemia High blood glucose, above 125 milligrams per 100 milliliters of blood.

hypoglycemia Low blood glucose, below 40 to 50 milligrams per 100 milliliters of blood.

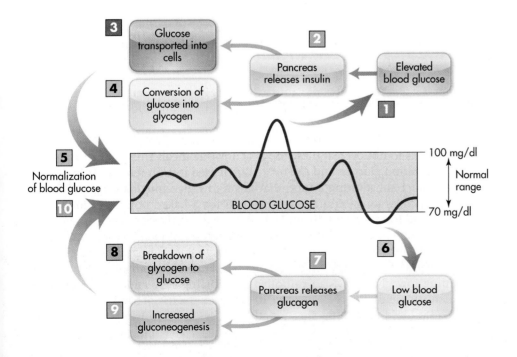

FIGURE 4-9 ▶ Regulation of blood glucose. Insulin and glucagon are key factors in controlling blood glucose. When blood glucose rises above the normal range of 70 to 90 milligrams per deciliter (mg/dl) ▢1, insulin is released ▢2 to lower it ▢3 and ▢4 blood glucose then falls back into the normal range ▢5. When blood glucose falls below the normal range ▢6, glucagon is released ▢7, which has the opposite effect of insulin ▢8, and ▢9 this then restores blood glucose to the normal range ▢10. Other hormones, such as epinephrine, norepinephrine, cortisol, and growth hormone, also contribute to blood glucose regulation.

See Nutrition and Your Health: Diabetes—When Blood Glucose Regulation Fails at the end of Chapter 4.

A term you might see on food labels is *net carbs*. Although this term is not FDA-approved, sometimes it is used to describe the carbohydrates that increase blood glucose. Fiber and sugar alcohol content are subtracted from the total carbohydrate content to yield net carbs because they have a negligible effect on blood glucose.

glycemic index (GI) The blood glucose response of a given food, compared to a standard (typically, glucose or white bread). Glycemic index is influenced by starch structure; fiber content; food processing; physical structure; and macronutrients in the meal, such as fat.

glycemic load (GL) The amount of carbohydrate in a serving of food multiplied by the glycemic index of that carbohydrate. The result is then divided by 100.

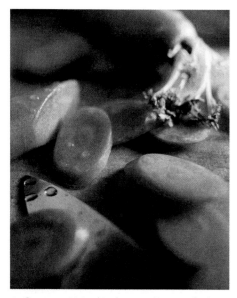

▲ Carrots, criticized in the popular press for having a high glycemic index (which isn't even true), actually contribute a low glycemic load to a diet.

The Glycemic Index and Glycemic Load of Carbohydrate Sources

Our bodies react uniquely to different sources of carbohydrates, such that a serving of a high-fiber food, such as baked beans, results in lower blood glucose levels compared to the same size serving of mashed potatoes. Why are we concerned with the effects of various foods on blood glucose? Foods that result in a high blood glucose elicit a large release of insulin from the pancreas. Chronically high insulin output leads to many deleterious effects on the body: high blood triglycerides, increased fat deposition in the adipose tissue, increased tendency for blood to clot, increased fat synthesis in the liver, and a more rapid return of hunger after a meal (insulin rapidly lowers the macronutrients in the blood as it stimulates their storage, signaling hunger). Over time, this increase in insulin output may cause the muscles to become resistant to the action of insulin, and eventually lead to type 2 diabetes in some people. Two food measurements have been developed that are useful in predicting the blood sugar response to various foods and for planning a diet to avoid hyperglycemia (high blood glucose).

The first of these tools is **glycemic index (GI)**. Glycemic index is a ratio of the blood glucose response to a given food compared to a standard (typically, glucose or white bread) (Table 4-4). Glycemic index is influenced by starch structure, fiber content, food processing, physical structure, and other macronutrients in the meal, such as fat. Foods with particularly high glycemic index values are potatoes, especially baking potatoes (due to higher amylopectin content compared to red potatoes), mashed potatoes (due to greater surface area exposed), short-grain white rice, honey, and jelly beans. A major shortcoming of glycemic index is that the measurement is based on a serving of food that would provide 50 grams of carbohydrate. As you can imagine, this amount of food may not reflect the amount typically consumed.

Another way of describing how different foods affect blood glucose (and insulin) levels is **glycemic load (GL)**. The glycemic load is more useful because it takes into account the glycemic index and the amount of carbohydrate consumed. Glycemic load, therefore, better reflects a food's effect on one's blood glucose than either number alone. To calculate the glycemic load of a food, the amount (in grams) of carbohydrate in a serving of the food is multiplied by the glycemic index of that food, and then divided by 100 (because glycemic index is a percentage). For example, vanilla wafers have a glycemic index of 77, and a small serving contains 15 grams of carbohydrate:

$$(\text{Glycemic Index} \times \text{Grams of Carbohydrate}) \div 100 = \text{Glycemic Load}$$
$$(77 \times 15) \div 100 = 12$$

Even though the glycemic index of vanilla wafers (77) is considered high, the glycemic load calculation shows that the impact of this food on blood glucose levels is fairly low (review Table 4-4).

There are many ways to address this problem of high glycemic load foods. The most important is to not overeat these foods at any one meal. This greatly minimizes their effects on blood glucose and the related increased insulin release. At least once per meal, consider substituting a food that has a low glycemic load for one with a higher value, such as long-grain rice or spaghetti for a baked potato. Combining a low glycemic load food, such as an apple, kidney beans, milk, or salad with dressing, with a high glycemic load food also reduces the effect on blood glucose. In addition, maintaining a healthy body weight and performing regular physical activity further reduces the effects of a high glycemic load diet (see Further Reading 9).

Substituting low glycemic load carbohydrates for high glycemic load foods can help in the treatment of diabetes; Chapter 10 discusses the use of foods with different glycemic load values in planning diets for athletes.

TABLE 4-4 Glycemic Index (GI) and Glycemic Load (GL) of Common Foods

Reference food glucose = 100
Low GI foods—below 55
Intermediate GI foods—between 55 and 70
High GI foods—more than 70

Low GL foods—below 15
Intermediate GL foods—between 15 and 20
High GL foods—more than 20

	Serving Size (grams)	Glycemic Index (GI)	Carbohydrate (grams)	Glycemic Load (GL)
Pastas/Grains				
White, long grain	1 cup	56	45	25
White, short grain	1 cup	72	53	38
Spaghetti	1 cup	41	40	16
Vegetables				
Carrots, boiled	1 cup	49	16	8
Sweet corn	1 cup	55	39	21
Potato, baked	1 cup	85	57	48
Dairy Foods				
Milk, skim	1 cup	32	12	4
Yogurt, low-fat	1 cup	33	17	6
Ice cream	1 cup	61	31	19
Legumes				
Baked beans	1 cup	48	54	26
Kidney beans	1 cup	27	38	10
Navy beans	1 cup	38	54	21
Sugars				
Honey	1 tsp	73	6	4
Sucrose	1 tsp	65	5	3
Fructose	1 tsp	23	5	1
Breads and Muffins				
Bagel	1 small	72	30	22
Whole-wheat bread	1 slice	69	13	9
White bread	1 slice	70	10	7
Fruits				
Apple	1 medium	38	22	8
Banana	1 medium	55	29	16
Orange	1 medium	44	15	7
Beverages				
Orange juice	1 cup	46	26	13
Gatorade	1 cup	78	15	12
Coca-Cola	1 cup	63	26	16
Snack Foods				
Potato chips	1 oz	54	15	8
Vanilla wafers	5 cookies	77	15	12
Jelly beans	1 oz	80	26	21

Source: Foster-Powell K. and others: International table of glycemic index and glycemic load. *American Journal of Clinical Nutrition* 76:5, 2002.

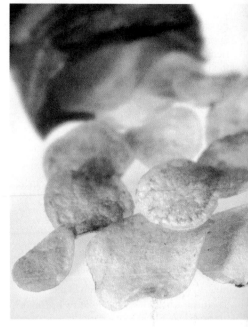

▲ A food such as potato chips, with a low glycemic index, can still have a high glycemic load if eaten in large portions.

You might wonder why the glycemic index and glycemic load of white bread and whole wheat are similar. This is because whole-wheat flour is typically so finely ground that it is quickly digested. Thus the effect of fiber in slowing digestion and related absorption of glucose is no longer present. Some experts suggest we focus more on minimally processed (e.g., coarsely ground, steel cut, or rolled) grains, such as with whole-wheat flour and oatmeal, to get the full benefits of these fiber sources in reducing blood glucose levels.

Recall from Chapter 2 that FDA has approved the following claim: "Diets rich in whole-grain foods and other plant foods and low in total fat, saturated fat, and cholesterol may decrease the risk for cardiovascular (heart) disease and certain cancers."

diverticula Pouches that protrude through the exterior wall of the large intestine.

hemorrhoid A pronounced swelling of a large vein, particularly veins found in the anal region.

diverticulosis The condition of having many diverticula in the large intestine.

diverticulitis An inflammation of the diverticula caused by acids produced by bacterial metabolism inside the diverticula.

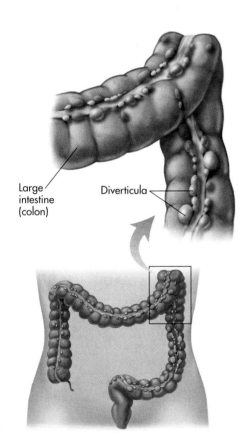

Large intestine (colon)   Diverticula

FIGURE 4-10 ▶ Diverticula in the large intestine. A low-fiber diet increases the risk of developing diverticula. About one-third of people over age 45 have diverticulosis, while two-thirds of people over 85 do.

CONCEPT CHECK

Carbohydrates provide glucose for the energy needs of red blood cells and parts of the brain and nervous system. Eating too little carbohydrates forces the body to make glucose using primarily amino acids from proteins found in muscles and other vital organs. A low glucose supply in cells also inhibits efficient metabolism of fats. Ketosis can then result.

Blood glucose concentration is maintained within a narrow range. When blood glucose rises after a meal, the hormone insulin is released in great amounts from the pancreas. Insulin acts to lower blood glucose by increasing glucose storage in the liver and glucose up-take by other body cells. If blood glucose falls during fasting, glucagon and other hormones increase the liver's release of glucose into the bloodstream to restore normal blood glucose concentrations. In a similar way, the hormone epinephrine can make more glucose available in response to stress. This balance in hormone activity helps maintain blood glucose within a healthy range.

4.8 Putting Fiber to Work

Promoting Bowel Health

Fiber supplies mass to the feces, making elimination much easier. This is especially true for insoluble fibers. When enough fiber is consumed, the stool is large and soft because many types of plant fibers attract water. The larger size stimulates the intestinal muscles to contract, which aids elimination. Consequently, less pressure is necessary to expel the stool.

When too little fiber is eaten, the opposite can occur: very little water is present in the feces, making it small and hard. Constipation may result, which forces one to exert excessive pressure in the large intestine during defecation. This high pressure can force parts of the large intestine (colon) wall out from between the surrounding bands of muscle, forming many small pouches called **diverticula** (Fig. 4-10). **Hemorrhoids** may also result from excessive straining during defecation (review Chapter 3).

Diverticula are asymptomatic in about 80% of affected people; that is, they are not noticeable. The asymptomatic form of this disease is called **diverticulosis**. If the diverticula become filled with food particles, such as hulls and seeds, they may eventually become inflamed and painful, a condition known as **diverticulitis**. Surprisingly, intake of fiber then should be reduced to limit further bacterial activity. Once the inflammation subsides, a high-fiber diet is resumed to ease stool elimination and reduce the risk of a future attack.

Over the past 30 years, many population studies have shown a link between increased fiber intake and a decrease in colon cancer development (see Further Reading 10). Most of the research on diet and colon cancer is focusing on the potential preventive effects of fruits, vegetables, whole-grain breads and cereals, and beans (rather than just fiber). Smoking, obesity in men, excessive alcohol use, starch- and sugar-rich foods, and processed meat intake are under study as potential causes of colon cancer. Overall, the health benefits to the colon that stem from a high-fiber diet are partially due to the nutrients that are commonly present in most high-fiber foods, such as vitamins, minerals, phytochemicals, and in some cases essential fatty acids. Thus it is more advisable to increase fiber intake using fiber-rich foods, rather than mostly relying on fiber supplements.

Reducing Obesity Risk

Aside from its role in maintaining bowel regularity, the consumption of fiber has many additional health benefits. A diet high in fiber likely controls weight and reduces the risk of developing obesity (see Further Reading 13). The bulky nature of high-fiber foods requires more time to chew and fills us up without yielding many calories. Increasing intake of foods rich in fiber is one strategy for feeling satisfied or full after a meal (review the discussion of energy density in Chapter 2). This is still another reason to question the low-carbohydrate diets—where is the whole-grain fiber going to come from?

Enhancing Blood Glucose Control

Consuming large amounts of viscous fibers, such as oat fiber, slows glucose absorption from the small intestine, and so contributes to better blood glucose regulation. This effect can be helpful in the treatment of diabetes. In fact, adults whose main carbohydrate source is low-fiber foods are much more likely to develop diabetes than those who have high-fiber diets.

Reducing Cholesterol Absorption

Recall that good sources of viscous fiber are apples, bananas, oranges, carrots, barley, oats, and kidney beans. A high intake of viscous fiber also inhibits absorption of cholesterol and cholesterol-rich bile acids from the small intestine, thereby reducing blood cholesterol and possibly reducing the risk of cardiovascular disease and gallstones. The beneficial bacteria in the large intestine degrade soluble fiber and produce certain fatty acids that probably also reduce cholesterol synthesis in the liver. In addition, the slower glucose absorption that occurs with diets high in viscous fiber is linked to a decrease in insulin release. One of the effects of insulin is to stimulate cholesterol synthesis in the liver, so this reduction in insulin may contribute to the ability of viscous fiber to lower blood cholesterol. Overall, a fiber-rich diet containing fruits, vegetables, beans, and whole-grain breads and cereals (including whole-grain breakfast cereals) is advocated as part of a strategy to reduce cardiovascular disease (coronary heart disease and stroke) risk. And again, this is something that a low-carbohydrate diet can't promise.

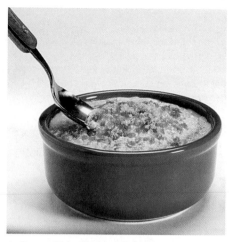

▲ Oatmeal is a rich source of viscous fiber. FDA allows a health claim for the benefits of oatmeal to lower blood cholesterol that arise from the effects of this viscous fiber.

CONCEPT CHECK

Fiber forms a vital part of the diet by adding mass to the stool, which eases elimination. Fiber-rich foods also help in weight control and reduce the risk of developing obesity and cardiovascular disease, and possibly colon cancer. Soluble fiber can also be useful for controlling blood glucose in patients with diabetes and in lowering blood cholesterol. Whole-grain breads and cereals, vegetables, beans, and fruits are excellent sources of fiber.

4.9 Carbohydrate Needs

Currently, recommendations for carbohydrate intake vary widely in the scientific literature and popular press. The RDA for carbohydrates is 130 grams per day for adults (see Further Reading 6). This is based on the amount needed to supply adequate glucose for the brain and nervous system, without having to rely on ketone bodies from incomplete fat breakdown as a calorie source. Somewhat exceeding this amount is fine; the Food and Nutrition Board recommends that carbohydrate intake should range from 45% to 65% of total calorie intake. The Nutrition Facts panel on food labels uses 60% of calorie intake as the standard for recommended carbohydrate intake. This would be 300 grams of carbohydrate when consuming a 2000-calorie diet.

North American adults consume about 180 to 330 grams of carbohydrates per day, which supply about 50% of calorie intake. Worldwide, however, carbohydrates account for about 70% of all calories consumed, and in some countries, up to 80% of the calories consumed. One recommendation on which almost all experts agree is that one's carbohydrate intake should be based primarily on fruits, vegetables, whole-grain breads and cereals, and beans, rather than on refined grains, potatoes, and sugar.

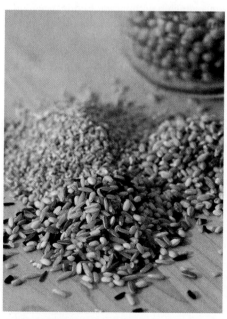

▲ The 2010 Dietary Guidelines define whole grain as the entire grain seed or kernel made of three components: bran, germ, and endosperm.

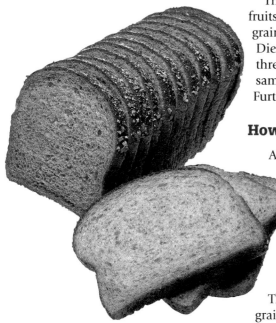

▲ Look for the term "whole-grain" or "whole-wheat" flour on the label for breads that are an excellent source of fiber.

The 2010 Dietary Guidelines for Americans recommend that we choose fiber-rich fruits, vegetables, and whole grains often. More specifically, three or more ounces of grains, roughly one-half of one's grains, should be whole. Remember that the 2010 Dietary Guidelines define whole grain as the entire grain seed or kernel made of three components: the bran, germ, and endosperm, which must be in nearly the same relative proportions as the original grain if cracked, crushed, or flaked (see Further Reading 14).

How Much Fiber Do We Need?

An Adequate Intake for fiber has been set based on the ability of fiber to reduce risk of cardiovascular disease (and likely many cases of diabetes). The Adequate Intake for fiber for adults is 25 grams per day for women and 38 grams per day for men. The goal is to provide at least 14 grams per 1000 kcal in a diet. After age 50, the Adequate Intake falls to 21 grams per day and 30 grams per day, respectively. The Daily Value used for fiber on food and supplement labels is 25 grams for a 2000 kcal diet. In North America, fiber intake averages 13 grams per day for women and 17 grams per day for men and the average whole-grain intake is less than one serving per day. This low intake is attributed to the lack of knowledge on the benefits of whole grains, and the inability to recognize whole-grain products at the time of purchase. Thus, most of us should increase our fiber intake. At least three servings of whole grains per day is recommended. Eating a high-fiber cereal (at least 3 grams of fiber per serving) for breakfast is one easy way to increase fiber intake (Fig. 4-11).

The "Rate Your Plate" exercise shows a diet containing 25 or 38 grams of fiber within moderate calorie intakes. Diets to meet the fiber recommendations are possible and enjoyable if you incorporate plenty of whole-wheat bread, fruits, vegetables, and beans. Use the "Rate Your Plate" exercise to estimate the fiber content of your diet. What is *your* fiber score?

The 2010 Dietary Guidelines for Americans provide the following recommendations regarding carbohydrate intake as part of a healthy eating pattern while staying within their calorie needs:

- Limit the consumption of foods that contain refined grains, especially refined grain foods that contain solid fats, added sugars, and sodium.
- Increase vegetable and fruit intake.
- Eat a variety of vegetables, especially dark-green and red and orange vegetables and beans and peas.
- Consume at least half of all grains as whole grains. Increase whole-grain intake by replacing refined grains with whole grains.
- Choose foods that provide more potassium, dietary fiber, calcium, and vitamin D, which are nutrients of concern in American diets. These foods include vegetables, fruits, whole grains, and milk and milk products.

MAKING DECISIONS

Whole Grains

When buying bread, if you see the name "wheat bread" on the label, do you think you are buying a whole-wheat product? Most people do. The flour is from the wheat plant, so manufacturers correctly list enriched white (refined) flour as wheat flour on food labels. However, if the label does not list "whole-wheat flour" first, then the product is not primarily a whole-wheat bread and thus does not contain as much fiber as it could. Careful reading of labels is important in the search for more fiber. Look especially for the term whole grains on the food label to ensure that you are getting a good source of natural fiber.

In the final analysis, keep in mind that any nutrient can lead to health problems when consumed in excess. High carbohydrate, high fiber, and low fat do not mean zero calories. Carbohydrates help moderate calorie intake in comparison with fats, but high-carbohydrate foods also contribute to total calorie intake.

4.10 Health Concerns Related to Carbohydrate Intake

Aside from the health risks related to ketosis, both excessive fiber and sugar intakes can pose health problems. Too much lactose in the diet is also a problem for some people.

Problems with High-Fiber Diets

Very high intakes of fiber—for example, 60 grams per day—can pose some health risks and therefore should be followed only under the guidance of a physician. Increased

Nutrition Facts

Serving Size .... 1 cup (55g/2.0 oz.)
Servings Per Container 10

Amount Per Serving	Cereal	Cereal with ½ Cup Vitamins A & D Skim Milk
Calories	170	210
Calories from Fat	10	10
	% Daily Value**	
Total Fat 1.0g*	2%	2%
Sat. Fat 0g	0%	0%
Trans Fat 0g		*
Cholesterol 0mg	0%	0%
Sodium 300mg	13%	15%
Potassium 340mg	10%	16%
Total Carbohydrate 43g	14%	16%
Dietary Fiber 7g	**28%**	**28%**
Sugars 16g		
Other Carbohydrate 20g		
Protein 4g		
Vitamin A	15%	20%
Vitamin C	20%	22%
Calcium	2%	15%
Iron	65%	65%
Vitamin D	10%	25%
Thiamin	25%	30%
Riboflavin	25%	35%
Niacin	25%	25%
Vitamin B$_6$	25%	25%
Folic acid	30%	30%
Vitamin B$_{12}$	25%	35%
Phosphorus	20%	30%
Magnesium	20%	25%
Zinc	25%	25%
Copper	10%	10%

*Amount in cereal. One half cup skim milk contributes an additional 40 calories, 65mg sodium, 6g total carbohydrate (6g sugars), and 4g protein.
**Percent Daily Values are based on a 2,000 calorie diet. Your daily values may be higher or lower depending on your calorie needs:

	Calories:	2,000	2,500
Total Fat	Less than	65g	80g
Sat Fat	Less than	20g	25g
Cholesterol	Less than	300mg	300mg
Sodium	Less than	2,400mg	2,400mg
Potassium		3,500mg	3,500mg
Total Carbohydrate		300g	375g
Dietary Fiber		25g	30g

Calories per gram:
Fat 9 • Carbohydrate 4 • Protein 4

*Intake of *trans* fat should be as low as possible.

Ingredients: Wheat bran with other parts of wheat, raisins, sugar, corn syrup, salt, malt flavoring, glycerin, iron, niacinamide, zinc oxide, pyridoxine hydrochloride (vitamin B₆), riboflavin (vitamin B₂), vitamin A palmitate, thiamin hydrochloride (vitamin B₁), folic acid, vitamin B₁₂, and vitamin D.

Nutrition Facts

Serving Size: ¾ Cup (30g)
Servings Per Package: About 17

Amount Per Serving	Cereal	Cereal With ½ Cup Skim Milk
Calories	170	210
Calories from Fat	0	5
	%Daily Value**	
Total Fat 0g*	0%	1%
Saturated Fat 0g	0%	1%
Trans Fat 0g		*
Cholesterol 0mg	0%	1%
Sodium 60mg	2%	4%
Potassium 80mg	2%	8%
Total Carbohydrate 35g	9%	11%
Dietary Fiber 1g	4%	4%
Sugars 20g		
Other Carbohydrate 13g		
Protein 3g		
Vitamin A	25%	30%
Vitamin C	0%	2%
Calcium	0%	15%
Iron	10%	10%
Vitamin D	10%	20%
Thiamin	25%	25%
Riboflavin	25%	35%
Niacin	25%	25%
Vitamin B$_6$	25%	25%
Folic acid	25%	25%
Vitamin B$_{12}$	25%	30%
Phosphorus	4%	15%
Magnesium	4%	8%
Zinc	10%	10%
Copper	2%	2%

*Amount in Cereal. One-half cup skim milk contributes an additional 65mg sodium, 6g total carbohydrate (6g sugars), and 4g protein.
**Percent Daily Values are based on a 2,000 calorie diet. Your daily values may be higher or lower depending on your calorie needs:

	Calories:	2,000	2,500
Total Fat	Less than	65g	80g
Sat. Fat	Less than	20g	25g
Cholesterol	Less than	300mg	300mg
Sodium	Less than	2,400mg	2,400mg
Potassium		3,500mg	3,500mg
Total Carbohydrate		300g	375g
Dietary Fiber		25g	30g

Calories per gram:
Fat 9 • Carbohydrate 4 • Protein 4

*Intake of *trans* fat should be as low as possible.

Ingredients: Wheat, Sugar, Corn Syrup, Honey, Caramel Color, Partially Hydrogenated Soybean Oil, Salt, Ferric Phosphate, Niacinamide (Niacin), Zinc Oxide, Vitamin A (Palmitate), Pyridoxine Hydrochloride (Vitamin B6), Riboflavin, Thiamin Mononitrate, Folic Acid (Folate), Vitamin B12 and Vitamin D.

FIGURE 4-11 ▶ Reading the Nutrition Facts on food labels helps us choose more nutritious foods. Based on the information from these nutrition labels, which cereal is the better choice for breakfast? Consider the amount of fiber in each cereal. Did the ingredient lists give you any clues? (Note: Ingredients are always listed in descending order by weight on a label.) When choosing a breakfast cereal, it is generally wise to focus on those that are rich sources of fiber. Sugar content can also be used for evaluation. However, sometimes this number does not reflect added sugar but simply the addition of fruits, such as raisins, complicating the evaluation.

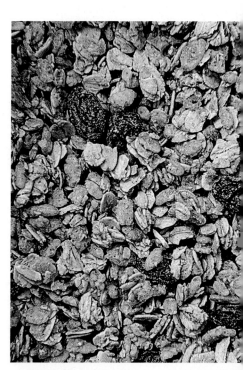

▲ Whole-grain foods, such as granola, are excellent sources of fiber.

fluid intake is extremely important with a high-fiber diet. Inadequate fluid intake can leave the stool very hard and painful to eliminate. In more severe cases, the combination of excess fiber and insufficient fluid may contribute to blockages in the intestine, which may require surgery.

Aside from problems with the passage of materials through the GI tract, a high-fiber diet may also decrease the availability of nutrients. Certain components of fiber may bind to essential minerals, keeping them from being absorbed. For example, when fiber is consumed in large amounts, zinc and iron absorption may be hindered. In children, a very high fiber intake may reduce overall calorie intake, because fiber can quickly fill a child's small stomach before food intake meets energy needs.

Problems with High-Sugar Diets

The main problems with consuming an excess amount of sugar are that it provides empty calories and increases the risk for dental decay.

Diet Quality Declines When Sugar Intake Is Excessive. Overcrowding the diet with sweet treats can leave little room for important, nutrient-dense foods, such as fruits and vegetables. Children and teenagers are at the highest risk for overconsuming empty calories in place of nutrients essential for growth. Many children and teenagers are drinking an excess of sugared soft drinks and other sugar-containing beverages and much less milk than ever before. This exchange of soft drinks for milk can compromise bone health because milk contains calcium and vitamin D, both essential for bone health.

Supersizing sugar-rich beverages is also a growing problem; for example, in the 1950s a typical serving size of a soft drink was a 6½-ounce bottle, and now a 20-ounce plastic bottle is a typical serving. This one change in serving size contributes 170 extra kcal of sugars to the diet. Most convenience stores now offer cups that will hold 64 ounces of soft drinks. Filling up on sugared soft drinks in place of foods is not a healthy practice, but enjoying an occasional soft drink or limiting intake to one 12-ounce serving a day is generally fine. Switching to diet soft drinks would spare the simple sugar calories but still lacks nutritional value except for the fluid.

The sugar found in cakes, cookies, and ice cream also supplies many extra calories that promote weight gain, unless an individual is physically active. Today's low-fat and fat-free snack products usually contain lots of added sugar to produce a product with an acceptable taste. The result is to produce a high-calorie food equal to or greater in calorie content than the high-fat food product it was designed to replace.

With regard to sugar intake, an upper limit of 25% of total calorie intake from "added sugars" has been set by the Food and Nutrition Board (sugars added to foods during processing and preparation). Diets that go beyond this upper limit are likely to be deficient in vitamins and minerals. The World Health Organization suggests that added sugars provide no more than 10% of total daily calorie intake.

A moderate intake of about 10% of calorie intake corresponds to a maximum of approximately 50 grams (or 12 tsp) of sugars per day, based on a 2000 kcal diet. Most of the sugars we eat come from foods and beverages to which sugar has been added during processing and/or manufacture. On average, North Americans eat about 82 grams of added sugars daily, amounting to about 16% of calorie intake. Major sources of added sugars include soft drinks; cakes; cookies; fruit drinks; and dairy desserts, such as ice cream (Fig. 4-12). Following the recommendation of having no more than 10% of added calories from sugars is easier if sweet desserts such as cakes, cookies, and ice cream (full and reduced fat) are consumed sparingly (Table 4-5).

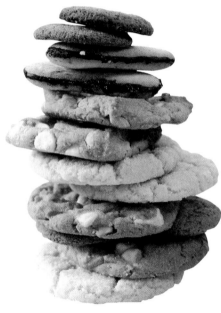

An excess intake of sugared soft drinks has recently been linked to a risk for both weight gain and type 2 diabetes in adults.

▲ Cookies and cakes are one of the top five carbohydrate sources for U.S. adults.

MAKING DECISIONS

Sugar and Hyperactivity

There is a widespread notion that high sugar intake by children causes hyperactivity, typically part of the syndrome called *attention deficit hyperactivity disorder (ADHD)*. However, most researchers find that sucrose may have the opposite effect. A high-carbohydrate meal, if also low in protein and fat, has a calming effect and induces sleep; this effect may be linked to changes in the synthesis of certain neurotransmitters in the brain, such as serotonin. If there is a problem, it is probably the excitement or tension in situations in which sugar-rich foods are served, such as at birthday parties and on Halloween.

TABLE 4-5 Suggestions for Reducing Simple-Sugar Intake

Many foods we enjoy are sweet. These should be eaten in moderation.

At the Supermarket

- Read ingredient labels. Identify all the added sugars in a product. Select items lower in total sugar when possible.
- Buy fresh fruits or fruits packed in water, juice, or light syrup rather than those packed in heavy syrup.
- Buy fewer foods that are high in sugar, such as prepared baked goods, candies, sugared cereals, sweet desserts, soft drinks, and fruit-flavored punches. Substitute vanilla wafers, graham crackers, bagels, English muffins, diet soft drinks, and other low-sugar alternatives.
- Buy reduced-fat microwave popcorn to replace candy for snacks.

In the Kitchen

- Reduce the sugar in foods prepared at home. Try new low-sugar recipes or adjust your own. Start by reducing the sugar gradually until you've decreased it by one-third or more.
- Experiment with spices, such as cinnamon, cardamom, coriander, nutmeg, ginger, and mace, to enhance the flavor of foods.
- Use home-prepared items with less sugar instead of commercially prepared ones that are higher in sugar.

At the Table

- Reduce your use of white and brown sugars, honey, molasses, syrups, jams, and jellies.
- Choose fewer foods high in sugar, such as prepared baked goods, candies, and sweet desserts.
- Reach for fresh fruit instead of cookies or candy for dessert and between-meal snacks.
- Add less sugar to foods—coffee, tea, cereal, and fruit. Cut back gradually to a quarter or half the amount. Consider using sugar alternatives to substitute for some sugar.
- Reduce the number of sugared soft drinks, punches, and fruit juices you drink. Substitute water, diet soft drinks, and whole fruits.

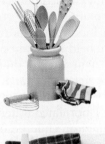
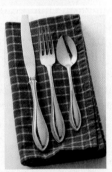

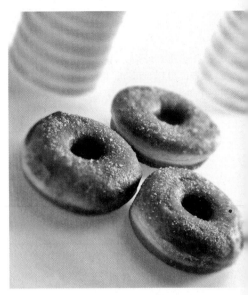

▲ Many foods we enjoy are sweet. These should be eaten in moderation.

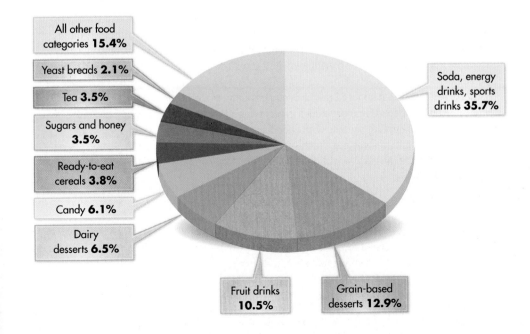

All other food categories **15.4%**

Yeast breads **2.1%**

Tea **3.5%**

Sugars and honey **3.5%**

Ready-to-eat cereals **3.8%**

Candy **6.1%**

Dairy desserts **6.5%**

Fruit drinks **10.5%**

Grain-based desserts **12.9%**

Soda, energy drinks, sports drinks **35.7%**

FIGURE 4-12 ▶ Sources of added sugars in the diets of the U.S. population ages 2 years and olders.

Sources: Dietary Guidelines for Americans Chapter Three.

National Cancer Institute. Sources of added sugars in the diets of the U.S. population ages 2 years and older, NHANES 2005–2006. Risk Factor Monitoring and Methods. Cancer Control and Population Sciences. http://riskfactor.cancer .gov/diet/foodsources/added_sugars/table5a .html. Accessed August 11, 2010.

dental caries Erosions in the surface of a tooth caused by acids made by bacteria as they metabolize sugars.

Dental Caries

Sugars in the diet (and starches readily fermented in the mouth, such as crackers and white bread) also increase the risk of developing **dental caries**. Recall that caries, also known as cavities, are formed when sugars and other carbohydrates are metabolized into acids by bacteria that live in the mouth. These acids dissolve the tooth enamel and underlying structure. Bacteria also use the sugars to make plaque, a sticky substance that both adheres acid-producing bacteria to teeth and diminishes the acid-neutralizing effect of saliva.

The worst offenders in terms of promoting dental caries are sticky and gummy foods high in sugars, such as caramel, because they stick to the teeth and supply the bacteria with a long-lived carbohydrate source. Frequent consumption of liquid sugar sources (e.g., fruit juices) can also cause dental caries. Snacking regularly on sugary foods is also likely to cause caries because it gives the bacteria on the teeth a steady source of carbohydrate from which to continually make acid. Sugared gum chewed between meals is a prime example of a poor dental habit. Still, sugar-containing foods are not the only foods that promote acid production by bacteria in the mouth. As mentioned, if starch-containing foods (e.g., crackers and bread) are held in the mouth for a long time, the starch will be broken down to sugars by enzymes in the mouth; bacteria can then produce acid from these sugars. Overall, the sugar and starch content of a food and its ability to remain in the mouth largely determine its potential to cause caries.

Fluoridated water and toothpaste have contributed to fewer dental caries in North American children over the past 20 years due to fluoride's tooth-strengthening effect (see Chapter 10). Research has also indicated that certain foods—such as cheese, peanuts, and sugar-free chewing gum—can help reduce the amount of acid on teeth. In addition, rinsing the mouth after meals and snacks reduces the acidity in the mouth. Certainly, good nutrition, habits that do not present an overwhelming challenge to oral health (e.g., chewing sugar-free gum), and routine visits to the dentist all contribute to improved dental health.

CRITICAL THINKING

John and Mike are identical twins who like the same games, sports, and foods. However, John likes to chew sugar-free gum and Mike doesn't. At their last dental visit, John had no cavities but Mike had two. Mike wants to know why John, who chews gum after eating, doesn't have cavities and he does. How would you explain this to him?

CONCEPT CHECK

The RDA for carbohydrate is 130 grams per day. The typical North American diet provides 180 to 330 grams per day. A reasonable goal is to have about half of our calorie intake coming from starch and our total carbohydrate intake making up about 60% of our calorie intake, with a range of 45% to 65%. This should allow for the recommended intake of 25 to 38 grams of fiber per day for women and men, respectively. High-fiber diets must be accompanied by adequate fluid intakes to avoid constipation and should be followed only under a physician's guidance.

North Americans eat about 82 grams of sugars added to foods each day. Most of these sugars are added to foods and beverages in processing. To reduce consumption of sugars, one must reduce consumption of items with added sugars, such as some baked goods, sweetened beverages, and presweetened ready-to-eat breakfast cereals. This is one practice that can help reduce the development of dental caries and likely improve diet quality and various aspects of health.

Diabetes—When Blood Glucose Regulation Fails

Improper regulation of blood glucose results in either hyperglycemia (high blood glucose) or hypoglycemia (low blood glucose) as noted in this chapter. High blood glucose is most commonly associated with diabetes (technically, *diabetes mellitus*), a disease that affects 6.5% of the North American population (see Further Reading 5). Of these, it is estimated one-third to one-half of these people do not know that they have the disease. Diabetes leads to about 200,000 deaths each year in North America. Diabetes is currently increasing in epidemic proportions in North America. New recommendations promote testing fasting blood glucose in adults over age 45 every 3 years to help diagnose the problem. Diabetes is diagnosed when one's fasting blood glucose is 126 milligrams per 100 milliliters of blood or greater. In contrast, low blood glucose is a much rarer condition.

Diabetes

There are two major forms of diabetes: **type 1** (formerly called insulin-dependent or juvenile-onset diabetes), and **type 2 diabetes** (formerly called non–insulin-dependent or adult-onset diabetes) (Table 4-6). The change in names to type 1 and type 2 diabetes stems from the fact that many type 2 diabetics eventually must also rely on insulin injections as a part of their treatment. In addition, many children today have type 2 diabetes. A third form, called gestational diabetes, occurs in some pregnant women (see Chapter 16). It is usually treated with an insulin regimen and diet and resolves after delivery of the baby. However, women who have gestational diabetes during pregnancy are at high risk for developing type 2 diabetes later in life.

Traditional symptoms of diabetes are excessive urination, excessive thirst, and excessive hunger. No one symptom is diagnostic of diabetes, and other

TABLE 4-6 Comparison of Type 1 and Type 2 Diabetes

	Type 1 Diabetes	Type 2 Diabetes
Occurrence	5%–10% of cases of diabetes	90% of cases of diabetes
Cause	Autoimmune attack on the pancreas	Insulin resistance
Risk Factors	Moderate genetic predisposition	Strong genetic predisposition Obesity and physical inactivity Ethnicity Metabolic Syndrome Pre-diabetes
Characteristics	Distinct symptoms (frequent thirst, hunger, and urination) Ketosis Weight loss	Mild symptoms, especially in early phases of the disease (fatigue and nighttime urination) Ketosis does not generally occur.
Treatment	Insulin Diet Exercise	Diet Exercise Oral medications to lower blood glucose Insulin (in advanced cases)
Complications	Cardiovascular disease Kidney disease Nerve disease Blindness Infections	Cardiovascular disease Kidney disease Nerve damage Blindness Infections
Monitoring	Blood glucose Urine ketones HbA1c*	Blood glucose HbA1c

*Hemoglobin Alc.

type 1 diabetes A form of diabetes prone to ketosis and that requires insulin therapy.

type 2 diabetes A form of diabetes characterized by insulin resistance and often associated with obesity. Insulin therapy can be used but is often not required.

symptoms—such as unexplained weight loss, exhaustion, blurred vision, tingling in hands and feet, frequent infections, poor wound healing, and impotence— often accompany traditional symptoms.

Type 1 Diabetes

Type 1 diabetes often begins in late childhood, around the age of 8 to 12 years, but can occur at any age. The disease runs in certain families, indicating a clear genetic link. Children usually are admitted to the hospital with abnormally high blood glucose after eating, as well as evidence of ketosis.

The onset of type 1 diabetes is generally associated with decreased release of insulin from the pancreas. As insulin in the blood declines, blood glucose increases, especially after eating. Figure 4-13 shows a typical glucose tolerance curve observed in a patient with this form of diabetes after consuming about 75 grams of glucose. When blood glucose levels are high, the kidneys let excess glucose spill into the urine, resulting in frequent urination of urine high in sugar.

A common clinical method to determine a person's success in controlling blood glucose is to measure glycated (also termed glycosylated) hemoglobin (hemoglobin A1c). Over time, blood glucose attaches to (glycates) hemoglobin in red blood cells and more so when blood glucose remains elevated. A hemoglobin A1c value of over 7% indicates poor blood glucose control. Maintaining near-normal hemoglobin A1c levels (6% or less) greatly reduces the risk of death and developing other diseases in people with diabetes. Elevated blood glucose also leads to glycation of other proteins and fats in the body, forming what are called advanced glycation endproducts (AGEs). These have been shown to be toxic to cells, especially those of the immune system and kidneys.

Most cases of type 1 diabetes begin with an immune system disorder, which causes destruction of the insulin-producing cells in the pancreas. Most likely, a virus or protein foreign to the body sets off the destruction. In response to their damage, the affected pancreatic cells release other proteins, which stimulate a more furious

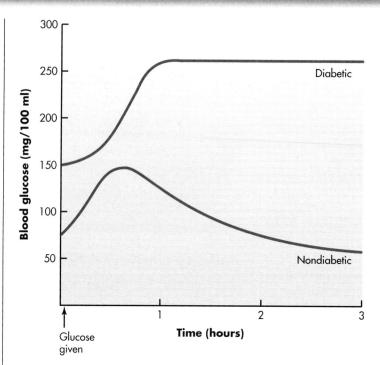

FIGURE 4-13 ▶ Glucose tolerance test. A comparison of blood glucose concentrations in untreated diabetic and healthy nondiabetic persons after consuming a 75 g test load of glucose.

attack. Eventually, the pancreas loses its ability to synthesize insulin, and the clinical stage of the disease begins. Consequently, early treatment to stop the immune-linked destruction in children may be important. Research into this area is ongoing.

Type 1 diabetes is treated primarily by insulin therapy, either with injections two to six times per day or with an insulin pump. The pump dispenses insulin at a steady rate into the body, with greater amounts delivered after each meal. Inhaled forms of insulin also are available. Dietary therapy includes three regular meals and one or more snacks (including one at bedtime) and having a regulated ratio of carbohydrate:protein:fat to maximize insulin action and minimize swings in blood glucose (see Further Reading 2 and 3 for more information on nutrition treatment of diabetes). If one does not eat often enough, the injected insulin can cause a severe drop in blood glucose or hypoglycemia, because it acts on whatever glucose is available. The diet should be moderate in simple carbohydrates, include ample fiber and polyunsaturated fat, but be low in both animal and *trans* fats, supply an amount of calories in balance with needs, and include fish twice a week.

▶ **Symptoms of Diabetes**

The symptoms of diabetes may occur suddenly, and include one or more of the following:

- Extreme thirst
- Frequent urination
- Drowsiness, lethargy
- Sudden vision changes
- Increased appetite
- Sudden weight loss
- Sugar in urine
- Fruity, sweet, or winelike odor on breath
- Heavy, labored breathing
- Stupor, unconsciousness

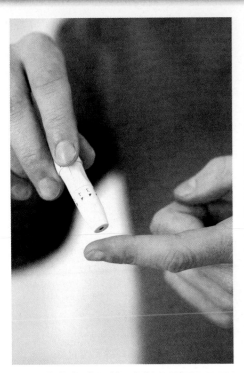

▲ Regularly checking blood glucose is part of diabetes therapy.

MAKING DECISIONS

Are You Prediabetic?

Often people with type 2 diabetes did not develop the disease suddenly. It may develop for years before symptoms are noticed. Prediabetes is a condition in which the concentration of blood glucose has drifts up higher than normal. By the time symptoms are noticeable, organs and tissues may be damaged. Simple tests of your fasting blood glucose level can determine if you are prediabetic. Early detection of diabetes risk can help prevent diabetes if you make lifestyle changes. If you have a family history of diabetes or if your habits (being physically inactive and overweight, and having a poor diet) put you at risk, it is fortunate to discover if your blood glucose is still in the prediabetic stage. Prediabetes, also called impaired fasting glucose, is diagnosed if the fasting blood glucose is 100–125 mg/dL.

Meeting magnesium needs is also helpful, as well as a moderate intake of coffee.

If a high carbohydrate intake raises triglycerides and cholesterol in the blood beyond desired ranges, carbohydrate intake can be reduced and replaced with unsaturated fat. Surprisingly, this change tends to reduce blood triglycerides and cholesterol. Chapter 5 discusses how to implement such a diet (as well as when certain related medications may be beneficial). Some consumption of sugars with meals is fine, as long as blood glucose regulation is preserved and the sugars replace other carbohydrates in the meal, so that undesirable weight gain does not take place.

The latest evidence suggests that diabetes essentially guarantees development of cardiovascular disease. Because people with diabetes (type 1, as well as type 2) are at a high risk for cardiovascular disease and related heart attacks, they should take an aspirin each day (generally 80 to 160 milligrams per day) if their physicians find no reason not to do so. Blood cholesterol lowering medications also may be prescribed. As discussed in Chapter 5, these practices reduce the risk of heart attack.

The hormone imbalances that occur in people with untreated type 1 diabetes—chiefly, not enough insulin—lead to mobilization of body fat, taken up by liver cells. Ketosis is the result because the fat is partially broken down to ketone bodies. Ketone bodies can rise excessively in the blood, eventually forcing ketone bodies into the urine. These pull sodium and potassium ions and water with them into the urine. This series of events also causes frequent urination and can contribute to a chain reaction that eventually leads to dehydration; ion imbalance; coma; and even death, especially in patients with poorly controlled type 1 diabetes. Treatment includes provision of insulin, fluids, and minerals such as sodium and potassium.

In addition to cardiovascular disease, other degenerative complications that result from poor blood glucose regulation, specifically long-term hyperglycemia, include blindness, kidney disease, and deterioration of nerves. The high blood sugar concentration physically deteriorates small blood vessels (capillaries) and nerves. When improper nerve stimulation

occurs in the intestinal tract, intermittent diarrhea and constipation result. Because of nerve deterioration in the extremities, many people with diabetes lose the sensation of pain associated with injuries or infections. They do not have as much pain, so they often delay treatment of hand or foot problems. This delay, combined with a rich environment for bacterial growth (bacteria thrive on glucose) sets the stage for damage and death of tissues in the extremities, sometimes leading to the need for amputation of feet and legs. Current research has shown that the development of blood vessel and nerve complications of diabetes can be slowed with aggressive treatment directed at keeping blood glucose within the normal range. The therapy poses some risks of its own, such as hypoglycemia, so it must be implemented under the close supervision of a physician.

A person with diabetes generally must work closely with a physician and registered dietitian to make the correct alterations in diet and medications and to perform physical activity safely. Physical activity enhances glucose uptake by muscles independent of insulin action, which in turn can lower blood glucose. This outcome is beneficial, but people with type 1 diabetes need to be aware of their blood glucose response to physical activity and compensate appropriately.

Type 2 Diabetes

Type 2 diabetes usually begins after age 40. This is the most common type of diabetes, accounting for about 90% of the cases diagnosed in North America. Minority populations such as Latino/Hispanic Americans, African Americans, Asian Americans, Native Americans, and those from Pacific Islands are at particular risk. As noted in the introduction, the overall number of people affected also is on the rise, primarily because of widespread inactivity and obesity in our population. There has been a substantial increase in type 2 diabetes in children, due mostly to an increase in overweight in this population (coupled with limited physical activity). Type 2 diabetes is also genetically linked, so family history is an important risk factor. However, the initial problem is not with the insulin-secreting cells of the pancreas. Instead, type 2 diabetes arises when the insulin receptors on the cell surfaces of certain body tissues, especially muscle tissue, become insulin resistant. In this case, blood glucose is not readily transferred into cells, so the person develops high blood glucose as a result of the glucose remaining in the bloodstream. The pancreas attempts to increase insulin output to compensate, but there is a limit to its ability to do this. Thus, rather than insufficient insulin production, there is an abundance of insulin, particularly during the onset of the disease. As the disease develops, pancreatic function can fail, leading to reduced insulin output. Because of the genetic link for type 2 diabetes, those who have a family history should schedule regular blood glucose tests and be careful to avoid risk factors such as obesity, inactivity, a diet rich in animal and *trans* fats, and simple carbohydrates.

Many cases of type 2 diabetes (about 80%) are associated with obesity (especially with fat located in the abdominal region), but high blood glucose is not directly caused by the obesity. In fact, some lean people also develop this type of diabetes. Obesity associated with oversized adipose cells increases the risk for insulin resistance by the body as more fat is added to these cells during weight gain.

Type 2 diabetes linked to obesity often disappears if the obesity is corrected. Achieving a healthy weight therefore should be a primary goal of treatment, but even limited weight loss can lead to better blood glucose regulation. Although many cases of type 2 diabetes can be relieved by reducing excess adipose tissue stores, many people are not able to lose weight. They remain affected with diabetes and may experience the degenerative complications seen in the type 1 form of the disease. Ketosis, however, is not usually seen in type 2 diabetes. Certain oral medications can also help control blood glucose. Adequate chromium intake is also important for blood glucose regulation (see Chapter 11). Patients with type 2 diabetes may experience decreased effectiveness of their treatments over time resulting in spikes in blood glucose after meals and weight gain. New classes of drugs that mimic gut hormones are helping diabetic patients overcome the chronic

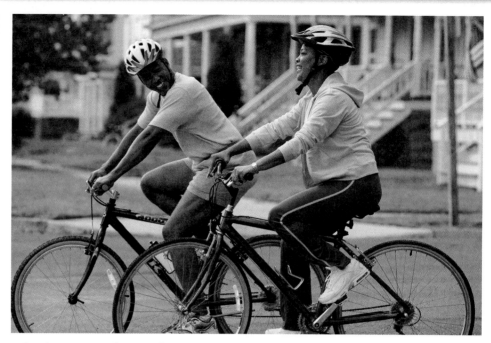

▲ Regular exercise is a key part of a plan to prevent (and control) type 2 diabetes (see Further Reading 8).

problems that conventional treatments alone have been unable to control.

Sometimes it may be necessary to provide insulin injections in type 2 diabetes because nothing else is able to control the disease. (This eventually becomes true in about half of all cases of type 2 diabetes.) Regular physical activity also helps the muscles take up more glucose. And regular meal patterns, with an emphasis on control of calorie intake and consumption of mostly fiber-rich carbohydrates, as well as regular fish intake, is important therapy. Nuts help fulfill the goal of increased fiber consumption. (An almost daily intake of nuts was even shown to reduce the risk of developing type 2 diabetes in one study.) Some sugar consumption is fine with meals, but again these must be substituted for other carbohydrates, not simply added to the meal plan. Distributing carbohydrates throughout the day is also important, as this helps minimize the high and low swings in blood glucose concentrations. Moderate alcohol use is acceptable (1 serving per day) and has been shown to substantially reduce heart attack risk in people with type 2 diabetes. Still, the person must be warned that alcohol can lead to hypoglycemia and that regular testing for this possibility is necessary. And, as mentioned

before, meeting magnesium needs and moderate coffee intake are also helpful.

People with type 2 diabetes who have high blood triglycerides should moderate their carbohydrate intake and increase their intake of unsaturated fat and fiber, as noted earlier for people with type 1 diabetes.

Hypoglycemia

As noted earlier, people with diabetes who are taking insulin sometimes have hypoglycemia if they do not eat frequently enough. Hypoglycemia can also develop in nondiabetic individuals. The two common forms of nondiabetic hypoglycemia are termed *reactive* and *fasting*.

Reactive hypoglycemia occurs 2 to 4 hours after eating a meal, especially a meal high in simple sugars. It results

▶ For more information on diabetes, consult the following websites: **www.diabetes.org** and **www.ndep.nih.gov**.

reactive hypoglycemia Low blood glucose that follows a meal high in simple sugars, with corresponding symptoms of irritability, headache, nervousness, sweating, and confusion; also called *postprandial hypoglycemia*.

in irritability, nervousness, headache, sweating, and confusion. The cause of reactive hypoglycemia is unclear, but it may be overproduction of insulin by the pancreas in response to rising blood glucose. In **fasting hypoglycemia**, blood glucose falls to low concentrations after fasting for about 8 hours to 1 day. It usually is caused by pancreatic cancer, which may lead to excessive insulin secretion. This form of hypoglycemia is rare.

The diagnosis of hypoglycemia requires the simultaneous presence of low blood glucose and the typical hypoglycemic symptoms. Blood glucose of 40 to

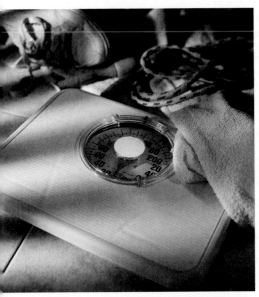

▲ Decreasing body weight and increasing physical activity are interventions to help prevent metabolic syndrome.

fasting hypoglycemia Low blood glucose that follows about a day of fasting.

metabolic syndrome A condition in which a person has poor blood glucose regulation, hypertension, increased blood triglycerides, and other health problems. This condition is usually accompanied by obesity, lack of physical activity, and a diet high in refined carbohydrates. Also called Syndrome X.

50 milligrams per 100 milliliters is suggestive, but just having low blood glucose after eating is not enough evidence to make the diagnosis of hypoglycemia. Although many people think they have hypoglycemia, few actually do.

It is normal for healthy people to have some hypoglycemic symptoms, such as irritability, headache, and shakiness, if they have not eaten for a prolonged period. If you sometimes have symptoms of hypoglycemia, you need to eat regular meals, make sure you have some protein and fat in each meal, and eat complex carbohydrates with ample soluble fiber. Avoid meals or snacks that contain little more than simple carbohydrates. This standard nutrition therapy is one we all could follow. If symptoms continue, try small protein-containing snacks or fruits and juice between meals. Fat, protein, and viscous fiber in the diet tend to moderate swings in blood glucose. Last, moderate caffeine and alcohol intake.

Metabolic Syndrome

Metabolic syndrome, also known as Syndrome X, is characterized by the occurrence of several risk factors for diabetes and cardiovascular disease. The precise definition and criteria for diagnosis have recently been debated by health scholars (see Further Readings 7 and 11). A person with metabolic syndrome has several or all of the following conditions: abdominal obesity (accumulation of fat around and within the midsection), high blood triglycerides, low HDL or "good" cholesterol, hypertension, high fasting blood glucose, increased blood clotting, and increased inflammation (Fig. 4-14). Each aspect of metabolic syndrome is a unique health problem with its own treatment. In metabolic syndrome, however, these risk factors are clustered together, making a person twice as likely to develop cardiovascular disease and five times more likely to develop diabetes.

It is generally accepted that one key element unifies all the aspects of metabolic syndrome: *insulin resistance.* As you learned in this chapter, insulin is a hormone that directs tissues to pull glucose out of the blood and into cells for storage or fuel. With insulin resistance, the pancreas

produces plenty of insulin, but the cells of the body do not respond to it effectively. Instead, excess glucose stays in the bloodstream. For a while the pancreas may be able to compensate for the resistance of cells to insulin by overproducing insulin. Over time, however, the pancreas is unable to keep up the accelerated insulin production and blood glucose levels remain elevated. With metabolic syndrome, blood glucose is not high enough to be classified as diabetes ($\geq$ 126 milligrams per deciliter), but without intervention, it is likely to get worse and eventually lead to diabetes.

Genetics and aging contribute to the development of insulin resistance and the other elements of metabolic syndrome, but environmental factors such as diet and activity play an important role. Obesity, particularly abdominal obesity, is highly related to insulin resistance. More than half of adults in the United States are overweight, 30% are obese, and these numbers continue to climb year after year. Increases in body weight among children and adolescents are of great concern because it places them at high risk for these health problems. This increase in body weight has precipitated a dramatic surge in cardiovascular disease and diabetes risk—an estimated 50 million Americans now have metabolic syndrome.

There is controversy among health professionals over whether to treat each risk factor uniquely or to attempt to integrate therapies to treat all the risk factors simultaneously. For example, the chief culprits contributing to the high blood triglycerides of metabolic syndrome are excessively large meals full of foods rich in simple sugars and refined starches and low in fiber, coupled with little physical activity. Nutrition and lifestyle changes are key strategies in addressing all of the unhealthy conditions of metabolic syndrome as a whole. Suggested interventions include:

- Decrease body weight. Even small improvements (e.g., 5% weight loss) for overweight and obese individuals can lessen disease risk. The most successful weight-loss and weight-maintenance programs include moderate dietary restriction combined with physical activity.

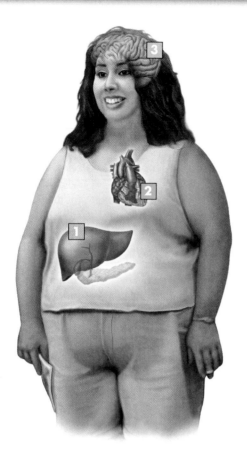

Metabolic Syndrome Risk Indicators

- **High blood pressure**
  130/85 mmHg or higher

- **Low HDL cholesterol**
  - Men with HDL level less than 40 mg/dl
  - Women with HDL level less than 50 mg/dl

- **Elevated glucose**
  Fasting level of 100 mg/dl or higher

- **Elevated triglycerides (blood fat)**
  150 mg/dl or higher

- **Abdominal obesity**
  - Men with waist circumference greater than 40 inches
  - Women with waist circumference greater than 35 inches

Medical Conditions Related to Metabolic Syndrome

1 Type 2 diabetes
Over time, insulin resistance can increase blood glucose levels, which can lead to type 2 diabetes.

2 Coronary artery disease
Elevated blood pressure and cholesterol levels can cause plaque to build up inside coronary arteries, which may eventually lead to a heart attack.

3 Stroke
Plaque buildup in arteries can lead to blood clots that prevent blood flow to the brain, causing damage to brain tissue.

FIGURE 4-14 ▶ For a patient to be diagnosed with metabolic syndrome, he or she must have three of the five risk factors listed above.

- Increase physical activity. To alleviate risks for chronic diseases, the 2010 Dietary Guidelines for Americans include a recommendation to do the equivalent of 150 minutes of moderate-intensity physical activity each week.
- Choose healthy fats. Limiting intakes of total fat, saturated fat, and *trans* fat are generally recommended for improving blood lipids. Including omega-3 fats, such as those found in fish and nuts, is another way to combat chronic disease.
- For those with particularly high risk for cardiovascular disease, medications may be warranted.

Case Study Problems with Milk Intake

Myeshia is a 19-year-old African-American female who recently read about the health benefits of calcium and decided to increase her intake of dairy products. To start, she drank a cup of 1% milk at lunch. Not long afterward, she experienced bloating, cramping, and increased gas production. She suspected that the culprit of this pain was the milk she consumed, especially because her parents and her sister complain of the same problem. She wanted to determine if other milk products were, in fact, the cause of her discomfort so the next day she substituted a cup of yogurt for the glass of milk at lunch. Subsequently, she did not have any pain.

Answer the following questions, and check your response in Appendix A.

1. Why did Myeshia believe that she was sensitive to milk?
2. What component of milk is likely causing the problems that Myeshia experiences after drinking milk?
3. Why does this component cause intestinal discomfort in some individuals?
4. What is the name of this condition?
5. What groups of people are most likely to experience this condition?
6. Why did consuming yogurt not cause the same effects for Myeshia?
7. Are there any other products on the market that can replace regular milk or otherwise alleviate symptoms for individuals with this problem?
8. Can people with this condition ever drink regular milk?
9. What nutrients may be inadequate in the diet if dairy products are not consumed?
10. Why do some individuals have trouble tolerating milk products during or immediately after an intestinal viral infection?

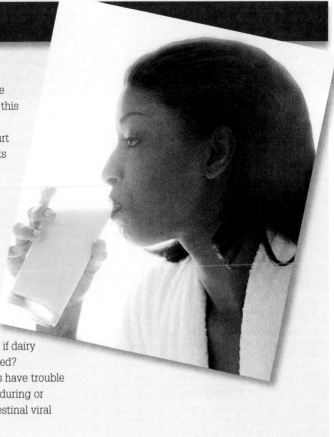

Summary (Numbers refer to numbered sections in the chapter.)

4.1 Carbohydrates are created in plants through photosynthesis. They are our main fuel source for body cells. Some carbohydrates promote health more than others.

4.2 The common monosaccharides in food are glucose, fructose, and galactose. Once these are absorbed from the small intestine and delivered to the liver, much of the fructose and galactose is converted to glucose.

The major disaccharides are sucrose (glucose + fructose), maltose (glucose + glucose), and lactose (glucose + galactose). When digested, these yield their component monosaccharides.

4.3 One major group of polysaccharides consists of storage forms of glucose: starches in plants and glycogen in humans. These can be broken down by human digestive enzymes, releasing the glucose units. The main plant starches—straight-chain amylose and branched-chain amylopectin—are digested by enzymes in the mouth and small intestine. In humans,

glycogen is synthesized in the liver and muscle tissue from glucose. Under the influence of hormones, liver glycogen is readily broken down to glucose, which can enter the bloodstream.

4.4 Fiber is composed primarily of the polysaccharides cellulose, hemicellulose, pectin, gum, and mucilage, as well as the noncarbohydrate lignins. These substances are not broken down by human digestive enzymes. However, soluble (also called viscous) fiber is fermented by bacteria in the large intestine.

4.5 Table sugar, honey, jelly, fruit, and plain baked potatoes are some of the most concentrated sources of carbohydrates. Other high-carbohydrate foods, such as pie and fat-free milk, are diluted by either fat or protein. Nutritive sweeteners in food include sucrose, high-fructose corn syrup, brown sugar, and maple syrup. Several alternative sweeteners are approved for use

by FDA: saccharin, aspartame, sucralose, neotame, acesulfame-K, and tagatose.

4.6 Some starch digestion occurs in the mouth. Carbohydrate digestion is completed in the small intestine. Some plant fibers are digested by the bacteria present in the large intestine; undigested plant fibers become part of the feces. Monosaccharides in the intestinal contents mostly follow an active absorption process. They are then transported via the portal vein that leads directly to the liver.

The ability to digest large amounts of lactose often diminishes with age. People in some ethnic groups are especially affected. This condition often develops early in childhood and is referred to as *lactose maldigestion*. Undigested lactose travels to the large intestine, resulting in such symptoms as abdominal gas, pain, and diarrhea. Most people with lactose maldigestion can tolerate cheese, yogurt, and moderate amounts of milk.

4.7 Carbohydrates provide calories (on average, 4 kcal per gram), protect against wasteful breakdown of food and body protein, and prevent ketosis. The RDA for carbohydrate is 130 grams per day. If carbohydrate intake is inadequate for the body's needs, protein is metabolized to provide glucose for energy needs. However, the price is loss of body protein, ketosis, and eventually a general body weakening. For this reason, low-carbohydrate diets are not recommended for extended periods.

Blood glucose concentration is regulated within a narrow range of 70 to 99 mg/dl. Insulin and glucagon are hormones that control blood glucose concentration. When we eat a meal, insulin promotes glucose uptake by cells. When fasting, glucagon promotes glucose release from glycogen stores in the liver.

4.8 Insoluble (also called nonfermentable) fiber provides mass to the feces, thus easing elimination. In high doses, soluble fiber can help control blood glucose in diabetic people and lower blood cholesterol.

4.9 Diets high in complex carbohydrates are encouraged as a replacement for high-fat diets. A goal of about half of calories as complex carbohydrates is a good one, with about 45% to 65% of total calories coming from carbohydrates in general. Foods to consume are whole-grain cereal products, pasta, legumes, fruits, and vegetables. Many of these foods are rich in fiber.

4.10 Moderating sugar intake, especially between meals, reduces the risk of dental caries. Alternative sweeteners, such as aspartame, aid in reducing intake of sugars.

N&YH Diabetes is characterized by a persistent high blood glucose concentration. A healthy diet and regular physical activity are helpful in treating both type 1 and type 2 diabetes. Insulin is the main medication employed—it is required in type 1 diabetes and may be used in type 2 diabetes.

Check Your Knowledge (Answers to the following questions are below.)

1. Dietary fiber
   a. raises blood cholesterol levels.
   b. speeds up transit time for food through the digestive tract.
   c. causes diverticulosis.
   d. causes constipation.

2. When the pancreas detects excess glucose, it releases the
   a. enzyme amylase.
   b. monosaccharide glucose.
   c. hormone insulin.
   d. hormone glucagon.

3. Cellulose is a(n)
   a. indigestible fiber.
   b. simple carbohydrate.
   c. energy-yielding nutrient.
   d. animal polysaccharide.

4. Digested white sugar is broken into _____ and _____.
   a. glucose, lactose
   b. glucose, fructose

   c. sucrose, maltose
   d. fructose, sucrose

5. Starch is a
   a. complex carbohydrate.
   b. fiber.
   c. simple carbohydrate.
   d. gluten.

6. Fiber content of the diet can be increased by adding
   a. fresh fruits.
   b. fish and poultry.
   c. eggs.
   d. whole grains and cereals.
   e. Both a and d.

7. Which form of diabetes is most common?
   a. type 1
   b. type 2
   c. type 3
   d. gestational

8. The recommended daily intake for fiber is approximately _____ grams.
   a. 5   c. 100
   b. 30   d. 450

9. Glucose, galactose, and fructose are
   a. disaccharides.
   b. sugar alcohols.
   c. monosaccharides.
   d. polysaccharides.

10. One of the components of metabolic syndrome is
    a. obesity.
    b. diabetes.
    c. low blood sugar.
    d. low blood pressure.

Answer Key: 1. b (LO 4.6), 2. c (LO 4.5), 3. a (LO 4.1), 4. b (LO 4.1), 5. a (LO 4.1), 6. e (LO 4.2), 7. b (LO 4.8), 8. b (LO 4.7), 9. c (LO 4.1), 10. b (LO 4.8)

Study Questions (Numbers refer to Learning Outcomes)

1. Why do we need carbohydrates in the diet? **(LO 4.3)**

2. What are the three major monosaccharides and the three major disaccharides? Describe how each plays a part in the human diet. **(LO 4.3)**

3. Why are some foods that are high in carbohydrates, such as cookies and fat-free milk, not considered to be concentrated sources of carbohydrates? **(LO 4.3)**

4. Describe the digestion of the various types of carbohydrates in the body. **(LO 4.3)**

5. Describe the reason why some people are unable to tolerate high intakes of milk. **(LO 4.3)**

6. List three alternatives to simple sugars for adding sweetness to the diet. **(LO 4.3)**

7. Outline the basic steps in blood glucose regulation, including the roles of insulin and glucagon. **(LO 4.3)**

8. What are the important roles that fiber plays in the diet? **(LO 4.3)**

9. Summarize current carbohydrate intake recommendations. **(LO 4.3)**

10. What, if any, are the proven ill effects of sugar in the diet? **(LO 4.3)**

What Would You Choose Recommendations

It is smart to reach for a carbohydrate-containing beverage when needing quick energy. Some of us also rely on caffeine in drinks to give us a boost. Many beverages on the market contain high concentrations of carbohydrate as "added sugar." This added sugar has recently been the subject of many debates because the consumption of added sugars, especially high-fructose corn syrup (HFCS), has been on the rise since 1970 and excessive sugar intake has been linked to several adverse health conditions. The major sources of added sugars are sodas, energy drinks, and sports drinks (review Fig. 4-12). Sugar intake has been of concern based on total consumption and source of the sugar.

Does the source of the added sugar matter? As we discussed in Chapter 4, the glucose and fructose in HFCS exist in free form, compared to their bound form in cane sugar, sucrose. Sucrose is quickly and completely digested to glucose and fructose in the small intestine so that nearly equal amounts of glucose and fructose are being absorbed from beverages containing HFCS and pure cane sugar. Once absorbed, fructose is more easily converted to and stored as fat than glucose. Researchers speculate that the extra 5% of fructose in HFCS may be responsible for increased body fatness. Also, fructose does not stimulate the release of chemical signals that help to regulate appetite, in the same way glucose does. Changes in appetite can dramatically affect how much of a particular sweetener is consumed. It is still unclear whether altering the type of sweetener in soft drinks will impact our nation's obesity epidemic.

The larger issue here is the abundance of empty calories supplied by soft drinks—regardless of whether these calories come from HFCS or pure cane sugar (sucrose). HFCS represents nearly 100% of sweeteners in all soft drinks, and since soft drink consumption has skyrocketed, so has HFCS consumption. Studies show that liquid calories do not promote satiety in the same way that food calories do. In other words, consuming 250 kcal of cola does not mean that you will feel full enough to eat one less slice of pizza to compensate for those extra kcal. Excess calories from any source will lead to weight gain over time.

Clearly, portion size is an issue. A 20-ounce bottle of regular cola contains about 68 grams (about 15 teaspoons) of sweeteners. This means that a soft drink sweetened with HFCS has 37 grams of fructose compared to 34 grams in a 20-ounce soft drink made with pure cane sugar. Both types of soft drink provide about 250 kcal. Is 3 grams of fructose a big deal? In terms of a soft drink, a 12-ounce soda, such as the Jones Root Beer Soda, will have proportionally less sugar (48 grams) due to its smaller volume. If you consume one soft drink per day or less, the type of sweetener is not likely to make a big difference. If you consume several soft drinks per day, you would be better off choosing a beverage that does not contain calories, such as diet cola or water.

Beverages, such as Coke Zero®, with artificial sweeteners such as aspartame, typically are calorie-free and therefore provide you with no energy when you need a boost. You may feel a temporary lift from the caffeine in some of these products. Water is the perfect drink to restore fluid losses and prevent dehydration but also contains no calories for energy.

Your best choice when needing a quick energy boost in this case is the low-fat chocolate milk. The chocolate milk not only

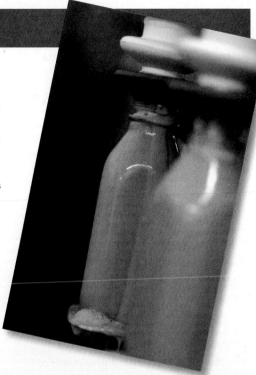

▲ Chocolate milk is a very nutritious beverage that provides protein, vitamins, and minerals, along with calories.

provides less sugar than the sodas on our list but is also the best source of total nutrition. Most convenience stores sell chocolate milk in pint bottles or ½-pint (8-ounce) cartons (similar to those served in school cafeterias). The 8-ounce carton of chocolate milk provides a good amount of calories (150 kcal) as well as 8 grams of protein, 2.5 grams of fat, and 25 grams of sugar. It also provides calcium (290 mg), vitamin A (490 IU), and vitamin D (2.8 micrograms), as well as other vitamins and minerals. A pint bottle (16 ounces) would provide twice the amount of calories and other nutrients. In addition, the chocolate provides a source of caffeine that you may be looking for.

Further Readings

1. ADA Reports: Position of the American Dietetic Association: Use of nutritive and nonnutritive sweeteners. *Journal of the American Dietetic Association* 104:225, 2004.

   When currently recommended diet practices are met, such as the Dietary Guidelines for Americans, use of some nutritive and nonnutritive sweeteners is acceptable. The text of the article explores in detail both classes of sweeteners, in turn supporting this overall conclusion.

2. American Diabetes Association: Nutrition recommendations and interventions for diabetes: A position statement of the American Diabetes Association. *Diabetes Care* 31 (suppl 1):S61, 2008.

   This article provides a comprehensive look at the treatment of diabetes. Goals for therapy and medical tools to help reach those goals are highlighted.

3. American Diabetes Association and American Dietetic Association: *Choose your foods: Exchange lists for diabetes.* 2008.

   This update of a booklet that has been in existence for more than 50 years is used as the basis for nutrition education for diabetes meal planning. Foods are grouped into general categories (or lists) that, per serving size, are similar in macronutrients and calories. Changes have been made so they are easier to use and foods within the lists have been updated.

4. Bray GA and others: Consumption of high-fructose corn syrup in beverages may play a role in the epidemic of obesity. *American Journal of Clinical Nutrition,* 79(4):537, 2004.

   The intake of high-fructose corn syrup (HFCS) was studied and compared to the development of obesity. The increase in HFCS use has paralleled the increase in obesity. Although differences in the digestion, absorption, and metabolism of fructose compared to glucose have been suggested as explanations for the relationship between HFCS and obesity, studies have been unable to separate the effects of the widely consumed sweetener from the impact of other environmental factors.

5. Cowie CC and others: Prevalence of diabetes and impaired fasting glucose in adults in the U.S. population. *Diabetes Care* 29:1263, 2006.

   The results of this study of the National Health And Nutrition Examination Survey (NHANES) suggest that 73 million Americans have diabetes or are at risk based on higher-than-normal blood glucose levels. The prevalence of diagnosed diabetes increased significantly over the last decade, and minority groups remain disproportionately affected. The overall prevalence of total diabetes in 1999–2002 was 9.3% (19.3 million), consisting of 6.5% diagnosed and 2.8% undiagnosed.

   The prevalence of diagnosed diabetes rose from 5.1% in 1988–1994 to 6.5% in 1999–2002. The prevalence of total diabetes was much greater (21.6%) in older individuals aged ≥ 65 years. Diagnosed diabetes was twice as prevalent in non-Hispanic blacks and Mexican-Americans compared with non-Hispanic whites.

6. Food and Nutrition Board: *Dietary reference intakes for energy, carbohydrate, fiber, fat, fatty acids, cholesterol, protein, and amino acids.* Washington, DC: National Academy Press, 2005.

   This report provides the latest guidance for macronutrient intakes. With regard to carbohydrate, the RDA has been set at 130 grams per day. Carbohydrate intake should range from 45% to 65% of calorie intake. Sugars added to foods should constitute no more than 25% of calorie intake.

7. Grundy SM: Does a diagnosis of metabolic syndrome have a value in clinical practice? *American Journal of Clinical Nutrition* 83:1248, 2006.

   The metabolic syndrome concept has led to the development of clinical guidelines by the World Health Organization and the National Cholesterol Education Program. These guidelines have been well accepted by medical professionals. This article reviews the new diagnosis of metabolic syndrome and discusses why organizations including the American Diabetes Association and many diabetes specialists have not embraced the clustering of its risk factors.

8. Hayes C, Kriska A: Role of physical activity in diabetes management and prevention. *Journal of the American Dietetic Association* 108:S19, 2008.

   Evidence supporting the important role of physical activity in the prevention and treatment of diabetes has accumulated. Despite the benefits of physical activity, many people are physically inactive. As the prevalence of overweight and obesity, prediabetes, and type 2 diabetes rises, physical inactivity has become an urgent public health concern. This article reviews research about physical activity/exercise in diabetes and summarizes the current exercise recommendations. This information can be used by health professionals to make safe and effective recommendations for integrating physical activity/exercise into plans for individuals with or at risk of developing diabetes.

9. McMillan-Price J and others: Comparison of 4 diets of varying glycemic load on weight loss and cardiovascular risk reduction in overweight and obese young adults. *Archives of Internal Medicine* 166:1466, 2006.

   In this study of 128 overweight or obese young adults, both high-protein and low-glycemic index diets increased body fat loss. Cardiovascular disease risk was decreased best with a high-carbohydrate, low-glycemic index diet.

10. Park Y and others: Dietary fiber intake and risk of colorectal cancer. *Journal of the American Medical Association* 294:2849, 2005.

    In this large analysis of pooled data from 13 prospective studies, dietary fiber was inversely associated with risk of colorectal cancer when data were adjusted for age. However, when other dietary risk factors (red meat, total milk, and alcohol intake) were accounted for, high-dietary fiber intake was not associated with a decreased risk of colorectal cancer. The authors conclude that a diet high in dietary fiber from whole plant foods can still be advised because this has been related to lower risks of other chronic conditions, including heart disease and diabetes.

11. Pastors JG: Metabolic syndrome—is obesity the culprit? *Today's Dietitian* 8(3):12, 2006.

    Metabolic syndrome, especially its link to obesity, has become better understood in recent years. This article reviews the role of obesity, the dilemmas of diagnosis, new diet and activity guidelines, and the need for a combination of therapeutic approaches for metabolic syndrome.

12. Savaiano DA and others: Lactose intolerance symptoms assessed by meta-analysis: A grain of truth that leads to exaggeration. *Journal of Nutrition* 136:1107, 2006.

    An analysis of the results of 21 studies of lactose intolerance revealed that lactose is not a major cause of symptoms for lactose maldigesters after a moderate intake of dairy foods equaling about 1 cup.

13. Slavin J and others: How fiber affects weight regulation. *Food Technology,* p. 34, February 2008.

    High-fiber diets are linked to lower body weight. This article discusses the effect of different fibers on satiety and food intake. Dietary fiber has intrinsic, hormonal, and intestinal effects that decrease food intake by promoting satiety. Examples of these effects include decreased gastric emptying and/or slowed energy and nutrient absorption.

14. Swann L: Educate your brain about whole grain. *Today's Dietitian* 8(6):36, 2006.

    The 2005 Dietary Guidelines recommend 3 or more ounces of whole-grain products per day. This equals about one-half of one's intake from the grain group. Recent surveys, however, have found that only 5% of American adults eat one-half of their grains as whole grains. This article discusses the need to better educate consumers about whole grain including better definitions and ways of measuring these foods.

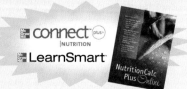

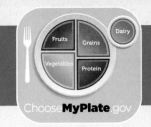

I. Estimate Your Fiber Intake

Review the sample menus shown in Table 4-7. The first menu contains 1600 kcal and 25 grams of fiber (AI for women); the second menu contains 2100 kcal and 38 grams of fiber (AI for men).

TABLE 4-7 Sample Menus Containing 1600 kcal with 25 g of Fiber and 2000 kcal with 38 g of Fiber*

Menu	25 g Fiber			38 g Fiber		
	Serving Size	Carbohydrate Content (g)	Fiber Content (g)	Serving Size	Carbohydrate Content (g)	Fiber Content (g)
Breakfast						
Muesli cereal	1 cup	60	6	1 cup	60	6
Raspberries	½ cup	11	2	½ cup	11	2
Whole-wheat toast	1 slice	13	2	2 slices	26	4
Margarine	1 tsp	0	0	1 tsp	0	0
Orange juice	1 cup	28	0	1 cup	28	0
1% milk	1 cup	24	0	1 cup	24	0
Coffee	1 cup	0	0	1 cup	0	0
Lunch						
Bean and vegetable burrito	2 small	50	4.5	3 small	75	7
Guacamole	¼ cup	5	4	¼ cup	5	4
Monterey Jack cheese	1 oz	0	0	1 oz	0	0
Pear (with skin)	1	25	4	1	25	4
Carrot sticks	—	—	—	¾ cup	6	3
Sparkling water	2 cups	0	0	2 cups	0	0
Dinner						
Grilled chicken (no skin)	3 oz	0	0	3 oz	0	0
Salad	½ cup red cabbage ½ cup romaine ¼ cup peach slices	7	3	½ cup red cabbage ½ cup romaine 1 cup peach slices	19	6
Toasted almonds	—	—	—	½ oz	3	2
Fat-free salad dressing	2 tbsp	0	0	2 tbsp	0	0
1% milk	1 cup	24	0	1 cup	24	0
Total		247	25		306	38

*The overall diet is based on MyPlate Breakdown of approximate energy content: carbohydrate 58%; protein 12%; fat 30%.

To roughly estimate your daily fiber consumption, determine the number of servings that you ate yesterday from each food category listed here. If you are not meeting your needs, how could you do so? Multiply the serving amount by the value listed and then add up the total amount of fiber.

Food	Servings	Grams
Vegetables (serving size: 1 cup raw leafy greens or 1/2 cup other vegetables)	_____ × 2	_____
Fruits (serving size: 1 whole fruit; 1/2 grapefruit; 1/2 cup berries or cubed fruit; 1/4 cup dried fruit)	_____ × 2.5	_____
Beans, lentils, split peas (serving size: 1/2 cup cooked)	_____ × 7	_____
Nuts, seeds (serving size: 1/4 cup; 2 tbsp peanut butter)	_____ × 2.5	_____
Whole grains (serving size: 1 slice whole-wheat bread; 1/2 cup whole-wheat pasta, brown rice, or other whole grain; 1/2 each bran or whole-grain muffin)	_____ × 2.5	_____
Refined grains (serving size: 1 slice bread, 1/2 cup pasta, rice, or other processed grains; and 1/2 each refined bagels or muffins)	_____ × 1	_____
Breakfast cereals (serving size: check package for serving size and amount of fiber per serving)	_____ × grams of fiber per serving	_____
Total Grams of Fiber =		_____

Adapted from Fiber: Strands of protection. *Consumer Reports on Health*, p. 1, August 1999.

How does your total fiber intake for yesterday compare with the general recommendation of 25 to 38 g of fiber per day for women and men, respectively? If you are not meeting your needs, how could you do so?

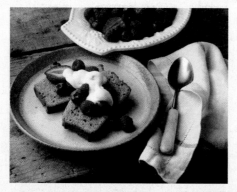

▲ This dessert is an excellent source of fiber from 2 slices of whole-wheat banana bread (7 grams) with ½ cup of berries (1.8 grams) and 2 ounces of yogurt for a total of 8.8 grams of fiber.

II. Can You Choose the Sandwich with the Most Fiber?

Assume the sandwiches on this blackboard are available at your local deli and sandwich shop. All of the sandwiches provide about 350 kcal. The fiber content ranges from about 1 gram to about 7.5 grams. Rank the sandwiches from highest amount of fiber to lowest amount; then check your answers at the bottom of the page.

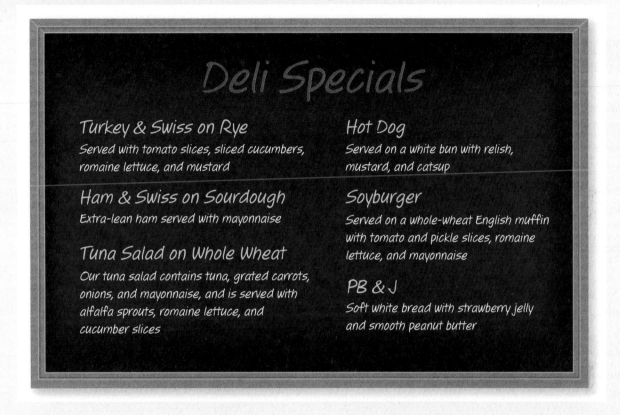

Deli Specials

Turkey & Swiss on Rye
Served with tomato slices, sliced cucumbers, romaine lettuce, and mustard

Ham & Swiss on Sourdough
Extra-lean ham served with mayonnaise

Tuna Salad on Whole Wheat
Our tuna salad contains tuna, grated carrots, onions, and mayonnaise, and is served with alfalfa sprouts, romaine lettuce, and cucumber slices

Hot Dog
Served on a white bun with relish, mustard, and catsup

Soyburger
Served on a whole-wheat English muffin with tomato and pickle slices, romaine lettuce, and mayonnaise

PB & J
Soft white bread with strawberry jelly and smooth peanut butter

Chapter 5 Lipids

Student Learning Outcomes

Chapter 5 is designed to allow you to:

5.1   Understand the common properties of lipids.

5.2   List four classes of lipids (fats) and the role of each in nutritional health. Distinguish between fatty acids and triglycerides.

5.3   Differentiate among saturated, monounsaturated, and polyunsaturated fatty acids in terms of structure and food sources.

5.4   Explain how lipids are digested and absorbed.

5.5   Name the classes of lipoproteins and classify them according to their functions.

5.6   Discuss the implications of various fats, including omega-3 fatty acids, with respect to cardiovascular disease.

5.7   List the function of lipids, including the two essential fatty acids.

5.8   Explain the roles of phospholipids in the body.

5.9   Discuss the functions of cholesterol in the body.

5.10 Explain the recommendations for fat intake.

5.11 Characterize the symptoms of cardiovascular disease and highlight some known risk factors.

What Would You Choose?

Several of your friends are getting together for a cookout and you have volunteered to be the grill master. Hamburgers will be the main "protein" portion of your meal. (Remember the size of that group on MyPlate?) You have heard that eating red meat is bad for your heart. Is all red meat bad for your heart? In the meat section of the grocery store, you see several varieties of ground beef. Which of the following types of ground beef would you choose for heart health?

a   Ground round

b   Ground chuck

c   Ground sirloin

d   Ground beef

 Think about your choice as you read Chapter 5, then see our recommendations at the end of the chapter. To learn more about ground beef choices, check out the Connect site: www.mcgrawhillconnect.com

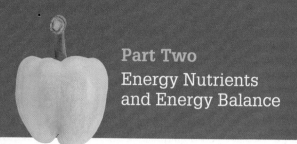

ipids contain more than twice the calories per gram (on average, 9 kcal) as proteins and carbohydrates (on average, 4 kcal each). Consumption of common solid fats also contributes to the risk of cardiovascular disease. As the comic in this chapter suggests, for these reasons, some concern about certain lipids is warranted, but lipids also play vital roles both in the body and in foods. Their presence in the diet is essential to good health, and in general, lipids such as those found in plant oils and fish, such as the salmon pictured here, should comprise 20% to 35% of an adult's total calorie intake.

Let's look at lipids in detail—their forms, functions, metabolism, and food sources. Chapter 5 will also look at the link between various lipids and the major "killer" disease in North America: cardiovascular disease, which involves the heart, including the coronary arteries (coronary heart disease), as well as other arteries in the body.

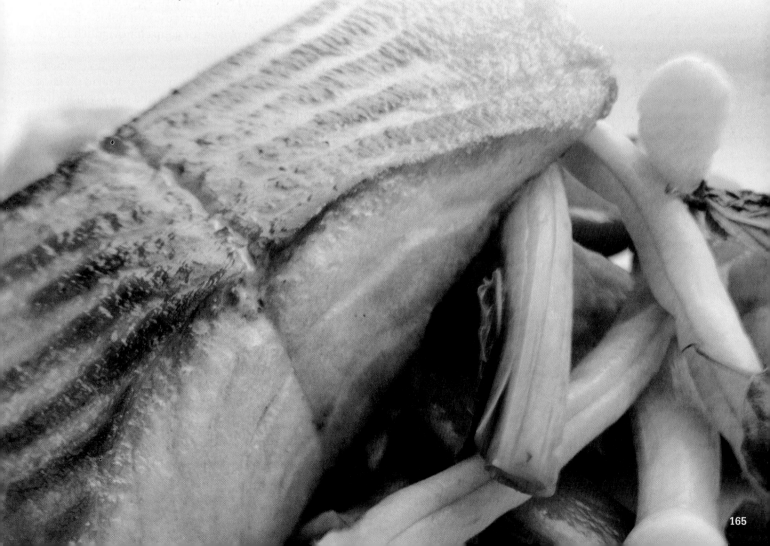

Refresh Your Memory

As you begin your study of lipids in Chapter 5, you may want to review:

- Legal definitions for various label descriptors, such as low fat and fat free in Chapter 2
- The concept of energy density in Chapter 2
- The processes of digestion and absorption in Chapter 3
- The metabolic syndrome in Chapter 4

5.1 Lipids: Common Properties

Humans need very little fat in their diet to maintain health. In fact, the body's need for the essential fatty acids can be met by daily consumption of about 2 to 4 tablespoons of plant oil incorporated into foods and consumption of fatty fish such as salmon or tuna at least twice weekly. If fish is not consumed, the essential fatty acids in canola oil, soybean oil, and walnuts contribute much of the same health benefits as those found in fish. Thus, one could follow a purely vegetarian diet containing about 10% of calories from fat and still maintain health. However, as long as animal fat, cholesterol, and other solid fat are minimized, fat intake can safely be higher than that 10% allotment. The Food and Nutrition Board suggests that fat intake can be as high as 35% of calories consumed for an adult (the Acceptable Macronutrient Distribution Range for fat is 20%–35% of calories consumed for adults). Some experts suggest that an intake as high as 40% of calories is appropriate. After learning more about lipids—fats, oils, and related compounds—in Chapter 5, you can decide for yourself how much fat you want to consume, as well as how to track your daily intake.

Lipids are a diverse group of chemical compounds. They share one main characteristic: They do not readily dissolve in water. Think of an oil and vinegar salad dressing. The oil is not soluble in the water-based vinegar; on standing, the two separate into distinct layers, with oil on top and vinegar on the bottom.

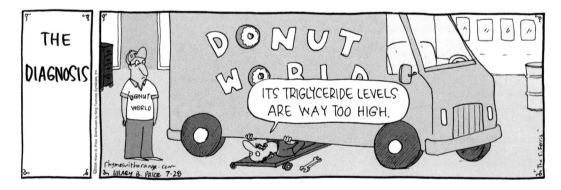

High fat, low fat, no fat—which is best? And why is there such a debate? Would it be easier just to avoid fat altogether? Doesn't a high-fat diet lead to obesity? To cardiovascular disease? Overall, which are the "best" fats, and why are French fries, "donuts," stick margarine, and crackers getting such a bad rap? Chapter 5 provides some answers.

5.2 Lipids: Main Types

The chemical structure of lipids is diverse. Lipids (mostly fats and oils) are composed primarily of the elements carbon and hydrogen; they contain fewer oxygen **atoms** than do carbohydrates. Lipids yield more calories per gram than do carbohydrates—on the average, 9 kcal per gram—because of this difference in composition. **Triglycerides** are the most common type of lipid found in the body and in foods. Each triglyceride molecule consists of three fatty acids bonded to **glycerol. Phospholipids** and **sterols,** including **cholesterol,** are also classified as lipids, although their structures can be quite different from the structure of triglycerides. All of these lipid compounds are described in Chapter 5.

Food experts, such as chefs, call lipids that are solid at room temperature *fats*, and lipids that are liquid *oils*. Most people use the word *fat* to refer to all lipids because they don't realize there is a difference. However, *lipid* is a generic term that includes triglycerides and many other substances. To simplify our discussion, Chapter 5 primarily uses the term *fat*. When necessary for clarity, the name of a specific lipid, such as cholesterol, will be used. This word use is consistent with the way many people use these terms.

Fatty Acids: The Simplest Form of Lipids

In the body and in foods, fatty acids are found in the main form of lipids, triglycerides. A fatty acid is basically a long chain of carbons bonded together and flanked by hydrogens. At one end of the molecule (the alpha end), is an **acid group.** At the other end (the omega end) is a **methyl group** (Fig. 5-1).

Fats in foods are not composed of a single type of fatty acid. Rather, each dietary fat, or triglyceride, is a complex mixture of many different fatty acids, the combination of which provides each food its unique taste and smell.

Fatty acids can be saturated or unsaturated. Chemically speaking, a carbon atom can form four bonds. Within the carbon chain of a fatty acid, the carbons bond to other carbons and to hydrogens. The carbons that make up the chain of a **saturated fatty acid** are all connected to each other by single bonds. This allows for the maximum number of hydrogens to be bound. Just as a sponge can be saturated (full) with water, a saturated fatty acid such as stearic acid is saturated with hydrogen (Fig. 5-1a).

Most fats high in saturated fatty acids, such as animal fats, remain solid at room temperature. A good example is the solid fat surrounding a piece of uncooked steak. Chicken fat, semisolid at room temperature, contains less saturated fat than beef fat. However, in some foods, saturated fats are suspended in liquid, such as the butterfat in whole milk, so the solid nature of these fats at room temperature is less apparent.

If the carbon chain of a fatty acid contains a double bond, those carbons in the chain have fewer bonds to share with hydrogen, and the chain is said to be *unsaturated*. A fatty acid with only one double bond is **monounsaturated** (Fig. 5-1b). Canola and olive oils contain a high percentage of monounsaturated fatty acids. Likewise, if two or more of the bonds between the carbons are double bonds, the fatty acid is even less saturated with hydrogens, and so it is **polyunsaturated** (Fig. 5-1c, d). Corn, soybean, sunflower, and safflower oils are rich in polyunsaturated fatty acids.

Unsaturated fatty acids can exist in two different structural forms, the *cis* and *trans* forms. In their natural form, monounsaturated and polyunsaturated fatty acids usually are in the *cis* form (Fig. 5-2). By definition, the resulting *cis* **fatty acid** has the hydrogens on the same side of the carbon-carbon double bond. During certain types of food processing (discussed later in this chapter), some hydrogens are

triglyceride The major form of lipid in the body and in food. It is composed of three fatty acids bonded to glycerol, an alcohol.

glycerol A three-carbon alcohol used to form triglycerides.

phospholipid Any of a class of fat-related substances that contain phosphorus, fatty acids, and a nitrogen-containing base. The phospholipids are an essential part of every cell.

sterol A compound containing a multi-ring (steroid) structure and a hydroxyl group (–OH). Cholesterol is a typical example.

cholesterol A waxy lipid found in all body cells. It has a structure containing multiple chemical rings that is found only in foods that contain animal products.

saturated fatty acid A fatty acid containing no carbon-carbon double bonds.

monounsaturated fatty acid A fatty acid containing one carbon-carbon double bond.

polyunsaturated fatty acid A fatty acid containing two or more carbon-carbon double bonds.

cis **fatty acid** A form of an unsaturated fatty acid that has the hydrogens lying on the same side of the carbon-carbon double bond.

acid group
$$-\overset{\overset{\displaystyle O}{\|}}{C}-OH$$

methyl group $-CH_3$

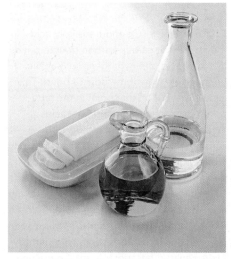

▲ Saturated fats, such as butter, are solid at room temperature, whereas unsaturated fats, such as olive and corn oil, are liquid at room temperature.

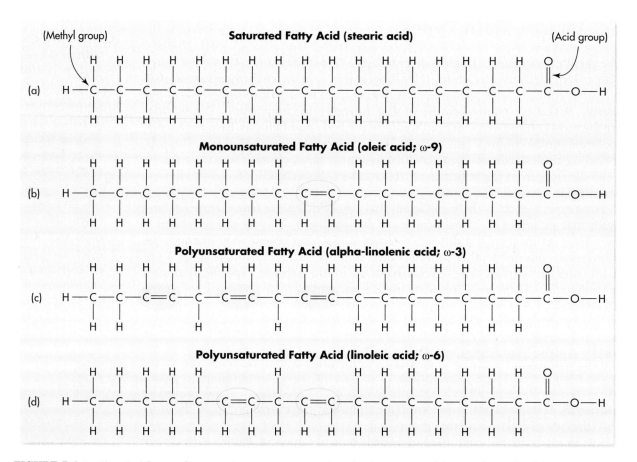

FIGURE 5-1 ▶ Chemical forms of saturated, monounsaturated, and polyunsaturated fatty acids. Each of the depicted fatty acids contains 18 carbons, but they differ from each other in the number and location of double bonds. The double bonds are shaded. The linear shape of saturated fatty acids, as shown in (a), allows them to pack tightly together and so form a solid at room temperature. In contrast, unsaturated fatty acids have "kinks" where double bonds interrupt the carbon chain (see Figure 5-2). Thus, unsaturated fatty acids pack together only loosely, and are usually liquid at room temperature.

FIGURE 5-2 ▶ *Cis* and *trans* fatty acids. In the *cis* form at carbon-carbon double bonds in a fatty acid, the hydrogens (in blue) lie on the same side of the double bond. This causes a "kink" at that point in the fatty acid, typical of unsaturated fatty acids in foods. In contrast, in the *trans* form at carbon-carbon double bonds in a fatty acid, the hydrogens lie across from each other at the double bond. This causes the fatty acid to exist in a linear form, like a saturated fatty acid. *Cis* fatty acids are much more common in foods than *trans* fatty acids. The latter are primarily found in foods containing partially-hydrogenated fats, notably stick margarine, shortening, and deep-fat fried foods.

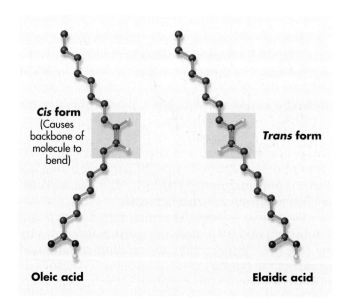

transferred to opposite sides of the carbon-carbon double bond, creating the *trans* form, or a *trans* **fatty acid.** As seen in Figure 5-2, the *cis* bond causes the fatty acid backbone to bend, whereas the *trans* bond allows the backbone to remain straighter. This makes it similar to the shape of a saturated fatty acid. The Food and Nutrition Board suggests limiting intake of *trans* fatty acids in processed foods (also referred to as *trans* fats) as much as possible. Later you will see why.

You may be surprised to learn that some *trans* fatty acids, known as conjugated linoleic acid (CLA), occur naturally. CLA is a family of derivatives of the fatty acid linoleic acid. The bacteria that live in the rumens of some animals (cows, sheep, and goats, for example) produce *trans* fatty acids that eventually appear in foods such as beef, milk, and butter. These naturally occurring *trans* fats are currently under study for possible health benefits, including prevention of cancer, decreasing body fat, and improvement in insulin levels in diabetics. About 20% of *trans* fatty acids in our diets come from this source. Dietary supplements of CLA are available but are highly variable in their quality.

Overall, a fat or an oil is classified as saturated, monounsaturated, or polyunsaturated based on the type of fatty acids present in the greatest concentration (Fig. 5-3). Fats in foods that contain primarily saturated fatty acids are solid at room temperature, especially if the fatty acids have long carbon chains (i.e., a **long-chain fatty acid**), as opposed to shorter versions. In contrast, fats containing primarily polyunsaturated or monounsaturated fatty acids (long chain or shorter) are usually liquid at room temperature. Almost all fatty acids in the body and in foods are long-chain varieties.

An important characteristic of unsaturated fatty acids is the location of the double bonds. If the first double bond starts three carbons from the methyl (omega) end of the fatty acid, it is an **omega-3 (ω-3) fatty acid** (review Fig. 5-1c). If the first double bond is located six carbons from the omega end, it is an **omega-6 (ω-6) fatty acid** (review Fig. 5-1d). Following this scheme, an omega-9 fatty acid has its first double bond starting at the ninth carbon from the methyl end (review Fig. 5-1b). In foods, **alpha-linolenic acid** is the major omega-3 fatty acid; **linoleic acid** is the major omega-6 fatty acid. These are also the **essential fatty acids** we need to consume (more on this in the later section about putting lipids to work in the body). **Oleic acid** is the major omega-9 fatty acid.

Triglycerides

Fats and oils in foods are mostly in the form of triglycerides. The same is true for fats found in body structures. Although some fatty acids are transported in the bloodstream attached to proteins, most fatty acids are formed into triglycerides by cells in the body.

As noted before, triglycerides contain a simple three-carbon alcohol, glycerol, which serves as a backbone for the three attached fatty acids (Fig. 5-4a). Removing one fatty acid from a triglyceride forms a **diglyceride.** Removing two fatty acids from a triglyceride forms a **monoglyceride.** Later you will see that before most dietary fats are absorbed in the small intestine, the two outer fatty acids are typically removed from the triglyceride. This produces a mixture of fatty acids and monoglycerides, absorbed into the intestinal cells. After absorption, the fatty acids and monoglycerides are mostly re-formed into triglycerides.

Phospholipids

Phospholipids are another class of lipid. Like triglycerides, they are built on a backbone of glycerol. However, at least one fatty acid is replaced with a compound containing phosphorus (and often other elements, such as nitrogen) (Fig. 5-4b).

trans fatty acid A form of an unsaturated fatty acid, usually a monounsaturated one when found in food, in which the hydrogens on both carbons forming the double bond lie on opposite sides of that bond.

long-chain fatty acid A fatty acid that contains 12 or more carbons.

omega-3 (ω-3) fatty acid An unsaturated fatty acid with the first double bond on the third carbon from the methyl end (—CH₃).

omega-6 (ω-6) fatty acid An unsaturated fatty acid with the first double bond on the sixth carbon from the methyl end (—CH₃).

alpha-linolenic acid An essential omega-3 fatty acid with 18 carbons and three double bonds.

linoleic acid An essential omega-6 fatty acid with 18 carbons and two double bonds.

essential fatty acids Fatty acids that must be supplied by the diet to maintain health. Currently, only linoleic acid and alpha-linolenic acid are classified as essential.

oleic acid An omega-9 fatty acid with 18 carbons and one double bond.

diglyceride A breakdown product of a triglyceride consisting of two fatty acids bonded to a glycerol backbone.

monoglyceride A breakdown product of a triglyceride consisting of one fatty acid attached to a glycerol backbone.

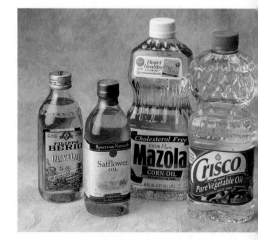

▲ Plant oils vary in their content of specific fatty acids. Oils similar in appearance may vary significantly in fatty acid composition. Olive and canola oils are rich in monounsaturated fat; olive oil has been awarded much attention in recent years. Canola oil, however, is a much less expensive choice of monounsaturated fat. Safflower oil is rich in polyunsaturated fat.

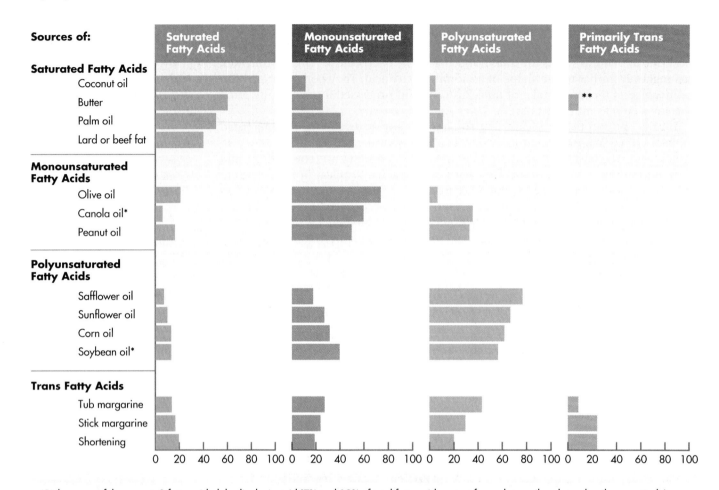

*Rich source of the omega-3 fatty acid alpha-linolenic acid (7% and 12% of total fatty acid content for soybean oil and canola oil, respectively).

**The natural *trans* fatty acids in butter are not harmful and may even have health-promoting properties, such as preventing certain forms of cancer.

FIGURE 5-3 ▶ Saturated, monounsaturated, polyunsaturated, and *trans* fatty acid composition of common fats and oils (expressed as % of all fatty acids in the product).

lecithin A group of compounds that are major components of cell membranes.

Many types of phospholipids exist in the body, especially in the brain. They form important parts of cell membranes. **Lecithin** is a common example of a phospholipid. Various forms are found in body cells and they participate in fat digestion, absorption, and transport. The body is able to produce all the phospholipids it needs. Even though lecithin is sold as a dietary supplement and is present as an additive in many foods, phospholipids such as this one are not essential components of the diet.

Sterols

Sterols are a class of lipids with a characteristic multi-ringed structure that makes them different from the other lipids already discussed (Fig. 5-4c). The most common example of a sterol is cholesterol. This waxy substance doesn't look like a triglyceride—it doesn't have a glycerol backbone or any fatty acids. Still, because it doesn't readily dissolve in water, it is a lipid. Among other functions, cholesterol is used to form certain hormones and bile acids and is incorporated into cell structures. The body can make all the cholesterol it needs.

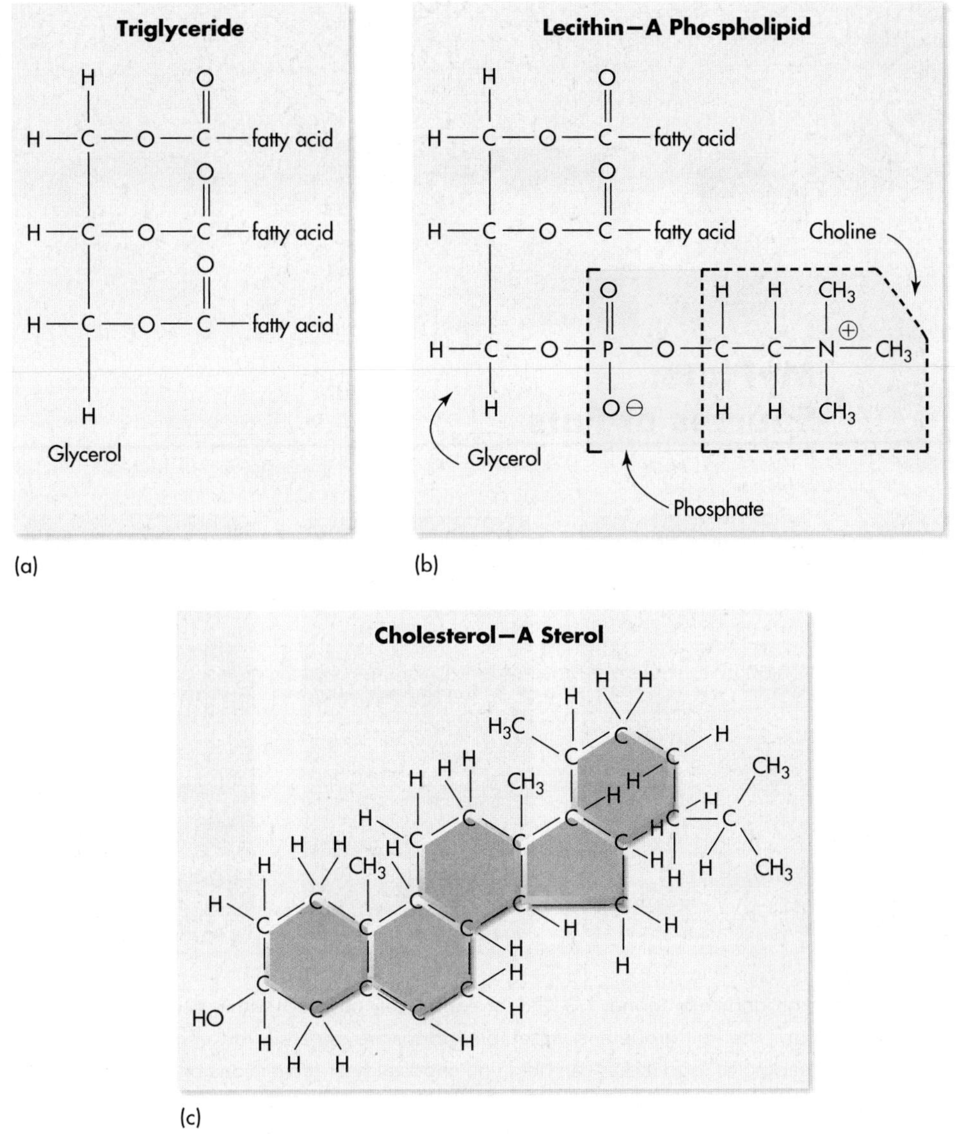

FIGURE 5-4 ▶ Chemical forms of common lipids: (a) triglyceride, (b) phospholipid (in this case, lecithin), and (c) sterol (in this case, cholesterol).

CONCEPT CHECK

Lipids are a group of compounds that do not dissolve readily in water. Included in this group are fatty acids, triglycerides, phospholipids, and sterols. Fatty acids can be distinguished from one another by the length of the carbon skeleton and the number and position of double bonds along that skeleton. Saturated fatty acids contain no double bonds within their carbon skeleton; that is, they are fully saturated with hydrogens. Monounsaturated fatty acids contain one carbon-carbon double bond, and polyunsaturated fatty acids contain two or more of these bonds. Certain omega-3 and omega-6 fatty acids are essential in the human diet.

Triglycerides are the major form of fat in the body and in foods. These consist of three fatty acids bonded to a glycerol backbone. Phospholipids are similar to triglycerides in structure, but at least one fatty acid is replaced by another compound containing phosphorus. Phospholipids play an important structural role in cell membranes. Sterols, another class of lipids, do not resemble either triglycerides or phospholipids, but instead have a multi-ringed structure. Cholesterol, one example of a sterol, forms parts of cells, some hormones, and bile acids. Whereas certain essential fatty acids (as components of triglycerides) are needed in the diet, the body produces all the triglycerides, phospholipids, and cholesterol it needs. Next we will discuss the sources of fat in foods (Fig. 5-5).

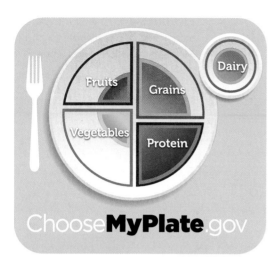
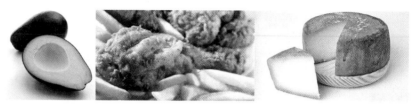

**MyPlate:
Sources of Fats**

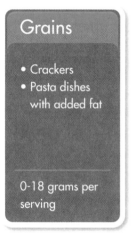
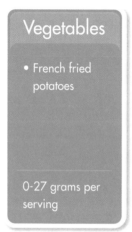
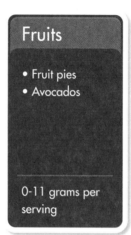
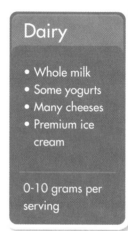
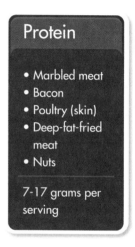

Grains
- Crackers
- Pasta dishes with added fat

0-18 grams per serving

Vegetables
- French fried potatoes

0-27 grams per serving

Fruits
- Fruit pies
- Avocados

0-11 grams per serving

Dairy
- Whole milk
- Some yogurts
- Many cheeses
- Premium ice cream

0-10 grams per serving

Protein
- Marbled meat
- Bacon
- Poultry (skin)
- Deep-fat-fried meat
- Nuts

7-17 grams per serving

FIGURE 5-5 ▶ Sources of fats from MyPlate. The fill of the background color (none, 1/3, 2/3, or completely covered) within each group in the plate indicates the average nutrient density for fat in that group. The fruit group and vegetable groups are generally low in fat. In the other groups, both high-fat and low-fat choices are available. Careful reading of food labels can help you choose lower-fat versions of some foods. In general, any type of frying adds significant amounts of fat to a product, as with French fries and fried chicken. With regard to physical activity, fats are a key fuel in prolonged events, such as long-distance cycling, long-distance running, and prolonged slow to brisk walking.

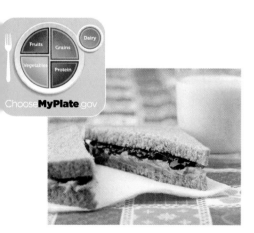

▲ This peanut butter (**protein**) and jelly (**fruit**) sandwich on whole-grain bread (**grain**) with low-fat milk (**dairy**) follows **MyPlate** guidelines well and provides a healthy source of plant fat from the peanut butter. Which section are we missing?

5.3 Fats and Oils in Foods

Lipids in the form of triglycerides are abundant in the North American diet. The foods highest in fat (and therefore energy dense) include salad oils and spreads such as butter, margarine, and mayonnaise. All of these foods contain close to 100% of calories as fat. In reduced-fat margarines, water replaces some of the fat. Whereas regular margarines are 80% fat by weight (11 grams per tablespoon), some reduced-fat margarines are as low as 30% fat by weight (4 grams per tablespoon). When used in recipes, the extra water added to these margarines can cause texture and volume changes in the finished product. Cookbooks can suggest alterations in recipes to compensate for the increased water content of these products.

Still considering the overall fat content, whole foods highest in fat include nuts, bologna, avocados, and bacon, which have about 80% of calories as fat. Next, peanut butter and cheddar cheese have about 75%. Marbled steak and hamburgers (ground chuck) have about 60%, and chocolate bars, ice cream, doughnuts, and whole milk have about 50% of calories as fat. Eggs, pumpkin pie, and cupcakes have 35%, as do lean cuts of meat, such as top round (and ground round) and sirloin. Bread contains about 15%. Finally, foods such as cornflakes, sugar, and fat-free milk have essentially no fat. Figure 5-6 shows examples of food sources of fat. Label reading is necessary to determine the true fat content of food.

The type of fat in food is important to consider along with the total amount of fat. Animal fats are the chief contributors of saturated fatty acids to the North American diet. About 40% to 60% of total fat in dairy and meat products is in the form of saturated fatty acids. In contrast, plant oils contain mostly unsaturated fatty acids, ranging from 73% to 94% of total fat. A moderate to high proportion of total fat (49% to 77%) is supplied by monounsaturated fatty acids in canola oil, olive oil, and peanut oil. Some animal fats are also good sources of monounsaturated fatty acids (30% to 47%) (review Fig. 5-3). Corn, cottonseed, sunflower, soybean, and safflower oils contain mostly polyunsaturated fatty acids (54% to 77%). These plant oils supply the majority of the linoleic and alpha-linolenic acid in the North American food supply.

Wheat germ, peanuts, egg yolk, soy beans, and organ meats are rich sources of phospholipids. Phospholipids such as lecithin, a component of egg yolks, are often added to salad dressing. Lecithin is used as an **emulsifier** in these and other products because of its ability to keep mixtures of lipids and water from separating (see Fig. 5-7). Emulsifiers are added to salad dressings to keep the vegetable oil suspended in water. Eggs added to cake batters likewise emulsify the fat with the milk.

Cholesterol is found only in animal foods. An egg yolk contains about 210 milligrams of cholesterol. Eggs are our main dietary source of cholesterol, along with

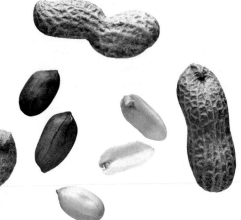

▲ Peanuts are a source of lecithins, as are wheat germ and egg yolks.

emulsifier A compound that can suspend fat in water by isolating individual fat droplets, using a shell of water molecules or other substances to prevent the fat from coalescing.

FIGURE 5-6 ▶ Food sources of fat compared to the American Heart Association (AHA) recommendation of 70 grams per day, or 30% of calories from fat for a 2100 kcal diet.

Food Sources of Fat

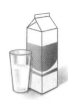

Food Item	Fat (grams)	Calories from Fat %	% AHA Recommendation
AHA Recommendation	70	30%	100%
T-bone steak, 3 ounces	17	66%	24%
Mixed nuts, 1 ounce	16	78%	23%
Canola oil, 1 tablespoon	14	100%	20%
Hamburger with bun, 1 each	12	39%	17%
Stick margarine, 1 tablespoon	12	100%	17%
Avocado, 1/2 cup	11	86%	16%
Cheddar cheese, 1 ounce	10	74%	14%
Whole milk, 1 cup	8	49%	11%
Chicken breast with skin, 3 ounces	7	36%	10%
Whole-milk yogurt, 8 ounces	7	28%	10%
Snack crackers, 1 ounce	7	45%	10%
Baked beans, 1/2 cup	7	31%	10%
M&M chocolate candies, 1 ounce	6	39%	9%
Flax seeds, 1 tablespoon	3	62%	4%
Fig Newton cookies, 2 each	3	23%	4%

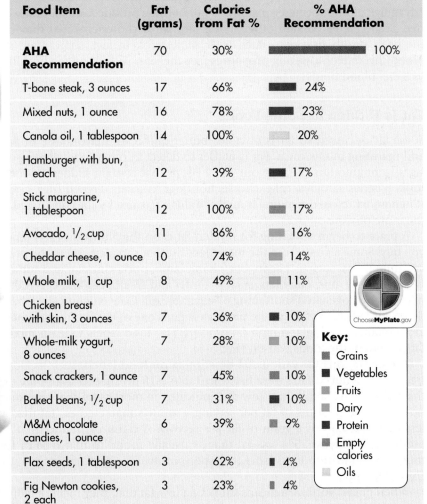

ChooseMyPlate.gov

Key:
- ■ Grains
- ■ Vegetables
- ■ Fruits
- ■ Dairy
- ■ Protein
- ■ Empty calories
- ■ Oils

FIGURE 5-7 ▶ Emulsifiers in action. Emulsifiers prevent many brands of salad dressings and other condiments from separating into layers of water and fat. Emulsifiers attract fatty acids inside and have a water-attracting group on the outside. Add them to salad dressing, shake well, and they hold the oil in the dressing away from the water. Emulsification is important in both food production and fat digestion/absorption.

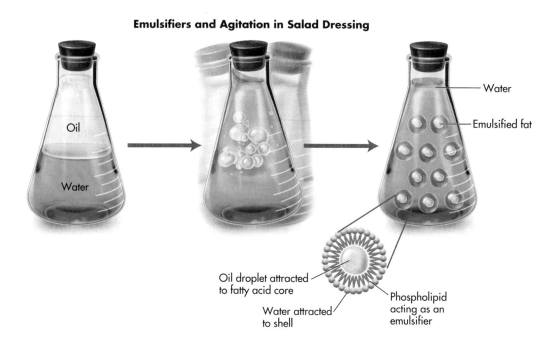

Emulsifiers and Agitation in Salad Dressing

Oil droplet attracted to fatty acid core

Water attracted to shell

Phospholipid acting as an emulsifier

Water

Emulsified fat

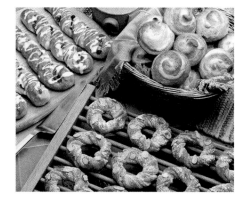

▲ The North American diet contains many high-fat foods—including typical pastry choices. Portion control with these foods is thus important, especially if one is trying to control calorie intake.

meats and whole milk. Manufacturers who advertise their brand of peanut butter, vegetable shortening, margarines, and vegetable oils as "cholesterol-free" are taking advantage of uninformed consumers—all of these products are naturally cholesterol-free. Some plants contain other sterols similar to cholesterol, but they do not pose the heart health risks associated with cholesterol. In fact, some plant sterols have blood cholesterol-lowering properties (see the later section on medical interventions to lower blood lipids).

Fat Is Hidden in Some Foods

Some fat discussed so far is obvious: butter on bread, mayonnaise in potato salad, and marbling in raw meat. Fat is harder to detect in other foods that also contribute significant amounts of fat to our diets. Foods that contain hidden fat include whole milk, pastries, cookies, cake, cheese, hot dogs, crackers, French fries, and ice cream. When we try to cut down on fat intake, hidden fats need to be considered, along with the more obvious sources.

A place to begin searching for hidden fat is on the Nutrition Facts labels of foods you buy. Some signals from the ingredient list that can alert you to the presence of fat are animal fats, such as bacon, beef, ham, lamb, pork, chicken, and turkey fats; lard; vegetable oils; nuts; dairy fats, such as butter and cream; egg and egg-yolk solids; and partially-hydrogenated shortening or vegetable oil. Conveniently, the label lists ingredients by order of weight in the product. If fat is one of the first ingredients listed, you are probably looking at a high-fat product. Use food labels to learn more about the fat content of the foods you eat (Fig. 5-8).

The definitions for various fat descriptors on food labels, such as "low-fat," "fat-free," and "reduced-fat," were listed in Table 2-11 in Chapter 2 and are reprinted in the margin here. Recall that "low-fat" indicates, in most cases, that a product contains no more than 3 grams of fat per serving. Products marketed as "fat-free" must have less than one-half of a gram of fat per serving. A claim of "reduced-fat" means the product has at least 25% less fat than is usually found in that type of food. When there is no Nutrition Facts label to inspect, controlling portion size is a good way to control fat intake.

When many North Americans think of a low-fat diet, they include reduced-fat versions of pastries, cookies, and cakes. When health professionals refer to a low-fat diet,

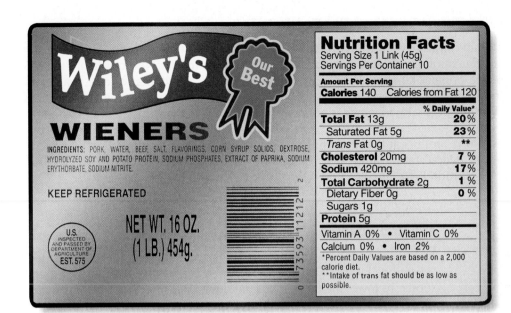

FIGURE 5-8 ▶ Reading labels helps locate hidden fat. Who would think that wieners (hot dogs) can contain about 85% of food calories as fat? Looking at the hot dog does not suggest that almost all of its food calories come from fat, but the label shows otherwise. Let's do the math: 13 grams total fat × 9 kcal per gram of fat = 120 kcal from fat; 120 kcal/140 kcal per link = 0.86 or 86% kcal from fat.

they often have a different plan in mind: focusing primarily on fruits, vegetables, and whole-grain breads and cereals. Whether to choose a fat-rich food should depend on how much fat you have eaten or will eat during that particular day. So, if you plan to eat high-fat foods at your evening meal, you could reduce your fat intake at a previous meal to balance overall fat intake for the day.

Fat in Food Provides Some Satiety, Flavor, and Texture

Fat in foods has generally been considered to be the most satiating of all the macro-nutrients. However, studies show that protein and carbohydrate probably lead to the most satiety (gram for gram). High-fat meals do provide satiety, but primarily because one consumes a lot of calories in the process. A high-fat meal is likely to be a high-calorie meal.

Various fats play important roles in foods, so much ingenuity must go into the production of reduced-fat products to preserve flavor and texture. In some cases, "fat-free" also means tasteless. Fat components in foods provide important textures and carry flavors. If you've ever eaten a high-fat yellow cheese or cream cheese, you probably agree that fat melting on the tongue feels good. The fat in reduced-fat and whole milk also gives body, which fat-free milk lacks. The most tender cuts of meat are high in fat, visible as the marbling of meat. In addition, many flavorings dissolve in fat. Heating spices in oil intensifies the flavors of an Indian curry or a Mexican dish, carried to the sensory cells that discriminate taste and smell in the mouth.

MAKING DECISIONS

Low-Fat Diets

A person who has been following a typical North American diet will probably need some time to adjust to the taste of a lower-fat diet. Emphasizing flavorful fruits, vegetables, and whole grains will help one to adapt to a low-fat diet. Interestingly, after an adjustment period, higher-fat foods may not be as palatable or may lead to gastrointestinal discomfort. For example, after switching from whole to 1% low-fat milk for a few weeks, whole milk begins to taste more like cream than milk. It is certainly possible to make the change from a higher-fat diet to a lower-fat diet. The benefits of weight control and reduced risk for several chronic diseases make the adjustment worth the effort.

▶ **Definitions for Nutrient Claims About Fat and Cholesterol on Food Labels**

Fat

- **Fat free:** less than 0.5 g of fat per serving

- **Saturated fat free:** less than 0.5 g per serving, and the level of *trans* fatty acids does not exceed 0.5 g per serving

- **Low fat:** 3 g or less per serving and, if the serving is 30 g or less or 2 tablespoons or less, per 50 g of the food. 2% milk can no longer be labeled low fat, as it exceeds 3 g per serving. *Reduced fat* will be the term used instead.

- **Low saturated fat:** 1 g or less per serving and not more than 15% of kcal from saturated fatty acids

- **Reduced or less fat:** at least 25% less per serving than reference food

- **Reduced or less saturated fat:** at least 25% less per serving than reference food

Cholesterol

- **Cholesterol free:** less than 2 milligrams (mg) of cholesterol and 2 g or less of saturated fat per serving

- **Low cholesterol:** 20 mg or less cholesterol and 2 g or less of saturated fat per serving and, if the serving is 30 g or less or 2 tablespoons or less, per 50 g of the food

- **Reduced or less cholesterol:** at least 25% less cholesterol and 2 g or less of saturated fat per serving than reference food

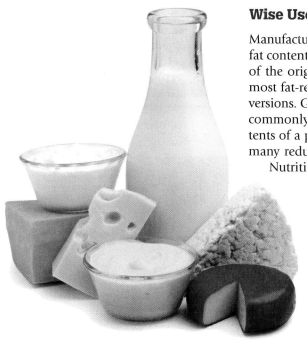

▲ Dairy products are a primary contributor of saturated fat to our diets.

Wise Use of Reduced-Fat Foods Is Important

Manufacturers have introduced reduced-fat versions of numerous food products. The fat content of these alternatives ranges from 0% in fat-free Fig Newtons to about 75% of the original fat content in other products. However, the total calorie content of most fat-reduced products is not substantially lower than that of their conventional versions. Generally, when fat is removed from a product, something must be added—commonly, sugars—in its place. It is difficult to reduce both the fat and sugar contents of a product at the same time and maintain flavor and texture. For this reason, many reduced-fat products (e.g., cakes and cookies) are still energy dense. Use the Nutrition Facts label to choose the portion size with the desired calories.

Fat-Replacement Strategies for Foods

To help consumers trim their fat intake and still enjoy the mouth feel sensations fat provides, food companies offer low-fat versions of many foods. To lower the fat in foods, manufacturers may replace some of the fat with water, protein (Dairy-Lo®), or forms of carbohydrates such as starch derivatives (Z-trim®), fiber (Maltrin®, Stellar™, Oatrim), and gums. Manufacturers also may use engineered fats, such as olestra (Olean®) and salatrim (Benefat®), that are made with fat and sucrose (table sugar) but that provide few or no calories because they cannot be digested and/or absorbed well.

So far, fat replacements have had little impact on our diets, partly because the currently approved forms are either not very versatile or not used extensively by manufacturers. In addition, fat replacements are not practical for use in the foods that provide the most fat in our diets—beef, cheese, whole milk, and pastries.

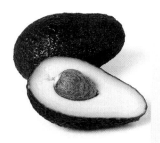

CONCEPT CHECK

Fat-dense foods—those with more than 60% of total calories as fat—include plant oils, butter, margarine, mayonnaise, nuts, bacon, avocados, peanut butter, cheddar cheese, steak, and hamburger. Of the foods we typically eat, cholesterol is found naturally only in those of animal origin, with eggs being a primary source. Emulsifiers, such as the phospholipids, lecithins, are added to salad dressings and other fat-rich products to keep the vegetable oils and other fats suspended in the water. Hidden fat exists in foods such as whole milk, pastries, cookies, cake, cheese, hot dogs, crackers, French fries, and ice cream. Fat has a variety of roles in foods, including that of contributing to flavor and texture. Fat also provides the pleasurable mouth feel of many of our favorite foods, intensifies the taste of many spices, and tenderizes many popular cuts of meat. Fat free doesn't mean calorie free; moderation in the use of reduced-fat products is still important.

CRITICAL THINKING

Allison has decided to start eating a low-fat diet. Allison has mentioned to you that all she needs to do is add less butter, oil, or margarine to her foods and she will dramatically lower her fat intake. How can you explain to Allison that she needs to be aware of the hidden fats in her diet as well?

Fat Rancidity Limits Shelf Life of Foods

Decomposing oils emit a disagreeable odor and taste sour and stale. Stale potato chips are a good example. The double bonds in unsaturated fatty acids break down, producing rancid by-products. Ultraviolet light, oxygen, and certain procedures can break double bonds and, in turn, destroy the structure of polyunsaturated fatty acids. Saturated fats and *trans* fats can much more readily resist these effects because they contain fewer carbon-carbon double bonds.

Rancidity is not a major problem for consumers because the odor and taste generally discourage us from eating enough to become sick. However, rancidity is a problem for manufacturers because it reduces a product's shelf life. To increase shelf life, manufacturers often add partially-hydrogenated plant oils to products. Foods most likely to become rancid are deep-fried foods and foods with a large amount of exposed surface. The fat in fish is also susceptible to rancidity because it is highly polyunsaturated.

Antioxidants such as vitamin E help protect foods against rancidity by guarding against fat breakdown. The vitamin E naturally occurring in plant oils reduces the breakdown of double bonds in fatty acids. When food manufacturers want to prevent rancidity in polyunsaturated fats, they often add the synthetic antioxidants **BHA** and **BHT** or vitamin C to products that contain fat such as salad dressings and cake mixes. Manufacturers also tightly seal products and use other methods to reduce oxygen levels inside packages.

Hydrogenation of Fatty Acids in Food Production Increases *Trans* Fatty Acid Content

As mentioned previously, most fats with long-chain saturated fatty acids are solid at room temperature, and those with unsaturated fatty acids are liquid at room temperature. In some kinds of food production, solid fats work better than liquid oils. In pie crust, for example, solid fats yield a flaky product, whereas crusts made with liquid oils tend to be greasy and more crumbly. If oils with unsaturated fatty acids are used to replace solid fats, they often must be made more saturated (with hydrogen), as this solidifies the vegetable oils into shortenings and margarines. Hydrogen is added by bubbling hydrogen gas under pressure into liquid vegetable oils in a process called **hydrogenation** (Fig. 5-9). The fatty acids aren't fully hydrogenated to the saturated fatty acid form, as this would make the product too hard and brittle. Partial hydrogenation—leaving some monounsaturated fatty acids—creates a semi-solid product.

The process of hydrogenation produces *trans* fatty acids as was described earlier in this chapter. Most natural monounsaturated and polyunsaturated fatty acids exist in the *cis* form, causing a bend in the carbon chain, whereas the straighter carbon forms of *trans* fat more closely resemble saturated fatty acids. This may be the mechanism

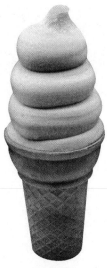

▲ Fat replacements such as gum fiber are typically seen in soft serve ice cream.

Canada has not approved the use of olestra in food products; the United States is the sole country that permits the use of this fat substitute in foods.

BHA, BHT Butylated hydroxyanisole and butylated hydroxytoluene—two common synthetic antioxidants added to foods.

hydrogenation The addition of hydrogen to a carbon-carbon double bond, producing a single carbon-carbon bond with two hydrogens attached to each carbon. Hydrogenation of unsaturated fatty acids in a vegetable oil increases its hardness, so this process is used to convert liquid oils into more solid fats, used in making margarine and shortening. *Trans* fatty acids are a by-product of hydrogenation of vegetable oils.

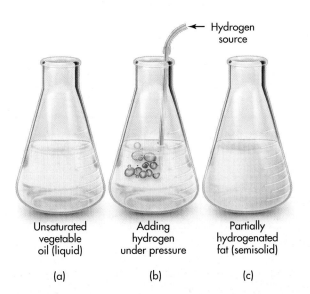

Hydrogen source

Unsaturated vegetable oil (liquid)
(a)

Adding hydrogen under pressure
(b)

Partially hydrogenated fat (semisolid)
(c)

FIGURE 5-9 ▶ How liquid oils become solid fats. (a) Unsaturated fatty acids are present in liquid form. (b) Hydrogens are added (hydrogenation), changing some carbon-carbon double bonds to single bonds and producing some *trans* fatty acids. (c) The partially hydrogenated product is likely to be used in margarine, shortening, or for deep-fat frying.

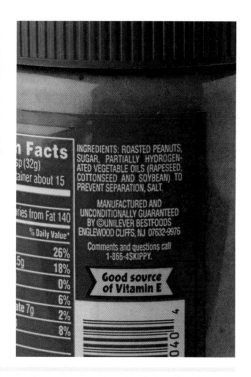

Peanut Butter: Is It "Good" Fat ?

At the grocery store, there are several brands of peanut butter on the shelf. The label on one brand of peanut butter indicates that the product is "cholesterol free," whereas none of the other brands make the same claim. A jar of "natural" peanut butter claims to have no hydrogenated fats. Which jar of peanut butter is best for heart health?

Cholesterol is a type of lipid that is only found in animal products. Therefore, all peanut butter is cholesterol free! Hydrogenated oils are used to increase shelf life of many products, including peanut butter. The process of hydrogenation can produce *trans* fats, which have many of the same detrimental health effects as saturated fat. *Trans* fats increase levels of "bad" blood cholesterol (LDL) and decrease "good" blood cholesterol (HDL). If hydrogenated oils appear in the list of ingredients as in the label shown here, there is a good chance the product contains *trans* fats. As you learned in Chapter 2, a product may claim to be free of *trans* fats as long as the product contains no more than 0.5 g of *trans* fats per serving. Therefore, the only guarantee to avoiding *trans* fat in peanut butter is to buy the "natural" peanut butter made from only peanuts.

whereby *trans* fat increases the risk for heart disease. Studies also indicate that *trans* fats increase overall inflammation in the body, which is not healthful. Thus, people should limit intake of partially-hydrogenated fat and thus *trans* fat. This may not be such a concern for the average person, as long as *trans* fat intake is not excessive and the diet is adequate in polyunsaturated fat. However, because *trans* fatty acids serve no particular role in maintaining body health, the latest Dietary Guidelines for Americans, the American Heart Association, and the Food and Nutrition Board each recommend minimal *trans* fat intake.

Not so long ago, public pressure persuaded manufacturers to eliminate the tropical oils rich in saturated fat (palm, palm olein, and coconut) from food processing. Partially-hydrogenated soybean oil—rich in *trans* fat—became the major replacement. Currently, *trans* fat intake in North America is estimated to contribute about 3% to 4% of total calories, amounting to 10 grams per day, on average. Table 5-1 lists typical sources.

FDA is now requiring the *trans* fat content of foods on food labels (review Fig. 5-8). The food labels in Canada also must list *trans* fat content. FDA hopes to make consumers more aware of the amounts of *trans* fat in foods as well as the negative health consequences associated with their excessive consumption. North American companies are already responding to this issue by creating products free of *trans* fat. For example, Promise, Smart Beat, and some Fleischmann's margarines are lower in or free of *trans* fat (less than 0.5 grams per serving) compared to typical margarines.

This addition of the *trans* fat listing on labels helps consumers at the supermarket, but when dining out, consumers are "left in the dark" as to which foods contain *trans* fat. Knowing which foods are low in *trans* fat when ordering at a restaurant is difficult because information about preparation methods and precise fat

TABLE 5-1 Main Sources of Fatty acids and Their State at Room Temperature

Type and Health Effects	Main Sources	State at Room Temperature
Saturated Fatty Acids Increase blood levels of cholesterol		
Long Chain	Lard; fat in beef, pork, and lamb	Solid
Medium and Short Chain	Milk fat (butter), coconut oil, palm oil, palm kernel oil	Soft or liquid
Monounsaturated Fatty Acids Decrease blood levels of cholesterol	Olive oil, canola oil, peanut oil	Liquid
Polyunsaturated Fatty Acids Decrease blood levels of cholesterol	Sunflower oil, corn oil, safflower oil, fish oil	Liquid
Essential Fatty Acids Omega 3: alpha–linolenic acid Reduces inflammation responses, blood clotting, and plasma triglycerides	Cold-water fish (salmon, tuna, sardines, mackerel), walnuts, flaxseed, hemp oil, canola oil, soybean oil	Liquid
Omega 6: Linoleic Acid Regulates blood pressure and increases blood clotting	Beef, poultry, safflower oil, sunflower oil, corn oil	Solid to liquid
***Trans* Fatty Acids** Increase blood cholesterol more than saturated fat	Margarine (squeeze, tub, stick), shortening	Soft to very solid

composition is rarely available. Many cities, including New York, Philadelphia, and Boston, have banned *trans* fat use in restaurants (see Further Reading 2). To minimize *trans* fat intake, a general guideline is to limit consumption of fried (especially deep-fat fried) food items, any pastries or flaky bread products (such as pie crusts, crackers, croissants, and biscuits), and cookies.

Until all foods are labeled with *trans* fat content, consumers can also make educated guesses on the *trans* fat content of foods by examining the list of ingredients on the food label. If partially-hydrogenated vegetable oil is one of the first three ingredients on the label, you can assume there is a significant amount of *trans* fat in the product.

Limiting *trans* fat at home is a much easier task. Most importantly, use little or no stick margarine or shortening. Instead, substitute vegetable oils and softer tub margarines (whose labels list vegetable oil or water as the first ingredient). Avoid deep-fat frying any food in shortening. Substitute baking, panfrying, broiling, steaming, grilling, or deep-fat frying in unhydrogenated vegetable oils. Replace nondairy creamers with reduced-fat or fat-free milk, since most nondairy creamers are rich in partially-hydrogenated vegetable oils. Finally, read the ingredients on food labels, using the previous tips to estimate *trans* fat content.

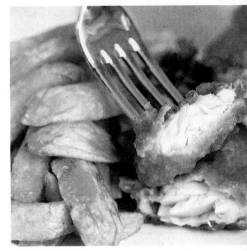

▲ Fried foods are a rich source of fat and *trans* fats. Reducing the intake of these foods can help lower blood lipid levels.

CONCEPT CHECK

Hydrogenation of unsaturated fatty acids is the process of adding hydrogen to carbon-carbon double bonds to produce single bonds. This results in the creation of some *trans* fatty acids. Hydrogenation changes vegetable oil to solid fat. It is wise to monitor *trans* fat intake, as this form of fat increases the risk for heart disease.

The carbon-carbon double bonds in polyunsaturated fatty acids are easily broken, yielding products responsible for rancidity. The presence of antioxidants, such as vitamin E in oils, naturally protects unsaturated fatty acids against oxidative destruction. Manufacturers can use hydrogenated fats and add natural or synthetic antioxidants to reduce the likelihood of rancidity.

5.4 Making Lipids Available for Body Use

It's no secret that fats and oils make foods more appealing. Their presence in foods adds flavor, lubrication, and texture. What happens to lipids once they are eaten? Let's take a closer look at the digestion, absorption, and physiological roles of lipids in the body.

Digestion

In the first phase of fat digestion, the stomach (and salivary glands to some extent) secretes **lipase.** This enzyme acts primarily on triglycerides that have fatty acids with short chain lengths, such as those found in butterfat. The action of salivary and stomach lipase, however, is usually dwarfed by that of the lipase enzyme released from the pancreas and active in the small intestine. Triglycerides and other lipids found in common vegetable oils and meats have longer chain lengths and are generally not digested until they reach the small intestine (Fig. 5-10).

In the small intestine, triglycerides are broken down by lipase into smaller products, namely monoglycerides (glycerol backbones with a single fatty acid attached) and fatty acids. Under the right circumstances, digestion is rapid and thorough. The "right" circumstances include the presence of bile from the gallbladder. Bile acids present in the bile act as emulsifiers on the digestive products of lipase action, suspending the monoglycerides and fatty acids in the watery digestive juices. This emulsification improves digestion and absorption because as large fat globules are broken down into smaller ones, the total surface area for lipase action increases (Fig. 5-11).

lipase Fat-digesting enzyme produced by the salivary glands, stomach, and pancreas.

FIGURE 5-10 ▶ A summary of fat digestion and absorption. Chapter 3 covered
general aspects of this process.

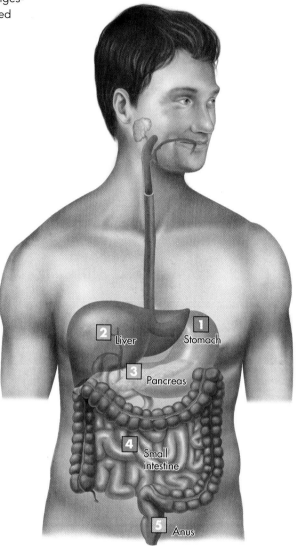

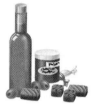

Fat Digestion and Absorption

1 Stomach: Only minor digestion of fat takes place in the stomach through the action of lipase enzymes.

2 Liver: The liver produces bile, stored in the gallbladder and released through the bile duct into the small intestine. Bile aids in fat digestion and absorption by emulsifying lipids in the digestive juices.

3 Pancreas: The pancreas secretes a mixture of enzymes, including lipase, into the small intestine.

4 Small intestine: The small intestine is the primary site for digestion and absorption of lipids. Once absorbed, long-chain fatty acids are packaged for transport through the lymph and bloodstream. (Shorter-chain fatty acids are absorbed directly into portal circulation.)

5 Large intestine: Less than 5% of ingested fat is normally excreted in the feces.

If the gallbladder is surgically removed
(e.g., in cases of gallstone formation),
bile will enter the small intestine directly
from the liver.

With regard to phospholipid digestion, certain enzymes from the pancreas and cells in the wall of the small intestine digest phospholipids. The eventual products are glycerol, fatty acids, and remaining parts. With regard to cholesterol digestion, any cholesterol with a fatty acid attached is broken down to free cholesterol and fatty acids by certain enzymes released from the pancreas.

MAKING DECISIONS

Bile Acids

During meals, bile acids circulate in a path that begins in the liver, goes on to the gallbladder, and then moves to the small intestine. After participating in fat digestion, most bile acids are absorbed and end up back at the liver. Approximately 98% of the bile acids are recycled. Only 1% to 2% ends up in the large intestine to be eliminated in the feces. Using medicines that block some of this reabsorption of bile acids is one way to treat high blood cholesterol. The liver takes cholesterol from the bloodstream to form replacement bile acids. Viscous fiber in the diet can also bind to bile acids to produce the same effect (see a later section on medical interventions related to cardiovascular disease for details).

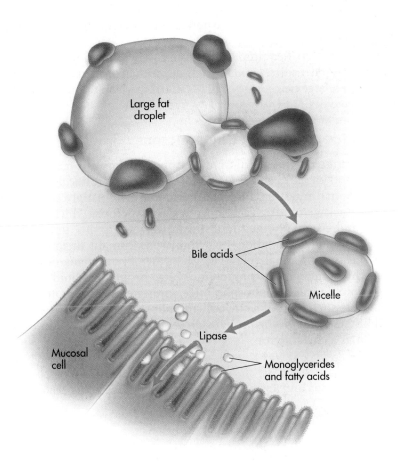

FIGURE 5-11 ▶ Bile acids mix with fats to form small droplets called micelles that facilitate the absorption of monoglycerides and fatty acids into the mucosal cells of the small intestine.

Absorption

The products of fat digestion in the small intestine are fatty acids and monoglycerides. These products diffuse into the absorptive cells of the small intestine. About 95% of dietary fat is absorbed in this way. The chain length of fatty acids affects the ultimate fate of fatty acids and monoglycerides after absorption. If the chain length of a fatty acid is less than 12 carbon atoms, it is water soluble and will therefore probably travel as such through the portal vein that connects directly to the liver. If the fatty acid is a more typical long-chain variety, it must be reformed into a triglyceride in the intestinal absorptive cell and eventually enter circulation via the lymphatic system (review Chapter 3 for an overview of this process).

CONCEPT CHECK

In the small intestine, a lipase enzyme released from the pancreas digests dietary triglycerides into monoglycerides (glycerol backbones with single fatty acids attached) and fatty acids. These breakdown products then diffuse into the absorptive cells of the small intestine. Long-chain fatty acids are transported through the lymphatic system, whereas fatty acids with shorter carbon chains are absorbed directly into the portal vein that connects directly to the liver. Other lipids are prepared for absorption by different enzymes.

5.5 Carrying Lipids in the Bloodstream

As noted earlier, fat and water don't mix easily. This incompatibility presents a challenge for the transport of fats through the watery media of the blood and lymph.

lipoprotein A compound found in the bloodstream containing a core of lipids with a shell composed of protein, phospholipid, and cholesterol.

chylomicron Lipoprotein made of dietary fats surrounded by a shell of cholesterol, phospholipids, and protein. Chylomicrons are formed in the absorptive cells of the small intestine after fat absorption and travel through the lymphatic system to the bloodstream.

Lipoproteins serve as vehicles for transport of lipids from the small intestine and liver to the body tissues (Table 5-2).

Lipoproteins are classified into four groups—chylomicrons, VLDL, LDL, and HDL—based on their densities. Lipids are less dense than proteins. Therefore, lipoproteins that contain a large percentage of lipids in comparison to protein are less dense than those depleted of lipids.

Dietary Fats Are Carried by Chylomicrons

As you learned in the previous section, digestion of dietary fats results in a mixture of glycerol, monoglycerides, and fatty acids. Once these products are absorbed by the cells of the small intestine, they are reassembled into triglycerides. Then, the intestinal cells package the triglycerides into **chylomicrons,** which enter the lymphatic system and eventually the bloodstream (review Fig. 3-5 in Chapter 3 for a depiction of lymphatic circulation). Chylomicrons contain dietary fat and originate only from the intestinal cells. Like the other lipoproteins described in the next section, chylomicrons are composed of large droplets of lipid surrounded by a thin, water-soluble shell of phospholipids, cholesterol, and protein (Fig. 5-12). The water-soluble shell around a chylomicron allows the lipid to float freely in the water-based blood. Some of the proteins present may also help other cells identify the lipoprotein as a chylomicron.

TABLE 5-2 Composition and Roles of the Major Lipoproteins in the Blood

Lipoprotein	Primary Component	Key Role
Chylomicron	Triglyceride	Carries dietary fat from the small intestine to cells
VLDL	Triglyceride	Carries lipids made and taken up by the liver to cells
LDL	Cholesterol	Carries cholesterol made by the liver and from other sources to cells
HDL	Protein	Contributes to cholesterol removal from cells and, in turn, excretion of it from the body

FIGURE 5-12 ▶ The structure of a lipoprotein, in this case an LDL. This structure allows fats to circulate in the water-based bloodstream. Various lipoproteins are found in the bloodstream. The primary component of LDL is cholesterol.

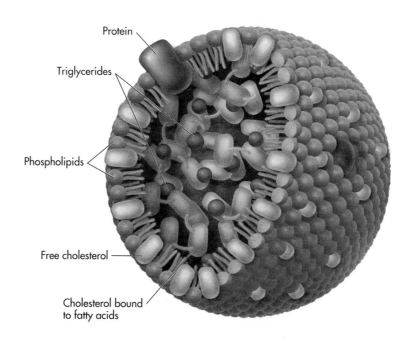

Protein

Triglycerides

Phospholipids

Free cholesterol

Cholesterol bound to fatty acids

Once a chylomicron enters the bloodstream, the triglycerides in its core are broken down into fatty acids and glycerol by an enzyme called **lipoprotein lipase,** attached to the inside walls of the blood vessels (Fig. 5-13). As soon as the fatty acids are released to the bloodstream, they are absorbed by cells in the vicinity, while much of the glycerol circulates back to the liver. Muscle cells can immediately use the absorbed fatty acids for fuel. Adipose cells, on the other hand, tend to re-form the fatty acids into triglycerides for storage. After triglycerides have been removed, a chylomicron remnant remains. Chylomicron remnants are removed from circulation by the liver and their components are recycled to make other lipoproteins and bile acids.

lipoprotein lipase An enzyme attached to the cells that form the inner lining of blood vessels; it breaks down triglycerides into free fatty acids and glycerol.

Other Lipoproteins Transport Lipids from the Liver to the Body Cells

The liver takes up various lipids from the blood. The liver also is the manufacturing site for lipids and cholesterol. The raw materials for lipid and cholesterol synthesis include free fatty acids taken up from the bloodstream, as well as carbon and hydrogen derived from carbohydrates, protein, and alcohol. The liver then must package these synthesized lipids as lipoproteins for transport in the blood to body tissues.

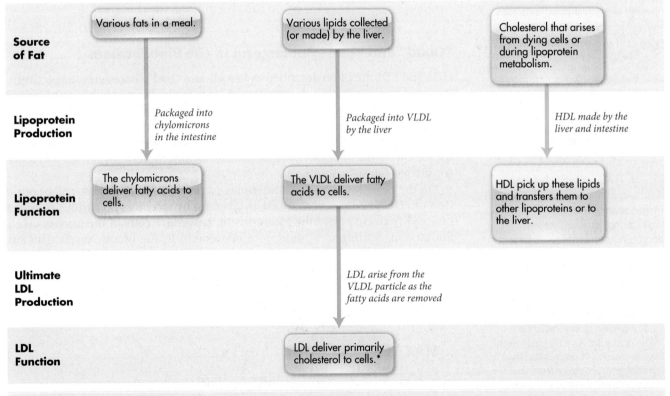

Source of Fat — Various fats in a meal. / Various lipids collected (or made) by the liver. / Cholesterol that arises from dying cells or during lipoprotein metabolism.

Lipoprotein Production — *Packaged into chylomicrons in the intestine* / *Packaged into VLDL by the liver* / *HDL made by the liver and intestine*

Lipoprotein Function — The chylomicrons deliver fatty acids to cells. / The VLDL deliver fatty acids to cells. / HDL pick up these lipids and transfers them to other lipoproteins or to the liver.

Ultimate LDL Production — *LDL arise from the VLDL particle as the fatty acids are removed*

LDL Function — LDL deliver primarily cholesterol to cells.*

* = Cholesterol not taken up by body cells can be taken up by scavenger cells in the arteries. The eventual cholesterol buildup leads to atherosclerosis.

VLDL = Very-Low-Density Lipoprotein

LDL = Low-Density Lipoprotein

HDL = High-Density Lipoprotein

FIGURE 5-13 ▶ Lipoprotein production and function. Chylomicrons carry absorbed fat to body cells. VLDL carries fat taken up from the bloodstream by the liver, as well as any fat made by the liver, to body cells. LDL arises from VLDL and carries mostly cholesterol to cells. HDL arises mostly from the liver and intestine. HDL carries cholesterol from cells to other lipoproteins and to the liver for excretion.

very-low-density lipoprotein (VLDL) The lipoprotein created in the liver that carries cholesterol and lipids that have been taken up or newly synthesized by the liver.

low-density lipoprotein (LDL) The lipoprotein in the blood containing primarily cholesterol; elevated LDL is strongly linked to cardiovascular disease risk.

high-density lipoprotein (HDL) The lipoprotein in the blood that picks up cholesterol from dying cells and other sources and transfers it to the other lipoproteins in the bloodstream, as well as directly to the liver; low HDL increases the risk for cardiovascular disease.

menopause The cessation of the menstrual cycle in women, usually beginning at about 50 years of age.

scavenger cells Specific form of white blood cells that can bury themselves in the artery wall and accumulate LDL. As these cells take up LDL, they contribute to the development of atherosclerosis.

atherosclerosis A buildup of fatty material (plaque) in the arteries, including those surrounding the heart.

See Nutrition and Your Health:
Lipids and Cardiovascular Disease
at the end of Chapter 5.

It appears that saturated fatty acids promote an increase in the amount of free cholesterol (not attached to fatty acids) in the liver, whereas unsaturated fatty acids do the opposite. As free cholesterol in the liver increases, it causes the liver to reduce cholesterol uptake from the bloodstream, contributing to elevated LDL in the blood. (*Trans* fatty acids are thought to act in the same ways as saturated fatty acids.)

First in our discussion of lipoproteins made by the liver are **very-low-density lipoproteins (VLDL).** These particles are composed of cholesterol and triglycerides surrounded by a water-soluble shell. VLDLs are rich in triglycerides and thus are very low in density. Once in the bloodstream, lipoprotein lipase on the inner surface of the blood vessels breaks down the triglyceride in the VLDL into fatty acids and glycerol. Fatty acids and glycerol are released into the bloodstream and taken up by the body cells.

As its triglycerides are released, the VLDL becomes proportionately denser. Much of what eventually remains of the VLDL fraction is then called **low-density lipoprotein (LDL)**; this is composed primarily of the remaining cholesterol. The primary function of LDL is to transport cholesterol to tissues. LDL particles are taken up from the bloodstream by specific receptors on cells, especially liver cells, and are then broken down. The cholesterol and protein components of LDL provide some of the building blocks necessary for cell growth and development, such as synthesis of cell membranes and hormones.

The final group of lipoproteins, **high-density lipoproteins (HDL),** is a critical and beneficial participant in this process of lipid transport. Its high proportion of protein makes it the densest lipoprotein. The liver and intestine produce most of the HDL in the blood. It roams the bloodstream, picking up cholesterol from dying cells and other sources. HDL donates the cholesterol primarily to other lipoproteins for transport back to the liver to be excreted. Some HDL travels directly back to the liver.

"Good" and "Bad" Cholesterol in the Bloodstream

HDL and LDL are often described as "good" and "bad" cholesterol, respectively. Many studies demonstrate that the amount of HDL in the bloodstream can closely predict the risk for cardiovascular disease. Risk increases with low HDL because little cholesterol is transported back to the liver and excreted. Women tend to have high amounts of HDL, especially before **menopause,** compared to men. High amounts of HDL slow the development of cardiovascular disease, so any cholesterol carried by HDL can be considered "good" cholesterol.

On the other hand, LDL is sometimes considered "bad" cholesterol. In our discussion of LDL, you learned that LDL is taken up by receptors on various cells. If LDL is not readily cleared from the bloodstream, **scavenger cells** in the arteries take up the lipoprotein, leading to a buildup of cholesterol in the blood vessels. This buildup, known as **atherosclerosis,** greatly increases the risk for cardiovascular disease (see the following Nutrition and Your Health section). LDL is only a problem when it is too high in the bloodstream because low amounts are needed as part of routine body functions.

MAKING DECISIONS

LDL Cholesterol

The cholesterol in foods is not designated as "good" or "bad." It is only after cholesterol has been made or processed by the liver that it shows up in the bloodstream as LDL or HDL. Dietary patterns can affect the metabolism of cholesterol, however. Diets low in saturated fat, *trans* fat, and cholesterol encourage the uptake of LDL by the liver, thereby removing LDL from the bloodstream and decreasing the ability of scavenger cells to form atherosclerotic plaques in the blood vessels. Likewise, diets high in saturated fat, *trans* fat, and cholesterol reduce the uptake of LDL by the liver, increasing cholesterol in the blood and the risk for cardiovascular disease. What foods in your diet are high in saturated fat, *trans* fat, or cholesterol?

CONCEPT CHECK

Lipids generally move through the bloodstream as part of lipoproteins. Dietary fats absorbed from the small intestine are packaged and transported as chylomicrons, whereas lipids synthesized in the liver are packaged as very-low-density lipoproteins (VLDL). Lipoprotein lipase removes triglycerides from the interiors of both chylomicrons and VLDL, breaking the triglycerides down into glycerol and fatty acids, which are taken up by tissues for energy needs or storage. What remains after the action of lipoprotein lipase are chylomicron remnants (from chylomicrons), the components of which are recycled by the liver, or low-density lipoproteins (LDL, from VLDL), rich in cholesterol. LDL is picked up by receptors on body cells, especially liver cells. Scavenger cells in the arteries may do the same, speeding the development of atherosclerosis. High-density lipoprotein (HDL), also produced in part by the liver, picks up cholesterol from cells and transports it primarily to other lipoproteins for eventual transport back to the liver. Risk factors for cardiovascular disease include an elevated level of LDL and/or low amounts of HDL in the blood.

5.6 Essential Functions of Fatty Acids

The various classes of lipids have diverse functions in the body. All are necessary for health, but, as mentioned earlier, many can be made by the body and therefore are not needed in our diet. Of all the classes of lipids, only certain polyunsaturated fatty acids are essential parts of a diet.

The Essential Fatty Acids

We must obtain linoleic acid (an omega-6 fatty acid) and alpha-linolenic acid (an omega-3 fatty acid) from foods to maintain health, so they are called *essential fatty acids* (Fig. 5-14). These omega-6 and omega-3 fatty acids form parts of vital body structures, perform important roles in immune system function and vision, help form cell membranes, and produce hormonelike compounds. Omega-6 and omega-3 fatty acids must be obtained through the diet because human cells lack the enzymes needed to produce these fatty acids. Other fatty acids, such as omega-9 fatty acids, can be synthesized in the body, and therefore are not essential components of the diet.

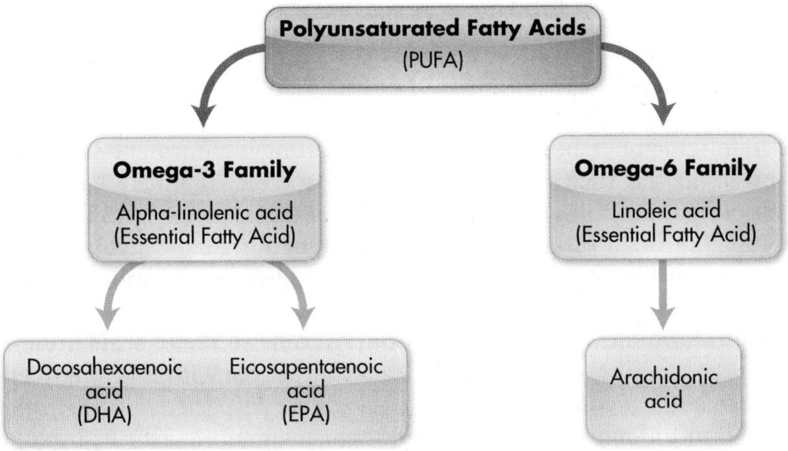

Omega-3 Fatty Acids in Fish (grams per 3 ounce serving)	
Atlantic salmon	1.8
Anchovy	1.7
Sardines	1.4
Rainbow trout	1.0
Coho salmon	0.9
Bluefish	0.8
Striped bass	0.8
Tuna, white, canned	0.7
Halibut	0.4
Catfish, channel	0.2

Recommended omega-3 fatty acid (alpha-linolenic acid) intake per day:	
Men	1.6 grams
Women	1.1 grams

FIGURE 5-14 ▶ The essential fatty acid (EFA) family. Linoleic acid and alpha-linolenic acid are available from dietary sources, and must be consumed as body synthesis does not take place. These are the essential fatty acids. The other fatty acids in this figure can be synthesized from the essential fatty acids.

eicosapentaenoic acid (EPA) An omega-3 fatty acid with 20 carbons and five carbon-carbon double bonds. It is present in large amounts in fatty fish and is slowly synthesized in the body from alpha-linolenic acid.

docosahexaenoic acid (DHA) An omega-3 fatty acid with 22 carbons and six carbon-carbon double bonds. It is present in large amounts in fatty fish and is slowly synthesized in the body from alpha-linolenic acid. DHA is especially present in the retina and brain.

arachidonic acid An omega-6 fatty acid made from linoleic acid with 20 carbon atoms and four carbon-carbon double bonds.

hemorrhagic stroke Damage to part of the brain resulting from rupture of a blood vessel and subsequent bleeding within or over the internal surface of the brain.

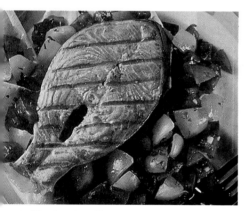

▲ The American Heart Association recommends eating fatty fish such as salmon at least twice a week. As a source of omega-3 fatty acids, fish is a heart-healthy alternative to other animal sources of protein, which can be high in saturated fat and cholesterol.

See Nutrition and Your Health: Lipids and Cardiovascular Disease at the end of Chapter 5.

Still, we need to consume only about 5% of our total calories per day from essential fatty acids. That corresponds to about 2 to 4 tablespoons of plant oil each day. We can easily get that much—from mayonnaise, salad dressings, and other foods—without much effort. Regular consumption of vegetables and whole-grain breads and cereals also helps to supply enough essential fatty acids.

Research also suggests that we include a regular intake of the omega-3 fatty acids, **eicosapentaenoic acid (EPA)** and **docosahexaenoic acid (DHA),** which can be made from alpha-linolenic acid. EPA and DHA are naturally high in fatty fish such as salmon, tuna, sardines, anchovies, striped bass, catfish, herring, mackerel, trout, or halibut. Consumption of one or more of these fish at least twice a week is recommended to obtain EPA and DHA. Additional sources of omega-3 fatty acids include canola and soybean oils, walnuts, flax seeds, mussels, crab, and shrimp (see Further Readings 4, 5, and 15).

MAKING DECISIONS

Mercury in Fish

Consumption of fatty fish at least twice a week is recommended as a good source of the omega-3 fatty acids. Some fish can be a source of mercury, toxic in high amounts, especially swordfish, shark, king mackerel, and tile fish (see Chapter 13). Albacore tuna also is a potential source, while other forms of tuna are much lower in mercury. Those fish low in mercury are salmon, sardines, bluefish, and herring. Shrimp is also low in mercury. For others, varying your choices rather than always eating the same species of fish and limiting overall intake to 12 ounces per week (on average 2 to 3 meals of fish or shellfish per week) is recommended to reduce mercury exposure, especially for pregnant women and children. Existing research indicates that the benefits of fish intake, especially in reducing the risk of cardiovascular disease, outweigh the possible risks of mercury contamination.

The recommendation to consume omega-3 fatty acids stems from the observation that compounds made from omega-3 fatty acids tend to decrease blood clotting and inflammatory processes in the body. The omega-6 fatty acids, notably **arachidonic acid** made from linoleic acid, generally increase clotting and inflammation, and saturated fatty acids also increase blood clotting.

Some studies show that people who eat fish at least twice a week (total weekly intake: 8 ounces [240 grams]) run lower risks for heart attack than do people who rarely eat fish. In these cases, the omega-3 fatty acids in fish oil are probably acting to reduce blood clotting. As will be covered in detail in the "Nutrition and Your Health" section, blood clots are part of the heart attack process. In addition, these omega-3 fatty acids have a favorable effect on heart rhythm. Consequently, the risk of heart attack decreases with the consumption of omega-3 fatty acids from fish, especially for people already at high risk.

We need to remember, however, that blood clotting is a normal body process. Certain groups of people, such as Eskimos in Greenland, eat so much seafood that their normal blood-clotting ability can be impaired. An excess of omega-3 fatty acid intake can allow uncontrolled bleeding and may cause **hemorrhagic stroke.** However, no increase in risk of stroke has been observed in studies using moderate amounts of omega-3 fatty acids.

Studies also have shown that large amounts of omega-3 fatty acids from fish (2 to 4 grams per day) can lower blood triglycerides in people with high triglyceride concentrations. In addition, these omega-3 fatty acids are suspected to be helpful in managing the pain of inflammation associated with rheumatoid arthritis by suppressing immune system responses. This may also help with certain behavioral disorders and cases of mild depression.

In some instances, fish oil capsules can be safely substituted for fish consumption if a person does not like fish. Generally, about 1 gram of omega-3 fatty acids (about three capsules) from fish oil per day is recommended, especially for people with evidence of cardiovascular disease. (Freezing fish oil capsules before consumption or using enteric coated capsules will reduce the fishy aftertaste.) The American Heart Association also recently suggested that fish oil supplements (providing 2 to 4 grams of omega-3 fatty acids per day) could be employed to treat elevated blood triglycerides, as previously noted. However, fish oil capsules should be limited for individuals who have bleeding disorders, take anticoagulant medications, or anticipate surgery, because they may increase risk of uncontrollable bleeding and hemorrhagic stroke. Thus for fish oil capsules, as well as other dietary supplements, it is important to follow a physician's recommendations. Remember that fish oil supplements are not regulated by the FDA. The quality of these supplements, therefore, is not standardized, and contaminants naturally present in the fish oil may not have been removed.

In summary, the regular consumption of fatty fish is advised. Consuming whole fish is thought to have greater benefits and be safer than using fish oil supplements. Fish is not only a rich source of omega-3 fatty acids, but is also a valuable source of protein and trace elements that may also provide protective effects for the cardiovascular system. Broiled or baked fish is recommended rather than fried fish because frying may decrease the ratio of omega-3 to omega-6 fatty acids and may produce *trans* fatty acids and oxidized lipid products that may increase cardiovascular disease risk.

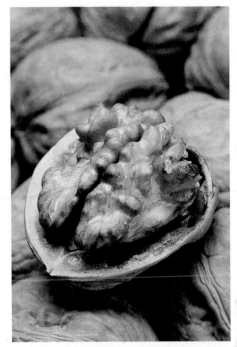

▲ Walnuts are one of the richest plant sources of the omega-3 fatty acid, alpha-linolenic acid, and are also a good source of plant sterols (see Further Reading 8).

MAKING DECISIONS

Flax Seeds or Walnuts?

Flax seeds and walnuts are getting attention today because they are rich vegetable sources of the omega-3 alpha-linolenic acid. About 2 tablespoons of flax seed per day is typically recommended if used as an omega-3 fatty acid source. Flax seeds can be purchased in many natural food stores rather inexpensively. These need to be chewed thoroughly or they will pass through the GI tract undigested. Many people find it easier to grind them in a coffee grinder before eating them. Flax seed oil is also available, but it turns **rancid** very quickly, especially if not refrigerated. Compared to other nuts and seeds, walnuts are one of the richest sources of alpha-linolenic acid (2.6 grams per 1-ounce serving or 14 walnut halves). The DRI for alpha-linolenic acid is 1.6 grams/day for men and 1.1 grams/day for women. In addition, walnuts are a rich source of plant sterols known to inhibit intestinal absorption of cholesterol.

CRITICAL THINKING

Advertisements often claim that fats are bad. Your classmate Mike asks, "If fats are so bad for us, why do we need to have any in our diets?" How would you answer him?

rancid Containing products of decomposed fatty acids that have an unpleasant flavor and odor.

total parenteral nutrition The intravenous feeding of all necessary nutrients, including the most basic forms of protein, carbohydrates, lipids, vitamins, minerals, and electrolytes.

Effects of a Deficiency of Essential Fatty Acids

If humans fail to consume enough essential fatty acids, their skin becomes flaky and itchy, and diarrhea and other symptoms such as infections often are seen. Growth and wound healing may be restricted. These signs of deficiency have been seen in people fed intravenously by **total parenteral nutrition** containing little or no fat for 2 to 3 weeks, as well as in infants receiving formulas low in fat. However, because our bodies need the equivalent of only about 2 to 4 tablespoons of plant oils a day, even a low fat diet will provide enough essential fatty acids if it follows a balanced plan such as MyPyramid and includes a serving of fatty fish at least twice a week.

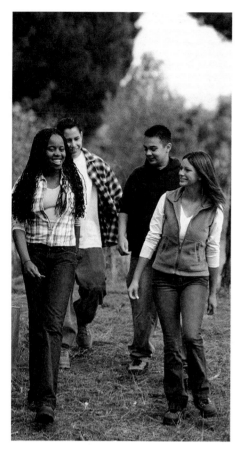

▲ When at rest or during light activity, the body uses mostly fatty acids for fuel.

Because humans can't make either omega-3 or omega-6 fatty acids, which perform vital functions in the body, they must be obtained from the diet and therefore are called essential fatty acids. Plant oils are generally rich in omega-6 fatty acids. Eating fatty fish at least twice a week is a good way to meet omega-3 fatty acid needs. Fish oil supplementation (about 1 gram per day of the related omega-3 fatty acids) is generally acceptable under a physician's guidance if a person does not like fish; however, people with certain medical conditions (e.g., taking anti-coagulant medications) should be cautious with use of fish oil supplements due to increased risk of hemorrhagic stroke. Essential fatty acid deficiency can occur after 2 to 3 weeks if fat is omitted from total parenteral nutrition solutions, which in turn can lead to skin disorders, diarrhea, and other health problems.

5.7 Broader Roles for Fatty Acids and Triglycerides in the Body

Many key functions of fat in the body require the use of fatty acids in the form of triglycerides. Triglycerides are used for energy storage, insulation, and transportation of fat-soluble vitamins.

Providing Energy

Triglycerides contained in the diet and stored in adipose tissue provide the fatty acids that are the main fuel for muscles while at rest and during light activity. Muscles use carbohydrate for fuel in addition to fatty acids supplied by triglycerides only in endurance exercise, such as long-distance running and cycling, or in short bursts of intense activity, such as a 200-meter run. Other body tissues also use fatty acids for energy needs. Overall, about half of the energy used by the entire body at rest and during light activity comes from fatty acids. When considering the whole-body, the use of fatty acids by skeletal and heart muscle is balanced by the use of glucose by the nervous system and red blood cells. Recall from Chapter 4 that cells need a supply of carbohydrate to efficiently process fatty acids for fuel. The details about how we burn fat as a fuel will be discussed in Chapter 7.

Storing Energy for Later Use

We store energy mainly in the form of triglycerides. The body's ability to store fat is essentially limitless. Its fat storage sites, adipose cells, can increase about 50 times in weight. If the amount of fat to be stored exceeds the ability of the existing cells to expand, the body can form new adipose cells.

An important advantage of using triglycerides to store energy in the body is that they are energy dense. Recall that these yield, on average, 9 kcal per gram, whereas proteins and carbohydrates yield only about 4 kcal per gram. In addition, triglycerides are chemically stable, so they are not likely to react with other cell constituents, making them a safe form for storing energy. Finally, when we store triglycerides in adipose cells, we store little else, especially water. Adipose cells contain about 80% lipid and only 20% water and protein. In contrast, imagine if we were to store energy as muscle tissue, which is about 73% water. Body weight linked to energy storage would increase dramatically. The same would be true if we stored energy primarily as glycogen, as about 3 grams of water are stored for every gram of glycogen.

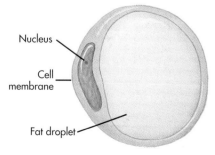

Nucleus

Cell membrane

Fat droplet

Adipose cell

Insulating and Protecting the Body

The insulating layer of fat just beneath the skin is made mostly of triglycerides. Fat tissue also surrounds and protects some organs—kidneys, for example—from injury. We usually don't notice the important insulating function of fat tissue, because we wear clothes and add more as needed. A layer of insulating fat is important in animals living in cold climates. Polar bears, walruses, and whales all build a thick layer of fat tissue around themselves to insulate against cold-weather environments. The extra fat also provides energy storage for times when food is scarce.

Transporting Fat-Soluble Vitamins

Triglycerides and other fats in food carry fat-soluble vitamins to the small intestine and aid their absorption. People who absorb fat poorly, such as those with the disease cystic fibrosis, are at risk for deficiencies of fat-soluble vitamins, especially vitamin K. A similar risk comes from taking mineral oil as a laxative at mealtimes. The body cannot digest or absorb mineral oil, so the undigested oil carries the fat-soluble vitamins from the meal into the feces, where they are eliminated. Unabsorbed fatty acids can bind minerals, such as calcium and magnesium, and draw them into the stool for elimination. This can harm mineral status (see Chapter 11). Recall that the main problem with the fat replacer, olestra, is that it can bind the fat-soluble vitamins and reduce their absorption.

5.8 Phospholipids in the Body

Many types of phospholipids exist in the body, especially in the brain. They form important parts of cell membranes. Phospholipids are found in body cells, and they participate in fat digestion in the intestine. Recall that the various forms of lecithin (discussed earlier) are common examples of phospholipids (review Fig. 5-4b).

Cell membranes are composed primarily of phospholipids. A cell membrane looks much like a sea of phospholipids with protein "islands" (Fig. 5-15). The proteins

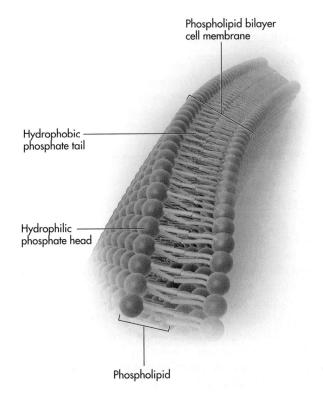

Phospholipid bilayer
cell membrane

Hydrophobic
phosphate tail

Hydrophilic
phosphate head

Phospholipid

FIGURE 5-15 ▶ Phospholipids are the main components of cell membranes, forming a double or bilayer of lipid.

form receptors for hormones, function as enzymes, and act as transporters for nutrients. The fatty acids on the phospholipids serve as a source of essential fatty acids for the cell. Some cholesterol is also present in the membrane.

In some foods, phospholipids function as emulsifiers (as covered earlier) allowing fat and water to mix. By breaking fat globules into small droplets, emulsifiers enable a fat to be suspended in water. They act as bridges between the oil and water that in turn lead to the formation of tiny oil droplets surrounded by thin shells of water. In an emulsified solution, such as salad dressing or mayonnaise, millions of tiny oil droplets are separated by shells of water (review Fig. 5-7).

The body's main emulsifiers are the lecithins and bile acids, produced by the liver and released into the small intestine via the gallbladder during digestion.

5.9 Cholesterol in the Body

Cholesterol plays many vital roles in the body. It forms part of some important hormones, such as estrogen, testosterone, and a form of the active vitamin D hormone. Cholesterol is also the building block of bile acids, needed for fat digestion. Finally, cholesterol is an essential structural component of cells and the outer layer of the lipoprotein particles that transport lipids in the blood. The cholesterol content of the heart, liver, kidney, and brain is high, reflecting its critical role in these organs.

About two-thirds of the cholesterol circulating through your body is made by body cells; the remaining one-third is consumed in the diet. Each day, our cells produce approximately 875 milligrams of cholesterol. Of the 875 milligrams of cholesterol made by the body, about 400 milligrams are used to make new bile acids to replenish those lost in the feces, and about 50 milligrams are used to make hormones. In addition to all the cholesterol cells make, we consume about 180 to 325 milligrams of cholesterol per day from animal-derived food products, with men consuming the higher amount compared to women. Absorption of cholesterol from food ranges from about 40% to 65%. The effect of blood cholesterol, especially LDL cholesterol, on cardiovascular disease risk will be discussed in the "Nutrition and Your Health" section.

See Nutrition and Your Health: Lipids and Cardiovascular Disease at the end of Chapter 5.

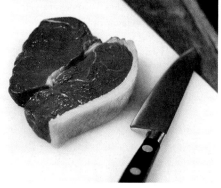

▲ Trimming the fat off meats can help reduce saturated fat intake. Limiting intake of meat that is highly marbled with fat (streaks of fat running through the lean) helps, too.

CONCEPT CHECK

Triglycerides are the major form of fat in the body. They are used for energy and stored in adipose tissue, they insulate and protect body organs, and they transport fat-soluble vitamins. Phospholipids are emulsifiers—compounds that can suspend fat in water. Phospholipids also form parts of cell membranes and various compounds in the body. Cholesterol, a sterol, forms part of cell membranes, hormones, and bile acids. If sufficient amounts are not consumed, the body makes what phospholipids and cholesterol it needs.

5.10 Recommendations for Fat Intake

There is no RDA for total fat intake for adults, although there is an Adequate Intake set for total fat for infants (see Chapter 15). The 2010 Dietary Guidelines for Americans recommendation and the Acceptable Macronutrient Distribution Range is that total fat intake should be 20% to 35% of total calories, which equates to 44 to 78 grams per day for a person who consumes 2000 kcal daily. The most specific recommendations for fat intake come from the American Heart Association (AHA) (see Further Reading 9). Many North Americans are at risk for developing cardiovascular disease, so AHA promotes dietary and lifestyle goals aimed at reducing this risk. The AHA diet and lifestyle goals for cardiovascular disease risk reduction for the general public are presented in Table 5-3. These goals include aiming for an overall healthy eating pattern; appropriate

TABLE 5-3 American Heart Association 2006 Diet and Lifestyle Goals for Cardiovascular Disease Risk Reduction

- Consume an overall healthy diet.

- Aim for a healthy body weight.

- Aim for recommended levels of low-density lipoprotein (LDL) cholesterol, high-density lipoprotein (HDL) cholesterol, and triglycerides.

- Aim for a normal blood pressure.

- Aim for a normal blood glucose level.

- Be physically active.

- Avoid use of and exposure to tobacco products.

From: Lichtenstein AH and others: Diet and lifestyle recommendations revision 2006. A scientific statement from the American Heart Association Nutrition Committee. *Circulation* 114:82, 2006.

body weight; and a desirable blood cholesterol profile, blood pressure, and blood glucose level. In Table 5-4, a more detailed list of recommendations is provided for those who currently are at high risk or have cardiovascular disease.

To reduce risk for cardiovascular disease, the AHA recommends that no more than 7% of total calories come from saturated fat and no more than 1% from *trans* fat. These are the primary fatty acids that raise LDL. In addition, cholesterol should amount to a maximum of 300 mg per day. Table 5-5 lists the cholesterol content of some foods. This often happens along with the reduction in saturated fat and *trans* fat intake. Table 5-6 is an example of a diet that adheres to 20% or 30% of calories as fat. Compare these recommendations to the actual dietary intake patterns of these fats by North Americans: 33% of calories from total fat, about 13% of calories from saturated fat, and 180 to 320 milligrams of cholesterol each day.

TABLE 5-4 American Heart Association 2006 Diet and Lifestyle Recommendations for Cardiovascular Disease Risk Reduction

- Balance calorie intake and physical activity to achieve or maintain a healthy body weight.

- Consume a diet rich in vegetables and fruits.

- Choose whole-grain, high-fiber foods.

- Consume fish, especially oily fish, at least twice a week.

- Limit your intake of saturated fat to less than 7% of energy, *trans* fat to less than 1% of energy, and cholesterol to less than 300 milligrams per day by
  — choosing lean meats and vegetable alternatives;
  — selecting fat-free (skim), 1%-fat, and low-fat dairy products; and
  — minimizing intake of partially-hydrogenated fats.

- Minimize your intake of beverages and foods with added sugars.

- Choose and prepare foods with little or no salt.

- If you consume alcohol, do so in moderation.

- When you eat food prepared outside of the home, follow the AHA Diet and Lifestyle Recommendations.

From: Lichtenstein AH and others: Diet and lifestyle recommendations revision 2006. A scientific statement from the American Heart Association Nutrition Committee. *Circulation* 114:82, 2006.

One goal of *Healthy People 2020* is to reduce consumption of saturated fat in the population ages 2 years and older to 9.5% of total calorie intake.

TABLE 5-5 Cholesterol Content of Foods

3 oz beef brains	2635 mg
3 oz beef liver	337 mg
1 large egg yolk*	209 mg
3 oz shrimp	166 mg
3 oz beef*	75 mg
3 oz pork	75 mg
3 oz chicken or turkey (white meat)*	75 mg
1 cup ice cream	63 mg
3 oz trout	60 mg
3 oz tuna	45 mg
3 oz hot dog	38 mg
1 oz cheddar cheese*	30 mg
1 cup whole milk*	24 mg
1 cup 1% milk	12 mg
1 cup fat-free milk	5 mg
1 large egg white	0 mg

*Leading dietary sources of cholesterol in American diets.

Some advice regarding fat intake from the 2010 Dietary Guidelines:

- Consume less than 10% of calories from saturated fatty acids by replacing them with monounsaturated and polyunsaturated fatty acids.

- Consume less than 300 mg per day of dietary cholesterol.

- Keep *trans* fatty acid consumption as low as possible by limiting foods that contain synthetic sources of *trans* fats, such as partially hydrogenated oils, and by limiting other solid fats.

- Reduce the intake of calories from solid fats and added sugars.

Continued

- Use oils to replace solid fats where possible.
- Limit the consumption of foods that contain refined grains, especially refined grain foods that contain solid fats, added sugars, and sodium.
- Replace protein foods that are higher in solid fats with choices that are lower in solid fats and calories and/or are sources of oils.
- Increase the amount and variety of seafood in place of same meat and poultry.
- Increase intake of fat-free or low-fat milk and milk products, such as milk, yogurt, cheese, or fortified soy beverages.

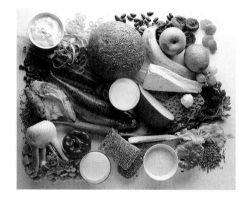

▲ **Whole grains** (shredded wheat, whole-wheat bread, oatmeal cookies, popcorn), **fruits** (orange juice, apple, banana, raisins), **vegetables** (carrots, lettuce, tomato), **lean meats** (roast beef, turkey, chicken), and **fat-free milk** are the primary components of the low-fat menus in Table 5-6.

The advice to consume 20% to 35% of calories as fat does not apply to infants and toddlers below the age of 2 years. These youngsters are forming new tissue that requires fat, especially in the brain, so their intake of fat and cholesterol should not be greatly restricted.

TABLE 5-6 Daily Menu Examples Containing 2000 kcal and 30% or 20% of Calories as Fat

30% of Calories as Fat		20% of Calories as Fat	
Food	Fat (grams)	Food	Fat (grams)
Breakfast			
Orange juice, 1 cup	0.5	Same	0.5
Shredded wheat, ¾ cup	0.5	Shredded wheat, 1 cup	0.7
Toasted bagel	1.1	Same	1.1
Tub margarine, 3 teaspoons	11.4	Tub margarine, 2 teaspoons	7.6
1% low-fat milk, 1 cup	2.5	Fat-free milk, 1 cup	0.6
Lunch			
Whole-wheat bread, 2 slices	2.4	Same	2.4
Roast beef, 2 ounces	4.9	Light turkey roll, 2 ounces	0.9
Mayonnaise, 3 teaspoons	11.0	Mayonnaise, 2 teaspoons	7.3
Lettuce	—	Same	—
Tomato	—	Same	—
Oatmeal cookie, 1	3.3	Oatmeal cookie, 2	6.6
Snack			
Apple	—	Same	—
Dinner			
Chicken tenders frozen meal	18.0	Fat-free chicken tenders	—
Carrots, ½ cup	—	Same	—
Dinner roll, 1	2.0	Same	2.0
Margarine, 1 teaspoon	3.8	Same	3.8
Banana	0.6	Same	0.6
1% low-fat milk, 1 cup	2.5	Fat-free milk, 1 cup	0.6
Snack			
Raisins, 2 teaspoons	—	Raisins, ½ cup	—
Air-popped popcorn, 3 cups	1.0	Air-popped popcorn, 6 cups	2.0
Margarine, 2 teaspoons	7.6	Same	7.6
Totals	**73.1**		**44.3**

The American Dietetic Association, the Dietitians of Canada (see Further Reading 1), the National Cholesterol Education Program (NCEP), and the Food and Nutrition Board are in agreement with the advice of the AHA. The 2010 Dietary Guidelines also support this advice. In addition to fat intake, controlling total calorie intake is also significant, as weight control is a vital component of cardiovascular disease prevention.

Regarding essential fatty acids, the Food and Nutrition Board has issued recommendations for both omega-6 and omega-3 fatty acids. The amounts listed in Table 5-7 work out to about 5% of calorie in-take for the total of both essential fatty acids. Infants and children have lower needs (again, see Chapter 15). Consumption of fish at least twice a week is one step toward meeting requirements for essential fatty acids.

The typical North American diet derives about 7% of calories from polyunsaturated fatty acids, and thus meets essential fatty acid needs. An upper limit of 10% of calorie intake as polyunsaturated fatty acids is often recommended, in part because the breakdown (oxidation) of those present in lipoproteins is linked to increased cholesterol deposition in the arteries (see the Nutrition and Your Health section in this chapter). Depression of immune function is also suspected to be caused by an excessive intake of polyunsaturated fatty acids.

TABLE 5-7 Food and Nutrition Board Recommendations for Omega-6 and Omega-3 Fatty Acids per Day

	Men (grams per day)	Women (grams per day)
Linoleic acid (omega-6)	17	12
Alpha-linolenic acid (omega-3)	1.6	1.1

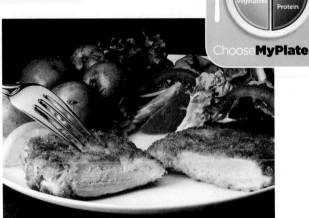

In recent years, the Mediterranean diet (see Newsworthy Nutrition in margin) has attracted a lot of attention as a result of lower rates of chronic diseases seen in people following such a diet plan. The major sources of fat in the Mediterranean diet include liberal amounts of olive oil compared to a small amount of animal fat (from animal flesh and dairy products). In contrast, major sources of fat in the typical North American diet include animal flesh, whole milk, pastries, cheese, margarine, and mayonnaise. While dietary fat sources definitely play a role in prevention of chronic disease, it is important to remember that other aspects of one's lifestyle also contribute to disease risk. People who follow a Mediterranean diet also tend to consume moderate alcohol (usually in the form of red wine, which contains many antioxidants), eat plenty of whole grains and few refined carbohydrates, and are also more physically active than typical North Americans.

An alternative plan for reduction of cardiovascular disease is Dr. Dean Ornish's purely vegetarian (**vegan**) diet plan (see Further Reading 12). This diet is very low in fat, including only a scant quantity of vegetable oil used in cooking and the small amount of oils present in plant foods. Individuals restricting fat intake to 20% of calories should be monitored by a physician, as the resulting increase in carbohydrate intake can increase blood triglycerides in some people, which is not a healthful change. Over time, however, the initial problem of high blood triglycerides on a low-fat diet may self-correct. Among people following the Ornish plan, blood triglycerides initially increased, but within a year, fell to normal values as long as they emphasized high-fiber carbohydrate sources, controlled (or improved) body weight, and followed a regular exercise program.

In summary, the general consensus among nutrition experts suggests that limitation of saturated fat, cholesterol, and *trans* fat intake should be the primary focus, and that the diet needs to contain some omega-3 and omega-6 fatty acids (Table 5-8). Furthermore, if fat intake exceeds 30% of total calories, the extra fat should come from monounsaturated fat.

▲ If you are looking to decrease the amount of saturated and *trans* fats in your diet, it is a good idea to opt for lower-fat substitutes for some of your current high-fat food choices. How do you think this meal compares with the fried meal on p. 179? How does it compare to MyPlate recommendations?

vegan A person who eats only plant foods.

NEWSWORTHY NUTRITION

Low-fat diet not necessary for weight loss

A low-fat, Mediterranean, or low-carbohydrate diet, was studied in moderately obese adults. Weight loss on the Mediterranean Diet (4.6 kg) and low-carbohydrate diet (5.5 kg) was greater than weight loss on the low-fat diet. This, along with the more favorable effects on lipids (low-carbohydrate diet) and on glycemic control (Mediterranean Diet), indicates they may be effective alternatives to low-fat diets.

Source: Shai I and others: Weight loss with a low-carbohydrate, Mediterranean, or low-fat diet. *New England Journal of Medicine* 359:229, 2008 (see Further Reading 14).

▣ connect PLUS NUTRITION **Check out the Connect site** www.mcgrawhillconnect.com **to further explore weight-loss diets.**

CONCEPT CHECK

There is no RDA for fat. We need about 5% of total calorie intake from plant oils to obtain the needed essential fatty acids. Eating fatty fish at least twice a week is also advised to supply omega-3 fatty acids. Many health-related agencies recommend a diet containing no more than 35% of calorie intake as fat, with no more than 7% to 10% of calorie intake as a combination of saturated fat and *trans* fat for the general public. Cholesterol intake should be limited to 200 to 300 milligrams per day. These practices help maintain a normal LDL value in the blood. The North American diet contains about 33% of calories as fat, with about 13% of calories as saturated fat and about 3% as *trans* fatty acids. Cholesterol intake varies from about 200 to 400 milligrams per day.

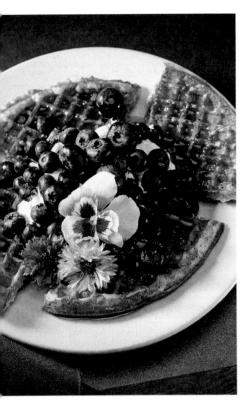

TABLE 5-8 Tips for Avoiding Too Much Fat, Saturated Fat, Cholesterol, and *Trans* Fat

	Eat Less of These Foods	Eat More of These Foods
Grains	• Pasta dishes with cheese or cream sauces • Croissants • Pastries • Doughnuts • Pie crust	• Whole-grain breads • Whole-grain pasta • Brown rice • Angel food cake • Animal or graham crackers • Air-popped popcorn
Vegetables	• French fries • Potato chips • Vegetables cooked in butter, cheese, or cream sauces	• Fresh, frozen, baked, or steamed vegetables
Fruit	• Fruit pies	• Fresh, frozen, or canned fruits
Dairy	• Whole milk • Ice cream • High-fat cheese • Cheesecake	• Fat-free and reduced-fat milk • Low-fat frozen desserts (e.g., yogurt, sherbet, ice milk) • Reduced-fat/part-skim cheese
Protein	• Bacon • Sausage • Organ meats (e.g., liver) • Egg yolks	• Fish • Skinless poultry • Lean cuts of meat (with fat trimmed away) • Soy products • Egg whites/egg substitutes
Oils	• Butter and stick margarine	• Canola oil or olive oil • Tub or liquid margarine (in small amounts)

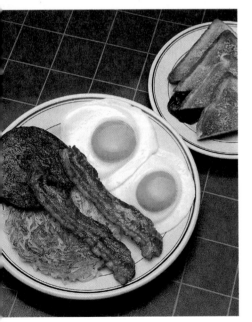

▲ To avoid too much saturated fat and cholesterol, for breakfast eat fewer foods like bacon, sausage, hash browns and whole eggs and more foods like whole-grain waffles and fresh fruit.

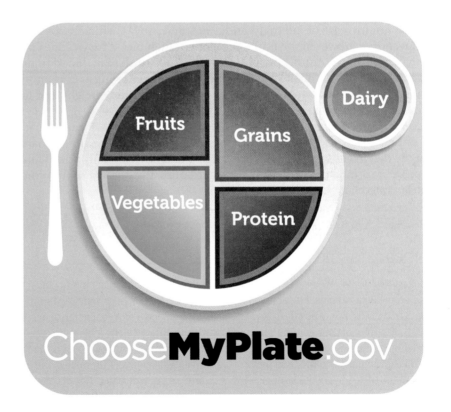

LIPIDS CONCEPT MAP

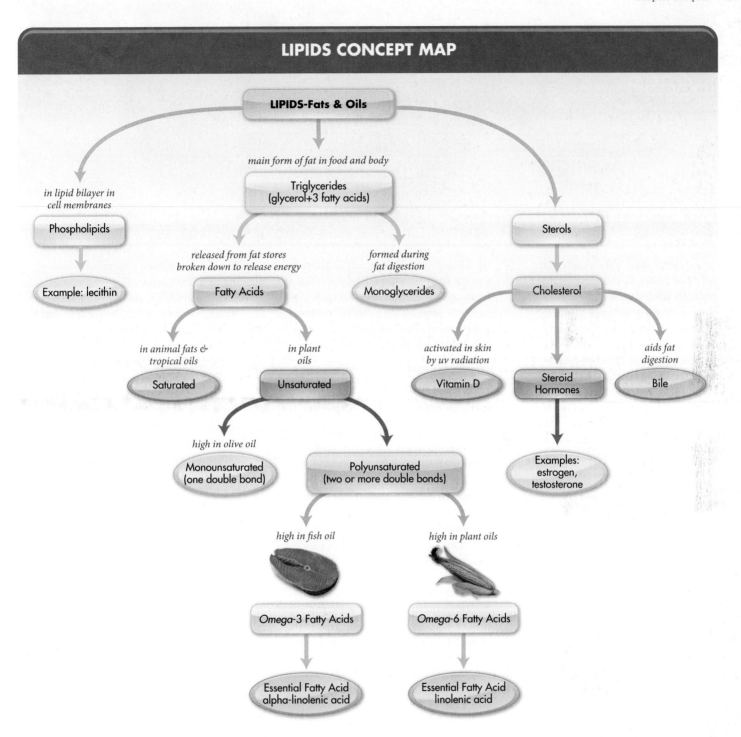

Lipids and Cardiovascular Disease

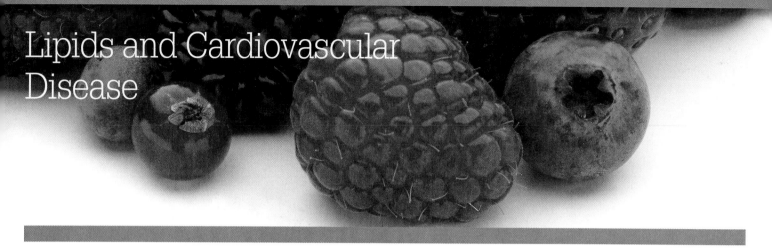

Cardiovascular disease is the major killer of North Americans. Cardiovascular disease typically involves the coronary arteries and, thus, frequently the term coronary heart disease (CHD) or coronary artery disease (CAD) is used. Each year about 500,000 people die of coronary heart disease in the United States, about 60% more than die of cancer. The figure rises to almost 1 million if strokes and other circulatory diseases are included in the global term *cardiovascular disease*. About 1.5 million people in the United States each year have a heart attack. The overall male-to-female ratio for cardiovascular disease is about 2:1. Women generally lag about 10 years behind men in developing

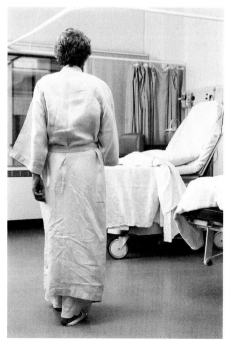

▲ Cardiovascular disease kills more women than any other disease—twice as many as does cancer.

the disease. Still, it eventually kills more women than any other disease—twice as many as does cancer. And, for each person in North America who dies of cardiovascular disease, 20 more (over 13 million people) have symptoms of the disease.

Development of Cardiovascular Disease

The symptoms of cardiovascular disease develop over many years and often do not become obvious until old age. Nonetheless, autopsies of young adults under 20 years of age have shown that many of them had atherosclerotic **plaque** in their arteries (Fig. 5-16). This finding indicates that plaque buildup can begin in childhood and continue throughout life, although it usually goes undetected for some time.

The typical forms of cardiovascular disease—coronary heart disease and strokes—are associated with inadequate blood circulation in the heart and brain related to buildup of this plaque. Blood supplies the heart muscle, brain, and other body organs with oxygen and nutrients. When blood flow via the coronary arteries surrounding the heart is interrupted, the heart muscle can be damaged. A heart attack, or **myocardial infarction,** may result (review Fig. 5-16). This may cause the heart to beat irregularly or to stop. About 25% of people do not survive their first heart attack. If blood flow to parts of the brain is interrupted long enough, part of the brain dies, causing a **cerebrovascular accident,** or stroke.

A heart attack can strike with the sudden force of a sledgehammer, with pain radiating up the neck or down the arm.

It can sneak up at night, masquerading as indigestion, with slight pain or pressure in the chest. Many times, the symptoms are so subtle in women that death occurs before she or the health professional realizes that a heart attack is taking place. If there is any suspicion at all that a heart attack is taking place, the person should first call 911 and then chew an aspirin (325 milligrams) thoroughly. Aspirin helps reduce the blood clotting that leads to a heart attack.

Continuous formation and breakdown of blood clots in the blood vessels is a normal process. However, in areas where plaques build up, blood clots are more likely to remain intact and then lead to a blockage, cutting off or diminishing the supply of blood to the heart (via the coronary arteries) or brain (via the carotid arteries). More than 95% of heart attacks are caused by such blood clots. Heart attacks generally are caused by total blockage of the coronary arteries due to a blood clot forming in an area of the artery already partially blocked by plaque. Disruption of the plaque may even lead to eventual clot formation.

plaque A cholesterol-rich substance deposited in the blood vessels; it contains various white blood cells, smooth muscle cells, various proteins, cholesterol and other lipids, and eventually calcium.

myocardial infarction Death of part of the heart muscle. Also termed a *heart attack.*

cerebrovascular accident (CVA) Death of part of the brain tissue due typically to a blood clot. Also termed a *stroke.*

> **Typical warning signs of a heart attack are:**

- Intense, prolonged chest pain or pressure, sometimes radiating to other parts of the upper body (men and women)
- Shortness of breath (men and women)
- Sweating (men and women)
- Nausea and vomiting (especially women)
- Dizziness (especially women)
- Weakness (men and women)
- Jaw, neck, and shoulder pain (especially women)
- Irregular heartbeat (men and women)

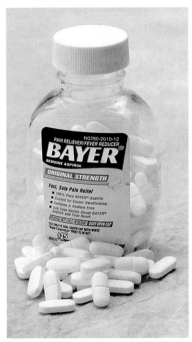

▲ At the first sign of a possible heart attack, the person should first call 911 and then thoroughly chew an aspirin.

> *Healthy People 2020* has set a goal of reducing death from coronary heart disease by 20%, compared with today's incidence.

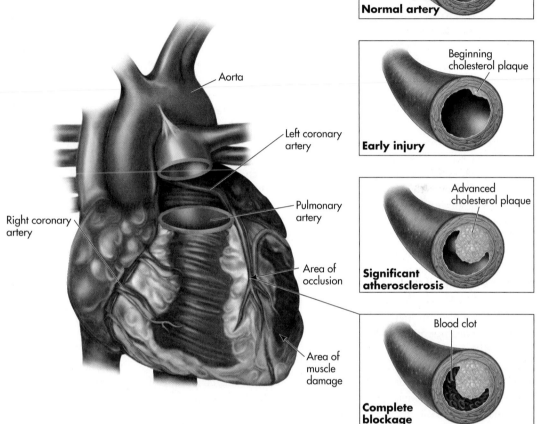

Cell lining (endothelium)

Muscle layer

Vessel opening

Normal artery

Beginning cholesterol plaque

Early injury

Advanced cholesterol plaque

Significant atherosclerosis

Blood clot

Complete blockage

Aorta

Left coronary artery

Pulmonary artery

Right coronary artery

Area of occlusion

Area of muscle damage

FIGURE 5-16 ▶ The road to a heart attack. Injury to an artery wall begins the process. This is followed by a progressive buildup of plaque in the artery walls. The heart attack represents the terminal phase of the process. Blockage of the left coronary artery by a blood clot is evident. The heart muscle served by the portion of the coronary artery beyond the point of blockage lacks oxygen and nutrients and is damaged and may die. This damage can lead to a significant drop in heart function and often total heart failure.

Atherosclerosis probably first develops to repair damage in a vessel lining. The damage that starts this process can be caused by smoking, diabetes, hypertension, LDL, and viral and bacterial infection. Ongoing inflammation in the blood vessel is also suspected to cause blood vessel damage. (A laboratory test for c-reactive protein in the blood is used to assess if inflammation is present.) (see Further Reading 3). Atherosclerosis can be seen in arteries throughout the body. The damage develops especially at points where an artery branches into two smaller vessels. A great deal of stress is placed on the vessel walls at these points due to changes in blood flow.

Once blood vessel damage has occurred, the next step in the development of atherosclerosis is the progression phase. This step is characterized by deposition of plaque at the site of initial damage. The rate of plaque buildup during the progression phase is directly related to the amount of LDL in the blood. The form of LDL that contributes to atherosclerosis is **oxidized** LDL (see Further Readings 6 and 10). This

oxidize In the most basic sense, the loss of an electron or gain of an oxygen by a chemical substance. This change typically alters the shape and/or function of the substance.

form is preferentially taken up by scavenger cells in the arterial wall. Nutrients and phytochemicals that have **antioxidant** properties may reduce LDL oxidation. Fruits and vegetables are particularly rich in these compounds. Eating fruits and vegetables regularly is one positive step we can make to reduce plaque buildup and slow the progression of cardiovascular disease. Some fruits and vegetables particularly helpful in this regard include legumes (beans), nuts, dried plums (prunes), raisins, berries, plums, apples, cherries, oranges, grapes, spinach, broccoli, red bell peppers, potatoes, and onions. Tea and coffee are also sources of antioxidants.

As plaque accumulates, arteries harden, narrow, and lose their elasticity. Affected arteries become further damaged as blood pumps through them and pressure increases. Finally, in the terminal phase, a clot or spasm in a plaque-clogged artery leads to a heart attack.

Factors that typically bring on a heart attack in a person already at risk include dehydration; acute emotional stress (such as firing an employee); strenuous physical activity when not otherwise physically fit (shoveling snow, for example); waking during the night or getting up in the morning (linked to an abrupt increase in stress); and consuming large, high-fat meals (increases blood clotting).

Risk Factors for Cardiovascular Disease

Many of us are free of the risk factors that contribute to rapid development of atherosclerosis. If so, the advice of health experts is to consume a balanced diet, perform regular physical activity, have a complete fasting lipoprotein analysis performed at age 20 or beyond, and reevaluate risk factors every 5 years.

For most people, however, the most likely risk factors are:

- **Total blood cholesterol over 200 milligrams per 100 milliliters of blood** (mg/dl; dl is short for deciliter or 100 milliliters). Risk is especially high when total cholesterol is at or over 240 mg/dl and LDL-cholesterol readings are over 130 to 160 mg/dl. (The terms LDL-cholesterol and HDL-cholesterol

are used when expressing the blood concentration because it is the cholesterol content of these lipoproteins that is measured.)

- **Smoking.** Smoking is the main cause of about 20% of cardiovascular disease deaths and generally negates the female advantage of later occurrence of the disease. A combination of smoking and oral contraceptive use increases the risk of cardiovascular disease in women even more. Smoking greatly increases the expression of a person's genetically linked risk for cardiovascular disease, even if one's blood lipids are low. Smoking also makes blood more likely to clot. Even secondhand smoke has been implicated as a risk factor.
- **Hypertension. Systolic blood pressure** over 139 (millimeters of mercury) and **diastolic blood pressure** over 89 indicate hypertension. Healthy blood pressure values are less than 120 and 80, respectively. (Treatment of hypertension is reviewed in Chapter 9.)
- **Diabetes.** Diabetes virtually guarantees development of cardiovascular disease and so puts a person with diabetes in the high-risk group. Insulin increases cholesterol synthesis in the liver, in turn increasing LDL in the bloodstream. This disease negates any female advantage.

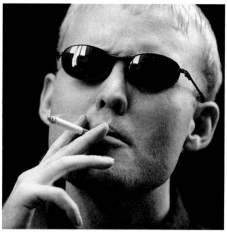

▲ Smoking is one of the four major risk factors for developing cardiovascular disease.

antioxidant Generally a compound that stops the damaging effects of reactive substances seeking an electron (i.e., oxidizing agents). This prevents breakdown (oxidizing) of substances in foods or the body, particularly lipids.

systolic blood pressure The pressure in the arterial blood vessels associated with the pumping of blood from the heart.

diastolic blood pressure The pressure in the arterial blood vessels when the heart is between beats.

MAKING DECISIONS

Antioxidant Supplements and Cardiovascular Disease

Are large doses of antioxidant vitamin supplements a reliable way to reduce LDL oxidation, and thereby prevent cardiovascular disease? Controversy about such dietary supplementation exists among the experts, as will be detailed in Chapter 10. The American Heart Association does not support use of antioxidant supplements (such as vitamin E) to reduce cardiovascular disease risk. This is because large-scale studies have shown no decrease in cardiovascular disease risk with use of antioxidant supplements. One study even showed a modest increase for heart failure in people with diabetes or otherwise at high risk for cardiovascular disease after taking antioxidant supplements. However, further trials of antioxidant supplementation (e.g., 600 IU of vitamin E every other day) for prevention of heart disease in men are ongoing. With regard to women, 600 IU of natural-source vitamin E taken every other day provided no overall benefit for major cardiovascular events (or cancer). More research is warranted, however, as a decrease in sudden cardiac death was seen in a subset of older women in this study. Some experts suggest daily vitamin E supplementation (100 IU to 400 IU) may be helpful for *preventing* cardiovascular disease, while other experts recommend against the practice. One thing is certain: any supplementation of vitamin E should be taken only under the guidance of a physician, because of interactions with vitamin K and anticlotting medications (and possibly high-dose aspirin use).

► For more information on cardiovascular disease, see the website of the American Heart Association at www.americanheart.org or the heart disease section of Healthfinder at www.healthfinder.gov/tours/heart.htm. This is a site created by the U.S. government for consumers. In addition, visit the website www.nhlbi.nih.gov/.

► *Healthy People 2020* has set a goal of reducing total blood cholesterol among adults from the average of 198 mg/dl to 178 mg/dl, as well as reducing the percentage of adults with high blood cholesterol from 15% to 13.5%.

► Cardiovascular Disease Risk Factors

- Total blood cholesterol > 200 mg/dl
- Smoking
- Hypertension
- Diabetes
- HDL cholesterol < 40 mg/dl
- Age: Men > 45 yr; Women > 55 yr
- Family history of cardiovascular disease
- Blood triglycerides > 200 mg/dl
- Obesity
- Inactivity

► Two approaches have been shown to cause reversal of atherosclerosis in the body. One employs a vegan diet and other lifestyle changes that are part of the Dr. Dean Ornish program. The other employs aggressive LDL lowering with medications.

► As noted earlier, aspirin in small doses reduces blood clotting. It is often used under a physician's guidance to treat people at risk for heart attack or stroke, especially if one has already occurred. About 80 to 160 milligrams per day is needed for such benefits. Individuals who may especially benefit from aspirin therapy are men over 40, smokers, postmenopausal women, and people with diabetes, hypertension, or a family history of cardiovascular disease.

Together, the previous four risk factors explain most cases of cardiovascular disease.

Other risk factors to consider:

- HDL-cholesterol under 40 mg/dl, especially when the ratio of total cholesterol to HDL-cholesterol is greater than 4:1 (3.5:1 or less is optimal). Women often have high values for HDL-cholesterol, and therefore it is important for this to be measured in women to establish cardiovascular disease risk. A value of 60 mg/dl or more is especially protective. Exercising for at least 45 minutes four times a week can increase HDL by about 5 mg/dl. Losing excess weight (especially around the waist) and avoiding smoking and overeating also help maintain or raise HDL, as does moderate alcohol consumption.
- Age. Men over 45 years and women over 55 years.
- Family history of cardiovascular disease, especially before age 50.
- Blood triglycerides 200 mg/dl or greater in the fasting state (less than 100 mg/dl is optimal).
- Obesity (especially fat accumulation in the waist). Typical weight gain seen in adults is a chief contributor to the increase in LDL seen with aging. Obesity also typically leads to insulin resistance, creating a diabetes-like state, and ultimately the disease itself. It also increases overall inflamation throughout the body.
- Inactivity. Exercise conditions the arteries to adapt to physical stress. Regular exercise also improves insulin action in the body. The corresponding reduction in insulin output leads to a reduction in lipoprotein synthesis in the liver. Both regular aerobic exercise and resistance exercise are recommended. A person with existing cardiovascular disease should seek physician approval before starting such a program, as should older adults.

Researchers are trying to unravel and quantify numerous other factors that may be linked to premature cardiovascular disease, such as the connection between inadequate intake of vitamin B-6, folate, and vitamin B-12, which can lead to increased

homocysteine in the blood. As noted, homocysteine may damage the cells lining the blood vessels, in turn promoting atherosclerosis. Studies show that supplementation with folic acid and B vitamins does not reduce risk of recurrent cardiovascular disease in patients that had previous heart attacks or had existing vascular diseases.

The term *risk factor* is not equivalent to cause of disease; nevertheless, the more of these risk factors one has, the greater the chances of ultimately developing cardiovascular disease. A good example is the **metabolic syndrome** (also called *Syndrome X)* discussed in Chapter 4. A person with the metabolic syndrome would have abdominal obesity, high blood triglycerides, low HDL-cholesterol, hypertension, poor blood glucose regulation (i.e., high fasting blood glucose), and increased blood clotting. This profile raises the risk for cardiovascular disease considerably. On a positive note, cardiovascular disease is rare in populations who have low LDL-cholesterol, normal blood pressure, and do not smoke or have diabetes. By minimizing these risk factors, as well as following the dietary recommendations of the American Heart Association on page 193 and staying physically active, one will most likely reduce many of the other controllable risk factors listed. In other words, develop and follow a total lifestyle plan. Medications may also be added to lower blood lipids, as discussed next. Finally, if a person has a family history of cardiovascular disease but the usual risk factors aren't present, a rarer defect might be the cause. In this case, having a detailed physical examination for other potential causes is advised.

Medical Interventions to Lower Blood Lipids

Some people need even more aggressive therapy added to their regimen of a diet and lifestyle overhaul to treat elevated blood lipids. The clearest indication for this more aggressive approach is in people who already have had a heart attack or have cardiovascular disease symptoms or diabetes.

Medications are the cornerstone of this more aggressive therapy. The National

Cholesterol Education Program in the United States has developed a formula based on age, total blood cholesterol, HDL-cholesterol, smoking history, and blood pressure to determine who needs such medications. Check out this formula at http://hp2010.nhlbihin.net/atpiii/calculator.asp?usertype=pub. This formula provides an estimate for having a heart attack in the next 10 years.

Medications work to lower LDL in one of two ways. Some reduce cholesterol synthesis in the liver. Such medicines are known as "statins" (e.g., atorvistatin [Lipitor]). The cost of treatment with one of these drugs can be from $1,600 or more per year, depending on the dose needed. These medications lead to problems in some people, and so require physician monitoring, especially of liver function. Another group of medications binds bile acids or the cholesterol that is part of bile secreted into the small intestine. This binding leads to their elimination in the feces and so requires the liver to synthesize new bile acids and/or cholesterol. The liver removes LDL from the blood to do this. Some of these medications taste gritty and therefore are not popular.

The current therapeutic goal for people with (or at high risk for) cardiovascular disease (Table 5-9) is to drive LDL down to less than 70 mg/dl.

The statin drug simvastatin (Zocor) has been combined with another drug (ezetimibe) and is marketed as Vytorin, a drug that will treat the two sources of cholesterol, "food and family." While the statin reduces the cholesterol made by the liver, the ezetimibe helps block the absorption of cholesterol from food.

A third group of drugs can be used to lower blood triglycerides by decreasing the triglyceride production of the liver. These include gemfibrozil (Lopid) and megadoses of the vitamin nicotinic acid. The use of nicotinic acid does result in pesky side effects, however, but these are typically manageable.

Other Possible Medical Therapies for Cardiovascular Disease

FDA has approved two margarines that have positive effects on blood cholesterol levels—Benecol and Take Control. These margarines contain plant stanols/sterols.

The plant stanols/sterols, also called phytosterols, work by reducing cholesterol absorption in the small intestine and lowering its return to the liver. The liver responds by taking up more cholesterol from the blood so it can continue to make bile acids. The studies done on the cholesterol-lowering effect of these margarines have found that 2 to 5 grams of plant stanols/sterols per day reduces total blood cholesterol by 8% to 10% and LDL-cholesterol by 9% to 14% (similar to what is seen with some cholesterol-lowering drugs). (see Further Readings 7, 11, and 13.)

Benecol is made from plant stanols extracted from wood pulp. It is sold as margarine and has been added to salad dressings. Take Control is made from plant sterols isolated from soybeans. The recommended amount for both is about 2 to 3 grams per day as part of at least two meals; this works out to about 1 or 2 tablespoons per day. Use would cost about $1.00 per day, as these margarines are more expensive than regular margarines.

In people who have borderline high total blood cholesterol (between 200 and 239 mg/dl), these margarines can be helpful in avoiding future drug therapy. Plant stanols/sterols have been made available in pill form as well. Remember that plant sterols are naturally present in nuts in high concentrations. Wheat germ, sesame seeds, pistachios, and sunflower seeds are some of the richest sources.

The two most common surgical treatments for coronary artery blockage are percutaneous transluminal coronary angioplasty (PTCA) and coronary artery bypass graft (CABG). PTCA involves the insertion of a balloon catheter into an artery. Once it is advanced to the area of the lesion, the balloon is expanded to crush the lesion. This method works best when only one vessel is blocked, and it may be held open with metal mesh, called a stent. CABG involves the removal and use of a saphenous vein, a large vein in the leg, or use of a mammary artery. The relocated vein is sewn to the main heart vessel (aorta) and then used to bypass the blocked artery. The procedure can be performed on one or more blockages.

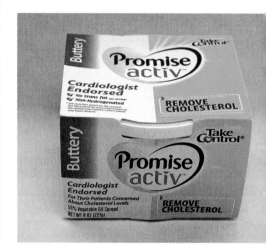

▲ Benecol and Take Control are margarines that are examples of "functional foods" because they contain added cholesterol-lowering plant stanols/sterols.

TABLE 5-9 Sorting Out One's Goals for Cardiovascular Disease Prevention/Treatment

Risk Class	This Is You If . . .	Your LDL (mg/dl) Goal
Very high	You have cardiovascular disease *and* other risk factors such as diabetes, obesity, smoking	Below 70
High	You have cardiovascular disease *or* diabetes *or* two or more risk factors for cardiovascular disease (e.g., smoking, hypertension)	Below 100
Moderately high	You have cardiovascular disease risks and an increased 10-year risk of developing a heart attack	100–130
Moderate	You have two or more risk factors and a marginal chance of developing cardiovascular disease in the next 10 years.	Below 130
Low	You have few or no cardiovascular disease risk factors	Below 160

Case Study Planning a Heart-Healthy Diet

Jackie is a 21-year-old health-conscious individual majoring in business. She recently learned that a diet high in saturated fat can contribute to high blood cholesterol and that exercise is beneficial for the heart. Jackie now takes a brisk 30-minute walk each morning before going to class, and she has started to cut as much fat out of her diet as she can, replacing it mostly with carbohydrates. A typical day for Jackie now begins with a bowl of Fruity Pebbles with 1 cup of skim milk and ½ cup of apple juice. For lunch, she might pack a turkey sandwich on white bread with lettuce, tomato, and mustard; a small package of fat-free pretzels; and a handful of reduced-fat vanilla wafers. Dinner could be a large portion of pasta with some olive oil and garlic mixed in, and a small iceberg lettuce salad with lemon juice squeezed over it. Her snacks are usually baked chips, low-fat cookies, fat-free frozen yogurt, or fat-free pretzels. She drinks diet soft drinks throughout the day as her main beverage.

Answer the following questions, and check your response in Appendix A.

1. Has Jackie made the best diet changes with regard to lowering blood cholesterol and maintaining heart health?
2. Is there much fat left in Jackie's new diet plan? Is it necessary for her to drastically lower her fat intake?
3. What types of fat should Jackie try to consume? Why are these types of fat the most desirable?
4. What types of foods has Jackie used to replace the fat in her diet?
5. What food groups are missing from her new diet plan? How many servings should she be including from these food groups?
6. Is Jackie's new exercise routine appropriate?

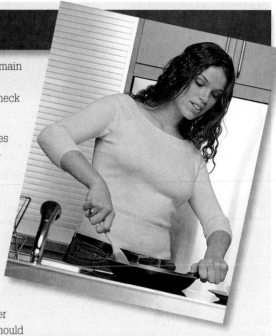

▲ Are there important food groups missing from Jackie's new diet plan?

Summary (Numbers refer to numbered sections in the chapter.)

5.1 Lipids are a group of compounds that do not dissolve in water. Fatty acids are the simplest form of lipid. There are three fatty acids on every triglyceride, the most common type of lipid found in the body and foods. Phospholipids and sterols are two other classes of lipids in food and our bodies.

5.2 Saturated fatty acids contain no carbon-carbon double bonds, monounsaturated fatty acids contain one carbon-carbon double bond, and polyunsaturated fatty acids contain two or more carbon-carbon double bonds in the carbon chain. In omega-3 polyunsaturated fatty acids, the first of the carbon-carbon double bonds is located three carbons from the methyl end of the carbon chain. In omega-6 polyunsaturated fatty acids, the first carbon-carbon double bond counting from the methyl end occurs at the sixth carbon. Both omega-3 and omega-6 fatty acids are essential fatty acids; these must be included in the diet to maintain health.

Triglycerides are formed from a glycerol backbone with three fatty acids. Triglycerides rich in long-chain saturated fatty acids tend to be solid at room temperature, whereas those rich in monounsaturated and polyunsaturated fatty acids are liquid at room temperature. Triglyceride is the major form of fat in both food and the body. It allows for efficient energy storage, protects certain organs, transports fat-soluble vitamins, and helps insulate the body.

5.3 Foods rich in fat include salad oils, butter, margarine, and mayonnaise. Nuts, bologna, avocados, and bacon are also high in fat, as are peanut butter and cheddar cheese. Steak and hamburger are moderate in fat content, as is whole milk. Many grain products, and fruits and vegetables in general, are low in fat.

Fats and oils have several functions as components of foods. Fats add flavor and texture to foods and provide some satiety after meals. Some phospholipids are used in foods as emulsifiers, which suspend fat in water. When fatty acids break down, food becomes rancid, resulting in a foul odor and unpleasant flavor.

Hydrogenation is the process of converting carbon-carbon double bonds into single bonds by adding hydrogen at the point of unsaturation. The partial-hydrogenation of fatty acids in vegetable oils changes the oils to semisolid fats and helps in food formulation and reduces rancidity. Hydrogenation also increases *trans* fatty acid content. High amounts of *trans* fat in the diet are discouraged, as these increase LDL and reduce HDL.

5.4 Fat digestion takes place primarily in the small intestine. Lipase enzyme released from the pancreas digests long-chain triglycerides into smaller breakdown products—namely, monoglycerides (glycerol backbones with single fatty acids attached) and fatty acids. The breakdown products are then taken up by the absorptive cells of the small intestine. These products are mostly remade into triglycerides and eventually enter the lymphatic system, in turn passing into the bloodstream.

5.5 Lipids are carried in the bloodstream by various lipoproteins, which consist of a central triglyceride core encased in a shell of protein, cholesterol, and phospholipid. Chylomicrons are released from intestinal cells and carry lipids arising from dietary intake. Very-low-density lipoprotein (VLDL) and low-density lipoprotein (LDL) carry lipids both taken up by and synthesized in the liver. High-density lipoprotein (HDL) picks up cholesterol from cells and facilitates its transport back to the liver.

5.6 The essential fatty acids are linoleic acid (an omega-6 fatty acid) and alpha-linolenic acid (on omega-3 fatty acid). Body cells can synthesize hormone-like compounds from both omega-3 and omega-6 fatty acids.

5.7 The compounds produced from omega-3 fatty acids tend to reduce blood clotting, blood pressure, and inflammatory responses in the body. Those produced from omega-6 fatty acids tend to increase blood clotting.

5.8 Phospholipids are derivatives of triglycerides in which one or two of the fatty acids are replaced by phosphorus-containing compounds. Phospholipids are important parts of cell membranes, and some act as efficient emulsifiers.

5.9 Cholesterol forms vital biological compounds, such as hormones, components of cell membranes, and bile acids. Cells in the body make cholesterol whether we eat it or not. It is not a necessary part of an adult's diet.

5.10 There is currently no RDA for fat for adults. Plant oils should contribute about 5% of total calories to achieve the Adequate Intakes proposed for essential fatty acids (linoleic acid and alpha-linolenic acid). Fatty fish are a rich source of omega-3 fatty acids and should be consumed at least twice a week.

Many health agencies and scientific groups suggest a fat intake of no more than 30% to 35% of total calories. Some health experts advocate an even further reduction to 20% of calorie intake for some people to maintain a normal LDL value, but such a diet requires professional guidance. Medications such as "statins" may be added also to lower LDL. If fat intake exceeds 30% of total calories, the diet should emphasize monounsaturated fat. The typical North American diet contains about 33% of total calories as fat.

N&YH In the blood, elevated amounts of LDL and low amounts of HDL are strong predictors of the risk for cardiovascular disease. Additional risk factors for the disease are smoking, hypertension, diabetes, obesity, and inactivity.

Check Your Knowledge (Answers to the following questions are below.)

1. Margarine usually is made by a process called _____, in which hydrogen atoms are added to carbon-carbon double bonds in the polyunsaturated fatty acids found in vegetable oils.
   a. saturation
   b. esterification
   c. isomerization
   d. hydrogenation

2. Essential fatty acids that cause a decrease in blood clotting are
   a. omega-3.
   b. omega-6.
   c. omega-9.
   d. prostacyclins.

3. Cholesterol is
   a. a dietary essential; the human body cannot synthesize it.
   b. found in foods of plant origin.
   c. an important part of human cell membranes and necessary to make some hormones.
   d. All of the above.

4. Which of the following groups of foods would be important sources of saturated fatty acids?
   a. olive oil, peanut oil, canola oil
   b. palm oil, palm kernel oil, coconut oil
   c. safflower oil, corn oil, soybean oil
   d. All of the above.

5. Lipoproteins are important for
   a. transport of fats in the blood and lymphatic system.
   b. synthesis of triglycerides.
   c. synthesis of adipose tissue.
   d. enzyme production.

6. Which of the following foods is the best source of omega-3 fatty acids?
   a. fatty fish
   b. peanut butter and jelly
   c. lard and shortenings
   d. beef and other red meats

7. Immediately after a meal, newly digested and absorbed dietary fats appear in the lymph, and then blood, as part of which of the following?
   a. LDL
   b. HDL
   c. chylomicrons
   d. cholesterol

8. High blood concentrations of _____ decrease the risk for cardiovascular disease.

   a. low-density lipoproteins
   b. chylomicrons
   c. high-density lipoproteins
   d. cholesterol

9. Phospholipids such as lecithin are used extensively in food preparation because they
   a. provide the agreeable feel of fat melting on the tongue.
   b. are excellent emulsifiers.
   c. provide important textural features.
   d. impart delicate flavors.

10. The main form of lipid found in the food we eat is
    a. cholesterol.
    b. phospholipids.
    c. triglycerides.
    d. plant sterols

Answers: 1. d (LO 5.3), 2. a (LO 5.6), 3. c (LO 5.9), 4. b (LO 5.3), 5. a (LO 5.5), 6. a (LO 5.6), 7. c (LO 5.5), 8. c (LO 5.5), 9. b (LO 5.8), 10. c (LO 5.2)

Study Questions (Numbers refer to Learning Outcomes)

1. Describe the chemical structures of saturated and polyunsaturated fatty acids and their different effects in both food and the human body. (LO 5.3)

2. Relate the need for omega-3 fatty acids in the diet to the recommendation to consume fatty fish at least twice a week. (LO 5.7)

3. Describe the structures, origins, and roles of the four major blood lipoproteins. (LO 5.5)

4. What are the recommendations from various health-care organizations regarding fat intake? What does this mean in terms of food choices? (LO 5.10)

5. What are two important attributes of fat in food? How are these different from the general functions of lipids in the human body? (LO 5.3)

6. Describe the significance of and possible uses for reduced-fat foods. (LO 5.10)

7. Does the total cholesterol concentration in the bloodstream tell the whole story with respect to cardiovascular disease risk? (LO 5.9)

8. List the four main risk factors for the development of cardiovascular disease. (LO 5.11)

9. What three lifestyle factors decrease the risk of cardiovascular disease development? (LO 5.11)

10. When are medications most needed in cardiovascular disease therapy, and how in general do the various classes of medications operate to reduce risk? (LO 5.11)

What Would You Choose Recommendations

With heart health in mind you will want to choose the ground meat with the lowest fat, saturated fat, and cholesterol. Check the Nutrition Facts label to compare the lipid content of various products. Look for cuts of meat with "round " or "loin" in the name for lowest fat content.

The USDA allows up to 30% fat (by weight) in raw ground beef, so the cut of beef makes a difference. Regular ground beef typically contains the most fat (about 20% to 30% fat). Next comes ground chuck (about 15% fat), followed by ground round (about 10% fat), and ground sirloin (about 3% fat). Table 5-10 shows a further breakdown of the fat content of varieties of ground beef. Based on this information, you can see that the ground sirloin will give you the leanest burgers.

The ground sirloin, however, will also be the most expensive variety of ground beef. You may, therefore, want to take advantage of the fact that ground beef loses a lot of fat during cooking—as much as 50% for the highest fat products. Typically, regular ground beef is the least expensive product. As the % lean increases, so does price. You can purchase the higher-fat regular ground beef and reduce the amount of fat in the final product by draining, blotting with paper towels, or rinsing under warm water.

For foods in which the ground beef will be shaped then cooked (e.g., hamburger patties, meatballs, or meatloaf), bake, grill, or broil the ground meat on a rack so that fat will drain from the product as it cooks, then let the cooked product rest on paper towels for 1 minute after cooking. For recipes that incorporate browned ground beef into a mixed dish (e.g., casseroles or spaghetti sauce), brown ground beef, crumbling as you cook, then blot with paper towels or rinse under warm water to achieve a final cooked product with nearly the same fat content as the ground round. Using the rinsing method, 100 grams (about 3.5 ounces) of ground beef yields a final product with just 4 grams of fat. Because a greater percentage of the starting product is lost during cooking, you will

TABLE 5-10 Calorie, Fat and Cholesterol Content of Types of Ground Beef

	Energy (kcal)	Total Fat(g)	Saturated Fat (g)	Cholesterol (mg)
Regular ground beef, 3.5 oz cooked	273	18	7	82
Ground chuck, 3.5 oz cooked	232	14	5	86
Ground round, 3.5 oz cooked	204	11	4	82
Ground sirloin, 3.5 oz cooked	164	6	3	76

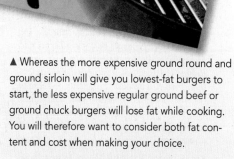

▲ Whereas the more expensive ground round and ground sirloin will give you lowest-fat burgers to start, the less expensive regular ground beef or ground chuck burgers will lose fat while cooking. You will therefore want to consider both fat content and cost when making your choice.

end up with less meat in the final product. However, this is not such a big deal because most Americans consume two to three times as much protein as they need. To further enhance the heart-healthiness of mixed dishes, replace some of that lost product with beans. Chili or tacos would be excellent recipes to try with this method.

Further Readings

1. ADA Reports: Position of the American Dietetic Association and Dietitians of Canada: Dietary fatty acids. *Journal of the American Dietetic Association* 107:1599, 2007.

   A diet is recommended that reduces fatty acids that increase risk of disease, while promoting fatty acids that benefit health. Dietary fat should provide 20% to 35% of energy and emphasize a reduction in saturated fatty acids and trans fatty acids and an increase in n-3 polyunsaturated fatty acids. A food-based approach should be used that includes fruits and vegetables, whole grains, legumes, nuts and seeds, lean protein, and fish. Nonhydrogenated margarines and oils are recommended such that unsaturated fatty acids are the predominant fat source in the diet.

2. Getz L: A burger and fries (hold the *trans* fats). *Today's Dietitian* 11(2):35, 2009.

   Several cities across the United States, including New York, Philadelphia, and Boston, have banned trans fat use in restaurants. Most eating establishments have willingly responded to the demand for healthier oils. It is important to remember that choosing trans fat-free foods does not necessarily make it a healthy choice.

3. Hansson GK: Inflammation, atherosclerosis, and coronary artery disease. *The New England Journal of Medicine* 352:1685, 2005.

   Excellent review of the role of inflammation in causing cardiovascular disease. Identifying atherosclerosis as an inflammatory disease offers new opportunities for the prevention and treatment of coronary artery disease.

4. He KA, Daviglus ML: A few more thoughts about fish and fish oil. *Journal of the American Dietetic Association* 105:428, 2005.

   Fish consumption has been shown to have beneficial effects on cardiovascular disease. Consuming whole fish is thought to have greater benefits and be safer than using fish oil supplements. Fish is not only a rich source of omega-3 fatty acids, but is also a valuable source of protein and trace elements that may also provide protective effects for the cardiovascular system. Broiled or baked fish is recommended rather than fried fish because frying may decrease the ratio of omega-3 to omega-6 fatty acids and may produce trans fatty acids and oxidized lipid products that may increase cardiovascular disease risk.

5. Kris-Etherton PM, Hill AM: n-3 fatty acids: Food or supplements? *Journal of the American Dietetic Association* 108:1125, 2008.

   A food-based approach is recommended for all fatty acids including the n-3 fatty acids. If an individual does not eat fish, the richest source of n-3 fatty acids, other options such as "designer" foods high in n-3 fatty acids, foods fortified with these fatty acids, or even supplements can be used. For vegans, algal supplements are an alternative source of DHA instead of fish or fish oil.

6. Kuller LH: Nutrition, lipids, and cardiovascular disease. *Nutrition Reviews* 64:S15, 2006.

   The development of coronary heart disease is discussed as an epidemic due to increased consumption of saturated fat and cholesterol, low intakes of polyunsaturated fat, and obesity. The risk of the disease is increased by hypertension, smoking, and diabetes. The careful monitoring and prevention of this disease beginning in young adults is important but expensive.

7. Lau VWY and others: Plant sterols are efficacious in lowering plasma LDL and non-HDL cholesterol in hypercholesterolemic type 2 diabetic and nondiabetic persons. *American Journal of Clinical Nutrition* 81:1351, 2005.

   Incorporation of plant sterols into a low-saturated-fat and low-cholesterol diet for persons at increased risk of CVD mortality could have a positive effect on reducing the mortality rate, including in those people with type 2 diabetes.

8. Lewis NM and others: The walnut: A nutritional nut case. *Today's Dietitian* 6(8):36, 2004.

   Compared to other nuts and seeds, walnuts are one of the richest sources of alpha-linolenic acid (2.6 grams per 1-ounce serving or 14 walnut halves). The DRI for alpha-linolenic acid is 1.6 grams/day for men and 1.1 grams/day for women. In addition, walnuts are a rich source of plant sterols known to inhibit intestinal absorption of cholesterol.

9. Lichtenstein AH and others: Diet and lifestyle recommendations revision 2006. A scientific statement from the American Heart Association Nutrition Committee. *Circulation* 114:82, 2006.

   The American Heart Association presents recommendations designed to reduce the risk of cardiovascular disease in the general population. Specific goals are presented and include consuming an overall healthy diet; to aim for a healthy body weight; recommended levels of low-density lipoprotein cholesterol, high-density lipoprotein cholesterol, and triglycerides; normal blood pressure; normal blood glucose level; being physically active; and avoiding the use of and exposure to tobacco products.

10. Meisinger C and others: Plasma oxidized low-density lipoprotein, a strong predictor for acute coronary heart disease events in apparently healthy, middle-aged men from the general population. *Circulation* 112:651, 2005.

    Elevated concentrations of oxidized low-density lipoprotein are predictive of future coronary heart disease events in apparently healthy men. Thus, oxidized LDL may represent a promising risk marker for clinical coronary heart disease complications and should be evaluated in further studies.

11. Micallef MA, Garg ML: The lipid-lowering effects of phytosterols and (n-3) polyunsaturated fatty acids are synergistic and complementary in hyperlipidemic men and women. *Journal of Nutrition* 138:1086, 2008.

    Phytosterols are plant compounds with structures similar to cholesterol. Some margarines and other products are enriched with phytosterols. Consuming phytosterols can reduce the intestinal absorption of cholesterol by 30% to 40%. Fish oils are rich in omega-3 polyunsaturated fatty acids (PUFA) and can reduce blood triglycerides and raise HDL-cholesterol. The combined effect of phytosterols and omega-3 PUFA on blood lipid profiles was studied in individuals with high blood lipids. The combined supplementation with phytosterols and omega-3 PUFA had synergistic and complementary lipid-lowering effects in men and women with high blood lipids, resulting in a reduction in plasma total and LDL-cholesterol concentrations, an increase in HDL-cholesterol concentration, and a decrease in plasma triglyceride concentration.

12. Palmer S: Fighting heart disease the Dean Ornish way. *Today's Dietitian* 2:48, 2009.

    The Ornish diet has been proven to prevent as well as reverse heart disease. Diet guidelines include eating no more than 10% of calories from fat from mostly a plant-based diet; consuming no more than 10 milligrams of cholesterol per day; and eating one serving of soy foods each day. Omega-3 fatty acids are recommended from supplements.

13. Phillips KM and others: Phytosterol composition of nuts and seeds commonly consumed in the United States. *Journal of Agriculture and Food Chemistry* 53:9436, 2005.

    This study set out to find the nuts and seeds that could provide the most heart-protective benefits. Of the 27 nuts and seeds analyzed, wheat germ and sesame seeds had the greatest concentration of phytosterols and Brazil nuts and walnuts ranked the lowest. Pistachio and sunflower seeds were the richest sources of phytosterols for products typically consumed as snack foods.

14. Shai I and others: Weight loss with a low-carbohydrate, Mediterranean, or low-fat diet. *The New England Journal of Medicine* 359:229, 2008.

Moderately obese adults (mean age, 52 years) were assigned to one of three diets: low-fat, restricted-calorie; Mediterranean, restricted-calorie; or low-carbohydrate, non-restricted-calorie, and studied for two years. The diet was monitored for various components, including amount and type of carbohydrates, fat, protein, and cholesterol. The mean weight loss among the 272 participants who remained on their diets was 3.3 kg for the low-fat group, 4.6 kg for the Mediterranean-diet group, and 5.5 kg for the low-carbohydrate group. The results indicate that Mediterranean and low-carbohydrate diets may be effective alternatives to low-fat diets. The more favorable effects on lipids (with the low-carbohydrate diet) and on glycemic control (with the Mediterranean diet) suggest that personal preferences and metabolic considerations might inform individualized tailoring of dietary interventions.

15. Wang C and others: n-3 fatty acids from fish or fish oil supplements, but not alpha-linolenic acid, benefit cardiovascular disease outcomes in primary- and secondary-prevention studies: A systematic review. *American Journal of Clinical Nutrition* 84:5, 2006.

This review of previous studies found that consumption of omega-3 fatty acids from fish or fish oil but not alpha-linolenic acid, significantly reduced all-cause mortality, myocardial infarction, cardiac and sudden death, or stroke.

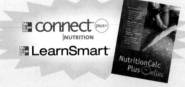

To get the most out of your study of nutrition, go to McGraw-Hill's online resources: Connect www.mcgrawhillconnect.com, where you will find NutritionCalc Plus, LearnSmart, and many other dynamic tools.

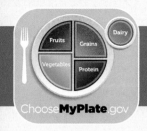
I. Is Your Diet High in Saturated and *Trans* Fat?

Instructions: In each row of the following list, circle your typical food selection from column A or B.

Column A		Column B
Bacon and eggs	or	Ready-to-eat whole-grain breakfast cereal
Doughnut or sweet roll	or	Whole-wheat roll, bagel, or bread
Breakfast sausage	or	Fruit
Whole milk	or	Reduced-fat, low-fat, or fat-free milk
Cheeseburger	or	Turkey sandwich, no cheese
French fries	or	Plain baked potato with salsa
Ground chuck	or	Ground round
Soup with cream base	or	Soup with broth base
Macaroni and cheese	or	Macaroni with marinara sauce
Cream/fruit pie	or	Graham crackers
Cream-filled cookies	or	Granola bar
Ice cream	or	Frozen yogurt, sherbet, or reduced-fat ice cream
Butter or stick margarine	or	Vegetable oils or soft margarine in a tub

Interpretation

The foods listed in column A tend to be high in saturated fat, *trans* fatty acids, cholesterol, and total fat. Those in column B generally are low in these dietary components. If you want to help reduce your risk of cardiovascular disease, choose more foods from column B and fewer from column A.

II. Applying the Nutrition Facts Label to Your Daily Food Choices

Imagine that you are at the supermarket looking for a quick snack to help you keep your energy up during afternoons. In the snack section, you settle on two choices (see labels a and b). Evaluate the products using the table on the left.

Compare the nutrients in each product by completing this list. For each serving, which product is lower in each of the following?

Calories	(a)	(b)	no difference
Calories from Fat	(a)	(b)	no difference
Total Fat	(a)	(b)	no difference
Saturated Fat	(a)	(b)	no difference
Trans Fat	(a)	(b)	no difference
Cholesterol	(a)	(b)	no difference
Sodium	(a)	(b)	no difference
Total Carbohydrates	(a)	(b)	no difference
Dietary Fiber	(a)	(b)	no difference
Sugars	(a)	(b)	no difference
Protein	(a)	(b)	no difference
Iron	(a)	(b)	no difference

Which package has more servings per container?

      (a)   (b)   no difference

Which of the two brands would you choose?

      (a)   (b)   no difference

What information on the Nutrition Facts labels contributed to your decision?

Nutrition Facts

Serving Size: 2 bars (42g)
Servings Per Container: 6

Amount Per Serving   **2 bars**
Calories 180   Calories from Fat 50

	% Daily Value*
Total Fat 6g	**9**%
Saturated Fat 0.5g	**3**%
Trans fat 0g	**
Cholesterol 0mg	**0**%
Sodium 160mg	**7**%
Total Carbohydrates 29g	**10**%
Dietary Fiber 2g	**8**%
Sugars 11g	
Protein 4g	
Iron	6%

Not a significant source of Vitamin A, Vitamin C, and calcium.

** Intake of *trans* fat should be as low as possible.

* Daily values are based on a 2,000 calorie diet. Your daily values may be higher or lower depending on your calorie needs:

** Intake should be as low as possible.

		Calories	2,000	2,500
Total Fat	Less than		65g	80g
Saturated Fat	Less than		20g	25g
Cholesterol	Less than		300mg	300mg
Sodium	Less than		2,400mg	2,400mg
Total Carbohydrates			300g	375g
Dietary Fiber			25g	30g

INGREDIENTS: WHOLE GRAIN ROLLED OATS, SUGAR, CANOLA OIL, CRISP RICE WITH SOY PROTEIN (RICE FLOUR, SOY PROTEIN CONCENTRATE, SUGAR, MALT, SALT), HONEY, BROWN SUGAR SYRUP, HIGH FRUCTOSE CORN SYRUP, SALT, SOY LECITHIN, BAKING SODA, NATURAL FLAVOR, PEANUT FLOUR, ALMOND FLOUR, HAZELNUT FLOUR, WALNUT FLOUR, PECAN FLOUR.

(a)

Nutrition Facts

Serving Size: 2 cookies (38g)
Servings Per Container: about 12

Amount Per Serving
Calories 180   Calories from Fat 70

	% Daily Value*
Total Fat 7g	**11**%
Saturated Fat 2g	**10**%
Trans fat 2g	**
Cholesterol 0mg	**0**%
Sodium 100mg	**4**%
Total Carbohydrate 26g	**9**%
Dietary Fiber 1g	**4**%
Sugars 12g	
Protein 2g	

Vitamin A 0%	•	Vitamin C 0%	
Calcium 0%	•	Iron	2%

** Intake of *trans* fat should be as low as possible.

* Daily values are based on a 2,000 calorie diet. Your daily values may be higher or lower depending on your calorie needs:

** Intake should be as low as possible.

		Calories	2,000	2,500
Total Fat	Less than		65g	80g
Saturated Fat	Less than		20g	25g
Cholesterol	Less than		300mg	300mg
Sodium	Less than		2,400mg	2,400mg
Total Carbohydrates			300g	375g
Dietary Fiber			25g	30g

Calories per gram: • Fat 9 • Carbohydrate 4 • Protein 4

INGREDIENTS: ENRICHED FLOUR (WHEAT FLOUR, NIACIN, REDUCED IRON, THIAMINE MONONITRATE, RIBOFLAVIN, FOLIC ACID), SUGAR, VEGETABLE OIL SHORTENING (PARTIALLY HYDROGENATED SOYBEAN, COCONUT, COTTONSEED, CORN AND/OR SAFFLOWER AND/OR CANOLA OIL), CORN SYRUP, HIGH FRUCTOSE CORN SYRUP, WHEY (A MILK INGREDIENT), CORN STARCH, SALT, SKIM MILK, LEAVENING (BAKING SODA, AMMONIUM BICARBONATE), ARTIFICIAL FLAVOR, SOYBEAN LECITHIN, COLOR (CONTAINING FD&C YELLOW #5 LAKE).

(b)

Chapter 6 Proteins

Student Learning Outcomes

Chapter 6 is designed to allow you to:

6.1 Distinguish between essential and nonessential amino acids and explain why adequate amounts of each of the essential amino acids are required for protein synthesis.

6.2 Describe how amino acids form proteins.

6.3 Distinguish between high-quality and low-quality proteins, identify examples of each, and describe the concept of complementary proteins.

6.4 Describe how protein is digested and absorbed in the body.

6.5 List the primary functions of protein in the body.

6.6 Calculate the RDA for protein for an adult when a healthy weight is given.

6.7 Describe what is meant by positive protein balance, negative protein balance, and protein equilibrium.

6.8 Describe how protein-calorie malnutrition eventually can lead to disease in the body.

6.9 Develop vegetarian diet plans that meet the body's nutritional needs.

What Would You Choose?

About 3 weeks ago, you started lifting weights at the student recreation center. You are disappointed that you have not seen the results you were anticipating. You can lift more now than you could when you started, but you were hoping to tone and define the muscles in your arms, back, and abs. Perhaps you need more protein. Bodybuilding magazines have numerous advertisements for protein and amino-acid supplements, but they are expensive. What would you choose as optimal nutrition to support your weight-training regimen?

a Take whey protein supplements.

b Take individual amino-acid supplements.

c Increase your consumption of animal protein.

d Consume a diet that provides 10% to 35% of calories from a variety of sources of protein.

 NUTRITION

Think about your choice as you read Chapter 6, then see our recommendations at the end of the chapter. To learn more about supplements and diet, check out the Connect site: www.mcgrawhillconnect.com

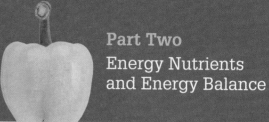

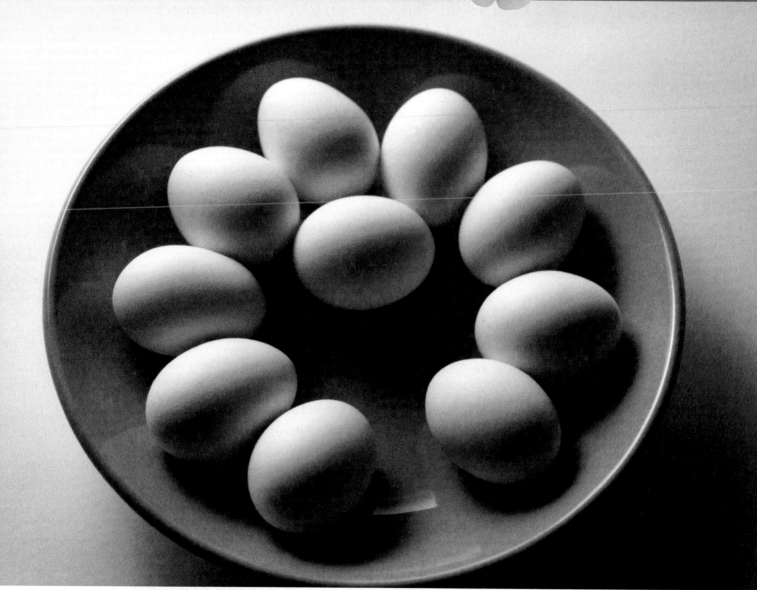

Consuming enough protein is vital for maintaining health. Proteins form important structures in the body, make up a key part of the blood, help regulate many body functions, and can fuel body cells.

North Americans generally eat more protein than is needed to maintain health. High-protein weight-loss diets have come and gone over the past 30 years. Our daily protein intake comes mostly from animal sources such as meat, poultry, fish, eggs, milk, and cheese. In contrast, in the developing world, diets can be deficient in protein.

Diets that are mostly vegetarian still predominate in much of Asia and areas of Africa, and, as suggested in the comic on the next page, some North Americans are currently adopting the practice. Plant sources of protein are worthy of more attention from North Americans. In the early 1900s, plant sources of proteins—nuts, seeds, and legumes—were consumed just as often as animal proteins. Over the years, though, plant proteins have been sidelined by meats. During this time, nuts have been viewed as high-fat foods, and beans have gotten the inferior reputation of "the poor man's meat." Contrary to these popular misconceptions, sources of plant proteins offer a wealth of nutritional benefits— from lowering blood cholesterol to preventing certain forms of cancer.

We could benefit from eating more plant sources of proteins. As shown in the comic in this chapter, it takes some knowledge to do so. It is possible— and desirable—to enjoy the benefits of animal and plant protein as we work toward the goal of meeting protein needs. This chapter takes a close look at protein, including the benefits of plant proteins in a diet. It will also examine vegetarian diets: their benefits and their risks, if not properly planned. Let's see why a detailed study of protein is worth your attention.

 ### Refresh Your Memory

As you begin your study of proteins in Chapter 6, you may want to review:

- Organization of the cell in Chapter 3
- The processes of digestion and absorption in Chapter 3
- The nervous system and immune system in Chapter 3
- The role of carbohydrates in sparing protein for energy in Chapter 4

FRANK & ERNEST® by Bob Thaves

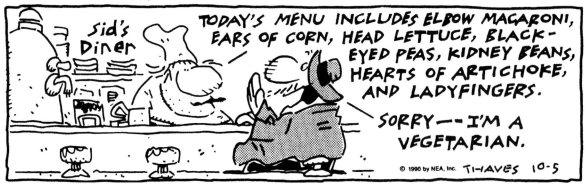

Can a vegetarian diet provide enough protein? What is prompting the growing interest in various forms of vegetarian diets? Why are plant protein sources, especially soy and nuts, gaining more attention? Should meat-eaters abandon that dietary practice? Chapter 6 provides some answers.

FRANK & ERNEST © United Features Syndicate. Reprinted by Permission.

6.1 Protein—An Introduction

Diets in the developed parts of the world, such as the United States and Canada, are typically rich in protein, and therefore a specific focus on eating enough protein is generally not needed. In the developing world, however, it is important to focus on protein in diet planning because diets in those areas of the world can be deficient in protein.

Thousands of substances in the body are made of proteins. Aside from water, proteins form the major part of lean body tissue, totaling about 17% of body weight. Amino acids—the building blocks for proteins—are unique in that they contain nitrogen along with carbon, oxygen, and hydrogen. Plants combine nitrogen from the soil with carbon and other elements to form amino acids. They then link these amino acids together to make proteins. We get the nitrogen we need by consuming dietary proteins. Proteins are thus an essential part of a diet because they supply nitrogen in a form we can readily use—namely, amino acids. Using simpler forms of nitrogen is, for the most part, impossible for humans.

Proteins are crucial to the regulation and maintenance of the body. Body functions such as blood clotting, fluid balance, hormone and enzyme production, visual processes, transport of many substances in the bloodstream, and cell repair require specific proteins. The body makes proteins in many configurations and sizes so that they can serve these greatly varied functions. Formation of these body proteins begins with amino acids from both the protein-containing foods we eat and those synthesized from other compounds within the body. Proteins can also be broken down to supply energy for the body—on average, 4 kcal per gram.

If you fail to consume an adequate amount of protein for weeks at a time, many metabolic processes slow down. This is because the body does not have enough amino acids available to build the proteins it needs. For example, the immune system no longer functions efficiently when it lacks key proteins, thereby increasing the risk of infections, disease, and death.

Amino Acids

Amino acids—the building blocks of proteins—are formed mostly of carbon, hydrogen, oxygen, and nitrogen. The following diagram shows the structure of a generic amino acid and also what one of the specific amino acids, glutamic acid, looks like. The amino acids have different chemical makeups, but all are slight variations of the generic amino acid pictured (see Appendix F). Each amino acid has an "acid" group; an "amino" group; and a "side" or R group specific to the amino acid.

The R group on some amino acids has a branched shape, like a tree. These so-called **branched-chain amino acids** are leucine, isoleucine, and valine (see Appendix F for the chemical structures of the amino acids). The branched-chain amino acids are the primary amino acids used by muscles for energy needs. This is one reason why proteins from milk (e.g., whey proteins) are popular with strength-training athletes (see Chapter 10 for details).

branched-chain amino acids Amino acids with a branching carbon backbone; these are leucine, isoleucine, and valine. All are essential amino acids.

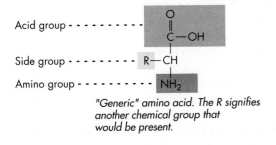

Acid group · · · · · · · · ·
Side group · · · · · · · · ·
Amino group · · · · · · · · ·

"Generic" amino acid. The R signifies another chemical group that would be present.

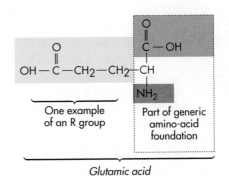

One example of an R group

Part of generic amino-acid foundation

Glutamic acid

TABLE 6-1 Classification of Amino Acids

Essential Amino Acids	Nonessential Amino Acids
Histidine	Alanine
Isoleucine*	Arginine
Leucine*	Asparagine
Lysine	Aspartic acid
Methionine	Cysteine
Phenylalanine	Glutamic acid
Threonine	Glutamine
Tryptophan	Glycine
Valine*	Proline
	Serine
	Tyrosine

*A branched-chain amino acid.

Your body needs to use 20 different amino acids to function (Table 6-1). Although all these commonly found amino acids are important, 11 are considered **nonessential** (also called *dispensable*) with respect to our diets. Human cells can produce these certain amino acids as long as the right ingredients are present—the key factor being nitrogen that is already part of another amino acid. Therefore it is not essential that these amino acids be in our diet.

The nine amino acids the body cannot make in sufficient amounts or at all are known as **essential** (also called *indispensable*)—they must be obtained from foods. This is because body cells either cannot make the needed carbon-based foundation of the amino acid, cannot put a nitrogen group on the needed carbon-based foundation, or just cannot do the whole process fast enough to meet body needs.

Eating a balanced diet can supply us with both the essential and nonessential amino-acid building blocks needed to maintain good health. Both nonessential and essential amino acids are present in foods that contain protein. If you don't eat enough essential amino acids, your body first struggles to conserve what essential amino acids it can. However, eventually your body progressively slows production of new proteins until at some point you will break protein down faster than you can make it. When that happens, health deteriorates.

The essential amino acid in smallest supply in a food or diet in relation to body needs becomes the limiting factor (called the **limiting amino acid**) because it limits the amount of protein the body can synthesize. For example, assume the letters of the alphabet represent the 20 or so different amino acids we consume. If *A* represents an essential amino acid, we need three of these letters to spell the hypothetical protein *BANANA*. If the body had a *B*, two *N*s, but only two *A*s, the "synthesis" of *BANANA* would not be possible. *A* would then be seen as the limiting amino acid.

Adults need only about 11% of their total protein requirement to be supplied by essential amino acids. Typical diets supply an average of 50% of protein as essential amino acids.

The estimated needs for essential amino acids for infants and preschool children are 40% of total protein intake; however, in later childhood the need drops to 20%.

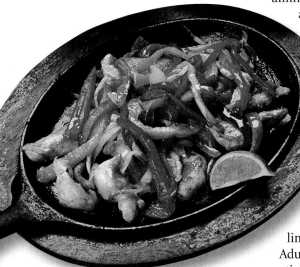

▲ When combined with vegetables, high-protein foods such as meats also help balance the amino-acid content of the diet.

Phenylketonuria

Some of the nonessential amino acids are also classed as conditionally essential. This means they must be made from essential amino acids if insufficient amounts are eaten. When that occurs, the body's supply of certain essential amino acids is depleted. Tyrosine is an example of a conditionally essential amino acid that can be made from the essential amino-acid phenylalanine.

The disease phenylketonuria (PKU) illustrates the importance of phenylalanine to make tyrosine. Recall from Chapter 4 that a person with PKU has a limited ability to metabolize the essential amino-acid phenylalanine. Normally, the body uses an enzyme to convert much of our dietary phenylalanine intake into tyrosine.

In PKU-diagnosed persons, the activity of the enzyme used in processing phenylalanine to tyrosine is insufficient. When the enzyme cannot synthesize enough tyrosine, both amino acids must be derived from foods. The point is that phenylalanine and tyrosine become *essential* in terms of dietary needs because the body can't produce enough tyrosine from phenylalanine. Phenylalanine levels in the blood increase because it is not converted to tyrosine. PKU is treated by limiting the consumption of phenylalanine with a special diet so that phenylalanine and its by-products do not rise to toxic concentrations in the body and cause the severe mental retardation seen in untreated PKU cases.

Rina is 7 months pregnant and has read about various tests that her baby will undergo when he or she is born. How can you explain to Rina the purpose and significance of one of those tests, the one that screens for PKU?

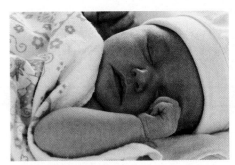

▲ Within the first few days of life all newborns are tested for phenylketonuria.

Diets designed for infants and young children need to take this into account to make sure enough proteins are present to yield a high-quality protein intake. Including some animal products in the diet, such as human milk or formula for infants, or cow's milk for children, helps ensure this. Otherwise, complementary amino acids from plant proteins should be consumed in each meal or within two subsequent meals. A major health risk for infants and children occurs in famine situations in which only one type of cereal grain is available, increasing the probability that one or more of the nine essential amino acids is lacking in the total diet. This is discussed further in a later section on protein-calorie malnutrition.

The human body uses 20 different amino acids from protein-containing foods. A healthy body can synthesize 11 of the amino acids, so it is not necessary to obtain all amino acids from foods—only nine of these must come from the diet and are therefore termed *essential (indispensable) amino acids*. The essential amino acid in smallest supply in a food in relation to body needs is called the limiting amino acid because it limits the amount of protein the body can synthesize.

6.2 Proteins—Amino Acids Bonded Together

Amino acids are linked together by chemical bonds—technically called **peptide bonds**—to form proteins. Although these bonds are difficult to break, acids, enzymes, and other agents are able to do so—for example, during digestion.

The body can synthesize many different proteins by linking together the 20 common types of amino acids with peptide bonds.

peptide bond A chemical bond formed between amino acids in a protein.

polypeptide A group of amino acids bonded together, from 50 to 2000 or more.

Protein Synthesis

Our discussion of protein synthesis, begins with DNA. DNA is present in the nucleus of the cell and contains coded instructions for protein synthesis (i.e., which specific amino acids are to be placed in a protein and in which order). Recall from Chapter 3 that DNA is a double-stranded molecule.

Protein synthesis in a cell, however, takes place in the cytoplasm, not in the nucleus. Thus, the DNA code used for synthesis of a specific protein must be transferred from the nucleus to the cytoplasm to allow for protein synthesis. This transfer is the job of messenger RNA (mRNA). Enzymes in the nucleus read the code on one segment (a gene) of one strand of the DNA and *transcribe* that information into a single-stranded mRNA molecule (Fig. 6-1). This mRNA undergoes processing and then it is ready to leave the nucleus.

Once in the cytoplasm, mRNA travels to the ribosomes. The ribosomes read the mRNA code and *translate* those instructions to produce a specific protein. Amino acids are added one at a time to the growing **polypeptide** chain according to the instructions on the mRNA. Another key participant in protein synthesis, transfer RNA (tRNA), is responsible for bringing the specific amino acids to the ribosomes as needed during protein synthesis (review Fig. 6-1). Energy input is required to add each amino acid to the chain, making protein synthesis "costly" in terms of calorie use.

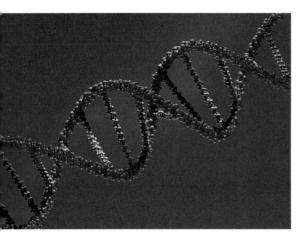

▲ Genes are present on DNA—a double-stranded helix. The cell nucleus contains most of the DNA in the body.

1 DNA contains the information necessary to produce proteins.

2 Transcription or copying of a segment of DNA results in mRNA, a copy of the information in DNA needed to make a protein.

3 The mRNA leaves the nucleus and goes to a ribosome.

4 Amino acids, the building blocks of proteins, are carried to the ribosome by tRNAs containing the code that matches that on the mRNA.

5 In the process of translation, the information contained in mRNA is used to determine the number, types, and arrangement of amino acids in the protein.

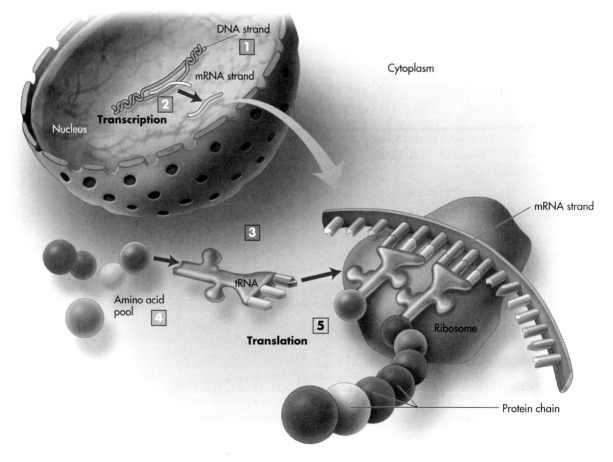

FIGURE 6-1 ▶ Protein synthesis (simplified). Once the mRNA is fully read, the amino acids have been connected into the polypeptide, which is released into the cytoplasm. It generally is then processed further to become a cell protein.

Once synthesis of a polypeptide is complete, it twists and folds into the appropriate three-dimensional structure of the intended protein. These structural changes occur based on specific interactions between the amino acids that make up the polypeptide chain (see the next section on protein organization for details). Some polypeptides, such as the hormone insulin, also undergo further changes in the cell before they are functional.

The important message in this discussion is the relationship between DNA and the proteins eventually produced by a cell. If the DNA code contains errors, an incorrect mRNA will be produced. The ribosomes will then read this incorrect message and an incorrect amino acid will be added and an incorrect polypeptide chain will be produced. As discussed in Chapter 3, genetic engineering may ultimately be able to correct many gene defects in humans, by placing the correct DNA code in the nucleus, so that the correct protein can be made by the ribosomes.

Protein Organization

As noted before, by bonding together various combinations of the 20 common types of amino acids, the body synthesizes thousands of different proteins. The sequential order of the amino acids then ultimately determines the protein's shape. The main point is that only correctly positioned amino acids can interact and fold properly to form the intended shape for the protein. The resulting unique, three-dimensional form goes on to dictate the function of each particular protein (Fig. 6-2). If it lacks the proper structure, a protein cannot function.

Sickle cell disease (also called **sickle cell anemia**) is one example of what happens when amino acids are out of order on a protein. North Americans of African descent are especially prone to this genetic disease. It occurs because of defects in the structure of the protein chains of hemoglobin, a protein that carries oxygen in red blood cells. In two of its four protein chains, an error in the amino-acid order occurs. This error produces a profound change in hemoglobin structure. It can no longer form the shape needed to carry oxygen efficiently inside the red blood cell. Instead of forming normal circular disks, the red blood cells collapse into crescent (or sickle) shapes (Fig. 6-3). Health deteriorates, and eventually episodes of severe pain in the bones and joints, abdominal pain, headaches, convulsions, and paralysis may occur.

These life-threatening symptoms are caused by a minute, but critical, error in the hemoglobin amino-acid order. Why does this error happen? It results from a defect in a person's genetic blueprint, DNA, inherited through one's parents. A defect in the DNA can dictate that a wrong amino acid will be built into the sequence of the body proteins. Many diseases, including cancer, stem from errors in the DNA code.

Denaturation of Proteins

Exposure to acid or alkaline substances, heat, or agitation can alter a protein's structure, leaving it uncoiled or otherwise deformed. This process of altering the three-dimensional structure of a protein is called **denaturation** (see Fig. 6-7 on p. 219). Changing a protein's shape often destroys its ability to function normally, such that it loses its biological activity.

Denaturation of proteins is useful for some body processes, especially digestion. The heat produced during cooking denatures some proteins. After food is ingested, the secretion of stomach acid denatures some bacterial proteins, plant hormones, many active enzymes, and other forms of proteins in foods, making it safer to eat. Digestion is also enhanced by denaturation because the unraveling increases exposure of the polypeptide chain to digestive enzymes. Denaturing proteins in some foods can also reduce their tendencies to cause allergic reactions.

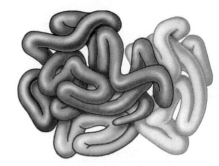

FIGURE 6-2 ▶ Protein organization. Proteins often form a coiled shape, as shown by this drawing of the blood protein hemoglobin. This shape is dictated by the order of the amino acids in the protein chain. To get an idea of its size, consider that each teaspoon (5 milliliters) of blood contains about 10^{18} hemoglobin molecules. One billion is 10^9.

sickle cell disease (sickle cell anemia) An illness that results from a malformation of the red blood cell because of an incorrect structure in part of its hemoglobin protein chains. The disease can lead to episodes of severe bone and joint pain, abdominal pain, headache, convulsions, paralysis, and even death.

denaturation Alteration of a protein's three-dimensional structure, usually because of treatment by heat, enzymes, acid or alkaline solutions, or agitation.

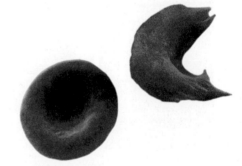

FIGURE 6-3 ▶ An example of the consequences of errors in DNA coding of proteins. (a) Normal red blood cell; (b) red blood cell from a person with sickle cell anemia—note its abnormal crescent (sicklelike) shape.

Recall that we need the essential amino acids that the proteins in the diet supply—not the proteins themselves. We dismantle ingested dietary proteins and use the amino-acid building blocks to assemble the proteins we need.

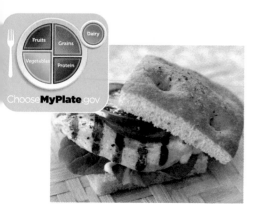

▲ This grilled chicken (protein) sandwich with lettuce and tomato (vegetables) on foccacia bread (grains) completes three section of MyPlate and provides a good source of protein. Which sections are missing?

CONCEPT CHECK

Amino acids are bonded together in specific sequences to form distinct proteins. DNA provides the directions for synthesizing these new proteins. Specifically, DNA directs the order of the amino acids on the protein. The amino-acid order within a protein determines its ultimate shape and function. Destroying the shape of a protein denatures it. Stomach acid, heat, and other factors can denature proteins, causing them to lose their biological activity. Proteins must be denatured during digestion so that amino acids are available for absorption.

6.3 Protein in Foods

Of the typical foods we eat, about 70% of our protein comes from animal sources (Fig. 6-4). The most nutrient-dense source of protein is water-packed tuna, which has 87% of calories as protein (Fig. 6-5). The top five contributors of protein to the North

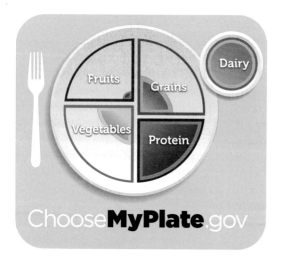

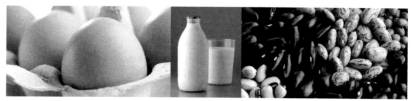

MyPlate: Sources of Protein

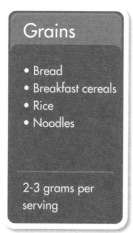

Grains
• Bread
• Breakfast cereals
• Rice
• Noodles
2-3 grams per serving

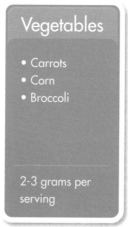

Vegetables
• Carrots
• Corn
• Broccoli
2-3 grams per serving

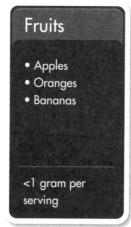

Fruits
• Apples
• Oranges
• Bananas
<1 gram per serving

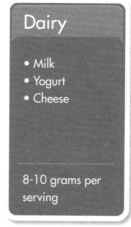

Dairy
• Milk
• Yogurt
• Cheese
8-10 grams per serving

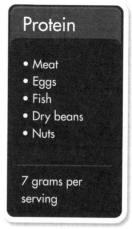

Protein
• Meat
• Eggs
• Fish
• Dry beans
• Nuts
7 grams per serving

FIGURE 6-4 ▶ Sources of protein from MyPlate. The fill of the background color (none, 1/3, 2/3, or completely covered) within each group on the plate indicates the average nutrient density for protein in that group. Overall, the dairy group and the protein group contain many foods that are nutrient-dense sources of protein. Based on serving sizes listed for MyPlate, the fruits group provides little or no protein (less than 1 gram per serving). Food choices from the vegetables group and grains group provide moderate amounts of protein (2 to 3 grams per serving). The dairy group provides much Protein (8 to 10 grams per serving), as does the protein group (7 grams per serving).

American diet are beef, poultry, milk, white bread, and cheese. In North America, meat and poultry consumption amounts to about 150 pounds per person per year. Worldwide, 35% of protein comes from animal sources. In Africa and East Asia, only about 20% of the protein eaten comes from animal sources.

Protein Quality of Foods

Animal and plant proteins can differ greatly in their proportions of essential and non-essential amino acids. Animal proteins contain ample amounts of all nine essential amino acids. (Gelatin—made from the animal protein collagen—is an exception because it loses one essential amino acid during processing and is low in other essential amino acids.) With the exception of soy protein, plant proteins don't match our need for essential amino acids as precisely as animal proteins. Many plant proteins, especially those found in grains, are low in one or more of the nine essential amino acids.

As you might expect, human tissue composition resembles animal tissue more than it does plant tissue. The similarities enable us to use proteins from any single animal source more efficiently to support human growth and maintenance than we do those from any single plant source. For this reason, animal proteins, except gelatin, are considered **high-quality** (also called **complete**) **proteins,** which contain the nine essential amino acids we need in sufficient amounts. Individual plant sources of proteins, except for soy beans, are considered **lower-quality** (also called **incomplete**) **proteins** because their amino-acid patterns can be quite different from ours. Thus, a single plant protein source, such as corn alone, cannot easily support body growth and maintenance. To obtain a sufficient amount of essential amino acids, a variety of plant proteins need to be consumed because each plant protein lacks adequate amounts of one or more essential amino acids.

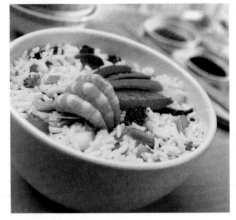

▲ Small amounts of animal protein in a meal easily add up to meet daily protein needs when mixed with grains and vegetables.

high-quality (complete) proteins
Dietary proteins that contain ample amounts of all nine essential amino acids.

lower-quality (incomplete) proteins
Dietary proteins that are low in or lack one or more essential amino acids.

Food Sources of Protein

FIGURE 6-5 ▶ Food sources of protein compared to the RDA of 56 grams for a 70 kg man.

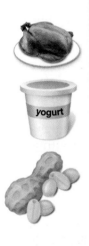

Food Item and Amount	Protein (grams)	% RDA
RDA	56*	100%
Canned tuna, 3 ounces	21.6	38.6%
Broiled chicken, 3 ounces	21.3	38%
Beef chuck, 3 ounces	15.3	27%
Yogurt, 1 cup	10.6	19%
Kidney beans, 1/2 cup	8.1	14.5%
1% low-fat milk, 1 cup	8.0	14%
Peanuts, 1 ounce	7.3	13%
Cheddar cheese, 1 ounce	7.0	12.5%
Egg, 1	5.5	10%
Cooked corn, 1/2 cup	2.7	5%
Seven grain bread, 1 slice	2.6	4.6%
White rice, 1/2 cup	2.1	4%
Pasta, 1 ounce	1.2	2%
Banana, 1	1.2	2%
* for 70 kg man		

Key:
■ Grains
■ Vegetables
■ Fruits
■ Dairy
■ Protein

When only lower-quality protein foods are consumed, enough of the essential amino acids needed for protein synthesis may not be obtained. Therefore, when compared to high-quality proteins, a greater amount of lower-quality protein is needed to meet the needs of protein synthesis. Moreover, once any of the nine essential amino acids in the plant protein we have eaten is used up, further protein synthesis becomes impossible. Because the depletion of just one of the essential amino acids prevents protein synthesis, the process illustrates the *all-or-none principle:* Either all essential amino acids are available or none can be used. The remaining amino acids would then be used for energy needs, or converted to carbohydrate or fat.

When two or more proteins combine to compensate for deficiencies in essential amino acid content in each protein, the proteins are called **complementary proteins.** Mixed diets generally provide high-quality protein because a complementary protein pattern results. Therefore, healthy adults should have little concern about balancing foods to yield the proteins needed to obtain enough of all nine essential amino acids. Even on plant-based diets, complementary proteins need not be consumed at the same meal by adults. Meeting amino-acid needs over the course of a day is a reasonable goal because there is a ready supply of amino acids from those present in body cells and in the blood (see Fig. 6-10 on page 224).

In general, plant sources of protein deserve more attention and use than they currently receive from many North Americans. Plant foods contribute fewer calories to the diet than most animal products and they supply an ample amount of protein, plus magnesium, plenty of fiber, and several other nutritional benefits (Fig. 6-6). The vegetable proteins we eat are a heart-healthy alternative to animal proteins because they contain no cholesterol and little saturated fat, aside from that added during processing or cooking. Legumes and nut sources of protein especially have received a lot of recent attention.

CRITICAL THINKING

Evan, a vegetarian, has heard of the "all-or-none principle" of protein synthesis but doesn't understand how this principle applies to protein synthesis in the body. He asks you, "How important is this nutritional concept for diet planning?" How would you answer his question?

A Closer Look at Plant Sources of Proteins

In proportion to the amount of calories they supply, plant foods provide not only protein, but also magnesium, fiber, folate, vitamin E, iron (absorption is increased by the vitamin C also present), zinc, and some calcium. In addition, phytochemicals from these foods are implicated in prevention of a wide variety of chronic diseases.

Nuts have a hard shell surrounding an edible kernel. Almonds, pistachios, walnuts, and pecans are some common examples. The defining characteristic of a nut is that it grows on a tree. (Peanuts, because they grow underground, are legumes.) Seeds (such as pumpkin, sesame, and sunflower seeds) differ from nuts in that seeds grow on vegetable or flowering plants, but they are similar to nuts in nutrient composition. In general, nuts and seeds supply 160 to 190 kcal, 6 to 10 grams of protein, and 14 to 19 grams of fat per 1 ounce serving. Although they are a dense source of calories, nuts and seeds make a powerful contribution to health when consumed in moderation.

Legumes are a plant family with pods that contain a single row of seeds. Besides peanuts, examples include garden and black-eyed peas, kidney beans, great northern beans, lentils, and soy beans. Dried varieties of the mature legume seeds—what we know as beans—also make an impressive contribution to the protein, vitamin, mineral, and fiber content of a meal. A one-half cup serving of legumes provides 100 to 150 kcal, 5 to 10 grams of protein, less than one gram of fat, and about 5 grams of fiber. Recall from Chapter 4 that consumption of beans can lead to intestinal gas because our bodies lack the enzymes to break down certain carbohydrates that beans contain. An over-the counter preparation called Beano® can greatly lessen symptoms if taken right before the meal. It is also helpful to soak dry beans in water, which

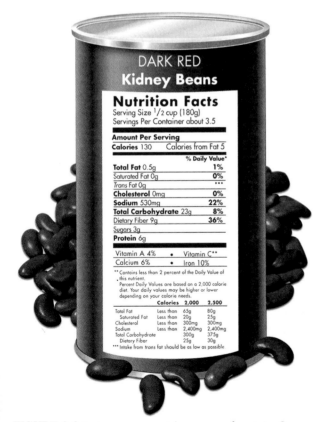

DARK RED
Kidney Beans

Nutrition Facts
Serving Size 1/2 cup (180g)
Servings Per Container about 3.5

Amount Per Serving
Calories 130   Calories from Fat 5

	% Daily Value*
Total Fat 0.5g	1%
Saturated Fat 0g	0%
Trans Fat 0g	***
Cholesterol 0mg	0%
Sodium 530mg	22%
Total Carbohydrate 23g	8%
Dietary Fiber 9g	36%
Sugars 3g	
Protein 6g	

Vitamin A 4%	•	Vitamin C**
Calcium 6%	•	Iron 10%

** Contains less than 2 percent of the Daily Value of this nutrient.
Percent Daily Values are based on a 2,000 calorie diet. Your daily values may be higher or lower depending on your calorie needs.

		Calories	2,000	2,500
Total Fat	Less than		65g	80g
Saturated Fat	Less than		20g	25g
Cholesterol	Less than		300mg	300mg
Sodium	Less than		2,400mg	2,400mg
Total Carbohydrate			300g	375g
Dietary Fiber			25g	30g

*** Intake from trans fat should be as low as possible

FIGURE 6-6 ▶ Legumes are rich sources of protein. One-half cup of these kidney beans has 6 grams of protein and meets about 10% of protein needs but contributes only about 5% of energy needs.

leaches the indigestible carbohydrates into the water so they can be disposed. However, intestinal gas is not harmful. In fact, fermentation products of ingestible carbohydrates promote the health of your colon (review Chapter 3 for more information on probiotics and prebiotics).

The impact of plant proteins on health will be discussed in the Nutrition and Your Health section at the end of this chapter.

MAKING DECISIONS

Soy and Nut Allergies

For some of us, food allergies from soy, peanuts and tree nuts (e.g., almonds and walnuts), and wheat are a concern. Overall, food allergies occur in up to 8% of children 4 years of age or younger and in up to 2% of adults. Eight foods account for 90% of food-related allergies; soy, peanuts, tree nuts, and wheat are four of these foods. (The other foods are milk, egg, fish, and shellfish.) The allergic reactions can range from a mild intolerance to fatal allergic reactions (see Chapter 15 for details). Current guidelines regarding plant sources of allergens advise that infants not be fed wheat products before 6 months of age. Children less than 3 years of age should not eat peanuts or tree nuts. In addition, any of the plant sources of allergens need to be avoided in children and adults who continue to experience such allergies (see Further Reading 11).

In sum, plant proteins are a nutritious alternative to animal proteins. They are inexpensive, versatile, tasty, add color to your plate, and benefit health beyond their contribution of protein to the diet. Simply adding these foods to your diet can lead to weight gain, but learning to substitute plant proteins in place of other less healthy foods is one way to reduce your risk for many diseases. Watch for news about additional research progress into this area.

See Nutrition and Your Health: Vegetarian and Plant-Based Diets at the end of Chapter 6.

6.4 Protein Digestion and Absorption

As with carbohydrate digestion, protein digestion begins with the cooking of food. Cooking unfolds (denatures) proteins (Fig. 6-7) and softens tough connective tissue in meat. Cooking also makes many protein-rich foods easier to chew and swallow and facilitates their breakdown during later digestion and absorption. As you will see in Chapter 13, cooking also makes many protein-rich foods, such as meats, eggs, fish, and poultry, much safer to eat.

Digestion

The enzymatic digestion of protein begins in the stomach (Fig. 6-8). Proteins are first denatured by stomach acid. **Pepsin**, a major stomach enzyme for digesting proteins, then goes to work on the unraveled polypeptide chains. Pepsin breaks the polypeptide into shorter chains of amino acids because it can break only a few of the many peptide bonds found in these large molecules. The release of pepsin is controlled by the hormone gastrin. Thinking about food or chewing food stimulates gastrin release in the stomach. Gastrin also strongly stimulates the stomach to produce acid.

The partially digested proteins move from the stomach into the small intestine along with the rest of the nutrients and other substances in a meal (chyme). Once in the small intestine, the partially digested proteins (and any fats accompanying them) trigger the release of the hormone cholecystokinin (CCK) from the walls of the small intestine. CCK, in turn, travels through the bloodstream to the pancreas where it causes the pancreas to release protein-splitting enzymes, such as **trypsin**. These digestive enzymes further divide the chains of amino acids into segments of two to three amino acids and some individual amino acids. Eventually, this mixture is digested

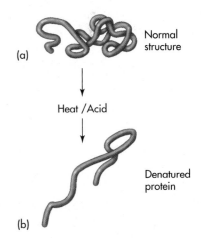

FIGURE 6-7 ▶ Denaturation. (a) Protein showing typical coiled state. (b) Protein is now partly uncoiled. This uncoiling can reduce biological activity and allow digestive enzymes to act on peptide bonds.

pepsin A protein-digesting enzyme produced by the stomach.

trypsin A protein-digesting enzyme secreted by the pancreas to act in the small intestine.

into amino acids, using other enzymes from the lining of the small intestine and enzymes present in the absorptive cells themselves.

Absorption

The short chains of amino acids and any individual amino acids in the small intestine are taken up by active transport into the absorptive cells lining the small intestine. Any remaining peptide bonds are broken down to yield individual amino acids inside the intestinal cells. They are water-soluble, so the amino acids travel to the liver via the portal vein, which drains absorbed nutrients from the intestinal tract. In the liver, individual amino acids can undergo several modifications, depending on the needs of the body. Individual amino acids may be combined into the proteins needed by the body; broken down for energy needs; released into the bloodstream; or converted to nonessential amino acids, glucose, or fat. With excess protein intake, amino acids are converted to fat as a last resort.

Except during infancy, it is uncommon for intact proteins to be absorbed from the digestive tract. In infants up to 4 to 5 months of age, the gastrointestinal tract is somewhat permeable to small proteins, so some whole proteins can be absorbed. Because proteins from some foods (e.g., cow's milk and egg whites) may predispose an infant to food allergies, pediatricians and registered dietitians recommend waiting until an infant is at least 6 to 12 months of age before introducing commonly allergenic foods (see Chapter 15 for details).

FIGURE 6-8 ▶ A summary of protein digestion and absorption. Enzymatic protein digestion begins in the stomach and ends in the absorptive cells of the small intestine, where any remaining short groupings of amino acids are broken down into single amino acids. Stomach acid and enzymes contribute to protein digestion. Absorption from the intestinal lumen into the absorptive cells requires energy input.

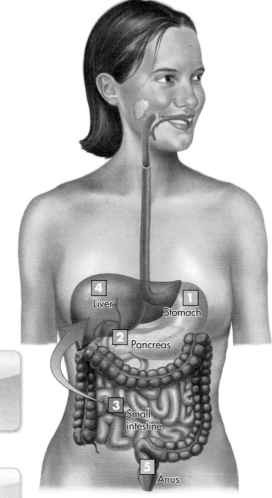

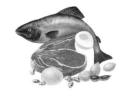

Protein Digestion and Absorption

1 Partial protein digestion by the enzyme pepsin and stomach acid.

2 Further digestion of polypeptides by enzymes released by the pancreas.

3 Final digestion of amino acid chains to single amino acids takes place mostly inside cells of the small intestine.

4 Amino acids absorbed into the portal vein and transported to the liver. From there they enter the general bloodstream.

5 Little dietary protein is present in feces.

Liver

Stomach

Pancreas

Small intestine

Anus

CONCEPT CHECK

Protein digestion begins with cooking, as proteins are denatured by heat. Once protein reaches the stomach, enzymes cleave proteins into smaller segments of amino acids. As food travels through the small intestine, protein breakdown products formed in the stomach are broken down further to individual amino acids or short segments of amino acids and taken up into the absorptive cells of the small intestine where final breakdown into amino acids occurs. The amino acids then travel to the liver via the portal vein.

6.5 Putting Proteins to Work in the Body

Proteins function in many crucial ways in human metabolism and in the formation of body structures. We rely on foods to supply the amino acids needed to form these proteins. However, only when we also eat enough carbohydrate and fat can food proteins be used most efficiently. If we don't consume enough calories to meet needs, some amino acids from proteins are broken down to produce energy, rendering them unavailable to build body proteins.

Producing Vital Body Structures

Every cell contains protein. Muscles, connective tissue, mucus, blood-clotting factors, transport proteins in the bloodstream, lipoproteins, enzymes, immune antibodies, some hormones, visual pigments, and the support structure inside bones are primarily made of protein. Excess protein in the diet doesn't enhance the synthesis of these body components, but eating too little protein can prevent it.

Most vital body proteins are in a constant state of breakdown, rebuilding, and repair. For example, the intestinal tract lining is constantly sloughed off. The digestive tract treats sloughed cells just like food particles, digesting them and absorbing their amino acids. In fact, most of the amino acids released throughout the body can be recycled to become part of the pool of amino acids available for synthesis of future proteins. Overall, **protein turnover** is a process by which a cell can respond to its changing environment by producing proteins that are needed and disassembling proteins that are not needed.

During any day, an adult makes and degrades about 250 grams of protein, recycling many of the amino acids. Relative to the 65 to 100 grams of protein typically consumed by adults in North America, recycled amino acids make an important contribution to total protein metabolism.

If a person's diet is low in protein for a long period, the processes of rebuilding and repairing body proteins will slow down. Over time, skeletal muscles; blood proteins; and vital organs, such as the heart and liver, will decrease in size or volume. Only the brain resists protein breakdown.

Maintaining Fluid Balance

Blood proteins help maintain body fluid balance. Normal blood pressure in the arteries forces blood into capillary beds. The blood fluid then moves from the **capillary beds** into the spaces between nearby cells (**extracellular spaces**) to provide nutrients to those cells (Fig. 6-9). Proteins in the bloodstream are too large however, to move out of the capillary beds into the tissues. The presence of these proteins in the capillary beds attracts the proper amount of fluid back to the blood, partially counteracting the force of blood pressure.

With an inadequate consumption of protein, the concentration of proteins in the bloodstream drops below normal. Excessive fluid then builds up in the surrounding tissues because the counteracting force produced by the smaller amount of blood proteins is too weak to pull enough of the fluid back from the tissues into the bloodstream. As

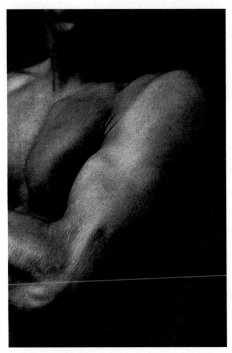

▲ Protein contributes to the structure and function of muscle.

protein turnover The process by which cells break down old proteins and resynthesize new proteins. In this way the cell will have the proteins it needs to function at that time.

capillary bed Network of one-cell-thick vessels that create a junction between arterial and venous circulation. It is here that gas and nutrient exchange occurs between body cells and the blood.

extracellular space The space outside cells; represents one-third of body fluid.

FIGURE 6-9 ▶ Blood proteins in relation to fluid balance. (a) Blood proteins are important for maintaining the body's fluid balance. (b) Without sufficient protein in the bloodstream, edema develops.

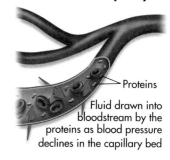

Arterial end of a capillary bed

Fluid forced into tissue spaces by blood pressure generated by pumping action of heart

Blood cells

Venous end of a capillary bed

Proteins

Fluid drawn into bloodstream by the proteins as blood pressure declines in the capillary bed

(a)

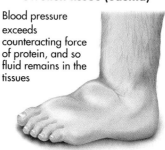

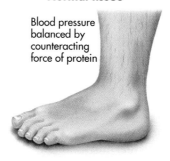

Normal tissue

Blood pressure balanced by counteracting force of protein

Swollen tissue (edema)

Blood pressure exceeds counteracting force of protein, and so fluid remains in the tissues

(b)

edema The buildup of excess fluid in extra-cellular spaces.

buffers Compounds that cause a solution to resist changes in acid-base conditions.

Neurotransmitters, released by nerve endings, are often derivatives of amino acids. This is true for dopamine and nor-epinephrine (both synthesized from the amino-acid tyrosine), and serotonin (synthesized from the amino-acid tryptophan).

The vitamin niacin can be made from the amino-acid tryptophan, illustrating another role of proteins.

fluids accumulate in the tissues, the tissues swell, causing **edema**. Edema may be a symptom of a variety of medical problems, so its cause must be identified. An important step in diagnosing the cause is to measure the concentration of blood proteins.

Contributing to Acid-Base Balance

Proteins help regulate acid-base balance in the blood. Proteins located in cell membranes pump chemical ions in and out of cells. The ion concentration that results from the pumping action, among other factors, keeps the blood slightly alkaline. In addition, some blood proteins are especially good **buffers** for the body. Buffers are compounds that maintain acid-base conditions within a narrow range.

Forming Hormones and Enzymes

Amino acids are required for the synthesis of many hormones—our internal body messengers. Some hormones, such as the thyroid hormones, are made from only one type of amino acid, tyrosine. Insulin, on the other hand, is a hormone composed of 51 total amino acids. Almost all enzymes are proteins or have a protein component.

Contributing to Immune Function

Proteins are a key component of the cells within the immune system. An example is the antibodies, proteins produced by one type of white blood cell. These antibodies can bind to foreign proteins in the body, an important step in removing invaders from the body. Without sufficient dietary protein, the immune system lacks the materials needed to function properly. For example, a low protein status can turn measles into a fatal disease for a malnourished child.

Forming Glucose

In Chapter 4 you learned that the body must maintain a fairly constant concentration of blood glucose to supply energy for the brain, red blood cells, and nervous tissue. At rest, the brain uses about 19% of the body's energy requirements, and it gets most

PROTEIN CONCEPT MAP

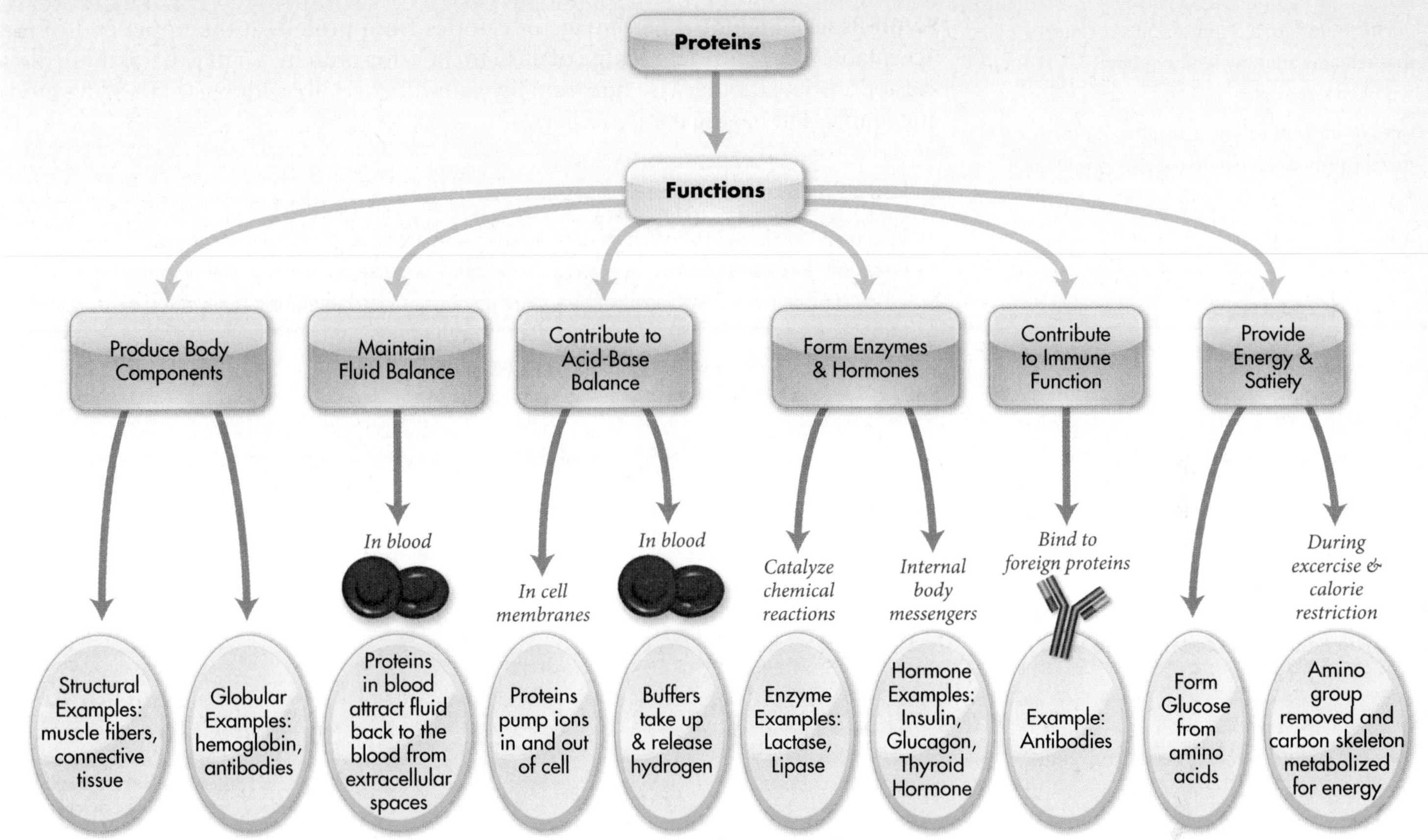

Proteins → **Functions**

- **Produce Body Components**
  - Structural Examples: muscle fibers, connective tissue
  - Globular Examples: hemoglobin, antibodies
- **Maintain Fluid Balance**
  - *In blood* — Proteins in blood attract fluid back to the blood from extracellular spaces
- **Contribute to Acid-Base Balance**
  - *In cell membranes* — Proteins pump ions in and out of cell
  - *In blood* — Buffers take up & release hydrogen
- **Form Enzymes & Hormones**
  - *Catalyze chemical reactions* — Enzyme Examples: Lactase, Lipase
  - *Internal body messengers* — Hormone Examples: Insulin, Glucagon, Thyroid Hormone
- **Contribute to Immune Function**
  - *Bind to foreign proteins* — Example: Antibodies
- **Provide Energy & Satiety**
  - Form Glucose from amino acids
  - *During excercise & calorie restriction* — Amino group removed and carbon skeleton metabolized for energy

of that energy from glucose. If you don't consume enough carbohydrate to supply the glucose, your liver (and kidneys, to a lesser extent) will be forced to make glucose from amino acids present in body tissues (Fig. 6-10).

Making some glucose from amino acids is normal. For example, when you skip breakfast and haven't eaten since 7 P.M. the preceding evening, glucose must be manufactured. In an extreme situation, however, such as in starvation, amino acids from muscle tissue are converted into glucose, which wastes muscle tissue and can produce edema.

Providing Energy

Proteins supply little energy for a weight-stable person. Two situations in which a person does use protein to meet energy needs are during prolonged exercise (see Chapter 10 for information about the use of amino acids for energy needs during exercise) and during calorie restriction, as with a weight-loss diet. In these cases, the amino group ($-NH_2$) from the amino acid is removed and the remaining carbon skeleton is metabolized for energy needs (Fig. 6-10). Still, under most conditions, cells primarily use fats and carbohydrates for energy needs. Although proteins contain the same amount of calories (on average, 4 kcal per gram) as carbohydrates, proteins are a costly source of calories, considering the amount of processing the liver and kidneys must perform to use this calorie source.

Contributing to Satiety

Compared to the other macronutrients, proteins provide the highest feeling of satiety after a meal. Thus, including some protein with each meal helps control overall

satiety A state in which there is no longer a desire to eat; a feeling of satisfaction.

pool The amount of a nutrient stored within the body that can be mobilized when needed.

carbon skeleton Amino-acid structure that remains after the amino group (—NH₂) has been removed.

urea Nitrogenous waste product of protein metabolism; major source of nitrogen in the urine, chemically NH₂—C—NH₂.

$$NH_2-\overset{\overset{\displaystyle O}{\|}}{C}-NH_2$$

food intake. Many experts warn against skimping on protein when trying to reduce energy intake to lose weight. Meeting protein needs is still important and exceeding needs somewhat may provide an additional benefit when dieting to lose weight (see Further Readings 7 and 8). Several effective weight-loss diets (e.g., Atkins, Zone, South Beach) include a percentage of calories from protein at the upper end of the Acceptable Macronutrient Range of 10% to 35% for protein. So in general these diets are appropriate if otherwise nutritionally sound, especially with regard to being moderate in fat and having enough fiber.

CONCEPT CHECK

Vital body constituents—such as muscle, connective tissue, blood transport proteins, enzymes, hormones, buffers, and immune factors—are mainly proteins. The degradation of existing proteins and synthesis of new proteins takes place constantly, amounting to a turnover rate of about 250 grams a day for the entire human body. Proteins can also be used for glucose and other fuel production and contributes to satiety.

FIGURE 6-10 ▶ Amino-acid metabolism. The amino-acid **pool** in a cell can be used to form body proteins, as well as a variety of other possible products. When the **carbon skeletons** of amino acids are metabolized to produce glucose or fat, ammonia (NH₃) is a resulting waste product. The ammonia is converted to **urea** and excreted in the urine.

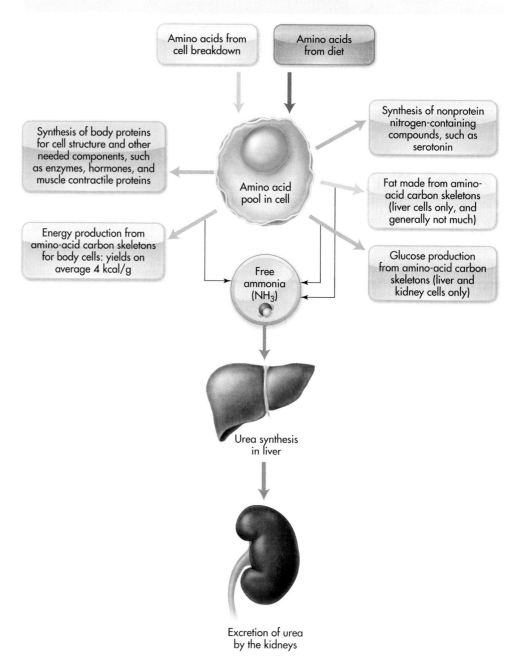

6.6 Protein Needs

How much protein (actually, amino acids) do we need to eat each day? People who aren't growing need to eat only enough protein to match whatever they lose daily from protein breakdown. The amount of breakdown can be determined by measuring the amount of urea and other nitrogen-containing compounds in the urine, as well as losses of protein from feces, skin, hair, nails, and so on. In short, people need to balance protein intake with such losses to maintain a state of **protein equilibrium,** also called *protein balance* (Fig. 6-11).

When a body is growing or recovering from an illness or injury, it needs a **positive protein balance** to supply the raw materials required to build new tissues. To achieve this, a person must eat more protein daily than he or she loses. In addition, the hormones insulin, growth hormone, and testosterone all stimulate positive protein balance. Resistance exercise (weight training) also enhances positive protein balance. Consuming less protein than needed leads to **negative protein balance,** such as when acute illness reduces the desire to eat and so one loses more protein than consumed.

For healthy people, the amount of dietary protein needed to maintain protein equilibrium (wherein intake equals losses) can be determined by increasing protein intake until it equals losses of protein and its related breakdown products (e.g., urea). Calorie needs must also be met so that amino acids are not diverted for such use.

Today, the best estimate for the amount of protein required for nearly all adults to maintain protein equilibrium is 0.8 grams of protein per kilogram of healthy

protein equilibrium A state in which protein intake is equal to related protein losses; the person is said to be in protein balance.

positive protein balance A state in which protein intake exceeds related protein losses, as is needed during times of growth.

negative protein balance A state in which protein intake is less than related protein losses, as is often seen during acute illness.

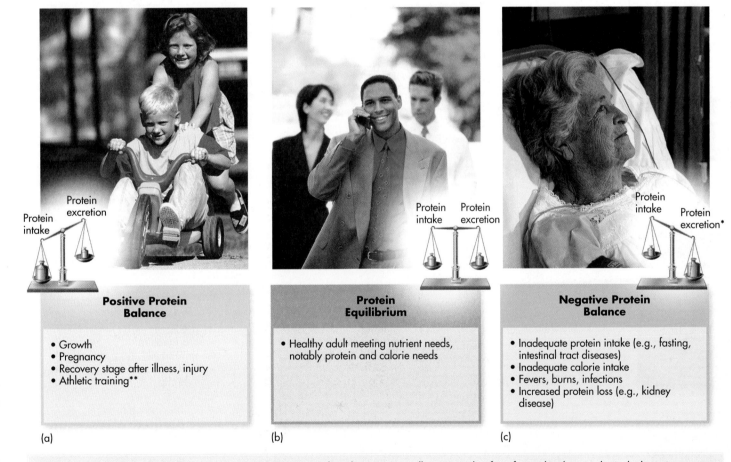

Positive Protein Balance

- Growth
- Pregnancy
- Recovery stage after illness, injury
- Athletic training**

Protein Equilibrium

- Healthy adult meeting nutrient needs, notably protein and calorie needs

Negative Protein Balance

- Inadequate protein intake (e.g., fasting, intestinal tract diseases)
- Inadequate calorie intake
- Fevers, burns, infections
- Increased protein loss (e.g., kidney disease)

(a)   (b)   (c)

*Based on losses of urea and other nitrogen-containing compounds in the urine, as well as protein lost from feces, skin, hair, nails, and other minor routes.
**Only when additional lean body mass is being gained. Nevertheless, the athlete is probably already eating enough protein to support this extra protein synthesis; protein supplements are not needed.

FIGURE 6-11 ▶ Protein balance in practical terms: (a) positive protein balance; (b) protein equilibrium; (c) negative protein balance.

The 2010 Dietary Guidlines for Americans in "**Food and Nutrients to Increase**," provide the following recommendatins regarding protein intake as part of healthy eating pattern and while staying within their calorie needs:

- Increase intake of fat-free or low-fat milk and milk product, such as milk, yogurt, cheese, or fortified soy beverages.

- Choose a variety of protein foods, which include seafood, lean meat and poultry, eggs, beans and peas, soy products, and unsalted nuts and seeds.

- Increase the amount and variety of seafood consumed by choosing seafood in place of some meat and poultry.

- Replace protein foods that are higher in solid fats with choices that are lower in solid fats and calories and/or are sources of oils.

body weight. This is the RDA for protein. Requirements are higher during periods of growth, such as pregnancy and infancy (see Chapters 14 and 15 for specific values for pregnant women, infants, and children). Healthy weight is used as a reference in the determination of protein needs because excess fat storage doesn't contribute much to protein needs (see Chapter 7 for insight into the concept of healthy weight). Calculations using this RDA are shown in the margin and estimate a requirement of about 56 grams of protein daily for a typical 70-kilogram (154-pound) man and about 46 grams of protein daily for a typical 57-kilogram (125-pound) woman.

The RDA for protein translates into about 10% of total calories. Many experts recommend up to 15% of total calories to provide more flexibility in diet planning, in turn allowing for the variety of protein-rich foods North Americans typically consume. Protein-rich foods are also part of the "Food and Nutritents to increase" in the 2010 Dietary Guidelines. As noted earlier, the Food and Nutrition Board has set an upper range for protein intake at 35% of calories consumed. It is easy to meet currently suggested daily protein needs (Table 6-2). On a daily basis, typical North American protein intakes are about 100 grams of protein for men and 65 grams for women. Thus, most of us consume much more protein than the RDA recommends because we like many high-protein foods and can afford to buy them. Our bodies cannot store excess protein once it is consumed, so the excess amino acids are converted to carbon skeletons that are turned into glucose or fat and then stored as fat or metabolized for energy needs (review Fig. 6-10).

TABLE 6-2 Protein Content of Sample Menus Containing 1600 kcal and 2000 kcal

Menu	1600 kcal		2000 kcal	
	Serving Size	Protein (g)	Serving Size	Protein (g)
Breakfast				
Low-fat granola	²/₃ cup	5	²/₃ cup	5
Blueberries	1 cup	1	1 cup	1
Fat-free (skim) milk	1 cup	8.5	1 cup	8.5
Coffee	1 cup	0	1 cup	0
Lunch				
Broiled chicken breast	3 oz	25	4 oz	33
Salad greens	3 cups	5	3 cups	5
Baked taco shell strips	½ cup	2	½ cup	2
Low-fat salad dressing	2 tbsp	0	2 tbsp	0
Fat-free (skim) milk	1 cup	8.5	1 cup	8.5
Dinner				
Yellow rice	1¼ cups	5	2½ cups	10
Shrimp	4 large	5	6 large	7
Mussels	4 medium	8	6 medium	12
Clams	5 small	12	10 small	24
Peas	¼ cup	4	½ cup	4
Sweet red pepper	¼ cup	0	½ cup	0
Snack				
Muffin	1 small	4	1 small	4
Swiss cheese	1 oz	7.5	1 oz	7.5
Banana	½ small	0.5	½ small	0.5
Total		101		132

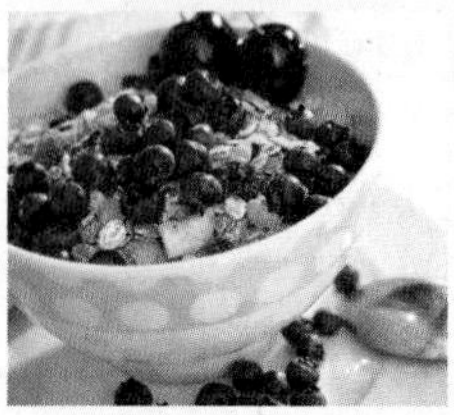

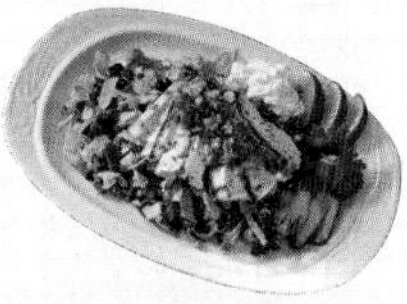

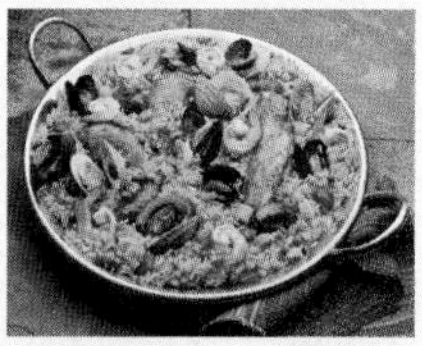

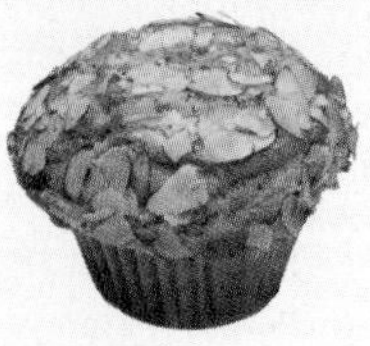

Mental stress, physical labor, and recreational weekend sports activities do not require an increase in the protein RDA. For some highly trained athletes, such as those participating in endurance or strength training, protein consumption may need to exceed the RDA. This is an area of debate in sports nutrition: the Food and Nutrition Board does not support an increased need, but some experts suggest an increase to about 1.7 grams per kilogram. Many North Americans already consume that much protein, especially men.

6.7 Does Eating a High-Protein Diet Harm You?

People frequently ask about the potential harm of protein intakes in excess of the RDA. Problems with diets that are high in protein foods primarily stem from the fact that they typically rely on animal sources of protein. Diets rich in animal products will most likely be simultaneously low in the beneficial substances found in plant sources, including fiber, some vitamins (e.g., folate), some minerals (e.g., magnesium), as well as phytochemicals, and high in substances such as saturated fat and cholesterol. A high animal-protein diet, therefore, is unlikely to follow the recommendations of the Dietary Guidelines for Americans or the Food and Nutrition Board in terms of reducing risk for cardiovascular disease.

Some, but not all, studies show that high-protein diets can increase calcium losses in urine. For people with adequate calcium intakes, little concern about this relationship is warranted, but keep in mind that calcium is commonly deficient in North American diets.

Meat is one of the richest sources of protein. Excessive intake of red meat, however, especially processed forms, is linked to colon cancer in population studies (see Further Reading 3). This association is still being studied (see Newsworthy Nutrition in margin), and there are several possible explanations for this connection. The curing agents used to process meats such as ham and salami may cause cancer. Substances that form during cooking of red meat at high temperatures may also cause cancer. The excessive fat or low-fiber contents of diets rich in red meat may also be a contributing factor. Because of these concerns, some nutrition experts suggest we focus more on poultry, fish, nuts, legumes, and seeds to meet protein needs. In addition, any red or other type of meat should be trimmed of all visible fat before grilling.

Some researchers have expressed concern that a high-protein intake may overburden the kidneys by forcing them to excrete the extra nitrogen as urea. Additionally, animal proteins may contribute to kidney stone formation in certain individuals. There is some support for limiting protein intake for people in the early stages of kidney disease, because low-protein diets somewhat slow the decline in kidney function. Laboratory animal studies show that moderate protein intakes that just meet nutritional needs preserve kidney function over time better than high-protein diets. Preserving kidney function is especially important for those who have diabetes, early signs of kidney disease, or only one functioning kidney, so a high-protein diet is not recommended for these people. High-protein diets increase urine output, in turn posing a risk for dehydration. This is a special concern for athletes (see Chapter 10).

Convert weight from pounds to kilograms:	154 pounds
	2.2 pounds/kilogram
	= 70 kilograms
	125 pounds
	2.2 pounds/kilogram
	= 57 kilograms

Calculate protein RDA:

$$70 \text{ kilograms} \times \frac{0.8 \text{ grams protein}}{\text{kilogram body weight}}$$
$$= 56 \text{ grams}$$

$$57 \text{ kilograms} \times \frac{0.8 \text{ grams protein}}{\text{kilogram body weight}}$$
$$= 46 \text{ grams}$$

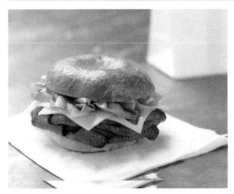

▲ Animal protein foods, such as the roast beef and swiss cheese on this bagel, are typically our main sources of protein in the North American diet.

NEWSWORTHY NUTRITION | **Link between colon cancer and recent fat, protein, and red meat consumption not supported**

The risk of distal colorectal cancer and the consumption of fat, protein, and red and processed meat was determined in whites and African-Americans. The diet was assessed for the previous 12 months in the 945 cases of colon cancer and 959 controls. No association was found between total, saturated, or monounsaturated fat intake and colon cancer risk; the percentages of calories from protein and red meat intake were both associated with a reduction (rather than increase) in risk of colon cancer, in whites. Although these results do not support the general hypotheses that fat, protein and red meat increase the risk of colon cancer, we must remember that the diet was only measured for 12 months prior to the study. A more long-term effect of these dietary factors, therefore, cannot be ruled out.

Source: Williams CD and others: Associations of red meat, fat, and protein intake with distal colorectal cancer risk. *Nutrition and Cancer* 62(6): 701, 2010 (see Further Reading 14).

▦ connect（NUTRITION） **Check out the Connect site** www.mcgrawhillconnect .com **to further explore diet and colorectal cancer.**

MAKING DECISIONS

Amino-Acid Supplements

Protein and amino-acid supplements are used primarily by athletes and dieters. Athletes use them hoping they will help build muscle. The branched-chain amino acids described earlier are especially popular with athletes looking to enhance their performance. Dieters have turned to these supplements hoping they will increase their weight loss. Although the right amount of protein in the diet will aid athletic performance and help in weight control, consuming this protein in the form of amino-acid supplements cannot be considered safe.

Earlier in this chapter, you learned that the body is designed to handle whole proteins as a dietary source of amino acids. When individual amino-acid supplements are taken, they can overwhelm the absorptive mechanisms in the small intestine, triggering amino-acid imbalances in the body. Imbalances occur because groups of chemically similar amino acids compete for absorption sites in the absorptive cells. For example, lysine and arginine are absorbed by the same transporter, so an excess of lysine can impair absorption of arginine. The amino acids most likely to cause toxicity when consumed in large amounts are methionine, cysteine, and histidine. Due to the potential for imbalances and toxicities of individual amino acids, the best advice to ensure adequacy is to stick to whole foods rather than supplements as sources of amino acids. Amino acids as such also have a disagreeable odor and flavor and are also much more expensive than food protein. In Canada the sale of individual amino acids to consumers is banned. Read more about this issue in the What Would You Choose Recommendations at the end of this chapter.

CONCEPT CHECK

The Recommended Dietary Allowance (RDA) for adults is 0.8 grams of protein per kilogram of healthy body weight. This is approximately 56 grams of protein daily for a 70-kilogram (156-pound) person. The average North American man consumes about 100 grams of protein daily, and a woman consumes about 65 grams. Thus, typically we eat more than enough protein to meet our needs. This even includes well-balanced vegetarian diets. Diets high in protein can compromise kidney health in people with diabetes and those with kidney disease, and animal protein sources likely increase cardiovascular disease and kidney stone risk when consumed in high amounts.

protein-calorie malnutrition (PCM)
A condition resulting from regularly consuming insufficient amounts of calories and protein. The deficiency eventually results in body wasting, primarily of lean tissue, and an increased susceptibility to infections.

kwashiorkor A disease occurring primarily in young children who have an existing disease and consume a marginal amount of calories and insufficient protein in relation to needs. The child generally suffers from infections and exhibits edema, poor growth, weakness, and an increased susceptibility to further illness.

marasmus A disease resulting from consuming a grossly insufficient amount of protein and calories; one of the diseases classed as protein-calorie malnutrition. Victims have little or no fat stores, little muscle mass, and poor strength. Death from infections is common.

6.8 Protein-Calorie Malnutrition

Protein deficiency is rarely an isolated condition and usually accompanies a deficiency of calories and other nutrients resulting from insufficient food intake. In the developed world, alcoholism can lead to cases of protein deficiency because of the low protein content of alcoholic beverages. Protein and calorie malnutrition is a significant problem in hospitals worldwide, affecting patients of all ages from infants to geriatric patients. Malnutrition can be caused by the illnesses or injuries for which the patients are admitted to the hospital and by the hospitalization itself (see Further Reading 4). In developing areas of the world, people often have diets low in calories and also in protein. This state of undernutrition stunts the growth of children and makes them more susceptible to disease throughout life. (Undernutrition is a main focus of Chapter 12.) People who consume too little protein calories can eventually develop **protein-calorie malnutrition (PCM),** also referred to as *protein-energy malnutrition (PEM).* In its milder form, it is difficult to tell if a person with PCM is consuming too little calories or protein, or both. When an inadequate intake of nutrients, including protein, is combined with an already existing disease, especially an infection, a form of malnutrition called **kwashiorkor** can develop. But if the nutrient deficiency—especially for calories—becomes severe, a deficiency disease called **marasmus** can result. Both conditions are seen primarily in children but also may develop in adults, even in those hospitalized in North America. These two conditions form the tip of the iceberg with respect to states of undernutrition, and symptoms of these two conditions can even be present in the same person (Fig. 6-12).

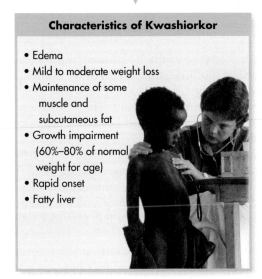

Severe protein (with moderate energy) deficit; often accompanied by infections or other diseases

Protein Energy Malnutrition

Severe energy and protein deficit

FIGURE 6-12 ▶ Classification of undernutrition in children.

Characteristics of Kwashiorkor

- Edema
- Mild to moderate weight loss
- Maintenance of some muscle and subcutaneous fat
- Growth impairment (60%–80% of normal weight for age)
- Rapid onset
- Fatty liver

Characteristics of Marasmus

- Severe weight loss
- Wasting of muscle and body fat (skin and bones appearance)
- Severe growth impairment (less than 60% of normal weight for age)
- Develops gradually

Kwashiorkor

Kwashiorkor is a word from Ghana that means "the disease that the first child gets when the new child comes." From birth, an infant in developing areas of the world is usually breastfed. Often by the time the child reaches 1 to 1.5 years of age, the mother is pregnant or has already given birth again, and the new child gets preference for breastfeeding. The older child's diet then abruptly changes from nutritious human milk to starchy roots and **gruels.** These foods have low-protein densities, compared with total energy. Additionally, the foods are usually full of plant fibers, often bulky, making it difficult for the child to consume enough to meet calorie needs. The child generally also has infections, which acutely raise calorie and protein needs. For these reasons, calorie needs of these children are met just barely, at best, and their protein consumption is grossly inadequate, especially in view of the increased amount needed to combat infections. Many vitamin and mineral needs are also far from being fulfilled. Famine victims face similar problems.

The major symptoms of kwashiorkor are apathy, diarrhea, listlessness, failure to grow and gain weight, and withdrawal from the environment. These symptoms complicate other diseases present. For example, a condition such as measles, a disease that normally makes a healthy child ill for only a week or so, can become severely debilitating and even fatal. Further symptoms of kwashiorkor are changes in hair color, potassium deficiency, flaky skin, fatty liver, reduced muscle mass, and massive edema in the abdomen and legs. The presence of edema in a child who has some subcutaneous fat (i.e., directly under the skin) is the hallmark of kwashiorkor (review Fig. 6-12). In addition, these children seldom move. If you pick them up, they don't cry. When you hold them, you feel the plumpness of edema, not muscle and fat tissue.

Many symptoms of kwashiorkor can be explained based on what we know about proteins. Proteins play important roles in fluid balance, lipoprotein transport, immune function, and production of tissues, such as skin, cells lining the GI tract, and hair. Children with an insufficient protein intake do not grow and mature normally.

If children with kwashiorkor are helped in time—if infections are treated and a diet ample in protein, calories, and other essential nutrients is provided—the disease

gruels A thin mixture of grains or legumes in milk or water.

Toxic products in moldy grains may also contribute to kwashiorkor.

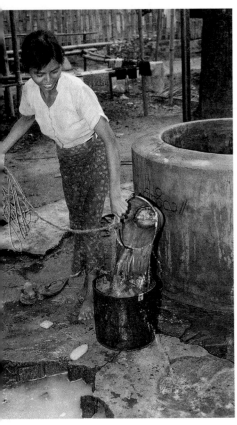

▲ Unsafe water supplies in developing countries contribute to the incidence of marasmus, particularly in bottle-fed infants.

preterm An infant born before 37 weeks of gestation; also referred to as premature.

process reverses. They begin to grow again and may even show no signs of their previous condition, except perhaps shortness of stature. Unfortunately, by the time many of these children reach a hospital or care center, they already have severe infections. Despite the best care, they still die. Or, if they survive, they return home only to become ill again.

Marasmus

Marasmus typically occurs as an infant slowly starves to death. It is caused by diets containing minimal amounts of calories, as well as too little protein and other nutrients. As previously noted, the condition is also commonly referred to as *protein-calorie malnutrition*, especially when experienced by older children and adults. The word *marasmus* means "to waste away," in Greek. Victims have a "skin-and-bones" appearance, with little or no subcutaneous fat (review Fig. 6-12).

Marasmus commonly develops in infants who either are not breastfed or have stopped breastfeeding in the early months. Often the weaning formula used is improperly prepared because of unsafe water and because the parents cannot afford sufficient infant formula for the child's needs. The latter problem may lead the parents to dilute the formula to provide more feedings, not realizing that this provides only more water for the infant.

Marasmus in infants commonly occurs in the large cities of poverty-stricken countries. When people are poor and sanitation is lacking, bottle feeding often leads to marasmus. In the cities, bottle feeding is often necessary because the infant must be cared for by others when the mother is working or away from home. An infant with marasmus requires large amounts of calories and protein—like a **preterm** infant—and, unless the child receives them, full recovery from the disease may never occur. The majority of brain growth occurs between conception and the child's first birthday. In fact, the brain is growing at its highest rate after birth. If the diet does not support brain growth during the first months of life, the brain may not grow to its full adult size. This reduced or retarded brain growth may lead to diminished intellectual function. Both kwashiorkor and marasmus plague infants and children; mortality rates in developing countries are often 10 to 20 times higher than in North America.

CONCEPT CHECK

Most undernutrition consists of mild deficits in calories, protein, and often other nutrients. If a person needs more nutrients because of disease and infection but does not consume enough calories and protein, a condition known as kwashiorkor can develop. The person suffers from edema and weakness. Children around age 2 are especially susceptible to kwashiorkor, particularly if they already have other diseases. Famine situations in which only starchy root products are available to eat contribute to this problem. Marasmus is a condition wherein people—infants, especially—starve to death. Symptoms include muscle wasting, absence of fat stores, and weakness. Both an adequate diet and the treatment of concurrent diseases must be promoted to regain and then maintain nutritional health.

Vegetarian and Plant-Based Diets

Vegetarianism has evolved over the centuries from a necessity into an option. Historically, vegetarianism was linked with specific philosophies and religions or with science. Today, about 1 in 40 adults in the United States (and about 1 in 25 in Canada) is a vegetarian. Vegetarian diets have evolved to include such new products as soy-based sloppy joes, chili, tacos, burgers, and more. In addition, cookbooks that feature the use of a variety of fruits, vegetables, and seasonings are enhancing food selection for vegetarians of all degrees.

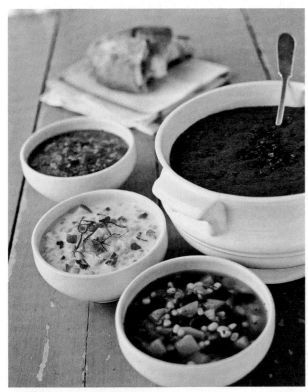

▲ Recipes for vegetarian and plant-based foods are widely available today. Soups are an excellent way to combine complementary plant proteins.

Vegetarianism is popular among college students. Fifteen percent of college students in one survey said they select vegetarian options at lunch or dinner on any given day. In response, dining services offer vegetarian options at every meal, such as pastas with meatless sauce and pizza. Many teenagers are also turning to vegetarianism. Many restaurants offer vegetarian meals in response to the growing number of its customers who want a vegetarian option when they eat out (see Further Reading 13). Many customers cite health and taste as reasons for choosing vegetarian meals.

As nutrition science has grown, new information has enabled the design of nutritionally adequate vegetarian diets. It is important for vegetarians to take advantage of this information because a diet of only plant-based foods has the potential to promote various nutrient deficiencies and substantial growth retardation in infants and children. People who choose a vegetarian diet can meet their nutritional needs by following a few basic rules and knowledgeably planning their diets.

Studies show that death rates from some chronic diseases, such as certain forms of cardiovascular disease, hypertention, many forms of cancer, type 2 diabetes, and obesity, are lower for vegetarians than for non-vegetarians. Vegetarians often live longer, as shown in religious groups that practice vegetarianism. Other aspects of healthful lifestyles, such as not smoking, abstaining from alcohol and drugs, and regular physical activity often go along with vegetarianism and probably partially account for the lower risks of chronic disease and longer lives seen in this population.

As you learned in Chapter 2, MyPlate and the 2010 Dietary Guidelines for Americans emphasize a plant-based diet of whole-grain breads and cereals, fruits, and vegetables. In addition, the American Institute for Cancer Research promotes "The New American Plate," which includes plant-based foods covering two-thirds (or more) of the plate and meat, fish, poultry, or lowfat dairy covering only one-third (or less) of the plate. Although these recommendations do allow the inclusion of animal products, they are definitely more "vegetarian-like" than typical North American diets.

Why Do People Become Vegetarians?

People choose vegetarianism for a variety of reasons including ethics, religion, economics, and health. Some believe that killing animals for food is unethical. Hindus and Trappist monks eat vegetarian meals as a practice of their religion. In North America, many Seventh Day Adventists base their practice of vegetarianism on biblical texts and believe it is a more healthful way to live.

Some advocates of vegetarianism base their food preference upon the inefficient use of animals as a source of protein. Forty percent of the world's grain production is used to raise meat-producing animals.

The New American Plate

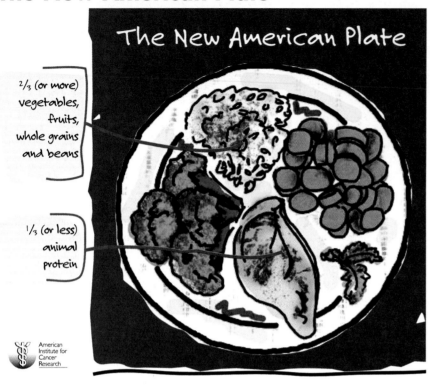

The New American Plate

⅔ (or more) vegetables, fruits, whole grains and beans

⅓ (or less) animal protein

American Institute for Cancer Research

Although animals that humans eat sometimes eat grasses that humans cannot digest, many also eat grains that humans can eat.

People might also practice vegetarianism because it limits saturated fat and cholesterol intake, while encouraging a high intake of complex carbohydrates, vitamins A, E, and C, carotenoids, magnesium, and fiber.

Good for Disease Prevention

Plant sources of proteins can positively impact heart health in several ways (see Further Readings 5, 6, 9, and 10). First, the plant foods we eat contain no cholesterol nor *trans* fat and little saturated fat. The major type of fats in plant foods are monounsaturated and polyunsaturated fats. Nuts in particular are high in monounsaturated fat, which helps to keep blood cholesterol low.

Beans and nuts contain soluble fiber, which binds to cholesterol in the small intestine and prevents it from being absorbed by the body. Also, due to the activity of some phytochemicals, foods made from soybeans can lower production of cholesterol by the body. The effect is modest (about a 2% to 6% drop). In 1999, the Food and Drug Administration allowed health claims for the cholesterol-lowering properties of soy foods, and in 2000, the American Heart Association recommended inclusion of some soy protein in the diets of people with high blood cholesterol. As noted in Chapter 2, to list a health claim for soy on the label, a food product must have at least 6.25 grams of soy protein and less than 3 grams of fat, 1 gram of saturated fat, and 20 milligrams of cholesterol per serving.

There are several other compounds in plant foods under study for their heart-protective roles. Some of the phytochemicals may help to prevent blood clots and relax the blood vessels. Nuts are an especially good source of nutrients implicated in heart health, including vitamin E, folate, magnesium, and copper. Frequent consumption of nuts (about 1 ounce of nuts five times per week) is associated with a decreased risk of cardiovascular disease. Recall from Chapter 2 that FDA also allows a provisional health claim to link nuts with a reduced risk of developing cardiovascular disease. As noted in Chapter 5, a vegan diet coupled with regular exercise and other lifestyle changes can lead to a reversal of atherosclerotic plaque in various arteries in the body.

Cancer-Fighting Agents

The numerous phytochemicals in plant foods are thought to aid in preventing cancers of the breast, prostate, and colon. Many of the proposed anticancer effects of foods containing plant protein are through antioxidant mechanisms.

Consumption of plant sources of proteins can aid in prevention of cardiovascular disease and cancer, but there are also other areas for future study. Some studies show that replacing animal proteins with plant proteins is beneficial for kidney health. However, because plant foods such as soy are high in oxalates, people with a history of kidney stones should probably limit intake of soy (see Chapter 8 for more about oxalates). Plants may be particularly good sources of protein for people with diabetes or impaired glucose tolerance because the high fiber content of plant foods leads to a slower increase in blood glucose (review Chapter 4 for a discussion of glycemic load). Frequent nut consumption may even reduce the risk of developing gallstones, obesity, and type 2 diabetes. A recent review of 18 studies concluded that soy consumption was associated with a 14% reduction in breast cancer risk, but several other studies have shown little benefit of soy in preventing many forms of cancer, in lowering blood cholesterol, contributing to bone maintenance in women after menopause, and in treating menopausal symptoms in women (see Further Readings 12 and 15).

Increasing Plant Proteins in Your Diet

Now that you've seen how much you can benefit from including plant proteins in your diet, here are some suggestions for putting the theory onto your plate:

- At your next cookout, try a veggie burger instead of a hamburger. These are usually made from beans and are available in the frozen foods section of the grocery store and come in a variety of delicious flavors. Many restaurants have added veggie burgers to their menus.
- Sprinkle sunflower seeds or chopped almonds on top of your salad to add taste and texture.
- Mix chopped walnuts into the batter of your banana bread to boost your intake of monounsaturated fats.
- Eat soy nuts (oil-roasted soybeans) as a great snack.
- Spread some peanut butter on your bagel instead of butter or cream cheese.
- Instead of having beef or chicken tacos for dinner, heat up a can of great northern beans in your skillet with one half of a packet of taco seasoning and chopped tomatoes. Use this as a filling in a tortilla shell.
- Consider using soy milk, especially if you have lactose malabsorption or lactose intolerance. Look for varieties fortified with calcium.

Food Planning for Vegetarians

There are a variety of vegetarian diet styles. **Vegans,** or "total vegetarians," eat only plant foods (and do not use animal products for other purposes, such as leather shoes or feather pillows). **Fruitarians** primarily eat fruits, nuts, honey, and vegetable oils. This plan is not recommended because it can lead to nutrient deficiencies in people of all ages. **Lactovegetarians** modify vegetarianism a bit—they include dairy products in their plant-based diet. **Lactoovovegetarians** modify the diet even further and eat dairy products and eggs, as well as plant foods. Including these animal products makes food planning easier because they are rich in some nutrients that are missing or minimal in plants, such as vitamin B-12 and calcium. The more variety in the diet, the easier it is to meet nutritional needs. Thus, the practice of eating no animal sources of food significantly separates the vegans and fruitarians from all other semivegetarian styles.

Most people who call themselves vegetarians consume at least some dairy products, if not all dairy products and eggs. A food-group plan has been developed for lactovegetarians and vegans (Table 6-3). This plan includes servings of nuts, grains, legumes, and seeds to help meet protein needs. There is also a vegetable group, a fruit group, and a milk group.

Vegan Diet Planning

Planning a vegan diet requires knowledge and creativity to yield high-quality protein and other key nutrients without animal products. Earlier in this chapter, you learned about complementing proteins, whereby the essential amino acids deficient in one protein source are supplied by those of another consumed at the same meal or the next (Fig. 6-13). Many legumes are deficient in the essential amino-acid methionine, while cereals are limited in lysine. Eating a combination of legumes and cereals, such as beans and rice, will supply the body with adequate amounts of all essential amino acids (Fig. 6-13). As for

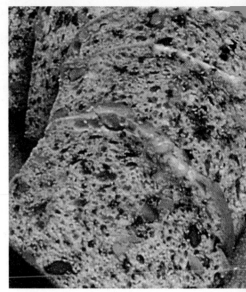

▲ Plant proteins, like those in walnuts, can be incorporated into one's diet in numerous ways, such as adding them to banana bread.

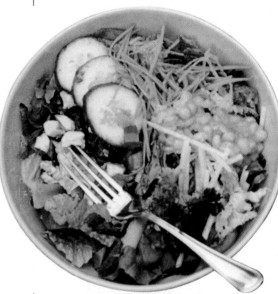

▲ A salad containing numerous types of vegetables and legumes is a healthy vegetarian choice.

vegan A person who eats only plant foods.

fruitarian A person who primarily eats fruits, nuts, honey, and vegetable oils.

lactovegetarian A person who consumes plant products and dairy products.

lactoovovegetarian A person who consumes plant products, dairy products, and eggs.

TABLE 6-3 Food Plan for Vegetarians Based on MyPlate

Food Group	MyPlate Servings Lactovegetarian[a]	Vegan[b]	Key Nutrients Supplied[c]
Grains	6–11	8–11	Protein, thiamin, niacin, folate, vitamin E, zinc, magnesium, iron, and fiber
Beans and other legumes	2–3	3	Protein, vitamin B-6, zinc, magnesium, and fiber
Nuts, seeds	2–3	3	Protein, vitamin E, and magnesium
Vegetables	3–5 (include 1 dark-green or leafy variety daily)	4–6 (include 1 dark-green or leafy variety daily)	Vitamin A, vitamin C, folate, vitamin K, potassium, and magnesium
Fruits	2–4	4	Vitamin A, vitamin C, and folate
Milk	3	_____	Protein, riboflavin, vitamin D, vitamin B-12, and calcium
Fortified soy milk	_____	3	Protein, riboflavin, vitamin D, vitamin B-12, and calcium

[a]This plan contains about 75 grams of protein in 1650 kcal.

[b]This plan contains about 79 grams of protein in 1800 kcal.

[c]One serving of vitamin- and mineral-enriched ready-to-eat breakfast cereal is recommended to meet possible nutrient gaps. Alternatively, a balanced multivitamin and mineral supplement can be used. Vegans also may benefit from the use of fortified soy milk to provide calcium, vitamin D, and vitamin B-12.

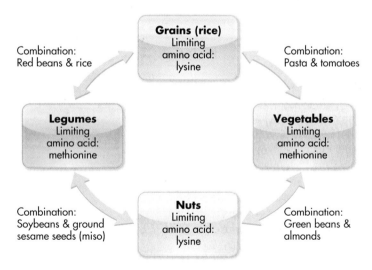

FIGURE 6-13 ▶ Plant group combinations in which the proteins complement each other in a meal based on their limiting amino acids.

any diet, variety is an especially important characteristic of a nutritious vegan diet.

Aside from amino acids, low intakes of certain micronutrients can be a problem for the vegan. At the forefront of nutritional concerns are riboflavin, vitamins D and B-12, iron, zinc, iodide, and calcium. The following dietary advice should be implemented. In addition, use of a balanced multivitamin and mineral supplement can help as well.

Riboflavin can be obtained from green leafy vegetables, whole grains, yeast, and legumes—components of most vegan diets. Alternate sources of vitamin D include fortified foods (e.g., margarine), as well as regular sun exposure (see Chapter 11).

Vitamin B-12 only occurs naturally in animal foods. Plants can contain soil or microbial contaminants that provide trace amounts of vitamin B-12, but these are negligible sources of the vitamin. Because the body can store vitamin B-12 for about 4 years, it may take a long time after removal of animal foods from the diet for a vitamin B-12 deficiency to surface. If dietary B-12 inadequacy persists, deficiency can lead to a form of anemia, nerve damage, and mental dysfunction. These deficiency consequences have been noted in the infants of vegetarian mothers whose breast milk was low in vitamin B-12. Vegans can prevent a vitamin B-12 deficiency by finding a reliable source of vitamin B-12,

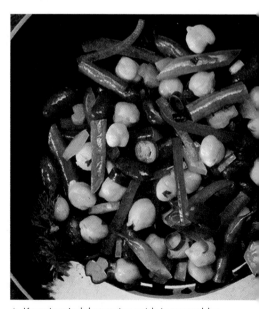

▲ Keep in mind that amino acids in vegetables are best used when a combination of sources is consumed.

such as fortified soybean milk, ready-to-eat breakfast cereals, and special yeast grown on media rich in vitamin B-12.

For iron, the vegan can consume whole grains (especially ready-to-eat breakfast cereals), dried fruits and nuts, and legumes. The iron in these foods is not absorbed as well as iron in animal foods. A good source of vitamin C helps with the absorption of iron so it is recommended that vitamin C be consumed with every meal that contains iron-rich plant foods. Cooking in iron pots and skillets can also add iron to the diet.

The vegan can find zinc in whole grains (especially ready-to-eat breakfast cereals), nuts, and legumes, but phytic acid and other substances in these foods limit zinc absorption. Breads are a good source of zinc because the leavening process (rising of the bread dough) reduces the influence of phytic acid. Iodized salt is a reliable source of iodide. It should be used instead of plain salt, both of which are found in U.S. supermarkets.

Of all nutrients, calcium is the most difficult to consume in sufficient quantities for vegans. Fortified foods including fortified soy milk, fortified orange juice, calcium-rich tofu (check the label), as well as certain ready-to-eat breakfast cereals and snacks are the vegan's best option for obtaining calcium. Green leafy vegetables and nuts also contain calcium, but the mineral is either not well absorbed or not very plentiful from these sources. Calcium supplements are another option (see Chapter 11). Special diet planning is always required, because even a multivitamin and mineral supplement will not supply enough calcium to meet the needs of the body.

Consuming adequate quantities of omega-3 fatty acids is yet another nutritional concern for vegetarians, especially vegans. Fish and fish oils, abundant sources of these

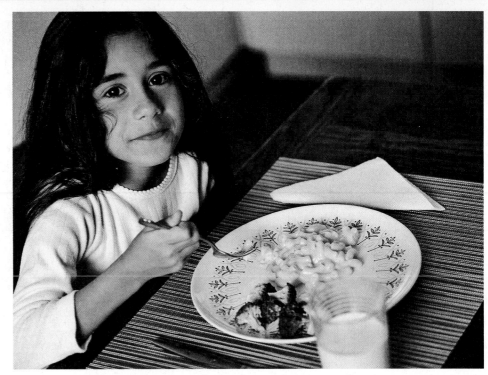

▲ Children can safely enjoy vegetarian and vegan diets as long as certain adjustments are made to meet their age-specific nutritional needs.

heart-healthy fats, are omitted from many types of vegetarian diets. Alternative plant sources of omega-3 fatty acids include canola oil, soybean oil, seaweed, microalgae, flax seeds, and walnuts.

Special Concerns for Infants and Children

Infants and children, notoriously picky eaters in the first place, are at highest risk for nutrient deficiencies as a result of improperly planned vegetarian and vegan diets. With the use of complementary proteins and good sources of problem nutrients just discussed, the calorie, protein, vitamin, and mineral needs of vegetarian and vegan infants and children can be met (see Further Reading 1). The most common nutritional concerns for infants and children following vegetarian and vegan diets are deficiencies of iron, vitamin B-12, vitamin D, and calcium.

Vegetarian and vegan diets tend to be high in bulky, high-fiber, low-calorie foods that cause a feeling of fullness. While this is a welcome advantage for adults, children have small stomach volume and relatively high nutrient needs compared to their size, and therefore may feel full before their calorie needs are met. For this reason, the fiber content of a child's diet may need to be decreased by replacing high-fiber sources with some refined grain products, fruit juices, and peeled fruit. Other concentrated sources of calories for vegetarian and vegan children include fortified soy milk, nuts, dried fruits, avocados, and cookies made with vegetable oils or tub margarine.

Case Study Planning a Vegetarian Diet

Jordan is a freshman in college. He lives in a campus residence hall and teaches martial arts in the afternoon. He eats two or three meals a day at the residence hall cafeteria and snacks between meals. Jordan and his roommate both decided to become vegetarians because they recently read a magazine article describing the health benefits of a vegetarian diet. Yesterday Jordan's vegetarian diet consisted of a Danish pastry for breakfast and a tomato-rice dish (no meat) with pretzels and a diet soft drink for lunch. In the afternoon, after his martial arts class, he had a milk shake and two cookies. At dinnertime he had a vegetarian sub sandwich consisting of lettuce, sprouts, tomatoes, cucumbers, and cheese, with two glasses of fruit punch. In the evening, he had a bowl of popcorn.

Answer the following questions, and check your response in Appendix A.

1. What type of health benefits can Jordan expect from following a well-planned vegetarian diet?
2. What is missing from Jordan's current diet plan in terms of foods that should be emphasized in a vegetarian diet?
3. Which nutrients are missing in this current diet plan?
4. Are there any food components in the current diet plan that should be minimized or avoided?
5. How could he improve his new diet at each meal and snack to meet his nutritional needs and avoid undesirable food components?

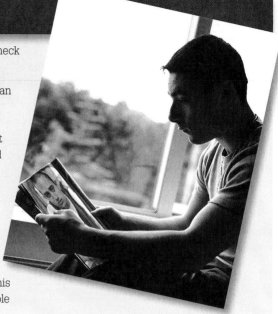

▲ Has Jordan planned a healthy and nutritious vegetarian diet?

Summary (Numbers refer to numbered sections in the chapter.)

6.1 Amino acids, the building blocks of proteins, contain a very usable form of nitrogen for humans. Of the 20 common types of amino acids found in food, nine must be consumed in food (essential) and the rest can be synthesized by the body (nonessential).

6.2 Individual amino acids are bonded together to form proteins. The sequential order of amino acids determines the protein's ultimate shape and function. This order is directed by DNA in the cell nucleus. Diseases such as sickle cell anemia can occur if the amino acids are incorrect on a polypeptide chain. When the three-dimensional shape of a protein is unfolded—denatured—by treatment with heat, acid or alkaline solutions, or other processes, the protein also loses its biological activity.

6.3 Almost all animal products are nutrient-dense sources of protein. The high quality of these proteins means that they can be easily converted into body proteins. Rich plant sources of protein, such as beans, are also available.

High-quality (complete) protein foods contain ample amounts of all nine essential amino acids. Furthermore, foods derived from animal sources provide high

biological value protein. Lower-quality (incomplete) protein foods lack sufficient amounts of one or more essential amino acids. This is typical of plant foods, especially cereal grains. Different types of plant foods eaten together often complement each other's amino-acid deficits, thereby providing high-quality protein in the diet.

6.4 Protein digestion begins in the stomach, dividing the proteins into breakdown products containing shorter polypeptide chains of amino acids. In the small intestine, these polypeptide chains eventually separate into amino acids in the absorptive cells. The free amino acids then travel via the portal vein that connects to the liver. Some then enter the bloodstream.

6.5 Important body components—such as muscles, connective tissue, transport proteins in the bloodstream, visual pigments, enzymes, some hormones, and immune cells—are made of proteins. These proteins are in a state of constant turnover. The carbon chains of proteins may be used to produce glucose (or fat) when necessary.

6.6 The protein RDA for adults is 0.8 grams per kilogram of healthy body weight. For a typical 70-kilogram (154-pound) person, this corresponds to 56 grams of

protein daily; for a 57-kilogram (125-pound) person, this corresponds to 46 grams per day. The North American diet generally supplies plenty of protein. Men typically consume about 100 grams of protein daily, and women consume closer to 65 grams. These usual protein intakes are also of sufficient quality to support body functions. This is even true for well-balanced vegetarian diets.

6.7 People need to balance protein intake with such losses to maintain a state of protein equilibrium, also called *protein balance.*

When a body is growing or recovering from an illness or injury, it needs a positive protein balance to supply the raw materials required to build new tissues. To achieve this, a person must eat more protein daily than he or she loses. Consuming less protein than needed leads to negative protein balance, such as when acute illness reduces the desire to eat and so one loses more protein than consumed.

6.8 Undernutrition can lead to protein-calorie malnutrition in the form of kwashiorkor or marasmus. Kwashiorkor results primarily from an inadequate calorie and protein intake in comparison with body needs, which often increase with concurrent disease and infection. Kwashiorkor often occurs when a child is weaned from human milk and fed mostly starchy gruels. Marasmus results from extreme starvation—a negligible intake of both protein and calories. Marasmus commonly occurs during famine, especially in infants.

N&YH Consumption of vegetarian and other plant-based diets provides many health benefits, including lower risks of chronic diseases including cardiovascular disease, diabetes, and certain cancers. The benefits associated with the plant-based diets appear to stem from the lower content of saturated fat and cholesterol and the higher amount of fiber, vitamins, minerals, and phytochemicals.

Check Your Knowledge (Answers to the following questions are below.)

1. The "instructions" for making proteins are located in the
   a. cell membrane.
   b. DNA and RNA genetic material.
   c. stomach.
   d. small intestine.

2. A nutrient that could easily be deficient in the diet of a vegan would be
   a. vitamin C.
   b. folic acid.
   c. calcium.
   d. All of the above.

3. If an essential amino acid is unavailable for protein synthesis, the
   a. cell will make the amino acid.
   b. synthesis of the protein will stop.
   c. cell will continue to attach amino acids to the protein.
   d. partially completed protein will be stored for later completion.

4. An example of protein complementation used in vegetarian diet planning would be the combination of
   a. cereal and milk.
   b. bacon and eggs.
   c. rice and beans.
   d. macaroni and cheese.

5. An individual who eats only plant food is referred to as a
   a. planetarium.
   b. vegan.
   c. lactovegetarian.
   d. ovovegetarian.

6. Which of the following groups accounts for the differences among amino acids?
   a. amine group
   b. side chain
   c. acid group
   d. keto group

7. Absorption of amino acids takes place in the
   a. stomach.
   b. liver.
   c. small intestine.
   d. large intestine.

8. Jack is not an athlete and weighs 176 pounds (80 kilograms). His RDA for protein would be _____ grams.
   a. 32
   b. 40
   c. 64
   d. 80

9. Which of the following is true about protein intake of people in the United States?
   a. Most do not consume enough protein.
   b. Most consume approximately the amount needed to balance losses.
   c. Athletes generally do not get enough protein without supplementation.
   d. Most consume more than is needed.

10. The basic building block of a protein is called a(n)
    a. fatty acid.
    b. monosaccharide.
    c. amino acid.
    d. gene.

Answers Key: 1. b (LO 6.2), 2. c (LO 6.3), 3. b (LO 6.2), 4. c (LO 6.9), 5. b (LO 6.9), 6. b (LO 6.1), 7. c (LO 6.4), 8. c (LO 6.6), 9. d (LO 6.7), 10. c (LO 6.1)

Study Questions (Numbers refer to Learning Outcomes)

1. Discuss the relative importance of essential and nonessential amino acids in the diet. Why is it important for essential amino acids lost from the body to be replaced in the diet? (LO 6.1)

2. Describe the concept of complementary proteins. (LO 6.3)

3. What is a limiting amino acid? Explain why this concept is a concern in a vegetarian diet. How can a vegetarian compensate for limiting amino acids in specific foods? (LO 6.9)

4. Briefly describe the organization of proteins. How can this organization be altered or damaged? What might be a result of damaged protein organization? (LO 6.2)

5. Describe four functions of proteins. Provide an example of how the structure of a protein relates to its function. (LO 6.5)

6. How are DNA and protein synthesis related? (LO 6.2)

7. What would be one health benefit of reducing high-protein intake(s) to RDA amounts for some people? (LO 6.6)

8. What characteristics of vegetable proteins could improve the North American diet? What foods would you include to provide a diet that has ample protein from both plant and animal sources but is moderate in fat? (LO 6.9)

9. Outline the major differences between kwashiorkor and marasmus. (LO 6.8)

10. What are the possible long-term effects of an inadequate intake of dietary protein among children between the ages of 6 months and 4 years? (LO 6.8)

What Would You Choose Recommendations

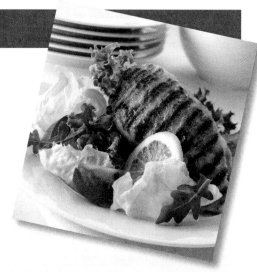

It is not a good idea to take individual amino-acid supplements. Your digestive tract is made to handle whole proteins—hydrochloric acid and enzymes break polypeptides into amino acids that can be absorbed by the cells of the small intestine. Taking large doses of one amino acid can impair the absorption and/or metabolism of other amino acids.

Whey protein, a by-product of cheese production from cow's milk, is considered to be a high-quality protein because it is easily digested and contains all of the essential amino acids. It is a source of the branched-chain amino acids, valine, leucine, and isoleucine. BCAAs can be used for fuel by exercising muscles and are particularly important for synthesizing muscle tissue. The rationale is that whey protein supports muscle recovery and anabolism after exercise.

Consuming adequate protein is important for muscle repair and synthesis, but consuming excessive protein from any source provides no advantage. Excess protein will be metabolized as fuel or stored as fat, not muscle. In fact, some excess subcutaneous fat is probably the reason you have not seen your toned muscles yet. Cutting back on calories or including more endurance exercise in your routine can help to reduce body weight and body fat as you tone your muscles. Animal protein, in particular, is often a source of excess total fat, saturated fat, and cholesterol. Not only will this hinder efforts at weight loss, but it is detrimental to heart health.

Americans typically consume two to three times as much protein as they actually need. The average American intake of 100 grams per day for men or 65 grams per day for women easily meets even the highest protein recommendations for resistance exercise (1.7 grams of protein per kilogram). Also, omnivorous diets and even appropriately planned vegan diets can supply ample amino acids to support muscle recovery and synthesis. Protein and amino

▲ This 4-ounce grilled chicken breast is an excellent choice, providing 38 grams of high-quality yet inexpensive lean protein.

acid supplements are expensive and may be detrimental to health. It is safer and more economical to focus on a diet that provides 10% to 35% of calories from a variety of lean sources of protein.

Further Readings

1. ADA Reports: Position of the American Dietetic Association and Dietitians of Canada: Vegetarian diets. *Journal of the American Dietetic Association* 109:1266, 2009.

   It is the position of the American Dietetic Association and Dietitians of Canada that appropriately planned vegetarian diets are healthful, nutritionally adequate, and provide health benefits in the prevention and treatment of certain diseases. Vegetarian diets are appropriate for all stages of the life cycle.

2. Barnard ND and others: A low-fat vegan diet improves glycemic control and cardiovascular risk factors in a randomized clinical trial in individuals with type 2 diabetes. *Diabetes Care* 29:1777, 2006.

   Improvements in glycemic (decreased hemoglobin A1C) and lipid (decreased LDL cholesterol) control were greater in type 2 diabetic patients that followed a low-fat vegan diet compared to a diet based on American Diabetes Association

   guidelines. In the vegan group, 43% of the subjects reduced their diabetes medications compared to 26% of the subjects on the ADA diet.

3. Chao A and others: Meat consumption and colorectal cancer. *Journal of the American Medical Association* 293:172, 2005.

   Diets rich in red meat, especially processed meat, increase the risk of colon cancer. Protein from poultry and fish, in contrast, does not pose the same risk.

4. Fessler TA: Malnutrition: A serious concern for hospitalized patients. *Today's Dietitian* 10(7): 44, 2008.

   Malnutrition continues to be a significant problem in hospitals worldwide, affecting patients of all ages from infants to geriatric patients. Malnutrition can be caused by the illnesses or injuries for which the patients are admitted to the hospital and by the hospitalization itself. This article outlines the need for prompt identification, treatment, and monitoring

   of malnourished patients among healthcare professionals.

5. Gardner CD and others: The effect of a plant-based diet on plasma lipids in hypercholesterolemic adults. *Annals of Internal Medicine* 142:725, 2005.

   Adding plant proteins to a diet already low in saturated fat and cholesterol provides additional benefits regarding lowering blood cholesterol. The authors emphasize the importance of including fruits, vegetables, legumes, and whole grains in a diet.

6. Key TJ and others: Health effects of vegetarian and vegan diets. *Proceedings of the Nutrition Society* 65:35, 2006.

   This study reviewed recent findings from large studies and summarizes the latest understanding of the health effects of vegetarian and vegan diets. Results indicated that vegetarians have a lower BMI and lower obesity rates than comparable nonvegetarians; total plasma cholesterol is lower in vegetarians that nonvegetarians; between vegetarians and nonvegetarians there is no significant differences in blood pressure; studies of vegetarians indicate a moderate reduction in mortality from ischemic heart disease; and studies showed no differences between vegetarians and nonvegetarians for colorectal cancer, breast cancer, prostate cancer, or total mortality.

7. Lejeune MP and others: Additional protein intake limits weight regain after weight loss in humans. *British Journal of Nutrition* 93:281, 2005.

   Adding 30 grams of protein per day to their usual diets helped people in this study limit weight regain after weight loss. The diet ended up 18% of calorie intake as protein, compared to 15% in the control group. This protein intake in the experimental group would not be considered excessive given an upper limit of 35% of calorie intake set by the Food and Nutrition Board.

8. Mangels R: Weight control the vegan way. *Vegetarian Journal* XXV(1), 2006.

   This article provides suggestions for vegans, or people interested in following a vegan diet, who want to lose weight. Two eating plans are included that were developed for people who are moderately active, spending 30 to 60 minutes daily in moderate physical activity. The first eating plan has approximately 1500 calories and is designed for women who want to lose 1 to 2 pounds per week. The second has about 1900 calories and is designed for men who want to lose 1 to 2 pounds per week. Protein foods include kidney beans, chickpeas, and other beans; tofu; lite or plain soymilk; nuts and nut butters; seitan (say-than, wheat meat); and meat analogs. Recipes are also included.

9. Newby PK: Risk of overweight and obesity among semivegetarian, lactovegetarian, and vegan women. *American Journal of Clinical Nutrition* 81:1267, 2005.

   Semivegetarian women in this study were less likely to be overweight and obese compared to omnivorous women. Consuming more plant foods and less animal products may help individuals control their weight.

10. Sacks FM and others: Soy protein, isoflavones, and cardiovascular health. An American Heart Association Science Advisory for Professionals From the Nutrition Committee. *Circulation* 113:1034, 2006.

    This scientific advisory evaluates recent work published on soy protein and its component isoflavones and their potential role in improving risk factors for cardiovascular disease. In the majority of studies, soy protein with isoflavones, as compared with milk or other proteins, decreased LDL cholesterol concentrations; the average effect was ~ 3% and no significant effects on HDL cholesterol, triglycerides, lipoprotein(a), or blood pressure were evident. The authors conclude that soy products should be beneficial to cardiovascular and overall health because of their high content of polyunsaturated fats, fiber, vitamins, and minerals and low content of saturated fat.

11. Taylor SL: Estimating prevalence of soy protein allergy. *The Soy Connection* 14(2):1, 2006.

    This article discusses the issue of soy protein allergy. Although soy protein has been designated one of the major allergens by the U.S. Food and Drug Administration, rigorous prevalence data for this allergy are not available, and indirect evidence suggests it occurs less frequently than other common allergens including shellfish, peanuts, tree nuts, and fish.

12. Trock BJ and others: Meta-analysis of soy intake and breast cancer risk. *Journal of the National Cancer Institute* 98(7):459, 2006.

    This study analyzed data from 18 previously published studies and concludes that consumption of soy foods among healthy women was associated with a significant reduction (14%) in breast cancer risk.

13. Who's the veggie-friendliest of them all? *Vegetarian Journal* XXVII, p. 14, 2008.

    The Vegetarian Resource Group evaluated the menus of the 400 largest restaurant chains in the United States. This article highlights the establishments that appeared to make the best effort at serving vegetarians of diverse needs. You can find more than 2000 veggie-friendly restaurants at their website www.vrg.org.

14. Williams CD and other: Associations of red meat, fat, and protein intake with distal colorectal cancer risk. *Nutrition and Cancer* 62(6):701, 2010.

    Studies suggest that red and processed meat consumption increase the risk of colon cancer. The risk of distal colorectal cancer (CRC) associated with red and processed meat, fat, and protein intakes was determined in whites and African-Americans. Dietary intake was assessed in 945 cases of distal CRC and in 959 controls in the previous 12 months. The results did not support the hypothesis that fat, protein, and red meat increase the risk of distal CRC. There was no association between total, saturated, or monounsaturated fat and distal CRC risk, and the percentages of energy from protein and red meat consumption were associated with a risk reduction (rather than increase).

15. Xiao CW: Health effects of soy protein and isoflavones in humans. *Journal of Nutrition* 138:1244S, 2008.

    The results of epidemiological and clinical studies have suggested that soy consumption may be associated with a lower incidence of certain chronic diseases and a reduction in the risk factors for cardiovascular disease. These results led to an FDA-approved food-labeling health claim for soy proteins in the prevention of coronary heart disease. This article reviews the evidence for health claims on the effects of soy protein and isoflavones in humans and concludes that the existing data are inconsistent or inadequate to support most of the suggested health benefits of consuming soy protein or ISF.

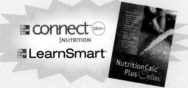

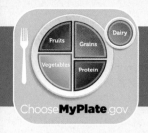

RATE YOUR PLATE

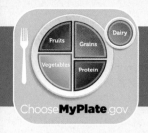

ChooseMyPlate.gov

I. Protein and the Vegetarian

Alana is excited about all the health benefits that might accompany a vegetarian diet. However, she is concerned that she will not consume enough protein to meet her needs. She is also concerned about possible vitamin and mineral deficiencies. Use NutritionCalc Plus or a food composition table to calculate her protein intake and see if her concerns are valid.

	Protein (g)
Breakfast Calcium fortified orange juice, 1 cup Soy milk, 1 cup Fortified bran flakes, 1 cup Banana, medium	
Snack Calcium-enriched granola bar	
Lunch GardenBurger, 4 oz Whole-wheat bun Mustard, 1 tbsp Soy cheese, 1 oz Apple, medium Green leaf lettuce, 1 ½ cups Peanuts, 1 oz Sunflower seeds, 1/4 cup Tomato slices, 2 Mushrooms, 3 Vinaigrette salad dressing, 2 tbsp Iced tea	
Dinner Kidney beans, ½ cup Brown rice, 3/4 cup Fortified margarine, 2 tbsp Mixed vegetables, 1/4 cup Hot tea	
Dessert Strawberries, ½ cup Angel food cake, 1 small slice Soy milk, ½ cup	
	TOTAL PROTEIN (grams) _____

Alana's diet contained 2150 kcal, with _____ grams (you fill in) of protein (Is this plenty for her?), 360 grams of carbohydrate, 57 grams of total dietary fat (only 9 grams of which came from saturated fat), and 50 grams of fiber. Her vitamin and mineral intake with respect to those of concern to vegetarians—vitamin B-12, vitamin D, calcium, iron, and zinc—met her needs.

II. Meeting Protein Needs When Dieting to Lose Weight

Your father has been steadily gaining weight for the last 30 years and now has developed hypertension and type 2 diabetes as a result. His physician recommends that he lose some weight by following an 1800 kcal diet. You know that it will be important for your father to meet protein needs as he tries to lose weight. Design a 1-day diet for him that contains about 20% of calorie intake as protein. Table 6-2 will provide some help. Will this diet meet his protein RDA? Does the diet look like a plan you could also follow?

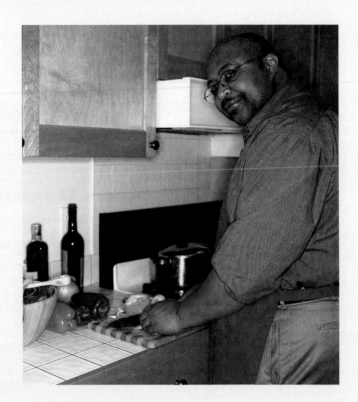

Chapter 7 Energy Balance and Weight Control

Student Learning Outcomes

Chapter 7 is designed to allow you to:

7.1 Describe energy balance and the uses of energy by the body.

7.2 Compare methods to determine energy use by the body.

7.3 Discuss methods for assessing body composition and determining whether body weight and composition are healthy.

7.4 Outline the risks to health posed by overweight and obesity.

7.5 Explain factors associated with the development of obesity.

7.6 List and discuss characteristics of a sound weight-loss program

7.7 Describe why reduced calorie intake is the main key to weight loss and maintenance.

7.8 Discuss why physical activity is a key to weight loss and especially important for later weight maintenance.

7.9 Describe why and how behavior modification fits into a weight-less program.

7.10 Outline the benefits and hazards of various weight-loss methods for severe obesity.

7.11 Discuss the causes and treatment of underweight.

7.12 Evaluate popular weight-reduction diets and determine which are unsafe, doomed to fail, or both.

What Would You Choose?

There are so many choices when it comes to controlling calorie intake. Is it possible to have dessert and still manage your weight? Consider the following frozen treats: regular ice cream, light ice cream, and frozen yogurt. Which of these desserts would you choose to cut back on calories? What information from the Nutrition Facts label is most helpful when it comes to weight management?

a Regular ice cream

b Light ice cream

c Frozen yogurt

 Think about your choice as you read Chapter 7, then see our recommendations at the end of the chapter. To learn more about controlling calorie intake, check out the Connect site: www.mcgrawhillconnect.com

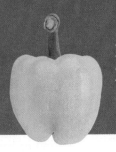
In the last 25 years (the years since most college students were born), there has been a dramatic increase in the percentage of individuals who are overweight or obese. The ranks of the obese are growing in North America and worldwide. Recall from Chapter 1 that an estimated 1 billion people in the world are overweight. This problem is increasing not only in the United States but also globally among affluent peoples and in developing countries where Westernized diets (high-fat, high-calorie) are increasing in popularity. Excess weight increases the likelihood of many health problems, such as cardiovascular disease, cancer, hypertension, strokes, certain bone and joint disorders, and type 2 diabetes, especially if a person performs minimal physical activity.

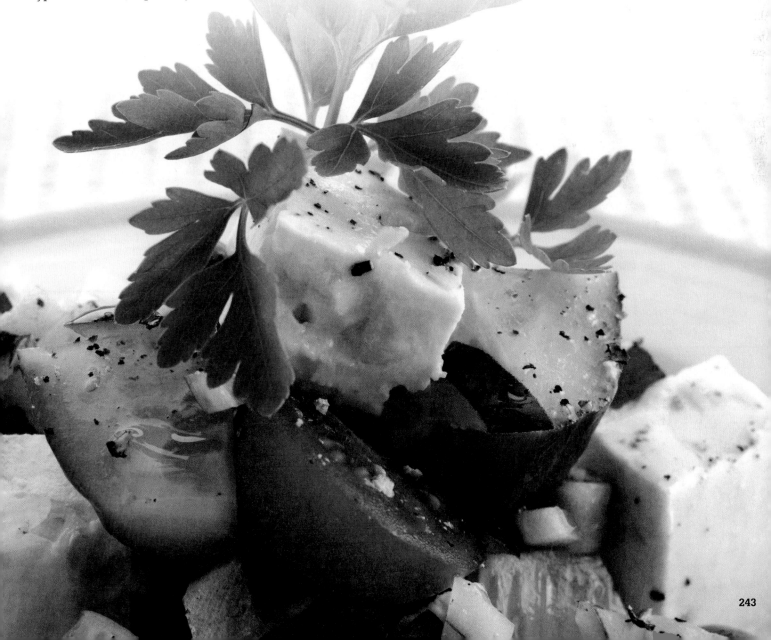

Currently, most weight-reduction efforts fizzle before bodies fall into a healthy weight range. As suggested in this chapter's comic, typical popular ("fad") diets are generally monotonous, ineffective, and confusing. They may even endanger some populations, such as children, teenagers, pregnant women, and people with various health disorders. A more logical approach to weight loss is straightforward: (1) eat less; (2) increase physical activity; and (3) change problematic eating behaviors.

A national commitment has begun from a variety of groups, including government agencies, the food industry, health professionals, and communities, to address the growing weight problem in North America. It has become obvious that, without this national effort to promote weight maintenance and effective new approaches to making our social environment more favorable to maintaining healthy weight, the current trends will not be reversed (Fig. 7-1) (see Futher Readings 3 and 9). Chapter 7 discusses these recommendations to help you understand obesity's causes, consequences, and potential treatments.

Refresh Your Memory

As you begin your study of weight control in Chapter 7, you may want to review:

- Biological and social influences of food intake in Chapter 1
- The concept of energy density and appropriate serving sizes for foods in Chapter 2
- The role of fiber in weight regulation in Chapter 4
- The fat content of various foods in Chapter 5
- The long-term risks of high-protein diets in Chapter 6

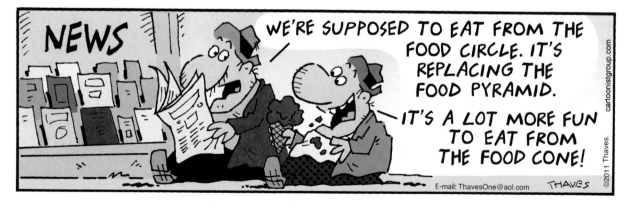

What components make up a successful diet plan? What constitutes a "fad" diet? Why are overweight and obesity growing problems worldwide? What might be the future consequences of this trend? Chapter 7 provides some answers.

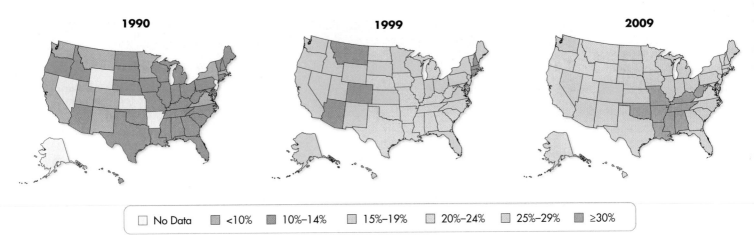

FIGURE 7-1 ▶ Obesity trends among U.S. adults: 1990, 1999, 2009 (BMI ≥ 30, or about 30 pounds overweight for 5′4″ person).

Source: CDC Behavioral Risk Factor Surveillance System.

7.1 Energy Balance

We begin this chapter with some good news and some bad news. The good news is that if you stay at a healthy body weight, you increase your chances of living a long and healthy life. The bad news is that currently 68% of all North American adults are overweight, significantly more than in the 1980s. Of those, about 50% (34% of the total population) are obese. There is a good chance that any of us could become part of those statistics if we do not pay attention to the prevention of significant weight gain in adulthood. Gaining more than 10 pounds or 2 inches in waist circumference are signals that a reevaluation of diet and lifestyle is in order.

There is no quick cure for overweight, despite what the advertisements claim. Successful weight loss comes from hard work and commitment. A combination of decreased calorie intake, increased physical activity, and behavior modification is considered to be the most reliable treatment for the overweight condition. And without a doubt, the prevention of the overweight condition in the first place is the most successful approach.

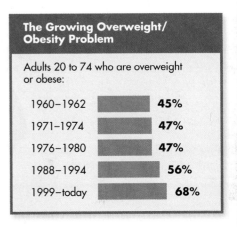

Positive and Negative Energy Balance

A healthy weight can result from paying more attention to the important concept of **energy balance.** Think of energy balance as an equation:

$$\underset{\text{(calories from food intake)}}{\text{Energy Input}} = \underset{\substack{\text{(metabolism; digestion, absorption, and transport} \\ \text{of nutrients; physical activity)}}}{\text{Energy Output}}$$

The balance of calories (measured in kcals) on the two sides of this equation can influence energy stores, especially the amount of triglyceride stored in adipose tissue (Fig. 7-2). Fat tissue contains about 3500 calories per pound. Therefore to lose 1 pound of fat per week, calorie intake must be decreased by about 500 calories per day. When energy input is greater than energy output, the result is **positive energy balance.** The excess calories consumed are stored, which results in weight gain. There are some situations in which positive energy balance is normal and healthy. During pregnancy, a surplus of calories supports the developing fetus. Infants and children require a positive energy balance for growth and development. In adults, however, even a small positive energy balance is usually in the form of fat storage rather than muscle and bone and, over time, can cause body weight to climb.

energy balance The state in which energy intake, in the form of food and beverages, matches the energy expended, primarily through basal metabolism and physical activity.

positive energy balance The state in which energy intake is greater than energy expended, generally resulting in weight gain.

FIGURE 7-2 ▶ A model for energy balance—input versus output. This figure depicts energy balance in practical terms.

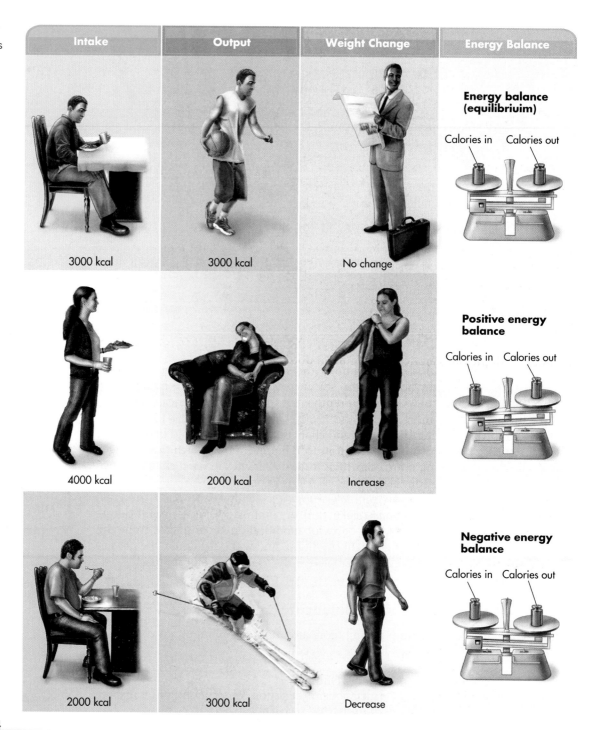

Intake	Output	Weight Change	Energy Balance
3000 kcal	3000 kcal	No change	**Energy balance (equilibriuim)** Calories in Calories out
4000 kcal	2000 kcal	Increase	**Positive energy balance** Calories in Calories out
2000 kcal	3000 kcal	Decrease	**Negative energy balance** Calories in Calories out

CRITICAL THINKING

As she gets closer to age 30, a 28-year-old classmate of yours has been thinking about the process of aging. One of the things she fears most as she gets older is gaining weight. How would you explain energy balance to her?

negative energy balance The state in which energy intake is less than energy expended, resulting in weight loss.

On the other hand, if energy input is less than energy output, there is a calorie deficit and **negative energy balance** results. A negative energy balance is necessary for successful weight loss. It is important to realize that during negative energy balance, weight loss involves a reduction in both lean and adipose tissue, not just "fat."

The maintenance of energy balance substantially contributes to health and well-being in adults by minimizing the risk of developing many common health problems. Adulthood is often a time of subtle increases in weight gain, which eventually turns into obesity if left unchecked. The process of aging does not cause weight gain; rather the problem stems from a pattern of excess food intake coupled with limited physical activity and slower metabolism. Let's look in detail at the factors that affect the energy balance equation.

Energy Intake

Energy needs are met by food intake, represented by the number of calories eaten each day. Determining the appropriate amount and type of food to match our energy needs is a challenge for many of us. Our desire to consume food and the ability of our bodies to use it efficiently are survival mechanisms that have evolved with humans. However, because of current North American food supplies and accessibility, many of us are now too successful in obtaining food energy. The abundant food supply has essentially replaced the need to store body fat. Given the wide availability of food in vending machines, drive-up windows, social gatherings, and fast-food restaurants—combined with *supersized* portions—it is no wonder that the average adult is 8 pounds heavier than just 10 years ago. In response to this cultural trend of food being widely available, "defensive eating" (i.e., making careful and conscious food choices, especially in regard to portion size) on a continual basis is important for many of us.

The number of calories in a food is determined with an instrument called a **bomb calorimeter.** This calorie determination is described in Figure 7-3. The bomb calorimeter measures the amount of calories coming from carbohydrate, fat, protein, and alcohol. Recall that carbohydrates yield about 4 kcal per gram, proteins yield about 4 kcal per gram, fats yield about 9 kcal per gram, and alcohol yields 7 kcal per gram. These energy figures have been adjusted for (1) our ability to digest the food and (2) substances in food, such as fibrous plant parts that burn in the bomb calorimeter but do not provide calories to the human body. The figures are then rounded to whole numbers. However, today it is also possible and more common to determine the calorie content of a food by quantifying its carbohydrate, protein, and fat (and possibly alcohol) content. Then the kcal per gram factors listed previously are used to calculate the total kcals. (Recall that Chapter 1 showed how to do this calculation.)

Energy Output

So far, some factors concerning energy intake have been discussed. Now let's look at the other side of the equation—energy output.

The body uses energy for three general purposes: basal metabolism; physical activity; and digestion, absorption, and processing of ingested nutrients. A fourth minor form of energy output, known as thermogenesis, refers to energy expended during fidgeting or shivering in response to cold (Fig. 7-4).

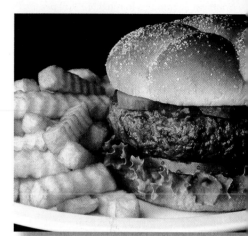

▲ The cultural trend of serving large quantities can easily lead to positive energy balance. Sharing your meal with another person is a good way to avoid overeating when served large portions.

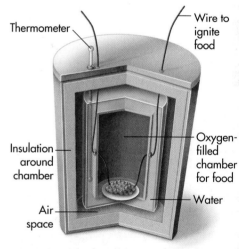

FIGURE 7-3 ▶ Bomb calorimeters measure calorie content by igniting and burning a dried portion of food. The burning food raises the temperature of the water surrounding the chamber holding the food. The increase in water temperature indicates the number of kilocalories in the food because 1 kilocalorie equals the amount of heat needed to raise the temperature of 1 kg of water by 1°C.

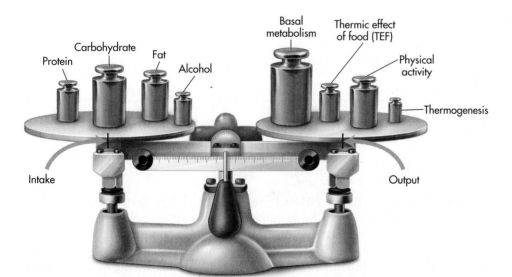

FIGURE 7-4 ▶ The components of energy intake and expenditure. This figure incorporates the major variables that influence energy balance. *Remember that alcohol is an additional source of energy for some of us.* The size of each component shows the relative contribution of that component to energy balance.

basal metabolism The minimal amount of calories the body uses to support itself in a fasting state when resting (e.g., 12 hours for both) and awake in a warm, quiet environment. It amounts to roughly 1 kcal per kilogram per hour for men and 0.9 kcal per kilogram per hour for women; these values are often referred to as *basal metabolic rate (BMR)*.

resting metabolism The amount of calories the body uses when the person has not eaten in 4 hours and is resting (e.g., 15 to 30 minutes) and awake in a warm, quiet environment. It is roughly 6% higher than basal metabolism due to the less strict criteria for the test; often referred to as *resting metabolic rate (RMR)*.

lean body mass Body weight minus fat storage weight equals lean body mass. This includes organs such as the brain, muscles, and liver, as well as bone and blood and other body fluids.

While a person is resting, the percentage of total energy use and corresponding energy use by various organs is approximately as follows:

Brain	19%	265 kcal/day
Skeletal muscle	18%	250 kcal/day
Liver	27%	380 kcal/day
Kidney	10%	140 kcal/day
Heart	7%	100 kcal/day
Other	19%	265 kcal/day

Basal Metabolism. **Basal metabolism** is expressed as basal metabolic rate (BMR) and represents the minimal amount of calories expended in a fasting state (for 12 hours or more) to keep a resting, awake body alive in a warm, quiet environment. For a sedentary person, basal metabolism accounts for about 60% to 70% of total energy use by the body. Some of the processes involved include the beating of the heart, respiration by the lungs, and the activity of other organs such as the liver, brain, and kidney. It does not include energy used for physical activity or digestion, absorption, and processing of recently consumed nutrients. If the person is not fasting or completely rested, the term **resting metabolism** is used and expressed as resting metabolic rate (RMR). An individual's RMR is typically 6% higher than his or her BMR.

To see how basal metabolism contributes to energy needs, consider a 130-pound woman. First, knowing that there are 2.2 pounds for every kilogram, convert her weight into metric units:

$$130 \text{ lbs} \div 2.2 \text{ lbs/kilograms} = 59 \text{ kilograms}$$

Then, using a rough estimate of basal metabolic rate of 0.9 kcal per kilogram per hour for an average female (1.0 kcal per kilogram per hour is used for an average male), calculate her basal metabolic rate:

$$59 \text{ kg} \times 0.9 \text{ kcal/kg} = 53 \text{ kcal per hour}$$

Finally, use this hourly basal metabolic rate to find her basal metabolic rate for an entire day:

$$53 \text{ kcal/hr} \times 24 \text{ hrs} = 1272 \text{ kcal}$$

These calculations give only an estimate of basal metabolism, as it can vary 25% to 30% among individuals. Factors that increase basal metabolism include:

- Greater **lean body mass**
- Larger body surface area per body volume
- Male gender (caused by greater lean body mass)
- Body temperature (fever or cold environmental conditions)
- Thyroid hormones
- Aspects of nervous system activity (release of norepinephrine)
- Pregnancy
- Caffeine and tobacco use (Using the practice of smoking to control body weight is not recommended as too many health risks are increased.)

Of those factors, the amount of lean body mass a person has is the most important one.

In contrast to factors that increase basal metabolism, a low calorie intake, such as that during an extreme diet regime, decreases basal metabolism by about 10% to 20% (about 150 to 300 kcal per day) as the body shifts into a conservation mode. This is a barrier to sustained weight loss during dieting that involves extremely low calorie diets. In addition, the effects of aging make weight maintenance a challenge. As lean body mass slowly and steadily decreases, basal metabolism declines 1% to 2% for each decade past the age of 30. However, because physical activity aids in maintenance of lean body mass, remaining active as one ages helps to preserve a high basal metabolism and, in turn, aids in weight control.

Energy for Physical Activity. Physical activity increases energy expenditure above and beyond basal energy needs by as much as 25% to 40%. In choosing to be active or inactive, we determine much of our total calorie expenditure for a day. Calorie expenditure from physical activity varies widely among people. For example, climbing stairs rather than riding the elevator, walking rather than driving to the store, and standing in a bus rather than sitting increase physical activity and, hence, energy use. The alarming incidence of and recent increase in obesity in North America are partially the result of our inactivity. Jobs demand less physical activity, and leisure time is often spent in front of a television or computer.

Thermic Effect of Food (TEF). In addition to basal metabolism and physical activity, the body uses energy to digest food, and absorb and further process the nutrients recently consumed. Energy used for these tasks is referred to as the **thermic effect of food (TEF).** TEF is similar to a sales tax—it is like being charged about 5% to 10% for the total amount of calories you eat to cover the cost of processing that food eaten. We may even recognize this increase in metabolism as a warming of the body during and right after a meal. Because of this "tax," you must eat between 105 and 110 kcal (5 to 10 kcal extra) for every 100 kcal needed for basal metabolism and physical activity. If your daily calorie intake was 3000 kcal, TEF would account for 150 to 300 kcal. As with other components of energy output, the total amount can vary somewhat among individuals.

Food composition influences TEF. For example, the TEF value for a protein-rich meal is 20% to 30% of the calories consumed and is higher than that of a carbohydrate-rich (5% to 10%) or fat-rich (0% to 3%) meal. This is because it takes more energy to metabolize amino acids into fat than to convert glucose into glycogen or transfer absorbed fat into adipose stores. In addition, large meals result in higher TEF values than the same amount of food eaten over many hours.

Thermogenesis. **Thermogenesis** represents the increase in nonvoluntary physical activity triggered by cold conditions or overeating. Some examples of nonvoluntary activities include shivering when cold, fidgeting, maintenance of muscle tone, and maintaining body posture when not lying down. Studies have shown that some people are able to resist weight gain from overfeeding by inducing thermogenesis, while others are not able to do so to a great extent.

The contribution of thermogenesis to overall calorie output is fairly small. The combination of basal metabolism and TEF accounts for 70% to 80% of energy used by a sedentary person. The remaining 20% to 30% is used mostly for physical activity, with a small amount used for thermogenesis.

Brown adipose tissue is a specialized form of adipose tissue that participates in thermogenesis. It is found in small amounts in infants. The brown appearance results from its rich blood flow. Brown adipose tissue contributes to thermogenesis by releasing some of the energy from energy-yielding nutrients into the environment as heat. In infants, brown adipose tissue contributes as much as 5% of body weight and is thought to be important for heat regulation. Hibernating animals also use brown adipose tissue to generate heat to withstand a long winter. Adults have very little brown adipose tissue, and its role in adulthood is unknown.

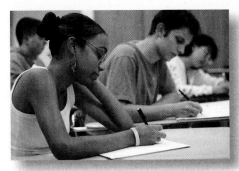
▲ Classwork leads to mental stress but puts little physical stress on the body. Hence, energy needs are only about 1.5 kcal per minute.

The TEF value for alcohol is 20%.

thermic effect of food (TEF) The increase in metabolism that occurs during the digestion, absorption, and metabolism of energy-yielding nutrients. This represents 5% to 10% of calories consumed.

thermogenesis This term encompasses the ability of humans to regulate body temperature within narrow limits (thermoregulation). Two visible examples of thermogenesis are fidgeting and shivering when cold.

brown adipose tissue A specialized form of adipose tissue that produces large amounts of heat by metabolizing energy-yielding nutrients without synthesizing much useful energy for the body. The unused energy is released as heat.

CONCEPT CHECK

Energy balance involves matching energy intake with energy output. Energy content of food is expressed in kcals and can be determined using a bomb calorimeter. This analysis yields the 4-9-4-7 estimates for the kcals in a gram of carbohydrate, fat, protein, and alcohol, respectively.

The body uses energy for four main purposes:

1. Basal metabolism (60% to 70% of total energy output) represents the minimal amount of calories needed to maintain the body at rest. Primary determinants of basal metabolic rate include quantity of lean body mass, amount of body surface, and thyroid hormone concentrations in the bloodstream.
2. Physical activity calorie expenditure (20% to 30% of total energy output) represents calorie use for total body cell metabolism above what is needed during rest.
3. Thermic effect of food (5% to 10% of total energy output) represents the calories needed to digest food and absorb and process nutrients recently consumed.
4. Thermogenesis (small, variable percentage of total energy output) includes nonvoluntary, heat-producing activities, such as fidgeting, as well as shivering when cold.

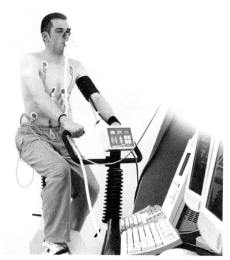

FIGURE 7-5 ▶ Indirect calorimetry measures oxygen intake and carbon dioxide output to determine energy expended during daily activities.

direct calorimetry A method of determining a body's energy use by measuring heat released from the body. An insulated chamber is usually used.

indirect calorimetry A method to measure energy use by the body by measuring oxygen uptake. Formulas are then used to convert this gas exchange value into energy use.

7.2 Determination of Energy Use by the Body

The amount of energy a body uses can be measured by both direct and indirect calorimetry or can be estimated based on height, weight, degree of physical activity, and age.

Direct and Indirect Calorimetry

Direct calorimetry measures the amount of body heat released by a person. The subject is put into an insulated chamber, often the size of a small bedroom, and body heat released raises the temperature of a layer of water surrounding the chamber. A kcal, as you recall, is related to the amount of heat required to raise the temperature of water. By measuring the water temperature in the direct calorimeter before and after the body releases heat, scientists can determine the energy expended.

Direct calorimetry works because almost all the energy used by the body eventually leaves as heat. However, few studies use direct calorimetry, mostly because of its expense and complexity.

The most commonly used method of **indirect calorimetry** measures the amount of oxygen a person consumes instead of measuring heat output (Fig. 7-5). A predictable relationship exists between the body's use of energy and oxygen. For example, when metabolizing a typical mixed diet of the energy-yielding nutrients, carbohydrate, fat, and protein, the human body uses 1 liter of oxygen to yield about 4.85 kcal of energy.

Instruments to measure oxygen consumption for indirect calorimetry are widely used. They can be mounted on carts and rolled up to a hospital bed or carried in backpacks while a person plays tennis or jogs. There are even newly developed handheld instruments (Body Gem). Tables showing energy costs of various forms of exercises rely on information gained from indirect calorimetry studies.

Estimates of Energy Needs

As covered in Chapter 2, the Food and Nutrition Board has published a number of formulas to estimate energy needs, called Estimated Energy Requirements (EERs). Those for adults are shown here (remember to do multiplication and division before addition and subtraction). (Formulas for pregnant women, lactating women, children, and teenagers, are listed in Chapters 14 and 15.) The calories used for basal metabolism are already factored into these formulas.

Estimated Energy Requirement Calculation for Men 19 Years and Older

$$\text{EER} = 662 - (9.53 \times \text{AGE}) + \text{PA} \times (15.91 \times \text{WT} + 539.6 \times \text{HT})$$

Estimated Energy Requirement Calculation for Women 19 Years and Older

$$\text{EER} = 354 - (6.91 \times \text{AGE}) + \text{PA} \times (9.36 \times \text{WT} + 726 \times \text{HT})$$

The variables in the formulas correspond to the following:

EER = Estimated Energy Requirement
AGE = age in years
PA = Physical Activity Estimate (see following table)
WT = weight in kilograms (pounds ÷ 2.2)
HT = height in meters (inches ÷ 39.4)

Physical Activity (PA) Estimates

Activity Level	PA (Men)	PA (Women)
Sedentary (e.g., no exercise)	1.00	1.00
Low activity (e.g., walks the equivalent of 2 miles per day at 3 to 4 mph)	1.11	1.12
Active (e.g., walks the equivalent of 7 miles per day at 3 to 4 mph)	1.25	1.27
Very active (e.g., walks the equivalent of 17 miles per day at 3 to 4 mph)	1.48	1.45

The following is a sample calculation for a man who is 25 years old, 5 feet, 9 inches (1.75 meters), 154 pounds (70 kilograms), and has an active lifestyle. His EER is:

$$EER = 662 - (9.53 \times 25) + 1.25 \times (15.91 \times 70 + 539.6 \times 1.75) = 2997 \text{ kcal}$$

The next equation is a sample calculation for a woman who is 25 years old, 5 feet, 4 inches (1.62 meters), 120 pounds (54.5 kilograms), and has an active lifestyle. Her EER is:

$$EER = 354 - (6.91 \times 25) + 1.27 \times (9.36 \times 54.5 + 726 \times 1.62) = 2323 \text{ kcal}$$

You have determined the man's EER to be about 3000 kcal and the woman's EER to be about 2300 kcal per day. Remember that this is only an estimate; many other factors, such as genetics and hormones, can affect actual energy needs.

A simple method of tracking your energy expenditure, and thus your energy needs, is to use the forms in Appendix E. Begin by taking an entire 24-hour period and listing all activities performed, including sleep. Record the number of minutes spent in each activity; the total should equal 1440 minutes (24 hours). Next record the energy cost for each activity in kcal per minute following the directions in Appendix E. Multiply the energy cost by the minutes. This gives the energy expended for each activity. Total all the kcal values. This gives your estimated energy expenditure for the day.

The www.ChooseMyPlate.gov website provides an interactive tool to estimate your calorie needs called Daily Food Plan. Figure 7-6 shows the range of activity levels and calorie recommendations for age and gender groups.

MyPlate Calorie Guidelines		
Children	**Sedentary** ⟶	**Active**
2–3 years	1000 ⟶	1400
Females	**Sedentary** ⟶	**Active**
4–8 years	1200 ⟶	1800
9–13	1400 ⟶	2200
14–18	1800 ⟶	2400
19–30	1800 ⟶	2400
31–50	1800 ⟶	2200
51+	1600 ⟶	2200
Males	**Sedentary** ⟶	**Active**
4–8 years	1200 ⟶	2000
9–13	1600 ⟶	2600
14–18	2000 ⟶	3200
19–30	2400 ⟶	3000
31–50	2200 ⟶	3000
51+	2000 ⟶	2800

FIGURE 7-6 ▶ MyPlate Calorie Guidelines for age and gender groups.

CONCEPT CHECK

Energy use by the body can be measured as heat given off by direct calorimetry or as oxygen used by indirect calorimetry. A person's Estimated Energy Requirement can be calculated based on the following factors: gender, height, weight, age, and amount of physical activity.

7.3 Estimation of a Healthy Weight

Numerous methods are used to establish what body weight should be, typically called *healthy weight*. Healthy weight is currently the preferred term to use for weight recommendations. Older terms, such as *ideal weight* and *desirable weight*, are subjective and are no longer used in medical literature. Several tables exist, generally based on weight for height. These tables arise from studies of large population groups. When applied to a population, they provide good estimates of weight associated with health and longevity. However, they do not necessarily indicate the healthiest body weight

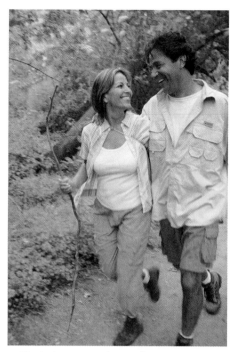

▲ Physical activity, such as walking, is an important component of our energy expenditure.

One BMI unit = 6 to 7 pounds

body mass index (BMI) Weight (in kilograms) divided by height (in meters) squared; a value of 25 and above indicates overweight and a value of 30 and above indicates obesity.

for each individual. For example, *athletes with large, lean body mass but low-fat content will have greater healthy weights than sedentary individuals.*

Overall, the individual, under a physician's guidance, should establish a "personal" healthy weight (or need for weight reduction) based on weight history, fat distribution patterns, family history of weight-related disease, and current health status. Indications that your weight is not healthy would include the following weight-related conditions:

- Hypertension
- Elevated LDL-cholesterol
- Family history of obesity, cardiovascular disease, or certain forms of cancer (e.g., uterus, colon)
- Pattern of fat distribution in the body
- Elevated blood glucose

This assessment points out how well the person is tolerating any existing excess weight. Thus, current height/weight standards are only a rough guide. On a more practical note, other questions can be pertinent: What is the least one has weighed as an adult for at least a year? What is the largest size clothing one would be happy with? What weight has one been able to maintain during previous diets without feeling constantly hungry? Furthermore, a healthy lifestyle may make a more important contribution to a person's health status than the number on the scale. Fit and overweight are not necessarily mutually exclusive (although not often seen together), and neither is thin synonymous with healthy if the person is not also physically active.

Body Mass Index (BMI)

For the past 50 years, weight-for-height tables issued by the Metropolitan Life Insurance Company have been the typical way healthy weight was established. These tables are organized by gender and frame size, predicting the weight range at a specific height that was associated with the greatest longevity. The latest table (issued in 1983) and methods for determining frame size can be found in Appendix G.

Currently, **body mass index (BMI)** is the preferred weight-for-height standard because it is the clinical measurement most closely related to body fat content (Fig. 7-7).

Body mass index is calculated as

$$\frac{\text{body weight (in kilograms)}}{\text{height}^2 \text{ (in meters)}}$$

An alternate method for calculating BMI is

$$\frac{\text{weight (pounds)} \times 703}{\text{height}^2 \text{ (inches)}}$$

Figure 7-8 lists the BMI for various heights and weights. A healthy weight for height is a BMI between 18.5 to 24.9. Health risks from excess weight may begin when the body mass index is 25 or more. What is your BMI? How much would your weight need to change to yield a BMI of 25? 30? These are general cutoff values for the presence of overweight and obesity, respectively. BMI offers another way to define obesity (Fig. 7-8).

| 30 to 39.9 | Obese | Increased health risk |
| 40 or greater | Severely obese | Major health risk (The number of North Americans falling into this category is increasing rapidly.) |

The concept of body mass index is convenient to use because the values apply to both men and women (i.e., gender neutral). However, any weight-for-height standard is a crude measure. Keep in mind, also, that a BMI of 25 to 29.9 is a marker of *overweight* (compared to a standard population) and not necessarily a marker of *overfat*. Many men (especially athletes) have a BMI greater than 25 because of extra muscle tissue. Also, very short adults (under 5 feet tall) may have high BMIs that may not reflect overweight or fatness. For this reason, BMI should be used only as a screening test for overweight or obesity. Even agreed upon weight standards for BMI are not for everyone. Adult BMIs should not be applied to children, still growing adolescents, frail older people, pregnant and lactating women, and highly muscular individuals. Pregnant women and children have unique BMI standards (see Chapters 14 and 15).

Still, overfat and overweight conditions generally appear together. The focus is on BMI in clinical settings mainly because this is easier to measure than total body fat.

Putting Healthy Weight into Perspective

Listening to the body for hunger cues, regularly eating a healthy diet, and remaining physically active (not to be overlooked) eventually helps one maintain an appropriate height/weight value. This concept will be further addressed in the upcoming discussion on treatment for obesity. Another school of thought is to let nature take its course with regard to body weight. Support for this proposal is that after weight is lost during dieting, people often regain their original weight plus more. The clearest idea regarding a healthy weight is that it is personal. Weight has to be considered in terms of health, not a mathematical calculation.

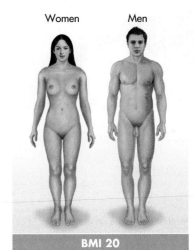

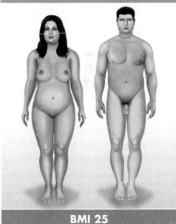

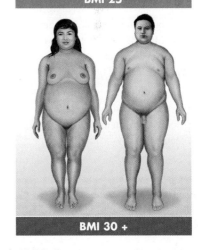

FIGURE 7-7 ▶ Estimates of body shapes at different BMI values.

Weight in pounds

Height	120	130	140	150	160	170	180	190	200	210	220	230	240	250
4'6"	29	31	34	36	39	41	43	46	48	51	53	56	58	60
4'8"	27	29	31	34	36	38	40	43	45	47	49	52	51	56
4'10"	25	27	29	31	34	36	38	40	42	44	46	48	50	52
5'0"	23	25	27	29	31	33	35	37	39	41	43	45	47	49
5'2"	22	24	26	29	29	31	33	35	37	38	40	42	44	46
5'4"	21	22	24	26	28	29	31	33	34	36	38	40	41	43
5'6"	19	21	23	24	26	27	29	31	32	34	36	37	39	40
5'8"	18	20	21	23	24	26	27	29	30	32	34	35	37	38
5'10"	17	19	20	22	23	24	26	27	29	30	32	33	35	36
6'0"	16	18	19	20	22	23	24	26	27	28	30	31	33	34
6'2"	15	17	18	19	21	22	23	24	26	27	28	30	31	32
6'4"	15	16	17	18	20	21	22	23	24	26	27	28	29	30
6'6"	14	15	16	17	19	20	21	22	23	24	25	27	28	29
6'8"	13	14	15	17	18	19	20	21	22	23	24	26	26	28

Height in feet and inches

☐ Healthy weight ☐ Overweight ☐ Obese

Developed by the National Center for Health Statistics in collaboration with the National Center for Chronic Disease Prevention and Health Promotion

FIGURE 7-8 ▶ Convenient height/weight table based on BMI. A healthy weight for height generally falls within a BMI range of 18.5 to 24.9 kilograms/meters^2.

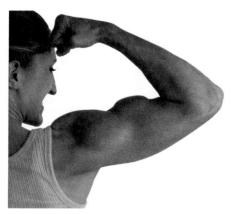

▲ A high BMI may not reflect overweight or fatness. Extra muscle tissue can result in a BMI greater than 25.

The total cost attributable to weight-related disease is about $147 billion annually in the United States. This is double what it was nearly a decade ago. Half of this cost is borne by the taxpayers through Medicare and Medicaid.

underwater weighing A method of estimating total body fat by weighing the individual on a standard scale and then weighing him or her again submerged in water. The difference between the two weights is used to estimate total body volume.

air displacement A method for estimating body composition that makes use of the volume of space taken up by a body inside a small chamber.

bioelectrical impedance The method to estimate total body fat that uses a low-energy electrical current. The more fat storage a person has, the more impedance (resistance) to electrical flow will be exhibited.

CONCEPT CHECK

Healthy body weight is generally determined in a clinical setting using a body mass index or another weight-for-height standard. The presence of existing weight-related diseases should be factored into the determination of healthy body weight. Total health history and lifestyle should be the major considerations when determining healthy weight.

7.4 Energy Imbalance

If calorie intake exceeds output over time, overweight (and often obesity) is a likely result. Often, health problems eventually follow (Table 7-1) (see Further Readings 1 and 12). As just discussed, BMI values can be used as a convenient clinical tool to estimate overweight (BMI ≥ 25), obesity (BMI ≥ 30), and severe obesity (BMI ≥ 40) in individuals greater than 20 years of age. Medical experts, however, recommend that an individual's diagnosis of obesity should not be based primarily on body weight but, rather, on the total amount of fat in the body, the location of body fat, and the presence or absence of weight-related medical problems.

Estimating Body Fat Content and Diagnosing Obesity

Body fat varies widely among individuals and can range from 2% to 70% of body weight. Desirable amounts of body fat are about 8% to 24% for men and 21% to 35% for women. Men with over 24% body fat and women with over about 35% body fat are considered obese. The higher range of body fat percentage for women is needed physiologically to maintain reproductive functions, including estrogen production.

To measure body fat content accurately using typical methods, both body weight and body volume of the person must be known. Body weight is easy to measure on a conventional scale. Of the typical methods used to estimate body volume, **underwater weighing** is the most accurate. This technique determines body volume using the difference between conventional body weight and body weight under water, along with the relative densities of fat tissue and lean tissue, and a specific mathematical formula. This procedure requires that an individual be totally submerged in a tank of water, with a trained technician directing the procedure (Fig. 7-9). **Air displacement** is another method of determining body volume. Body volume is quantified by measuring the space a person takes up inside a measurement chamber, such as the BodPod (Fig. 7-10). A less accurate method to measure body volume is to submerge a person in a tank and observe the level of the water before and after submersion. The volume of the displaced water is then calculated.

Once body volume is known, it can be used along with body weight in the following equation to calculate body density. Then using body density, body fat content finally can be determined.

$$\text{Body density} = \frac{\text{body weight}}{\text{body volume}}$$
$$\%\text{ body fat} = (495 \div \text{body density}) - 450$$

For example, assume that the individual in the underwater weighing tank in Figure 7-9 has a body density of 1.06 grams per centimeter[3]. We can use the second formula to calculate that he has 17% body fat ([495 ÷ 1.06] − 450 = 17).

Skinfold thickness is also a common anthropometric method to estimate total body fat content, although there are some limits to its accuracy. Clinicians use calipers to measure the fat layer directly under the skin at multiple sites and then plug these values into a mathematical formula (Fig. 7-11).

The technique of **bioelectrical impedance** is also used to estimate body fat content. The instrument sends a painless, low-energy electrical current to and from the

TABLE 7-1 Health Problems Associated with Excess Body Fat

Health Problem	Partially Attributable To
Surgical risk	Increased anesthesia needs, as well as greater risk of wound infections (the latter is linked to a decrease in immune function)
Pulmonary disease and sleep disorders	Excess weight over lungs and pharynx
Type 2 diabetes	Enlarged adipose cells, which poorly bind insulin and poorly respond to the message insulin sends to the cell; less synthesis of factors that aid insulin action, and greater synthesis of factors by adipose cells that lessen insulin action
Hypertension	Increased miles of blood vessels found in the adipose tissue, increased blood volume, and increased resistance to blood flow related to hormones made by adipose cells
Cardiovascular disease (e.g., coronary heart disease and stroke)	Increases in LDL-cholesterol and triglyceride values, low HDL-cholesterol, decreased physical activity, and increased synthesis of blood clotting and inflamatory factors by enlarged adipose cells. A greater risk for heart failure is also seen, due in part to altered heart rhythm.
Bone and joint disorders (including gout)	Excess pressure put on knee, ankle, and hip joints
Gallstones	Increased cholesterol content of bile
Skin disorders	Trapping of moisture and microorganisms in tissue folds
Various cancers, such as in the kidney, gall-bladder, colon and rectum, uterus (women), and prostate gland (men)	Estrogen production by adipose cells; animal studies suggest excess calorie intake encourages tumor development
Shorter stature (in some forms of obesity)	Earlier onset of puberty
Pregnancy risks	More difficult delivery, increased number of birth defects, and increased needs for anesthesia
Reduced physical agility and increased risk of accidents and falls	Excess weight that impairs movement
Menstrual irregularities and infertility	Hormones produced by adipose cells, such as estrogen
Vision problems	Cataracts and other eye disorders are more often present
Premature death	A variety of risk factors for disease listed in this table
Infections	Reduced immune system activity
Liver damage and eventual failure	Excess fat accumulation in the liver
Erectile dysfunction in men	Low-grade inflammation caused by excess fat mass and reduced function of the cells lining the blood vessels associated with being overweight

The greater the degree of obesity, the more likely and the more serious these health problems generally become. They are much more likely to appear in people who show an upper-body fat distribution pattern and/or are greater than twice healthy body weight.

body via wires and electrode patches to estimate body fat. This estimation is based on the assumption that adipose tissue resists electrical flow more than lean tissue because it has a lower electrolyte and water content than lean tissue. More adipose tissue therefore means proportionately greater electrical resistance. Within a few seconds, bioelectrical impedance analyzers convert body electrical resistance into an approximate estimate of total body fat, as long as body hydration status is normal (Fig. 7-12). Body composition monitors, better known as body fat calculators, that use bioelectric impedence are now available for home use. These machines are similar in shape and use to bathroom scales but their main purpose is to measure body fat. A current passes easily through conductive foot pads and/or handheld electrodes. These in-home devices will hopefully encourage people to be less concerned with what they weigh than whether their weight comes from fat or muscle.

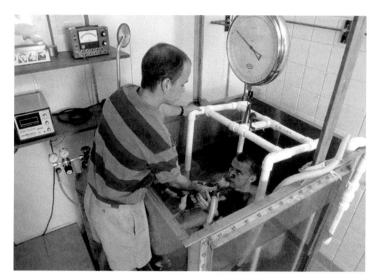

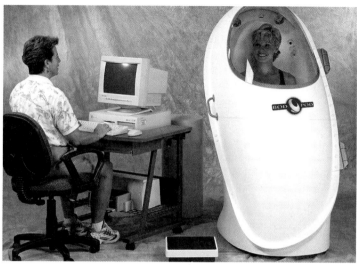

FIGURE 7-9 ▶ Underwater weighing. In this technique, the subject exhales as much air as possible and then holds his or her breath and bends over at the waist. Once the subject is totally submerged, the underwater weight is recorded. Using this value, body volume can be calculated.

FIGURE 7-10 ▶ BodPod. This device determines body volume based on the volume of displaced air, measured as a person sits in a sealed chamber for a few minutes.

FIGURE 7-11 ▶ Skinfold measurements. Using proper technique and calibrated equipment, skinfold measurements around the body can be used to predict body fat content in about 10 minutes. Measurements are made at several locations including the triceps (photo and drawing) skinfolds.

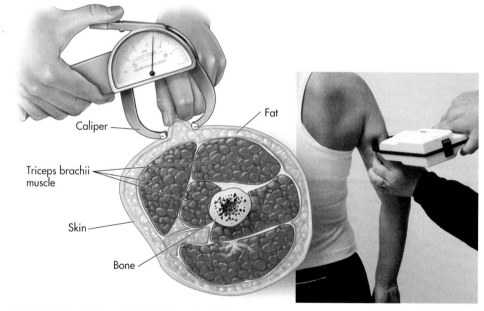

FIGURE 7-12 ▶ Bioelectrical impedance estimates total body fat in less than 5 minutes and is based on the principle that body fat resists the flow of electricity, since it is low in water and electrolytes. The degree of resistance to electrical flow is used to estimate body fatness.

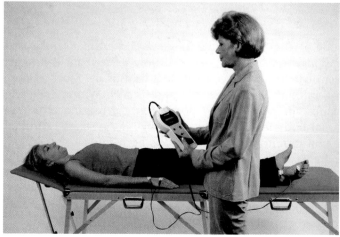

A more advanced determination of body fat content can be made using **dual energy X-ray absorptiometry (DEXA)**. DEXA is considered the most accurate way to determine body fat, but the equipment is expensive and not widely available for this use. This X-ray system allows the clinician to separate body weight into three separate components—fat, fat-free soft tissue, and bone mineral. The usual whole-body scan requires about 5 to 20 minutes and the dose of radiation is less than a chest X ray. An assessment of bone mineral density and the risk of osteoporosis also can be made using this method (Fig. 7-13).

Another method to assess body fat is to measure total-body electrical conductance (TOBEC) when placed in an electromagnetic field. Still another method, convenient and inexpensive, but not very accurate is **near-infrared reactance.** This method exposes the bicep muscle to a beam of near-infrared light and assesses the interactions of the light beam with fat and lean tissues in the upper arm after only 2 seconds.

In summary, although the DEXA is considered most accurate, the underwater weighing and air displacement methods of body fat estimation are also accurate because both body weight and body volume are measured. The adaptation of the bioelectrical impedence technology for in-home use is also a useful tool, providing valuable information about whether weight gain is coming from fat or muscle.

Using Body Fat Distribution to Further Evaluate Obesity

In addition to the amount of fat we store, the location of that body fat is an important predictor of health risks. Some people store fat in upper-body areas, whereas others store fat lower on the body. Excess fat in either location generally spells trouble, but each storage space also has its unique risks. **Upper-body obesity,** characterized by a large abdomen, is more often related to cardiovascular disease, hypertension, and type 2 diabetes. Whereas other adipose cells empty fat into general blood circulation, the fat released from abdominal adipose cells goes directly to the liver, by way of the portal vein. This process likely interferes with the liver's ability to use insulin and negatively affects lipoprotein metabolism by the liver. These abdominal adipose cells also make substances that increase insulin resistance, blood clotting, blood vessel constriction, and inflammation in the body. These changes can lead to long-term health problems.

High blood testosterone (primarily a male hormone) levels apparently encourage upper-body obesity, as does a diet with a high glycemic load, alcohol intake, and smoking. This characteristic male pattern of fat storage is also called android obesity and is commonly known as the apple shape (large abdomen [pot belly] and small buttocks and thighs). Upper-body obesity is assessed by measuring the waist at the widest point just above the hips when relaxed. A waist circumference more than 40 inches (102 centimeters) in men and more than 35 inches (88 centimeters) in women indicates upper-body obesity (Fig. 7-14). If BMI is also 25 or more, health risks are significantly increased.

Estrogen and progesterone (primarily female hormones) encourage lower-body fat storage and **lower-body (gynecoid or gynoid) obesity**—the typical female pattern. The small abdomen and much larger buttocks and thighs give a pearlike appearance. Fat deposited in the lower body is not mobilized as easily as the other type and often resists being shed. After menopause, blood estrogen falls, encouraging upper-body fat distribution.

dual energy X-ray absorptiometry (DEXA) A highly accurate method of measuring body composition and bone mass and density using multiple low-energy X rays.

upper-body obesity The type of obesity in which fat is stored primarily in the abdominal area; defined as a waist circumference more than 40 inches (102 centimeters) in men and more than 35 inches (89 centimeters) in women; closely associated with a high risk for cardiovascular disease, hypertension, and type 2 diabetes. Also known as android obesity.

lower-body obesity The type of obesity in which fat storage is primarily located in the buttocks and thigh area. Also known as gynoid or gynecoid obesity.

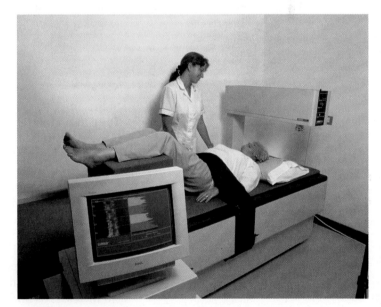

FIGURE 7-13 ▶ Dual energy X-ray absorptiometry (DEXA). This method measures body fat by passing small doses of radiation through the body. The radiation reacts differently with fat, lean tissue, or bone allowing these components to be quantified. The scanner arm moves from head to toe and in doing so can determine body fat as well as bone density. DEXA is currently considered the most accurate method for determining body fat (as long as the person can fit under the arm of the instrument). The radiation dose is minimal.

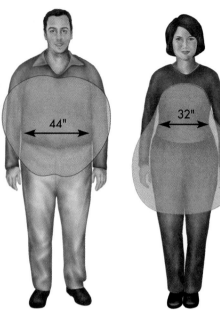

Upper-body fat distribution (android: apple shape)

Lower-body fat distribution (gynoid: pear shape)

FIGURE 7-14 ▶ Body fat stored primarily in the upper-body (android) form brings higher risks of ill health associated with obesity than does lower-body (gynoid) fat. The woman's waist circumference of 32 inches and the man's waist circumference of 44 inches indicate that the man has upper-body fat distribution but the woman does not, based on a cutoff of 35 inches for women and 40 inches for men.

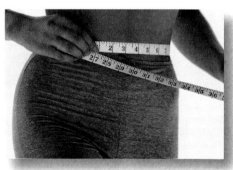

▲ Waist circumference is an important measure of weight-related health risk.

identical twins Two offspring that develop from a single ovum and sperm and, consequently, have the same genetic makeup.

CONCEPT CHECK

Overweight and obesity typically are associated with excessive body fat storage. The risk of health problems related to being overweight especially increases under the following conditions:

- A man's percentage of body fat exceeds 25%; a woman's exceeds about 35%.
- Excess fat is primarily stored in the upper-body region.
- Body mass index (BMI) is 30 or more (calculated as weight in kilograms divided by height squared in meters).

However, these are merely guidelines. A more individualized approach to assessment is warranted as long as a person is following a healthy lifestyle and has no existing health problems.

Body fat content can be estimated using a variety of methods such as underwater weighing, air displacement, skinfold thickness, bioelectrical impedance, and DEXA. Fat storage distribution further specifies an obese state as either upper-body or lower-body. Obesity leads to an increased risk for cardiovascular disease, some types of cancer, hypertension, type 2 diabetes, certain bone and joint disorders, and some digestive disorders. The risks for some of these diseases are greater with upper-body fat storage.

7.5 Why Some People Are Obese—Nature Versus Nurture

Both genetic (nature) and environmental (nurture) factors can increase the risk for obesity (Table 7-2). The eventual location of fat storage is strongly influenced by genetics. Consider the possibility that obesity is nurture allowing nature to express itself. Some obese people begin life with a slower basal metabolism; maintain an inactive lifestyle; and consume highly-refined, calorie-dense diets. These people in turn are nurtured into gaining weight, promoting their natural tendency toward obesity.

Still, genes do not fully control destiny. With increased physical activity and decreased food consumption, even those with a genetic tendency toward obesity can attain a healthier body weight.

How Does Nature Contribute to Obesity?

Studies in pairs of **identical twins** give us some insight into the contribution of nature to obesity. Even when identical twins are raised apart, they tend to show similar weight gain patterns, both in overall weight and body fat distribution. It appears that nurture—eating habits and nutrition, which varies between twins raised apart—has less to do with obesity than nature does. In fact, research suggests that genes account for up to 70% of weight differences between people. A child with no obese parent has only a 10% chance of becoming obese. When a child has one obese parent (common in our society), that risk advances up to 40%, and with two obese parents, it soars to 80%. Our genes help determine metabolic rate, fuel use, and differences in brain chemistry—all of which affect body weight.

We also inherit specific body types. Tall, thin people appear to have an inherently easier time maintaining healthy body weight. This is probably because basal metabolism increases as body surface increases, and therefore taller people use more calories than shorter people, even at rest.

Many of us probably have inherited a thrifty metabolism that enables us to store fat more readily than the typical human, so that we require fewer calories to get through the day. In earlier times, when food supplies were scarce, a thrifty metabolism would have been a built-in safeguard against starvation. Now, with a general abundance of food, people operating in this low gear require much physical activity and wise food choices to prevent obesity. If you think you are prone to weight gain, you likely have inherited a thrifty metabolism.

TABLE 7-2 What Encourages Excess Body Fat Stores and Obesity?

Factor	How Fat Storage is Affected
Age	Excess body fat is more common in adults and middle-age individuals.
Menopause	Increase in abdominal fat deposition is typical.
Gender	Females have more fat.
Positive energy balance	Over a long period promotes storage of fat.
Composition of diet	Excess calorie intake from fat, alcohol, and calorie dense (sugary, fat-rich) foods contributes to obesity.
Physical activity	Low physical activity ("couch potato") leads to positive energy balance and body fat storage.
Basal metabolism	A low BMR is linked to weight gain.
Thermic effect of food	Low for some obesity cases.
Increased hunger sensations	Some people have trouble resisting the abundant availability of food, which is likely linked to the activity of various brain chemicals.
Ratio of fat to lean tissue	A high ratio of fat mass to lean body mass is correlated with weight gain.
Fat uptake by adipose tissue	This is high in some obese individuals and remains high (perhaps even increases) with weight loss.
Variety of social and behavioral factors	Obesity is associated with socioeconomic status; familial conditions; network of friends; busy lifestyles that discourage balanced meals; binge eating; easy availability of inexpensive, "supersized" high-fat food; pattern of leisure activities; television time; smoking cessation; excessive alcohol intake; and number of meals eaten away from home.
Undetermined genetic characteristics	These affect components of energy balance, particularly energy expenditure, the deposition of the energy surplus as adipose tissue or as lean tissue, and the relative proportion of fat and carbohydrate used by the body.
Race	In some ethnic groups, higher body weight may be more socially acceptable.
Certain medications	Food intake increases.
Childbearing	Women may not lose all weight gained in pregnancy.
National region	Regional differences, such as high-fat diets and sedentary lifestyles in the Midwest and areas of the South, lead to geographically different rates of obesity.

Does the Body Have a Set Point for Weight?

The **set-point** theory of weight maintenance proposes that humans have a genetically predetermined body weight or body fat content, which the body closely regulates. Some research suggests that the **hypothalamus** region of the brain monitors the amount of body fat in humans and tries to keep that amount constant over time. The hypothalamus has two sites—the feeding center and the satiety center—that play a role in regulating hunger. The hormone **leptin** forms a communication link between adipose cells and the brain, which allows for some weight regulation.

Several physiological changes that occur during calorie reduction and weight loss also endorse the set-point theory (see Further Reading 2). For example, when calorie intake is reduced, the blood concentration of thyroid hormones falls, which slows basal metabolism. In addition, as weight is lost, the calorie cost of weight-bearing activity decreases, so that an activity that burned 100 kcal before weight loss may only burn 80 kcal after weight loss. Furthermore, with weight loss, the body becomes more efficient at storing fat by increasing the activity of the enzyme *lipoprotein lipase*, which takes fat into cells. All of these changes protect the body from losing weight.

If a person overeats, in the short run, basal metabolism tends to increase. This causes some resistance to weight gain. However, in the long run, resistance to weight

set point Often refers to the close regulation of body weight. It is not known what cells control this set point or how it functions in weight regulation. There is evidence, however, that mechanisms exist that help regulate weight.

hypothalamus A region at the base of the brain that contains cells that play a role in the regulation of hunger, respiration, body temperature, and other body functions.

leptin A harmone made by adipose tissue in proportion to total fat stores in the body that influences long-term regulation of fat mass. Leptin also influences reproductive functions, as well as other body processes, such as release of the hormone insulin.

▶ Studies in identical twins give us insight into the genetic contribution to obesity.

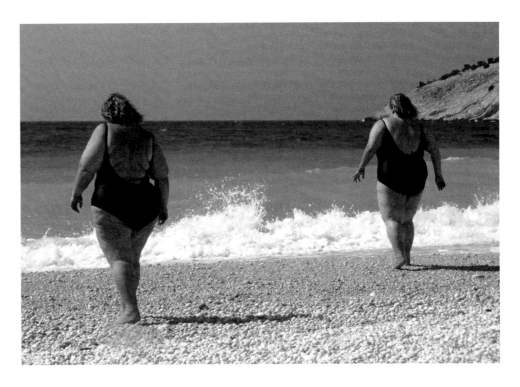

gain is much less than resistance to weight loss. When a person gains weight and stays at that weight for a while, the body tends to establish a new set point.

Opponents of the set-point theory argue that weight does not remain constant throughout adulthood—the average person gains weight slowly, at least until old age. Also, if an individual is placed in a different social, emotional, or physical environment, weight can be altered and maintained markedly higher or lower. These arguments suggest that humans, rather than having a set point determined by genetics or the number of adipose cells, settle into a particular stable weight based on their circumstances, often regarded as a "settling point."

The size-acceptance nondiet movement, "Health at Every Size," indirectly refers to a set point for weight by defining healthy weight as the natural weight the body adopts, given a healthy diet and meaningful levels of physical activity. Overall, the set point is weaker in preventing weight gain than in preventing weight loss. Even with a set point helping us, the odds are in favor of eventual weight gain unless we devote effort to a healthy lifestyle.

▼ Body weight is influenced by many factors related to both nature and nurture. We resemble our parents because of the genes we have inherited, as well as the lifestyle habits, including diet, that we have learned from them.

Does Nurture Have a Role?

Some would argue that body weight similarities between family members stem more from learned behaviors rather than genetic similarities. Even couples, who have no genetic link, may behave similarly toward food and eventually assume similar degrees of leanness or fatness. Proponents of nurture pose that environmental factors, such as high-fat diets and inactivity, literally shape us. This seems likely when we consider that our gene pool has not changed much in the past 50 years, whereas according to the U.S. Centers for Disease Control and Prevention the ranks of obese people have grown in epidemic proportions over the last 25 years.

Adult obesity in women is often rooted in childhood obesity. In addition, relative inactivity and periods of stress or boredom, as well as excess weight gain during pregnancy, contribute to female obesity. (Chapter 14 notes that breastfeeding one's infant contributes to loss of some of the excess fat associated with pregnancy.) These patterns

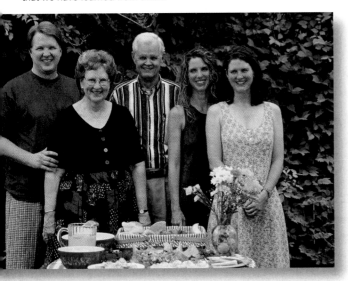

suggest both social and genetic links. Male obesity, however, is not strongly linked to childhood obesity and, instead, tends to appear after age 30. This powerful and prevalent pattern suggests a primary role of nurture in obesity, with less genetic influence.

Is poverty associated with obesity? Ironically, the answer is often yes. North Americans of lower socioeconomic status, especially females, are more likely to be obese than those in upper socioeconomic groups. Several social and behavioral factors promote fat storage. These factors include lower socioeconomic status, overweight friends and family, a cultural/ethnic group that prefers higher body weight, a lifestyle that discourages healthy meals and adequate exercise, easy availability of inexpensive high-calorie food, limited access to fresh fruits and vegetables, excessive television viewing, smoking cessation, lack of adequate sleep, emotional stress, and meals frequently eaten away from home.

7.6 Treatment of Overweight and Obesity

Treatment of overweight and obesity should be long-term, similar to that for any chronic disease. Treatments require long-term lifestyle changes, rather than a quick fix promoted by many popular (also called fad) diet books. We often view a "diet" as something one goes on temporarily, only to resume prior (typically poor) habits once satisfactory results have been achieved. This is a big reason that so many people regain lost weight. Instead, an emphasis on healthy, active living with acceptable dietary modifications will promote weight loss and later weight maintenance.

What to Look for in a Sound Weight-Loss Plan

A dieter can develop a plan of action by seeking advice from a health professional, such as a registered dietitian, or by using the interactive tools at www.ChooseMyPlate.gov. Either way, a sound weight-loss program (Fig. 7-15) should especially include these components:

1. Control of calorie intake. One recommendation is to decrease calorie intake by 100 kcal per day (and increase physical activity by 100 kcal per day). This should allow for slow and steady weight loss.
2. Increased physical activity.
3. Acknowledgment that maintenance of a healthy weight requires lifelong changes in habits, not a short-term weight-loss period.

A one-sided approach that focuses only on restricting calories is a difficult plan of action. Instead, adding physical activity and an appropriate psychological component

MAKING DECISIONS

Losing Body Fat

Rapid weight loss cannot consist primarily of fat loss because a high calorie deficit is needed to lose a large amount of adipose tissue. Adipose tissue, mostly fat, contains about 3500 kcal per pound. Weight loss, however, includes adipose tissue plus lean tissues that support it and represents approximately 3300 kcal per pound (about 7.2 kcal per gram). Therefore, to lose 1 pound of adipose tissue per week, calorie intake must be decreased by approximately 500 kcal per day, or physical activity must be increased by 500 kcal per day. Alternately, a combination of both strategies can be used. Diets that promise 10 to 15 pounds of weight loss per week cannot ensure that the weight loss is from adipose tissue stores alone. How many calories would need to be eliminated from the diet per day to lose 10 pounds per week? Is it possible to subtract enough calories from one's daily intake to lose that amount of adipose tissue? Lean tissue and water, rather than adipose tissue, account for the major part of the weight lost during these dramatic weight-loss programs.

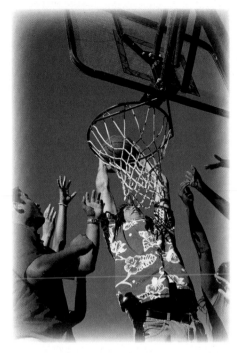

▲ Student life is often full of physical activity. This is not necessarily true for a person's later working life; hence, weight gain is a strong possibility.

▶ **Weight Status objectives from** *Healthy People 2020*

- Increase by 10% the proportion of adults who are at a healthy weight.
  - Target for 2020: 33.9%
  - Baseline in 2005–08: 30.8%
- Reduce by 10% the proportion of adults who are obese.
  - Target for 2020: 30.6%
  - Baseline in 2005–08: 34.0%
- Reduce by 10% the proportion of children and adolescents, 2 to 19 years, who are considered obese.
  - Target for 2020: 14.6%
  - Baseline in 2005–08: 16.2%
- Prevent inappropriate weight gain in youth and adults.

As you read brochures, articles, or research reports about specific diet plans, look beyond the weight loss promoted by the diet's advocate to see if the reported weight loss was maintained. If the weight-maintenance aspect was missing, then the program was not successful.

FIGURE 7-15 ▶ Characteristics of a sound weight-loss diet. Use this checklist to evaluate any new diet plan before putting it into practice.

The 2010 Dietary Guidelines for Americans provide the following recommendations regarding "Balancing Calories to Manage Weight" as part of healthy eating pattern and while staying within their calories need:

- Prevent and/or reduce overweight and obesity through improved eating and physical activity behaviors.

- Control total calorie intake to manage body weight. For people who are overweight or obese, this will mean consuming fewer calories from foods and beverages.

- Increase physical activity and reduce time spent in sedentary behaviors.

- Maintain appropriate calorie balance during each stage of life—childhood, adolescence, adulthood, pregnancy and breastfeeding, and older age.

RATE OF LOSS

☐ Encourages slow and steady weight loss, rather than rapid weight loss, to promote lasting weight
☐ Sets goal of 1 pound of fat loss per week
☐ Includes a period of weight maintenance for a few months after 10% of body weight is lost
☐ Evaluates need for further dieting before more weight loss begins

FLEXIBILITY

☐ Supports participation in normal activities (e.g., parties, restaurants)
☐ Adapts to individual habits and tastes

INTAKE

☐ Meets nutrient needs (except for energy needs)
☐ Includes common foods, with no foods being promoted as magical or special
☐ Recommends a fortified ready-to-eat breakfast cereal or balanced multivitamin/mineral supplement, especially when intake is less than 1600 kcal per day
☐ Uses MyPlate as a pattern for food choices

BEHAVIOR MODIFICATION

☐ Focuses on maintenance of healthy lifestyle (and weight) for a lifetime
☐ Promotes reasonable changes that can be maintained
☐ Encourages social support
☐ Includes plans for relapse, so that one does not quit after a setback
☐ Promotes changes that control problem eating behaviors

OVERALL HEALTH

☐ Requires screening by a physician for people with existing health problems, those over 40 (men) to 50 (women) years of age who plan to increase physical activity substantially, and those who plan to lose weight rapidly
☐ Encourages regular physical activity, sufficient sleep, stress reduction, and other healthy changes in lifestyle
☐ Addresses underlying psychological weight issues, such as depression or marital stress

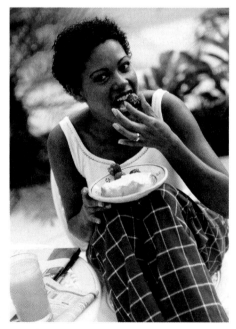

▲ Making a commitment to a healthier diet and lifestyle can be a challenge for many individuals. A sound weight-loss plan, however, does not require you to completely avoid certain favorite foods. Practical strategies include substituting lower-calorie choices, choosing high-calorie treats less often, and limiting portion sizes.

will contribute to success in weight loss and eventual weight maintenance (Fig. 7-16). From the 2010 Dietary Guidelines for Americans section on weight management, the key recommendations for those who need to lose weight is to aim for a slow, steady weight loss by decreasing calorie intake while maintaining an adequate nutrient intake and increasing physical activity.

Weight Loss in Perspective

These principles point to the importance of preventing obesity. This concept has wide support because conquering the disorder is so difficult. Public health strategies to address the current obesity problem must speak to all age groups. There is a particular need to focus on children and adolescents because patterns of excess weight and sedentary lifestyle developed during youth may form the basis for a lifetime

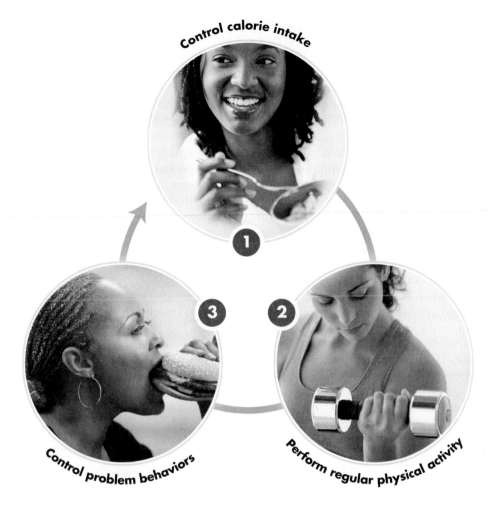

FIGURE 7-16 ▶ Weight-loss triad. The key to weight loss and maintenance can be thought of as a triad, which consists of three parts: (1) controlling calorie intake, (2) performing regular physical activity, and (3) controlling problem behaviors. The three parts of the triad support each other in that without one part of the triad, weight loss and later maintenance become unlikely.

For more information on weight control, obesity, and nutrition, visit the Weight-Control Information Network (WIN) at http://win.niddk.nih.gov/index.htm or call 800-WIN-8098. Complete guidelines for weight management are available at www.nhlbi.nih.gov/guidelines/index .htm. Other websites include www .caloriecontrol.org, www.weight.com, www.obesity.org, and www.cyberdiet .com.

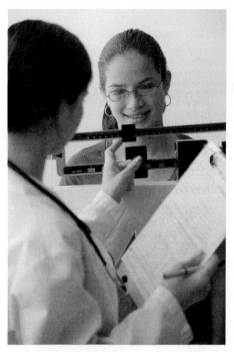

▲ Slow, steady weight loss is one of the characteristics of a sound weight-loss program.

CONCEPT CHECK

Obesity is a chronic disease that necessitates lifelong treatment. Emphasis should be placed especially on preventing obesity, because overcoming this disorder is difficult. Appropriate weight-loss programs have the following characteristics in common: (1) They meet nutritional needs; (2) they can adjust to accommodate habits and tastes; (3) they emphasize readily obtainable foods; (4) they promote changing habits that discourage overeating; (5) they encourage regular physical activity; and (6) they help change obesity-promoting beliefs and rally healthy social support.

of weight-related illness and increased mortality. In the adult population, attention should be directed toward weight maintenance and increased physical activity.

7.7 Control of Calorie Intake—The Main Key to Weight Loss and Weight Maintenance

A goal of losing 1 pound or so of stored fat per week may require limiting calorie intake to 1200 kcal per day for women and 1500 kcal for men. The calorie allowance could also be higher for very active people. Keep in mind that, in our sedentary society, decreasing calorie intake is vital because it is difficult to burn much energy without ample physical activity. With regard to consuming fewer calories, some experts

For interactive dietary and physical activity tools, check out the Food Tracker and Food Planner at www.ChooseMyPlate.gov.

suggest consuming less fat (especially saturated fat and *trans* fat), while others suggest consuming less carbohydrate, especially refined (high glycemic load) carbohydrate sources. Protein intakes in excess of what is typically needed by adults are also receiving attention. Using all these approaches simultaneously is fine. At this time, the low-fat, high-fiber approaches have been the most successful in long-term studies. A recent report (see Newsworthy Nutrition) confirms that the kinds of food we eat have a large effect on weight gain over the years. Finding what works for an individual is a process of trial and error. The notion that any type of diet promotes significantly greater calorie use by the body is unfounded (see Further Readings 13, 14, and 15).

One way for a dieter to monitor calorie intake at the start of a weight-loss program is by reading labels. Label reading is important, because many foods are more energy dense than people suppose (Fig. 7-17). Another method is to write down food intake for 24 hours (Appendix E) and then calculate calorie intake from the food table in the textbook supplement or by using your diet-analysis software. With knowledge of current calorie intake, future food choices can be adjusted as needed. People often underestimate portion size when recording food intake, so measuring cups and a food scale can help.

The Food Tracker at www.ChooseMyPlate.gov is an interactive online dietary and physical activity assessment tool that tracks the food calories you eat and compares them to the energy you expend in physical activity. The Food Planner is an interactive online tool for planning menus based on your personal ChooseMyPlate goals. Table 7-3 shows how to start reducing calorie intake. As you should realize, it is best to consider healthy eating a lifestyle change, rather than a weight-loss plan. Also, liquids deserve attention, because liquid calories do not stimulate satiety mechanisms to the same extent as solid foods. The corresponding advice from experts is to use beverages that have few or no calories and limit sugar-sweetened beverages.

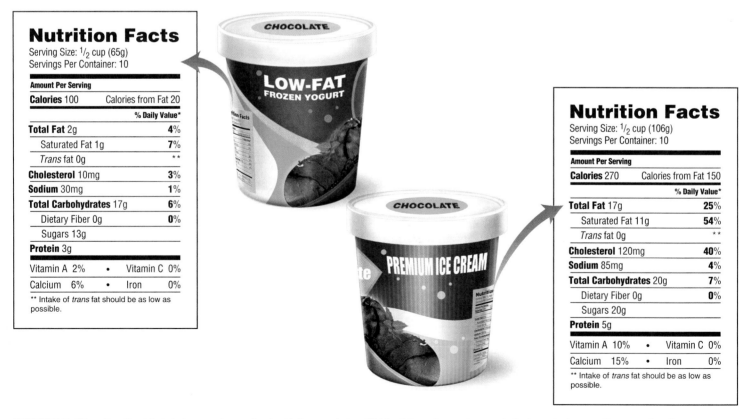

Nutrition Facts

Serving Size: ¹/₂ cup (65g)
Servings Per Container: 10

Amount Per Serving	
Calories 100	Calories from Fat 20

	% Daily Value*
Total Fat 2g	4%
Saturated Fat 1g	7%
Trans fat 0g	**
Cholesterol 10mg	3%
Sodium 30mg	1%
Total Carbohydrates 17g	6%
Dietary Fiber 0g	0%
Sugars 13g	
Protein 3g	

Vitamin A 2%	•	Vitamin C 0%
Calcium 6%	•	Iron 0%

** Intake of *trans* fat should be as low as possible.

Nutrition Facts

Serving Size: ¹/₂ cup (106g)
Servings Per Container: 10

Amount Per Serving	
Calories 270	Calories from Fat 150

	% Daily Value*
Total Fat 17g	25%
Saturated Fat 11g	54%
Trans fat 0g	**
Cholesterol 120mg	40%
Sodium 85mg	4%
Total Carbohydrates 20g	7%
Dietary Fiber 0g	0%
Sugars 20g	
Protein 5g	

Vitamin A 10%	•	Vitamin C 0%
Calcium 15%	•	Iron 0%

** Intake of *trans* fat should be as low as possible.

FIGURE 7-17 ▶ Reading labels helps you choose foods with fewer calories. Which of these frozen desserts is the best choice, per ½ cup serving, for a person on a weight-loss diet? The % Daily Values are based on a 2000 kcal diet. Read more about these dessert choices in What Would You Choose Recommendations.

TABLE 7-3 Lowering kcal: Point of Purchase and Consumption Decisions

Instead of	Try	Number of kcal Saved
3 oz well-marbled meat (prime rib)	3 oz lean meat (eye of round)	140
½ chicken breast, batter-fried	½ chicken breast, broiled with lemon	175
½ cup home-fried potatoes	1 medium baked potato	65
½ cup green bean-mushroom casserole	½ cup cooked green beans	50
½ cup potato salad	1 cup raw vegetable salad	140
½ cup pineapple chunks in heavy syrup	½ cup pineapple chunks canned in juice	25
2 tbsp bottled French dressing	2 tbsp low-calorie French dressing	150
⅛ 9-inch apple pie	1 baked apple, unsweetened	308
3 oatmeal-raisin cookies	1 oatmeal-raisin cookie	125
½ cup ice cream	½ cup ice milk	45
1 danish pastry	½ English muffin	150
1 cup sugar-coated corn flakes	1 cup plain corn flakes	60
1 cup whole milk	1 cup 1% low-fat milk	45
1 oz bag potato chips	1 cup plain popcorn	120
$\frac{1}{12}$ 8-inch white layer cake with chocolate frosting	$\frac{1}{12}$ angel food cake, 10-inch tube	185
12-fluid-ounce cola	12-fluid-ounce diet cola	150

7.8 Regular Physical Activity—A Second Key to Weight Loss and Especially Important for Later Weight Maintenance

Regular physical activity is important for everyone, especially those trying to lose weight or maintain a lower body weight. Calorie burning is enhanced both during and after physical activity. Therefore, activity greatly complements a reduction in calorie intake for weight loss. Many of us rarely do more than sit, stand, and sleep. More calories are used during physical activity than at rest. Expending only 100 to 300 extra kcal per day above and beyond normal daily activity, while controlling calorie intake, can lead to a steady weight loss. Furthermore, physical activity has so many other benefits, including a boost for overall self-esteem. A Key Recommendation from the 2010 Dietary Guidelines is to increase physical activity and reduce time spent in sedentary behaviors. The Dietary Guidelines point to the 2008 Physical Activity Guidelines for Americans for specific recommendations. Weight management, as well as other health outcomes including diseases and risk factors for disease, was considered in developing the Physical Activity Guidelines. Although some adults will need a higher level of physical activity than others, it is recommended that adults should do the equivalent of 150 minutes of moderate-intensity aerobic activity each week to achieve and maintain a healthy body weight. Some may need more than the equivalent of 300 minutes per week of moderate-intensity activity.

Adding any of the activities in Table 7-4 to one's lifestyle can increase calorie use. Duration and regular performance, rather than intensity, are the keys to success with this approach to weight loss. One should search for activities that can be continued over time. In this regard, walking vigorously 3 miles per day can be as helpful as

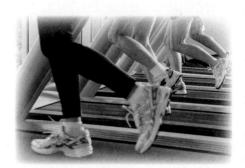

▲ Physical activity complements any diet plan.

TABLE 7-4 Approximate Calorie Costs of Various Activities and Specific Calorie Costs Projected for a 150-Pound (68-Kilogram) Person

Activity	kcal per kilogram per Hour	Total kcal per Hour	Activity	kcal per kilogram per Hour	Total kcal per Hour
Aerobics—heavy	8.0	544	Horseback riding	5.1	346
Aerobics—medium	5.0	340	Ice skating (10 mph)	5.8	394
Aerobics—light	3.0	204	Jogging—medium	9.0	612
Backpacking	9.0	612	Jogging—slow	7.0	476
Basketball—vigorous	10.0	680	Lying—at ease	1.3	89
Bowling	3.9	265	Racquetball—social	8.0	544
Calisthenics—heavy	8.0	544	Roller skating	5.1	346
Calisthenics—light	4.0	272	Running or jogging (10 mph)	13.2	897
Canoeing (2.5 mph)	3.3	224	Skiing downhill (10 mph)	8.8	598
Cleaning (female)	3.7	253	Sleeping	1.2	80
Cleaning (male)	3.5	236	Swimming (.25 mph)	4.4	299
Cooking	2.8	190	Tennis	6.1	414
Cycling (13 mph)	9.7	659	Volleyball	5.1	346
Cycling (5.5 mph)	3.0	204	Walking (3.75 mph)	4.4	299
Dressing/showering	1.6	106	Walking (2.5 mph)	3.0	204
Driving	1.7	117	Water skiing	7.0	476
Eating (sitting)	1.4	93	Weight lifting—heavy	9.0	612
Food shopping	3.6	245	Weight lifting—light	4.0	272
Football—touch	7.0	476	Window cleaning	3.5	240
Golf (using power cart)	3.6	244	Writing (sitting)	1.7	118

The values in Table 7-4 refer to total energy expenditure, including that needed to perform the physical activity, plus that needed for basal metabolism, the thermic effect of food, and thermogenesis. Use your diet-analysis software for your personal estimate.

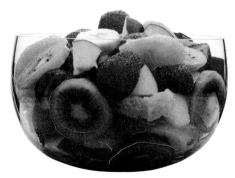

▲ Fruit is a great low-cal snack—high in nutrient density and low in calories.

aerobic dancing or jogging, if it is maintained. Moreover, activities of lighter intensity are less likely to lead to injuries. Some resistance exercises (weight training) also should be added to increase lean body mass and, in turn, fat use (see Chapter 10). As lean muscle mass increases, so will one's overall metabolic rate. An added benefit of including exercise in a weight-reduction program is maintenance of bone health.

Unfortunately, opportunities to expend calories in our daily lives are diminishing as technology systematically eliminates almost every reason to move our muscles. The easiest way to increase physical activity is to make it an enjoyable part of a daily routine. To start, one might pack a pair of athletic shoes and walk around the parking lot before coming home after school or work every day. Other ideas are avoiding elevators in favor of stairs and parking the car farther away from the shopping mall.

A pedometer is an inexpensive device that monitors activity as steps. A recommended goal for activity is to take at least 10,000 steps per day—typically we take half that many or less. A pedometer tracks this activity. Calorie counters, such as the Bodybugg, are new devices that track calorie expenditures throughout the day. The counters calculate calories by measuring heart rate, sweat rate, or heat loss and production. Like pedometers, calorie counters can motivate users to do more activity.

7.9 Behavior Modification—A Third Strategy for Weight Loss and Management

Controlling calorie intake also means modifying *problem* behaviors. Only the dieter can decide what behaviors are preventing calorie control. What events cause us to start (or stop) eating? What factors influence food choices?

The 2010 Dietary Guidelines identify the following behaviors as having the strongest evidence related to body weight:

- Focus on the total number of calories consumed.
- Monitor food intake.
- When eating out, choose smaller portions or lower-calorie options.
- Prepare, serve, and consume smaller portions of foods and beverages, especially those high in calories.
- Eat a nutrient-dense breakfast.
- Limit screen time.

Chain-breaking, stimulus control, cognitive restructuring, contingency management, and *self-monitoring* are behavior modification strategies used by psychologists that (Table 7-5) help place the problem in perspective and organize the intervention into manageable steps.

Chain-breaking separates behaviors that tend to occur together—for example, snacking on chips while watching television. Although these activities do not have to occur together, they often do. Dieters may need to break the chain reaction (see Rate Your Plate at the end of this chapter for more details).

Stimulus control puts us in charge of temptations. Options include pushing tempting food to the back of the refrigerator, removing fat-laden snacks from the kitchen counter, and avoiding the path by the vending machines. Provide a positive stimulus by keeping low-fat snacks available to satisfy hunger/appetite.

Cognitive restructuring changes our frame of mind. For example, after a hard day, avoid using alcohol or comfort foods as quick relief for stress. Instead, plan for healthful, relaxing activities for stress reduction. For example, take a walk around the neighborhood or have a satisfying talk with a friend.

Labeling some foods as "off limits" sets up an internal struggle to resist the urge to eat that food. This hopeless battle can keep us feeling deprived. We lose the fight. Managing food choices with the principle of moderation is best. If a favorite food becomes troublesome, place it off limits only temporarily, until it can be enjoyed in moderation.

Contingency management prepares one for situations that may trigger overeating (e.g., when snacks are served at a party) or hinder physical activity (e.g., rain).

A **self-monitoring** record can reveal patterns—such as unconscious overeating—that may explain problem eating habits. This record can encourage new habits that will counteract unwanted behaviors. Obesity experts note that this is the key behavioral tool to use in any weight-loss program (see Further Readings 4 and 6). See the margin for a list of free online tools available for self-monitoring.

Overall, it's important to address specific problems, such as snacking, compulsive eating, and mealtime overeating. Behavior Modification principles (review Table 7-5) are critical components of weight reduction and maintenance. Without them it is difficult to make lifelong lifestyle changes needed to meet weight-control goals.

Relapse Prevention Is Important

Preventing relapse is thought to be the hardest part of weight control—even harder than losing weight. A dieter needs to plan for lapses, not overreact, and take charge immediately. Change responses such as "I ate that cookie; I'm a failure" to "I ate that cookie, but I did well to stop after only one!" When dieters lapse from their diet plan, newly learned food habits should steer them back toward the plan. Without a strong behavioral program for **relapse prevention** in place, a lapse frequently turns into a relapse and a potential collapse. Once a pattern of poor food choices begins, dieters may feel

The motivation to lose weight and keep it off generally comes with a proverbial "flip of the switch," in which the desire to lose weight finally becomes more important than the desire to overeat.

chain-breaking Breaking the link between two or more behaviors that encourage overeating, such as snacking while watching television.

stimulus control Altering the environment to minimize the stimuli for eating—for example, removing foods from sight and storing them in kitchen cabinets.

cognitive restructuring Changing one's frame of mind regarding eating—for example, instead of using a difficult day as an excuse to overeat, substituting other pleasures for rewards, such as a relaxing walk with a friend.

contingency management Forming a plan of action to respond to a situation in which overeating is likely, such as when snacks are within arm's reach at a party.

self-monitoring Tracking foods eaten and conditions affecting eating; actions are usually recorded in a diary, along with location, time, and state of mind. This is a tool to help people understand more about their eating habits.

relapse prevention A series of strategies used to help prevent and cope with weight-control lapses, such as recognizing high-risk situations and deciding beforehand on appropriate responses.

Food and Activity Tracking
Here are some websites where you can record your food and physical activity online for free:

www.fitday.com
http://www.livestrong.com
www.mypyramidtracker.gov
http://nutritiondata.self.com
www.sparkpeople.com

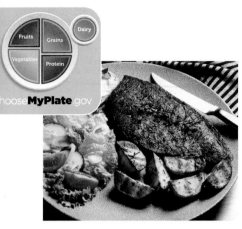

▲ Large portions of food, such as this steak, provide us with many opportunities to overeat. It takes much perseverance to eat sensibly. How do the portion sizes shown here compare to those recommended on MyPlate?

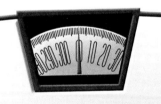

Successful weight losers and maintainers from the National Weight Control Registry:

- Eat a low-fat, high-carbohydrate diet (on average 25% of calorie intake as fat).
- Eat breakfast almost every day.
- Self-monitor by regularly weighing oneself and keeping a food journal.
- Exercise for about 1 hour per day.
- Eat at restaurants only once or twice per week.

Other recent studies support this approach, especially the last four characteristics.

TABLE 7-5 Behavior Modification Principles for Weight Loss

Shopping
1. Shop for food after eating—buy nutritious foods.
2. Shop from a list; limit purchases of irresistible "problem" foods. Shopping for fresh foods around the perimeter of the store first helps.
3. Avoid ready-to-eat foods.
4. Put off food shopping until absolutely necessary.

Plans
1. Plan to limit food intake as needed.
2. Substitute periods of physical activity for snacking.
3. Eat meals and snacks at scheduled times; don't skip meals.

Activities
1. Store food out of sight, preferably in the freezer, to discourage impulsive eating.
2. Eat all food in a "dining" area.
3. Keep serving dishes off the table, especially dishes of sauces and gravies.
4. Use smaller dishes and utensils.

Holidays and Parties
1. Drink fewer alcoholic beverages.
2. Plan eating behavior before parties.
3. Eat a low-calorie snack before parties.
4. Practice polite ways to decline food.
5. Don't get discouraged by an occasional setback.

Eating Behavior
1. Put fork down between mouthfuls.
2. Chew thoroughly before taking the next bite.
3. Leave some food on the plate.
4. Pause in the middle of the meal.
5. Do nothing else while eating (for example, reading, watching television).

Reward
1. Plan specific rewards for specific behavior (behavioral contracts).
2. Solicit help from family and friends and suggest how they can help you. Encourage family and friends to provide this help in the form of praise and material rewards.
3. Use self-monitoring records as basis for rewards.

Self-Monitoring
1. Note the time and place of eating.
2. List the type and amount of food eaten.
3. Record who is present and how you feel.
4. Use the diet diary to identify problem areas.

Cognitive Restructuring
1. Avoid setting unreasonable goals.
2. Think about progress, not shortcomings.
3. Avoid imperatives such as *always* and *never*.
4. Counter negative thoughts with positive restatements.

Portion Control
1. Make substitutions, such as a regular hamburger instead of a "quarter pounder" or cucumbers instead of croutons in salads.
2. Think small. Order the entrée and share it with another person. Order a cup of soup instead of a bowl or an appetizer in place of an entrée.
3. Use a doggie bag. Ask your server to put half the entrée in a doggie bag before bringing it to the table.

As we said at the start of this chapter, many of us need to become "defensive eaters." Know when to refuse food after satiety registers, and reduce portion sizes.

failure and stray farther from the plan. As the relapse lengthens, the diet plan collapses, and falls short of the weight-loss goal. Losing weight is difficult. Overall, maintenance of weight loss is fostered by the "3 Ms": motivation, movement, and monitoring.

Social Support Aids Behavioral Change

Healthy social support is helpful in weight control. Helping others understand how they can be supportive can make weight control easier. Family and friends can provide praise and encouragement. A registered dietitian or other weight-control professional can keep dieters accountable and help them learn from difficult situations. Long-term contact with a professional can be helpful for later weight maintenance. Groups of individuals attempting to lose weight or maintain losses can provide empathetic support.

Societal Efforts to Reduce Obesity

The incidence of obesity in the United States is now considered an epidemic. Improvement in the health of our nation requires an approach that includes many sectors. Although we ultimately make our own choices at an individual level, partnerships, programs, and policies that support healthy eating and active living must be coordinated. The 2010 Dietary Guidelines' Call to Action includes three guiding principles:

1. Ensure that all Americans have access to nutritious foods and opportunities for physical activity.
2. Facilitate individual behavior change through environmental strategies.
3. Set the stage for lifelong healthy eating, physical activity, and weight-management behaviors.

Public, private, and nonprofit organizations have begun to work together to address and reverse this public health crisis. For example, the U.S. Food and Drug Administration has brought together leaders from industry, government, academia, and the public health community to seek solutions to the obesity epidemic by making changes in foods eaten outside the home (restaurant and carry-out foods). These groups have collaborated and made recommendations to support the consumer's ability to manage calorie intake. Recommendations include "social marketing" programs that promote healthy eating and active living.

CONCEPT CHECK

Increasing physical activity in daily life should be part of any weight-loss plan. Daily activity, such as walking and stair climbing, is recommended. Behavior Modification can improve conditions for losing weight. One key step is to break behavior chains that encourage overeating, such as snacking while watching television. Another tactic is to modify the environment to reduce temptation; for example, put foods into cupboards to keep them out of sight. In addition, rethinking attitudes about eating—for example, substituting pleasures other than food as a reward for coping with a stressful day—can be important for altering undesirable behavior. Advanced planning to prevent and deal with lapses is vital, as is rallying healthy social support. Finally, careful observation and recording of eating habits can reveal subtle cues that lead to overeating. Overall, weight loss and maintenance are fostered by controlling calorie intake, performing regular physical activity, and modifying "problem" behaviors.

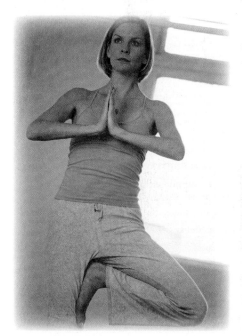

▲ Individuals who successfully maintain their weight loss employ a variety of strategies to cope with the stresses and challenges of changing problem behaviors.

7.10 Professional Help for Weight Loss

The first professional to see for advice about a weight-loss program is one's family physician. Doctors are best equipped to assess overall health and the appropriateness of weight loss. The physician may then recommend a registered dietitian for a specific weight-loss plan and answers to diet-related questions. Registered dietitians are uniquely qualified to help design a weight-loss plan because they understand both food composition and the psychological importance of food. Exercise physiologists can provide advice about programs to increase physical activity. The expense for such

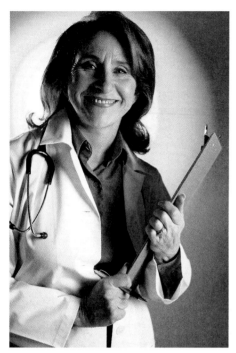

▲ All weight loss programs should begin with a visit to your family physician.

amphetamine A group of medications that induce stimulation of the central nervous system and have other effects in the body. Abuse is linked to physical and psychological dependence.

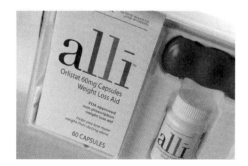

professional interventions is tax deductible in the United States in some cases (see a tax advisor) and often covered by health insurance plans if prescribed by a physician.

Many communities have a variety of weight-loss organizations. These include self-help groups, such as Take Off Pounds Sensibly and Weight Watchers. Other programs, such as Jenny Craig and Physicians' Weight Loss Center, are less desirable for the average dieter. Often, the employees are not registered dietitians or other appropriately trained health professionals. These programs also tend to be expensive because of their requirements for intense counseling or mandatory diet foods and supplements. In addition, the Federal Trade Commission has charged these and other commercial diet-program companies with misleading consumers through unsubstantiated weight-loss claims and deceptive testimonials.

North Americans are willing to try almost anything to shed unwanted pounds. Operation Waistline is a program designed by the U.S. Federal Trade Commission to terminate fraudulent claims being made by weight-loss charlatans with regard to diet products. The program hopes to put an end to the $6 billion spent annually in the United States on counterfeit products. The Enforma Natural Products Corporation had to pay $10 million in response to false claims for its "Fat Trapper" product.

Medications for Weight Loss

Candidates for medications for obesity include those with a BMI of 30 or more, or a BMI of 27 to 29.9 with weight-related health conditions, such as type 2 diabetes, cardiovascular disease, hypertension, or excess waist circumference; those with no contraindications to use the medication; and those ready to undertake lifestyle change. Drug therapy alone has not been found to be successful. Success with medications has been shown only in those who also modify their behavior, decrease calorie intake, and increase physical activity. In addition, if a person has not lost at least 4.4 pounds (2 kilograms) after 4 weeks, it is not likely that the person will benefit from further use of the medication.

Three main classes of medications have been used. An **amphetamine**-like medication (phenteramine [Fastin or Ionamin]) prolongs the activity of epinephrine and norepinephrine in the brain. This therapy is effective for some people in the short run but has not yet been proven effective in the long run. Most state medical boards limit use of this drug to 12 weeks unless the person is participating in a medical study using the product. The medication should not be used in pregnant or nursing women or those under 18 years of age.

The second class of medication approved by FDA for weight loss and the only weight-loss medication approved for long-term use is orlistat (Xenical). This medication reduces fat digestion by about 30% by inhibiting lipase enzyme action in the small intestine (Fig. 7-18). This cuts absorption of dietary fat by one-third for about 2 hours when taken along with a meal containing fat. This malabsorbed fat is deposited in the feces. *Fat intake has to be controlled,* however, because large amounts of fat in the feces cause numerous side effects, such as gas, bloating, and oily discharge. Interestingly, orlistat use can remind the person to follow a fat-controlled diet, as the symptoms resulting from consuming a high-fat meal are unpleasant and develop quickly. Orlistat is taken with each meal containing fat. The malabsorbed fat also carries fat-soluble vitamins into the feces, so the person taking orlistat must take a multivitamin and mineral supplement at bedtime. In this way, any micronutrients not absorbed during the day can be replaced; fat malabsorption from the dinner meal will not greatly influence micronutrient absorption in the late evening. A low-dose form of orlistat (alli™) is now available over the counter without a prescription.

Sibutramine (Meridia) is a third class of medication that was approved by FDA for weight loss and was available until October 2010. It enhances both norepinephrine and serotonin activity in the brain by reducing reuptake of these neurotransmitters by nerve cells. The neurotransmitters then remain active in the brain for

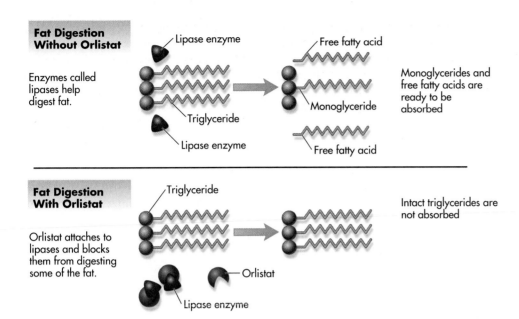

Fat Digestion Without Orlistat

Enzymes called lipases help digest fat.

Lipase enzyme

Triglyceride

Lipase enzyme

Free fatty acid

Monoglyceride

Free fatty acid

Monoglycerides and free fatty acids are ready to be absorbed

Fat Digestion With Orlistat

Orlistat attaches to lipases and blocks them from digesting some of the fat.

Triglyceride

Orlistat

Lipase enzyme

Intact triglycerides are not absorbed

FIGURE 7-18 ▶ Orlistat is a weight-loss drug that works in the digestive system to block digestion of about one-third of the fat in the food we eat. A low-dose form of this drug (alli™) is now available without a prescription.

a longer time and so prolong a sense of reduced hunger. The main effect is to moderately reduce appetite so that people eat less. Production of subutramine was voluntarily stopped at the request of FDA and based on increased risk of heart attacks and strokes observed in people taking sibutramine. Read more about this study in Newsworthy Nutrition.

Drug companies are working on many other types of medications and hopes that some of these will prove to be safe and effective for weight loss. In addition, physicians may prescribe medications not approved for weight loss but that have weight loss as a side effect. Certain antidepressants are an example. Such an application is termed *off-label*, because the product label does not include weight loss as an FDA-approved use. Over-the-counter medications and supplements are widely marketed as miracle cures for obesity, but in some cases, they do more harm than good (see Further Reading 11). Today more than ever, let the buyer beware concerning any purported weight-loss aid not prescribed by a physician.

Overall, in skilled hands, prescription medications can aid weight loss in some instances. However, they do not replace the need for reducing calorie intake, modifying "problem" behaviors, and increasing physical activity, both during and after therapy. Often, any weight loss during drug treatment can be attributed mostly to the individual's hard work at balancing calorie intake with calorie output.

Treatment of Severe Obesity

Severe (morbid) obesity, having a BMI greater than or equal to 40 or weighing at least 100 pounds over healthy body weight (or twice one's healthy body weight), requires professional treatment. Because of the serious health implications of severe obesity, drastic measures may be necessary. Such treatments are recommended only when traditional diets and medications fail. Drastic weight-loss procedures are not without side effects, both physical and psychological, making careful monitoring by a physician a necessity.

very-low-calorie diet (VLCD) Known also as *protein-sparing modified fast (PSMF)*, this diet allows a person 400 to 800 kcal per day, often in liquid form. Of this, 120 to 480 kcal is carbohydrate, and the rest is mostly high-quality protein.

bariatrics The medical specialty focusing on the treatment of obesity.

adjustable gastric banding A restrictive procedure in which the opening from the esophagus to the stomach is reduced by a hollow gastric band.

gastroplasty Gastric bypass surgery performed on the stomach to limit its volume to approximately 30 milliliters. Also referred to as stomach stapling.

Very-Low-Calorie Diets. If more traditional diet changes have failed, treating severe obesity with a **very-low-calorie diet (VLCD)** is possible, especially if the person has obesity-related diseases that are not well controlled (e.g., hypertension, type 2 diabetes). Some researchers believe that people with body weight greater than 30% above their healthy weight are appropriate candidates. VLCD programs are offered almost exclusively by medical centers or clinics since careful monitoring by a physician is crucial throughout this very restrictive form of weight loss. Major health risks include heart problems and gallstones. Optifast is one such commercial program. In general, the diet allows a person to consume only 400 to 800 kcal per day, often in liquid form. (These diets were previously known as protein-sparing modified fasts.) Of this amount, about 30 to 120 grams (120 to 480 kcal) is carbohydrate. The rest is high-quality protein, in the amount of about 70 to 100 grams per day (280 to 400 kcal). This low carbohydrate intake often causes ketosis, which may decrease hunger. However, the main reasons for weight loss are the minimal energy consumption and the absence of food choice. About 3 to 4 pounds can be lost per week; men tend to lose at a faster rate than women. When physical activity and resistance training augment this diet, a greater loss of adipose tissue occurs.

Weight regain remains a nagging problem, especially without a behavioral and physical activity component. If behavioral therapy and physical activity supplement a long-term support program, maintenance of the weight loss is more likely but still difficult. Any program under consideration should include a maintenance plan. Today, antiobesity medications also may be included in this phase of the program.

Bariatric Surgery. **Bariatrics** is the medical specialty focusing on the treatment of obesity. Bariatric surgery is only considered for people with severe obesity and includes operations aimed at promoting weight loss. Two types of bariatric operations are now common and effective (see Further Readings 7 and 10). Both procedures can be performed using an open (8- to 10-inch) incision in the middle of the abdomen or a laparoscopic approach in which several smaller (½- to 2-inch) incisions are used that allow cameras and instruments to enter the abdomen. **Adjustable gastric banding** (also known as the lap-band procedure) is a restrictive procedure in which the opening from the esophagus to the stomach is reduced by a hollow gastric band. This creates a small pouch and a narrow passage into the rest of the stomach and thus decreases the amount of food that can be eaten comfortably. The band can be inflated or deflated via an access port placed just under the skin. Studies have demonstrated that adjustable gastric banding is more effective long term than a very low-calorie diet (500 kcal) for people who are about 50 pounds overweight.

Gastric bypass (also called **gastroplasty** or stomach stapling) is another bariatric surgical procedure used for treating severe obesity. The most common and effective approach (the Roux-en-Y gastric bypass procedure) works by reducing the stomach capacity to about 30 milliliters (the volume of one egg or shot glass) and bypassing a short segment of the upper small intestine (Fig. 7-19). Weight loss is promoted mainly because overeating of solid foods is now less likely due to rapid satiety and discomfort or vomiting after overeating. About 75% of people with severe obesity eventually lose 50% or more of excess body weight with this method. In addition, the surgery's success at long-term maintenance often leads to dramatic health improvements, such as reduced blood pressure and elimination of type 2 diabetes. Risks of the surgery include bleeding, blood clots, hernias, and severe infections. In the long run, nutrient deficiencies can develop if the person is not adequately treated in the years following the surgery. Anemia and bone loss might then be the result. Risk of death from this demanding surgery can be as high as 2% (less risk with experienced surgeons).

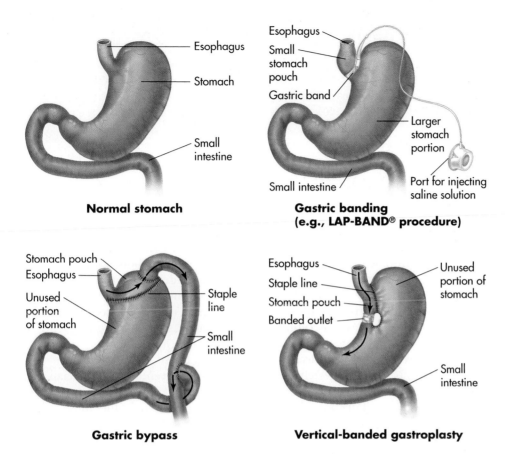

Normal stomach

Gastric banding (e.g., LAP-BAND® procedure)

Gastric bypass

Vertical-banded gastroplasty

FIGURE 7-19 ▶ The most common forms of gastroplasty for treating severe obesity. The gastric bypass is the most effective method. In banded gastroplasty, the band prevents expansion of the outlet for the stomach pouch.

Patient selection criteria for bariatric surgery include:

- BMI should be greater than 40.
- BMI between 35 and 40 is considered when there are serious obesity-related health concerns.
- Obesity must be present for a minimum of 5 years, with several nonsurgical attempts to lose weight.
- There should be no history of alcoholism or major untreated psychiatric disorders.

The person also must consider that the surgery is costly and may not be covered by medical insurance. The average cost for gastric bypass produres is $18,000 to $35,000 and for adjustable gastric banding is $17,000 to $30,000. In addition, follow-up surgery is often needed after weight loss to correct stretched skin, previously filled with fat. Furthermore, the surgery necessitates major lifestyle changes, such as the need to plan frequent, small meals. Therefore, the dieter who has chosen this drastic approach to weight loss faces months of difficult adjustments.

MAKING DECISIONS

Lipectomy

Spot-reducing by using diet and physical activity is not possible. "Problem" local fat deposits can be reduced in size, however, using suction lipectomy. Lipectomy or liposuction means surgical removal of fat. A pencil-thin tube is inserted into an incision in the skin, and the fat tissue, such as that in the buttocks and thigh area, is suctioned. This procedure carries some risks, such as infection; lasting depressions in the skin; and blood clots, which can lead to kidney failure and sometimes death. The procedure is designed to help a person lose about 4 to 8 pounds per treatment. Cost is about $1800 per site; total costs range as high as $2600 to $9000.

7.11 Treatment of Underweight

underweight A body mass index below 18.5. The cutoff is less precise than for obesity because this condition has been less studied.

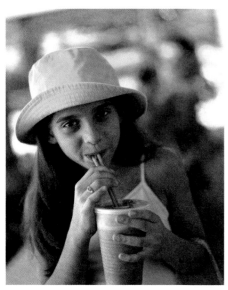

▲ Underweight people should increase their consumption of calorie-dense foods, such as smoothies, that are also loaded with nutrients.

Underweight is defined by a BMI less than 18.5 and can be caused by a variety of factors, such as cancer, infectious disease (e.g., tuberculosis), digestive tract disorders (e.g., chronic inflammatory bowel disease), and excessive dieting or physical activity. Genetic background may also lead to a higher resting metabolic rate, a slight body frame, or both. Health problems associated with underweight include the loss of menstrual function, low bone mass, complications with pregnancy and surgery, and slow recovery after illness. Significant underweight is also associated with increased death rates, especially when combined with cigarette smoking. We frequently hear about the risks of obesity, but seldom of underweight. In our culture, being underweight is much more socially acceptable than being obese.

Sometimes being underweight requires medical intervention. A physician should be consulted first to rule out hormonal imbalances; depression; cancer; infectious disease; digestive tract disorders; excessive physical activity; and other hidden disease, such as a serious eating disorder (see Chapter 11 for a detailed discussion of eating disorders).

The causes of underweight are not altogether different from the causes of obesity. Internal and external satiety-signal irregularities, the rate of metabolism, hereditary tendencies, and psychological traits can all contribute to underweight.

In growing children, the high demand for calories to support physical activity and growth can cause underweight. During growth spurts in adolescence, active children may not take the time to consume enough calories to support their needs. Moreover, gaining weight can be a formidable task for an underweight person. An extra 500 kcal per day may be required to gain weight, even at a slow pace, in part because of the increased expenditure of energy in thermogenesis. In contrast to the weight loser, the weight gainer may need to increase portion sizes.

When underweight requires a specific intervention, one approach for treating adults is to gradually increase their consumption of calorie-dense foods, especially those high in vegetable fat. Italian cheeses, nuts, and granola can be good calorie sources with low saturated-fat content. Dried fruit and bananas are good fruit choices. If eaten at the end of a meal, they don't cause early satiety. The same advice applies to salads and soups. Underweight people should replace such foods as diet soft drinks with good calorie sources, such as fruit juices and smoothies.

Encouraging a regular meal and snack schedule also aids in weight gain and maintenance. Sometimes underweight people have experienced stress at work or have been too busy to eat. Making regular meals a priority may not only help them attain an appropriate weight but also help with digestive disorders, such as constipation, sometimes associated with irregular eating times.

Excessively physically active people can reduce activity. If their weight remains low, they can add muscle mass through a resistance training (weight-lifting) program, but they must also increase their calorie intake to support that physical activity. Otherwise, weight gain will be hindered.

If these efforts fail to help a person achieve a healthy weight, they should at least prevent the health problems associated with being underweight. After achieving that, they may have to accept their lean frames.

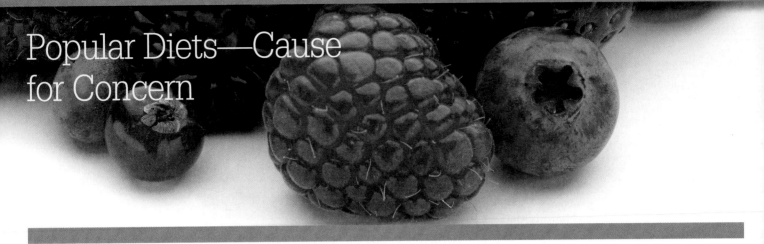

Popular Diets—Cause for Concern

Many overweight people try to help themselves by using the latest popular (also called fad) diet book. But, as you will see, most of these diets do not help, and some can actually harm those who follow them (Table 7-6). Research has shown that early dieting and other unhealthful weight control practices in adolescents lead to an increased risk of weight gain, overweight, and eating disorders.

Recently, weight-loss experts came together at the request of the USDA to evaluate weight-loss diets. They came to this conclusion: Forget these fads when it comes to dieting. Most of the popular diets are nutritionally inadequate and include certain foods that people would not normally choose to consume in large amounts. The experts stated that eating less of one's favorite foods and becoming more physically active can be much more effective when trying to implement a weight-loss diet. People need a plan they can live with in the long run so that weight control becomes permanent. The goal should be weight control over a lifetime, not immediate weight loss. Every popular diet leads to some immediate weight loss simply because daily in-take is monitored and monotonous food choices are typically part of the plan. A well-known example of the effectiveness of monotony contributing to weight loss is the experience of Jared Fogle. He ate primarily Subway sandwiches for 11 months and lost 245 pounds. He notes however that this is not a miracle diet—it takes a lot of hard work to lead to the success he experienced. There are also many other examples where diet monotony has led to weight loss. Overall, a traditional moderate diet coupled with regular physical activity is adequate for weight loss.

People on diets often fall within a healthy BMI of 18.5 to 25. Rather than worrying about weight loss, these individuals should be focusing on a healthy lifestyle that allows for weight maintenance. Incorporating necessary lifestyle changes and learning to accept one's particular body characteristics should be the overriding goals.

The dieting mania can be viewed as mostly a social problem, stemming from unrealistic weight expectations (especially for women) and lack of appreciation for the natural variety in body shape and weight. Not every woman can look like a fashion model, nor can every man look like a Greek god, but all of us can strive for good health and, if physically possible, an active lifestyle.

The size-acceptance nondiet movement, "Health at Every Size," has attempted to shift the paradigm away from the use of "popular" weight loss diets. The goals of the movement are all independent of body weight and include improvement of self-image, normalization of eating behavior, and increase in physical activity.

How to Recognize an Unreliable Diet

The criteria for evaluating weight-loss programs with regard to their safety and effectiveness were discussed previously (review Fig. 7-15). In contrast, unreliable diets typically share some common characteristics:

1. They promote quick weight loss. This is the primary temptation that the dieter falls for. As mentioned, this initial weight loss primarily results from water loss and lean muscle mass depletion.

2. They limit food selections and dictate specific rituals, such as eating only fruit for breakfast or cabbage soup every day.

3. They use testimonials from famous people and tie the diet to well-known cities, such as Beverly Hills and South Beach.

4. They bill themselves as cure-alls. These diets claim to work for everyone, whatever the type of obesity or the person's specific strengths and weaknesses.

5. They often recommend expensive supplements.

6. No attempts are made to change eating habits permanently. Dieters follow the diet until the desired weight is reached and then revert to old eating habits—they are told, for example, to eat rice for a month, lose weight, and then return to old habits.

7. They are generally critical of and skeptical about the scientific community. The lack of a quick fix from medical and dietetic professionals has led some of the public to seek advice from those who appear to have the answer.

8. They claim that there is no need to exercise.

Probably the cruelest characteristic of these diets is that they essentially guarantee failure for the dieter. The diets are not designed for permanent weight loss. Habits are not changed, and the food selection is so limited that the person cannot follow the diet in the long run. Although dieters assume they have lost fat, they have lost mostly muscle and other lean tissue mass. As soon as they begin

TABLE 7-6 Summary of Popular Diet Approaches to Weight Control

Approach	Examples*	Characteristics	Dietitian's Review
Moderate calorie restriction	• *Dieting for Dummies* (2003) • *Dieting with the Duchess* (2000) • *Dr. Phil's Ultimate Weight Solution* (2003, 2005) • Flat Belly Diet (2008) • Jenny Craig (1980s) • *Picture Perfect Weight Loss* (2003) • Slim-fast (1980s) • *Sonoma Diet* (2005) • *Volumetrics* (2000) • *Wedding Dress Diet* (2000) • Weight Watchers (1960s) • You on a Diet (2006)	• Generally 1200 to 1800 kcal per day • Moderate fat intake • Reasonable balance of macronutrients • Encourage exercise • May use behavioral approach	These diets are acceptable if a multivitamin and mineral supplement is used and permission of family physician is granted.
Carbohydrate focused	• *Carbohydrate Addicts Diet* (1993, 2001) • *Dr. Atkin's Diet Revolution* (1973, 2002) • *Dr. Gott's No Flour, No Sugar Diet* (2006) • *Eat, Drink & Weigh Less* (2006) • *G.I. (Glycemic Index) Diet* (2003) • *Healthy for Life* (2005) • *New Glucose Revolution* (2002) • Nutrisystem (2003) • *South Beach Diet* (especially initial phases) (2003) • *Sugar Busters Diet* (1998, 2003) • *Zone Diet* (1995)	• Restricted carbohydrate diets generally advise consumption of less than 100 grams of carbohydrate per day • Some plans focus on carbohydrate choices (e.g., choosing low rather than high glycemic index foods)	Selecting high-fiber, whole-grain sources of carbohydrates is an advisable practice for weight control and prevention of several chronic diseases. However, severe carbohydrate restriction may lead to ketosis, reduced exercise capacity (due to poor glycogen stores in the muscles), excessive animal fat intake, constipation, headaches, halitosis (bad breath), and muscle cramps. Severe carbohydrate restriction is not a nutritionally sound, long-term, weight-loss solution.
Low fat	• *20/30 Fat and Fiber Diet Plan* (2000) • *Complete Hip and Thigh Diet* (1989, 1999) • *Eat More, Weigh Less* (1993, 2001) • *Fit or Fat* (1977, 2005) • *Foods That Cause You to Lose Weight* (1992, 2003) • McDougall Program (1983, 1995) • Pritikin Diet (1984, 1995) • *Rice Diet Solution* (2005) • *T-Factor Diet* (1989, 2001) • Okinawa Program (2002)	• Generally less than 20% of calories from fat • Limited (or elimination of) animal protein sources; also limited plant oils, nuts, seeds	Low-fat diet plans are not necessarily to be avoided, but certain aspects may be unacceptable. Some potentially negative outcomes include flatulence, poor mineral absorption (from excess fiber intake), and a sense of deprivation (due to limited food choices).
Novelty diets	• *17-Day Diet* (2011) • *3-Hour Diet* (2005) • *Beverly Hills Diet* (1981, 1996) • Cabbage-Soup Diet (2004) • *Eat Right 4 Your Type* (1996) • Fat Smash Diet (2006) • *Fit for Life* (1987, 2001) • *Metabolic Typing Diet* (2002) • *New Hilton Head Metabolism Diet* (1983, 1996) • *Ultrametabolism* (2006) • *Weigh Down Diet* (2002)	• Promote certain nutrients, foods, or combinations of foods as having unique, magical, or previously undiscovered qualities	Novelty diets are usually not nutritionally balanced, thus malnutrition is a possible result. Also, failure to make long-term changes may lead to relapse, and unrealistic food choices lead to possible bingeing.

*Dates listed are original release date followed by most recent release date, if applicable.

eating normally again, much of the lost tissue is replaced. In a matter of weeks, most of the lost weight is back. The dieter appears to have failed, when actually the diet has failed. The gain and loss cycle is called weight cycling or "yo-yo" dieting. This whole scenario can add more blame and guilt, challenging the self-worth of the dieter. It can also come with some health costs, such as increased upper-body fat deposition. If someone needs help losing weight, professional help is advised. It is unfortunate that current trends suggest that people are spending more time and money on "quick fixes" rather than on such professional help.

Types of Popular Diets

Low- or Restricted-Carbohydrate Approaches

Low-carbohydrate diets have recently been the most popular diets. The low-carbohydrate intake leads to less glycogen synthesis, and therefore less water in the body (about 3 grams of water are stored per gram of glycogen). As discussed in Chapter 4, a very-low-carbohydrate intake also forces the liver to produce needed glucose. The source of carbons for this glucose is mostly proteins from tissues such as muscle resulting in loss of protein tissue, about 72% water. Essential ions, such as potassium are also lost in the urine. With the loss of glycogen stores, lean tissue and water, the dieter loses weight very rapidly. When a normal diet is resumed, the protein tissue is rebuilt and the weight is regained.

Although low-carbohydrate diets work in the short run primarily because they limit total food intake, recent results indicate that low-carbohydrate diets may be effective alternatives to low-fat diets. In a recent 2-year study published in the New England Journal of Medicine, moderately obese adults on a low-carbohydrate diet lost and kept off about 12 pounds, compared to 10 pounds for those following the traditional Mediterranean diet, and 7 pounds for those on a restricted-fat plan.

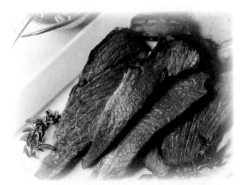

▲ In time, the very-low-carbohydrate, high-protein diets typically leave a person wanting more variety in meals, and so the diets are abandoned. Dropout rates are high on these diets.

The most popular diet using a low-carbohydrate approach is the Dr. Atkins' New Diet Revolution. More moderate approaches are found in the various Zone diets (40% of calorie intake as carbohydrate), Sugar Busters diet, and the South Beach diet (especially initial phases).

Carbohydrate-Focused Diets

Several recent diets, including Sugar Busters the Glucose Revolution, and Eat, Drink and Weigh Less, do not restrict carbohydrates, but rather emphasize the "good" carbohydrates in place of the "bad" or "harmful" ones. These diets recommend eating plenty of fruits, vegetables, whole grains, and cutting out simple sugars and processed grains. The carbohydrate-focused diets rely largely on low glycemic index and low glycemic load foods. In theory, these foods will cause a slow, steady rise in blood sugar, which will help control hunger.

Low-Fat Approaches

The very-low-fat diets contain approximately 5% to 10% of calories as fat and are very high in carbohydrates. The most notable are the Pritikin Diet and the Dr. Dean Ornish "Eat More, Weigh Less" diet plans. This approach is not harmful for healthy adults, but it is difficult to follow. People are quickly bored with this type of diet because they cannot eat many of their favorite foods. These dieters eat primarily grains, fruits, and vegetables, which most people cannot do for very long. Eventually, the person wants some foods higher in fat or protein. These diets are just too different from the typical North American diet for many adults to follow consistently, but may be acceptable for some people.

Novelty Diets

A variety of diets are built on gimmicks. Some novelty diets emphasize one food or food group and exclude almost all others. A rice diet was designed in the 1940s to lower blood pressure; now it has resurfaced as a weight-loss diet. The first phase consists of eating only rice and fruit. On the Beverly Hills Diet, you eat mostly fruit.

The rationale behind these diets is that you can eat only rice or fruit for just so long before becoming bored and, in theory, reducing your calorie intake. However,

chances are that you will abandon the diet entirely before losing much weight.

The most questionable of the novelty diets propose that "food gets stuck in your body." Fit for Life, the Beverly Hills Diet, and Eat Great, Lose Weight are examples. The supposition is that food gets stuck in the intestine, putrefies, and creates toxins, which invade the blood and cause disease. In response, recommendations are to not consume meat with potatoes or to consume fruits only after noon. These recommendations make no physiological sense.

Meal Replacements

Meal replacements come in many forms, including beverages or formulas, frozen or shelf-stable entrees, and meal or snack bars. Most meal replacements are fortified with vitamins and minerals and are appropriate to replace one or two regular meals or snacks per day. Although they are not a "magic bullet" for weight loss, they have been shown to help some people lose weight. Advantages of these convenient products are that they provide portion- and calorie-controlled foods that can serve as a visual education on appropriate portion sizes.

Quackery Is Characteristic of Many Popular Diets

Many popular diets fall under the category of quackery—people taking advantage of others. They usually involve a product or service that costs a considerable amount of money. Often, those offering the product or service don't realize that they are promoting quackery, because they were victims themselves. For example, they tried the product and by pure coincidence it worked for them, so they wish to sell it to all their friends and relatives.

Numerous other gimmicks for weight loss have come and gone and are likely to resurface. If in the future an important aid for weight loss is discovered, you can feel confident that major journals, such as the *Journal of the American Dietetic Association*, the *Journal of the American Medical Association*, or *The New England Journal of Medicine*, will report it. You don't need to rely on paperback books, infomercials, billboards, or newspaper advertisements for information about weight loss.

Case Study Choosing a Weight-Loss Program

Joe has a hectic schedule. During the day he works full-time at a warehouse distribution center filling orders. At night, three times a week, he attends class at the local community college in pursuit of computer certification. On weekends he likes to watch sports on TV, spend time with family and friends, and study. Joe has little time to think about what he eats—convenience rules. He stops for coffee and a pastry on his way to work, has a burger or pizza for lunch at a quick service restaurant, and for dinner picks up fried chicken or fish at the drive-through on his way to class. Unfortunately, over the past few years Joe's weight has been climbing. Watching a game on television a few nights ago, he saw an infomercial for a product that promises he can eat large portions of tasty foods but not gain weight. A famous actor supports the claim that this product allows one to eat at will and not gain weight. This claim is tempting to Joe.

Answer the following questions, and check your response in Appendix A.

1. Has Joe been experiencing positive or negative energy balance over the past few years?
2. What aspects of Joe's lifestyle (other than diet) are causing this effect on his energy balance? What changes could Joe make in his habits to promote weight loss or maintenance?
3. What changes could Joe make in his diet that would promote weight loss or maintenance?
4. Why should Joe be skeptical of the claims he heard about the weight-loss product in the infomercial?
5. What advice can you offer Joe for evaluation of weight-loss programs?

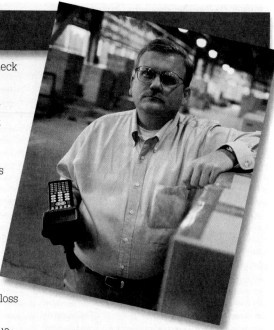

▲ What changes can Joe make in his daily routine and diet to stop his weight gain?

Summary (Numbers refer to numbered sections in the chapter.)

7.1 Energy balance considers energy intake and energy output. Negative energy balance occurs when energy output surpasses energy intake, resulting in weight loss. Positive energy balance occurs when calorie intake is greater than output, resulting in weight gain.

Basal metabolism, the thermic effect of food, physical activity, and thermogenesis account for total energy use by the body. Basal metabolism, which represents the minimum amount of calories required to keep the resting, awake body alive, is primarily affected by lean body mass, surface area, and thyroid hormone concentrations. Physical activity is energy use above that expended at rest. The thermic effect of food describes the increase in metabolism that facilitates digestion, absorption, and processing of the nutrients recently consumed. Thermogenesis is heat production caused by shivering when cold, fidgeting, and other stimuli. In a sedentary person, about 70% to 80% of energy use is accounted for by basal metabolism and the thermic effect of food.

7.2 Energy use by the body can be measured as heat given off by direct calorimetry or as oxygen used by indirect calorimetry. A person's Estimated Energy

Requirement can be calculated based on the following factors: gender, height, weight, age, and amount physical activity.

7.3 A person of healthy weight shows good health and performs daily activities without weight-related problems. A body mass index (weight in kilograms ÷ height² in meters) of 18.5 to 25 is one measure of healthy weight. A healthy weight is best determined in conjunction with a thorough health evaluation by a physician. A body mass index of 25 to 29.9 represents overweight. Obesity is defined as a total body fat percentage over 25% (men) or 35% (women) or a body mass index of 30 or more.

7.4 If calorie intake exceeds output, an energy imbalance occurs that results in overweight. Fat distribution greatly determines health risks from obesity. Upper-body fat storage, as measured by a waist circumference greater than 40 inches (102 centimeters) for men or 35 inches (88 centimeters) for women typically results in higher risks of hypertension, cardiovascular disease, and type 2 diabetes than does lower-body fat storage.

7.5 Both genetic (nature) and environmental (nurture) factors can increase the risk of obesity. The set-point theory pro-

poses that we have a genetically predetermined body weight or body fat content, which the body regulates.

7.6 A sound weight-loss program meets the dieter's nutritional needs by emphasizing a wide variety of low-calorie, bulky foods; adapts to the dieter's habits; consists of readily obtainable foods; strives to change poor eating habits; stresses regular physical activity; and stipulates the supervision by a physician if weight is to be lost rapidly or if the person is over the age of 40 (men) or 50 (women) and plans to perform substantially greater physical activity than usual.

7.7 A pound of adipose tissue contains about 3500 kcal. Loss or gain of a pound of adipose tissue—the fat itself plus lean support tissue—represents approximately 3300 kcal. Thus, if energy output exceeds calorie intake by about 500 kcal per day, a pound of adipose tissue can be lost per week.

7.8 Physical activity as part of a weight-loss program should be focused on duration rather than intensity. Ideally, vigorous activity for 60 minutes should be part of each day to prevent adult weight gain.

7.9 Behavior modification is a vital part of a weight-loss program because the dieter may have many habits that discourage weight maintenance. Specific behavior modification techniques, such as stimulus control and self-monitoring, can be used to help change problem behavior.

7.10 Medications to blunt appetite, such as phenteramine (Fastin), can aid weight-reduction strategies. Orlistat (Xenical) reduces fat absorption from a meal when taken with the meal. Weight-loss drugs are reserved for those who are obese or have weight-related problems, and they must be administered under close physician supervision.

The treatment of severe obesity may include surgery to reduce stomach volume to approximately 30 milliliters (1 ounce) or very-low-calorie diets containing 400 to 800 kcal per day. Both of these measures should be reserved for people who have failed at more conservative approaches to weight loss. They also require close medical supervision.

7.11 Underweight can be caused by a variety of factors, such as excessive physical activity and genetic background. Sometimes being underweight requires medical attention. A physician should be consulted first

to rule out underlying disease. The underweight person may need to increase portion sizes and learn to like calorie-dense foods. In addition, encouraging a regular meal and snack schedule aids in weight gain, as well as weight maintenance.

N&YH Many overweight people try popular diets that most often are not helpful and may actually be harmful. Unreliable diets typically share some common characteristics, including promoting quick weight loss, limiting food selections, using testimonials as proof, and requiring no exercise.

Check Your Knowledge (Answers to the following questions are below.)

1. Decreasing energy intake by about 500 kcal per day would mean a loss of 1 pound of body fat stores in _____ days.
   a. 2
   b. 7
   c. 10
   d. 14

2. Thermic effect of food represents the energy cost of
   a. chewing food.
   b. peristalsis
   c. basal metabolism.
   d. digesting, absorbing, and packaging nutrients.

3. A well-designed diet should
   a. increase physical activity.
   b. alter problem behaviors.
   c. reduce energy intake.
   d. All of the above.

4. All of the following factors are associated with a higher basal metabolic rate *except*
   a. stress.
   b. starvation.
   c. fever.
   d. pregnancy.

5. The intent of bariatric surgery is to
   a. limit stomach volume.
   b. speed transit time.
   c. surgically remove adipose tissue.
   d. prevent snacking.

6. Basal metabolism
   a. represents about 30% of total energy expenditure.
   b. is energy used to maintain heartbeat, respiration, and other basic functions and daily activities.
   c. represents about 60% to 70% of total calories used by the body during a day.
   d. includes energy to digest food.

7. Dr. Atkins' New Diet Revolution, The Zone, and the South Beach Diet are all examples of low- _____ diets.
   a. fat
   b. carbohydrate
   c. protein
   d. fiber

8. Probably the most important reason for obesity today in the United States is
   a. watching TV.
   b. snacking practices.
   c. inactivity.
   d. eating French fries.

9. The major goal for weight reduction in the treatment of obesity is the loss of
   a. weight.
   b. body fat.
   c. body water.
   d. body protein.

10. For most adults, the greatest portion of their energy expenditure is for
    a. physical activity.
    b. sleeping.
    c. basal metabolism.
    d. the thermic effect of food.

Answers: 1. b (LO 7.6), 2. d (LO 7.2), 3. d (LO 7.6), 4. b (LO 7.1), 5. a (LO 7.10), 6. c (LO 7.1), 7. b (LO 7.12), 8. c (LO 7.5), 9. b (LO 7.6), 10. c (LO 7.1)

Study Questions (Numbers refer to Learning Outcomes)

1. After reexamining the nature and nurture aspects of weight control, propose two hypotheses for the development of obesity. **(LO 7.5)**

2. Propose two hypotheses for the development of obesity, based on the four contributors to energy expenditure. **(LO 7.1)**

3. Define a healthy weight in a way that makes the most sense to you. **(LO 7.3)**

4. Describe a practical method to define obesity in a clinical setting. **(LO 7.3)**

5. What are the two most convincing pieces of evidence that both genetic and environmental factors play significant roles in the development of obesity? **(LO 7.5)**

6. List three health problems that obese people typically face and a reason that each problem arises. **(LO 7.4)**

7. What are three key characteristics of a sound weight-loss program? **(LO 7.6)**

8. Why is the claim for quick, effortless weight loss by any method always misleading? **(LO 7.6)**

9. Define the term *behavior modification*. Relate it to the terms *stimulus control, self-monitoring, chain-breaking, relapse prevention,* and *cognitive restructuring*. Give examples of each. **(LO 7.9)**

10. Why should obesity treatment be viewed as a lifelong commitment rather than a short episode of weight loss? **(LO 7.12)**

What Would You Choose Recommendations

Regular varieties of ice cream contain at least 10% milk fat by weight and are therefore a source of fat, saturated fat, and cholesterol. The milk fat gives the product the smooth, creamy texture for which ice cream is famous. You can see that the regular ice cream in the choices provided has 180 kcal, 10 grams of fat, 6 grams of saturated fat, and 65 mg of cholesterol. The sugar content is 19 grams—some of this comes from natural milk sugar (lactose), and some sugar is added for flavor.

Premium ice cream varieties, such as those you would find in an ice cream shop, may have up 300 kcal, 18 grams of fat, and 30 grams of sugar per ½-cup serving! That's equivalent to 4 teaspoons of butter and 7 teaspoons of sugar. Such decadent treats can be enjoyed in moderation, but are best reserved for special occasions.

Reduced-fat, low-fat, light, or fat-free varieties of ice cream have less than 10% milk fat. This can be accomplished by starting with lower-fat milk, using gelatin instead of eggs, using fat replacers incorporating more air into the product (e.g., "churned"), or any combination thereof. "Reduced fat" means the product has at least 25% less fat than the original product. "Low fat" sets the standard at 3 grams of fat or less per ½-cup serving. "Light" ice cream has at least 50% less fat than the original product. "Fat free" signifies 0.5 grams of fat or less per ½-cup serving. The brand shown here is "light"—it contains

lower fat and sugar than the regular ice cream. It has 110 kcal, 3 grams of fat, 2 grams of saturated fat, 10 mg cholesterol, and 14 grams of sugar per serving. For weight-management purposes, this saves you 70 kcals, 7 grams of fat, and 5 grams of sugar per serving compared to regular ice cream. Reducing the fat content of ice cream might also reduce the creamy texture, but for most reduced-fat, low-fat, and light products, the change is barely noticeable.

Frozen yogurt is not always a lower-calorie option than ice cream. It does not have to comply with the same 10% milk fat standard as ice cream does, so there may be a wide range of fat and sugar content. This brand of frozen yogurt has 180 kcal, 3 grams of fat, 1 gram of saturated fat, and 45 mg cholesterol—very similar to the regular ice cream. The product is marketed as "low fat"— and it does only contain 3 grams of fat per ½-cup serving—but there are still 22 grams of sugar. This is a great example of how low fat does not necessarily mean low calorie.

Serving size is the most important part of the Nutrition Facts panel when it comes to calorie control. No matter how low the calorie, fat, and sugar content are, if you consume multiple servings of any product, you are likely to take in too many calories.

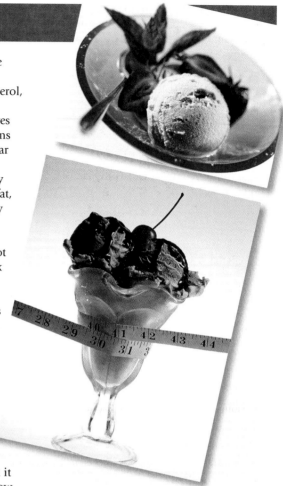

▲ One serving (one scoop) of ice cream with berries is a lower-calorie choice than several scoops with chocolate sauce and cherry.

NUTRITION FACTS		
Kroger Private Selection—Country Made Vanilla Ice Cream		
Serving: 1/2 cup		
Calories	180	Sodium	45 mg
Total Fat	10 g	Potassium	0 g
Saturated	6 g	Total Carbs	19 g
Polyunsaturated	0 g	Dietary Fiber	0 g
Monounsaturated	0 g	Sugars	19 g
Trans	0 g	Protein	6 g
Cholesterol	65 mg		
Vitamin A	8%	Calcium	10%
Vitamin C	2%	Iron	2%

*Percent Daily Values are based on a 2000 calorie diet. Your daily values may be higher or lower depending on your calories needs.

NUTRITION FACTS		
Kroger Deluxe—Vanilla Bean Light Ice Cream		
Serving: 1/2 cup		
Calories	110	Sodium	50 mg
Total Fat	3 g	Potassium	0 g
Saturated	2 g	Total Carbs	17 g
Polyunsaturated	0 g	Dietary Fiber	0 g
Monounsaturated	0 g	Sugars	14 g
Trans	0 g	Protein	3 g
Cholesterol	10 mg		
Vitamin A	6%	Calcium	10%
Vitamin C	2%	Iron	0%

*Percent Daily Values are based on a 2000 calorie diet. Your daily values may be higher or lower depending on your calories needs.

NUTRITION FACTS		
Haagen-Dazs—Yogurt Frozen Low Fat Vanilla		
Serving: 1/2 cup		
Calories	180	Sodium	45 mg
Total Fat	3 g	Potassium	0 g
Saturated	1 g	Total Carbs	30 g
Polyunsaturated	0 g	Dietary Fiber	0 g
Monounsaturated	0 g	Sugars	22 g
Trans	0 g	Protein	9 g
Cholesterol	45 mg		
Vitamin A	2%	Calcium	20%
Vitamin C	0%	Iron	0%

*Percent Daily Values are based on a 2000 calorie diet. Your daily values may be higher or lower depending on your calories needs.

Further Readings

1. Adams KF and others: Overweight, obesity, and mortality in a large prospective cohort of persons 50 to 71 years old. *The New England Journal of Medicine* 355:763, 2006.

    Excess body weight during midlife was associated with an increased risk of death. Risk of death increased by 20% to 40% among overweight persons and by two to three times among obese persons.

2. Blackburn GL, Corliss J: *Break Through Your Set Point.* New York: Harper Collins, 2007.

    This book outlines strategies for "breaking through" weight-loss plateaus by working with the body's natural tendency to stay at a fixed weight. The key is slow, gradual weight loss, followed by a 6-month period of holding steady at your new weight.

3. Flegal KM and others: Prevalence and trends in obesity among U.S. adults, 1999–2008. *Journals of the American Medical Association* 303(3):235, 2010.

    In the United States adult obesity rates have increased significantly. In the late 1970s, 15% of adults were obese compared to 34% in 2008.

4. Hollis JF and others: Weight loss during the intensive intervention phase of the weight-loss maintenance trial. *American Journal of Preventive Medicine* 35:118, 2008.

    Overweight or obese participants lost an average of 12 pounds. Keeping a daily record of food and physical activity helped them succeed suggesting that the willingness to record your eating habits could lead to a healthier weight.

5. James WPT and others: Effect of sibutramine on cardiovascular outcomes in overweight and obese subjects. *New England Journal of Medicine* 363(10):905, 2010.

    Sibutramine (Meridia) was withdrawn from the market in October 2010 based primarily on results from the SCOUT study (Sibutramine Cardiovascular OUTcomes Trial). Among subjects who were receiving long-term sibutramine treatment (~3.4 years), those with preexisting cardiovascular conditions had an increased risk of nonfatal heart attacks and stroke. More than 90% of the 10,000 patients in the study had underlying cardiovascular disease and therefore should not have received sibutramine. It was concluded that sibutramine should not be used in patients with preexisting cardiovascular disease.

6. Kruger J and others: Dietary and physical activity behaviors among adults successful at weight-loss maintenance. *International Journal of Behavioral Nutrition and Physical Activity* 3:17, 2006.

    Strategies practiced more frequently by successful weight losers included weighing oneself, planning meals, tracking fat and calories, exercising 30 or more minutes daily, and adding physical activity to their daily routines.

7. Madan AT, Orth WD: Vitamin and trace mineral levels after laparoscopic gastric bypass. *Obesity Surgery* 16:603, 2006.

    Vitamin and mineral deficiencies are thought to be a common long-term outcome of bariatric surgery. In this study, of 100 patients who underwent laparoscopic Roux-en-Y gastric bypass, most vitamins and minerals were slightly lower at 1-year postoperative. Significant decreases were observed only for vitamin D and selenium.

8. Mozaffarian D and others: Changes in diet and lifestyle and long-term weight gain in women and men. *New England Journal of Medicine* 364:2392, 2011.

    Relationships between lifestyle factors and weight change were evaluated. Subjects gained an average of 3.35 pounds every 4 years, adding up to 20 pounds in 20 years. Those with the greatest increase in physical activity gained 1.76 fewer pounds. The kind of foods eaten had a larger effect than changes in physical activity. Weight gained was associated with greater intake of French fries, potato chips, potatoes, sugar-sweetened beverages, unprocessed red meats, and processed meats. Foods that resulted in weight loss or no gain were fruits, vegetables, whole grains, yogurt, and nuts. Results show how small changes in eating, exercise, and other habits can result in large changes in body weight over the years.

9. National Center for Chronic Disease Prevention and Health Promotion: *Obesity: Halting the Epidemic by Making Health Easier.* Center for Disease Control and Prevention, Department of Health and Human Services, 2009. www.cdc.gov/nccdphp/dnpa.

    In the United States, obesity rates did not increase significantly between 2003–2004 and 2005–2006. Increased awareness of obesity as a national health problem, innovative policy and environmental changes in communities, work sites, and schools, and increased exercise and reduced consumption of high-calorie and fatty foods have likely led to this leveling of rates.

10. O'Brien PE and others: Treatment of mild to moderate obesity with laparoscopic adjustable gastric banding or an intensive medical program: A randomized trial. *Annals of Internal Medicine* 144:625, 2006.

    Surgical patients lost weight more rapidly and also had greater improvement in the metabolic syndrome and quality of life.

11. Robb M, Robb N: Tiny pills, big promises. *Today's Diet & Nutrition* 4(4):58, 2008.

    Information is provided about the latest dietary aids/diet pills for weight loss. Diet pills rely on one of three strategies: suppressing appetite, boosting metabolism, or blocking absorption of fats or carbohydrates. Each strategy is reviewed.

12. See R and others: The association of differing measures of overweight and obesity with prevalent atherosclerosis: the Dallas Heart Study. *Journal of American College of Cardiologists* 50:752, 2007.

    A study of associations between different measures of obesity (body mass index, waist circumference, and waist-to-hip ratio) and atherosclerosis found that waist-to-hip ratio was more strongly associated with atherosclerosis than body mass index or waist circumference. These results indicate that apple-shaped people are at greater risk for obesity-related diseases and heart attack than pear-shaped ones.

13. Shai I and others: Weight loss with a low-carbohydrate, Mediterranean, or low-fat diet. *New England Journal of Medicine* 359:229, 2008.

    Moderately obese adults were assigned to either a low-fat Mediterranean or low-carbohydrate diet, and studied for 2 years. Participants on the low-carbohydrate diet lost and kept off about 12 pounds; those on the Mediterranean Diet, kept off a 10-pounds weight loss; and those on the restricted-fat plan kept off 7 pounds. The results indicate that Mediterranean and low-carbohydrate diets may be effective alternatives to low-fat diets.

14. Slavin J and others: How fiber affects weight regulation. *Food Technology*, p. 34, February 2008.

    Dietary fiber has intrinsic, hormonal, and intestinal effects that decrease food intake by promoting satiety. Effects include decreased gastric emptying and/or slowed energy and nutrient absorption.

15. Svetkey LP and others: Comparison of strategies for sustaining weight loss: The weight-loss maintenance randomized controlled trial. *Journal of the American Medical Association* 299:1139, 2008.

    Participants weighed an average of 213 pounds, followed the Dietary Approaches to Stop Hypertension (DASH) diet for 6 months, and were encouraged to do 180 minutes of moderate exercise a week. Average weight loss was 19 pounds. After 2 ½ years, dieters kept more weight off if they reported to a nutrition counselor every month.

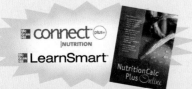

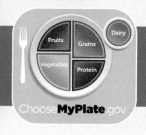

RATE YOUR PLATE

I. A Close Look at Your Weight Status

Determine the following two indices of your body status: body mass index and waist circumference.

Body Mass Index (BMI)

Record your weight in pounds: _____ pounds
Divide your weight in pounds by 2.2 to determine your weight in kilograms: _____ kilograms
Record your height in inches: _____ in
Divide your height in inches by 39.4 to determine your height in meters: _____ meters
Calculate your BMI using the following formula:
BMI = weight (kilograms)/height^2 (meters)
BMI = _____ kg/ _____ m^2 = _____

Waist Circumference

Use a tape measure to measure the circumference of your waist (at the umbilicus with stomach muscles relaxed). Circumference of waist (umbilicus) = _____ in

Interpretation

1. When BMI is greater than 25, health risks from obesity often begin. It is especially advisable to consider weight loss if your BMI exceeds 30. Does yours exceed 25 (or 30)?

   Yes _____ No _____

2. When a person has a BMI greater than 25 and a waist circumference of more than 40 inches (102 centimeters) in men or 35 inches (88 centimeters) in women, there is an increased risk of cardiovascular disease, hypertension, and type 2 diabetes. Does your waist circumference exceed the standard for your gender?

   Yes _____ No _____

3. Do you feel you need to pursue a program of weight loss?

   Yes _____ No _____

Application

From what you have learned in Chapter 7, what can you do to change your patterns of eating and physical activity to lose weight and help ensure maintenance of any loss?

_____

_____

_____

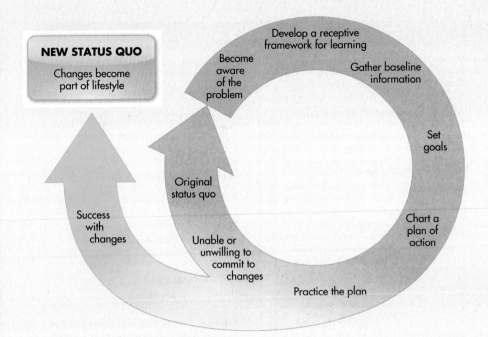

II. An Action Plan to Change or Maintain Weight Status

Now that you have assessed your current weight status, do you feel that you would like to make some changes? Following is a step-by-step guide to behavioral change. This process can be useful even for those satisfied with their current weight, as it can be applied to changing exercise habits, self-esteem, and a variety of other behaviors (Fig. 7-20).

Becoming Aware of the Problem

By calculating your current weight status, you have already become aware of the problem, if one exists. From here, it is important to find out more information about the cause of the problem and whether it is worth working toward a change.

1. What are the factors that most influence your eating habits? Do you eat due to stress, boredom, or depression? Is volume of food your problem, or do you eat mainly the wrong foods for you? Take some time to assess the root causes of your eating habits.

2. Once you have more information about your specific eating practices, you must decide if it is worth changing these practices. A benefits and costs analysis can be a useful tool in evaluating whether it is worth your effort to make life changes. Use the following example as a guide for listing benefits and costs pertinent to your situation (Fig. 7-21).

Setting Goals

What can we accomplish, and how long will it take? Setting a realistic, achievable goal and allowing a reasonable amount of time to pursue it increase the likelihood of success.

1. Begin by determining the outcome you would like to achieve. If you are trying to change your eating behaviors to be more healthy, list your reasons for doing so (e.g., overall health, weight loss, self-esteem).

    Overall goal:

    _____

    _____

FIGURE 7-21 ▶ Benefits and costs analysis applied to increasing physical activity. This process helps put behavior change into the context of total lifestyle.

Benefits and Costs Analysis

1 Benefits of changing eating habits?

What do you expect to get, now or later, that you want?
What may you avoid that would be unpleasant?

feel better physically and psychologically
look better

2 Benefits of not changing eating habits?

What do you get to do that you enjoy doing?
What do you avoid having to do?

no need for planning
can eat without feeling guilty

3 Costs involved in changing eating habits?

What do you have to do that you don't want to do?
What do you have to stop doing that you would rather continue doing?

take time to plan meals and shop
must give up some food volume

4 Costs of not changing eating habits?

What unpleasant or undesirable effects are you likely to experience now or in the future?
What are you likely to lose?

creeping weight gain
low self-esteem and poor health

Reasons to pursue goal:

_____

_____

_____

2. Now list several steps that will be necessary to achieve your goal. Keep in mind, however, that it is generally best to change only a few specific behaviors at first—walking briskly for 60 minutes each day, reducing fat intake, using more whole-grain products, and not eating after 7 P.M. Attempting small and perhaps easier dietary changes first reduces the scope of the problem and increases the likelihood of success.

Steps toward achieving goal:

1. _____

2. _____

3. _____

If you are having trouble deciphering the steps needed to achieve your goal, health professionals are an excellent resource for aid in planning.

Measuring Commitment

Now that you have collected information and know what is required to reach your goal, you must ask yourself, "Can I do this?" Commitment is an essential component in the success of behavioral change. Be honest with yourself. Permanent change is not quick or easy. Once you have decided that you have the commitment required to see this through, continue on to the following sections.

Making It Official with a Contract

Drawing up a behavioral contract often adds incentive to follow through with a plan. The contract could list goal behaviors and objectives, milestones for measuring progress, and regular rewards for meeting the terms of the contract. After finishing a contract, you should sign it in the presence of some friends. This encourages commitment.

Initially, plans should reward positive behaviors, and then they should focus on positive results. Positive behaviors, such as regular physical activity, eventually lead to positive outcomes, such as increased stamina.

Figure 7-22 is a sample contract for increasing physical activity. Keep in mind that this sample contract is only a suggestion; you can add your ideas as well.

Psyching Yourself Up

Once your contract is in place, you need to psych yourself up. Discouragement from peers and your temptations to stray from your plan need to be anticipated. Psyching yourself up can enable you to progress toward your goals in spite of others' attitudes and

Name *Alan Young*

Goal
I agree to *ride my exercise bike*
　　　　　　　　　(specify behavior)

under the following circumstances *for 30 minutes, 4 times per week*
in the evening　　(specify where, when, how much, etc.)

Substitute behavior and/or reinforcement schedule *I will reinforce myself if I've achieved my goal after a month with a weekend off campus with my roommate.*

Environmental planning
In order to help me do this, I am going to (1) arrange my physical and social environment by *buying a new portable CD player*

and (2) control my internal environment (thoughts, images) by *coordinating riding the bike with the first T.V. watching I do in the evening*

Reinforcements
Reinforcements provided by me daily or weekly (if contract is kept):
I will buy myself a new piece of clothing for off campus trip

Reinforcements provided by others daily or weekly (if contract is kept):
at the end of a month if I've completed my goal my parents will buy me a fitness club membership for winter.

Social support
Behavior change is more likely to take place when other people support you. During the quarter/semester please meet with the other person at least three times to discuss your progress.
The name of my "significant helper" is: *Mr. and Mrs. Young*

This contract should include:
1. Baseline data (one week)
2. Well-defined goal
3. Simple method for charting progress (diary, counter, charts, etc.)
4. Reinforcements (immediate and long-term)
5. Evaluation method (summary of experiences, success, and/or new learnings about self).

FIGURE 7-22 ▶ Alan's behavior contract. Completing such a contract can help generate commitment to behavior change. What would your contract look like?

opinions. Almost everyone benefits from some assertiveness training when it comes to changing behaviors. The following are a few suggestions. Can you think of any others?

- No one's feelings should be hurt if you say, "No, thank you," firmly and repeatedly when others try to dissuade you from a plan. Tell them you have new diet behavior and your needs are important.

- You don't have to eat a lot to accommodate anyone—your mother, business clients, or the chef. For example, at a party with friends, you may feel you have to eat a lot to participate, but you don't. Another trap is ordering a lot just because someone else is paying for the meal.

- Learn ways to handle put-downs—inadvertent or conscious. An effective response can be to communicate feelings honestly, without hostility. Tell criticizers that they have annoyed or offended you, that you are working to change your habits and would really like understanding and support from them.

Practicing the Plan

Once you've set up a plan, the next step is to implement it. Start with a trial of at least 6 to 8 weeks. Thinking of a lifetime commitment can be overwhelming. Aim for a total duration of 6 months of new activities before giving up. We may have to persuade ourselves more than once of the value of continuing the program. The following are some suggestions to help keep a plan on track:

- *Focus on reducing but not necessarily extinguishing undesirable behaviors.* For example, it's usually unrealistic to say, "I'll never eat a certain food again." It's better to say, "I won't eat that *problem* food as often as before."

- *Monitor progress.* Note your progress in a diary and reward yourself according to your contract. While conquering some habits and seeing improvement, you may find yourself quite encouraged, even enthusiastic, about your plan of action. That can give you the impetus to move ahead with the program.

- *Control environments.* In the early phases of behavioral change, try to avoid problem situations, such as parties, coffee breaks, and favorite restaurants. Once new habits are firmly established, you can probably more successfully resist the temptations of these environments.

Reevaluating and Preventing Relapse

After practicing a program for several weeks to months, it is important to reassess the original plan. In addition, you may now be able to pinpoint other problem areas for which you need to plan appropriately.

1. Begin by taking a close and critical look at your original plan. Does it lead to the goals you set? Are there any new steps toward your goal that you feel capable of adding to your contract? Do you need new reinforcements? It may even be necessary to make a new contract. For permanent change, it is worth this time of reassessment.

2. In practicing your plan over the past weeks or months, you have likely experienced relapses. What triggered these relapses? To prevent a total retreat to your old habits, it is important to set up a plan for such relapses. You can do this by identifying high-risk situations, rehearsing a response, and remembering your goals.

You may have noticed a behavior chain in some of your relapses. That is, the relapse may stem from a series of interconnected habitual activities. The way to break the chain is to first identify the activities, pinpoint the weak links, break those links, and substitute other behaviors. Figure 7-23 illustrates a sample behavior chain and a substitute activities list. Consider compiling a list based on your behavior chains.

Epilogue

If you have used the activities in this section, you are well on your way to permanent behavioral change. Recall that this exercise can be used for a variety of desired changes, including quitting smoking, increasing physical activity, and improving study habits. It is by no means an easy process, but the results can be well worth the effort. Overall, the keys to success are motivation (keeping the problem in the forefront of your mind), having a plan of action, securing the resources and skills needed for success, and looking for help from family, friends, or a group.

SUBSTITUTE ACTIVITIES

Pleasant activities
1. *Singing / washing hair*
2. *Reading comics / biking*
3. *Sewing / calling a friend*

Necessary activities
1. *Ironing*
2. *Vacuuming*
3. *Straightening apartment*

Situations when used
1. *Wanted ice cream – delayed with bath*
2. *Wanted wheat thins – cleaned up apt.*
3. *Wanted snack – went for walk*
4. *Wanted cookies – did dishes first*
5. *Saw leftovers – went for bike ride*
6. *Tempted by cookies – set timer*
7. *Wanted snack – read comics*

BEHAVIOR CHAIN

Identify the links in your eating response chain on the following diagram.
Draw a line through the chain where it was interrupted. Add the link you
substituted and the new chain of behavior this substitution started.

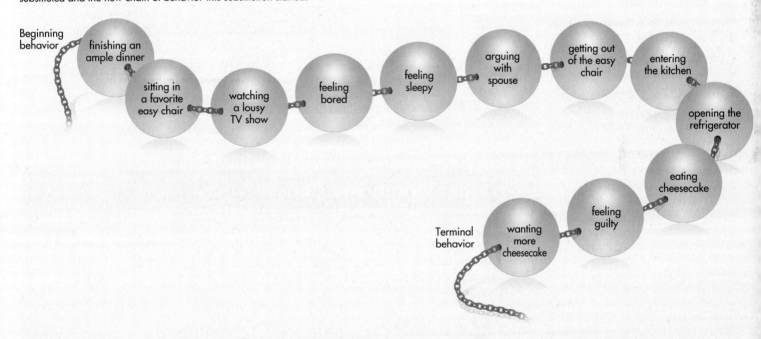

FIGURE 7-23 ▶ Identifying behavior chains. This is a good tool for understanding more about your habits and pinpointing ways
to change unwanted habits. The earlier in the chain you substitute a nonfood link, the easier it is to intervene. Four types of behaviors can be substituted in an ongoing behavior chain.

1. Fun activities (taking a walk, reading a book)
2. Necessary activities (cleaning a room, balancing your checkbook)
3. Incompatible activities (taking a shower)
4. Urge-delaying activities (setting a kitchen timer for 20 minutes before allowing yourself to eat)

Using activities to interrupt behavior patterns that lead to inappropriate eating (or inactivity) can be a powerful means of changing habits.

Chapter 8 Overview of The Micronutrients

Student Learning Outcomes

Chapter 8 is designed to allow you to:

8.1 Define the terms *vitamin* and *mineral* and list characteristics of each.

8.2 Classify the vitamins according to whether they are fat soluble or water soluble.

8.3 Classify the minerals as major, trace, or ultratrace.

8.4 Discuss the digestion, absorption, and storage of micronutrients, particularly as these processes relate to risk of toxicity.

8.5 Explain how food-handling practices, conditions of the body, dietary components, and other factors influence the availability of micronutrients from food.

8.6 Summarize the basic functional roles of micronutrients, providing two examples of micronutrients that participate in each role.

8.7 Discuss the roles of choline in human health.

What Would You Choose?

You heard an advertisement for a B-complex supplement that stated B vitamins will help "unlock the energy in foods." You have been feeling kind of tired lately and wonder if a B-complex supplement would give you more energy. In your health-food store, you find many options. Which of the following would you choose?

a A supplement with 50 milligrams of several B vitamins

b A supplement with 150 milligrams of several B vitamins

c A supplement with coenzyme forms of B vitamins

d None of these

 Think about your choice as you read Chapter 8, then see our recommendations at the end of the chapter. To learn more about dietary supplements, check out the Connect site: www.mcgrawhillconnect.com

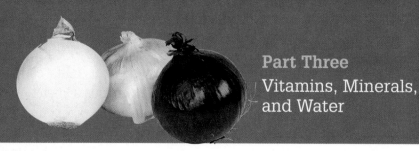
Can food be medicine? Consider the following examples:

- Fatigue, bleeding gums, bruising, and scaly skin—these are the symptoms of **scurvy,** which plagued seamen during long ocean voyages until 1753, when James Lind, a physician in the British navy, found that consumption of citrus fruits could prevent this disease.

- An epidemic of **rickets** occurred among children in post-Industrial-Revolution Britain during the late eighteenth century. They suffered from bone pain; frequent fractures; weakness; and deformities, such as bowed legs. In 1922, cod-liver oil was determined to be an effective treatment.

- First noted in medical literature in the mid-sixteenth century, **chlorosis** was a disorder characterized by a green skin color, extreme weakness, and poor appetite. Chlorosis was mainly described among adolescent women, so some physicians of the era declared it to be a hysterical condition. In the early 1700s, the British physician Thomas Sydenham prescribed that afflicted women should drink "mineral water impregnated with the Iron Mine."

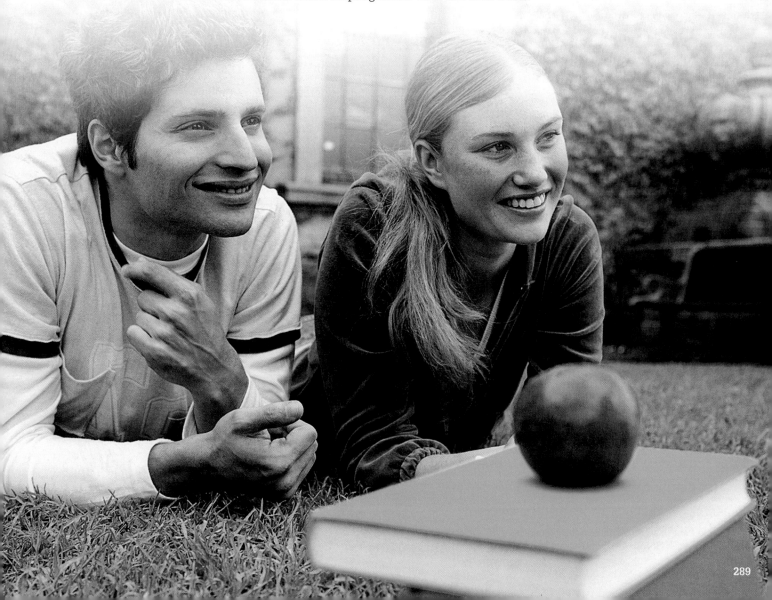

scurvy The vitamin C deficiency disease characterized by weakness, fatigue, slow wound healing, opening of previously healed wounds, bone pain, fractures, sore and bleeding gums, diarrhea, and pinpoint hemorrhages on the skin.

rickets A disease characterized by poor mineralization of newly synthesized bones because of low calcium content. Arising in infants and children, this deficiency is caused by insufficient amounts of the vitamin D hormone in the body.

chlorosis In traditional medical terminology, a form of iron-deficiency anemia characterized by pale or greenish skin, weakness, fatigue, and shortness of breath. In modern medical literature, chlorosis is termed hypochromic anemia.

micronutrient A nutrient needed in milligram or microgram quantities in a diet.

vitamin Compound needed in small amounts in the diet to help regulate and support chemical reactions and processes in the body. Contains carbon.

How do citrus fruits, cod-liver oil, and mineral water prevent or cure such serious ailments? As nutrition science has evolved, the discovery of essential compounds in the foods we eat has overturned old misconceptions about the origins of some diseases. These essential compounds are collectively known as **micronutrients**. Citrus fruits, sure cures for scurvy, contain vitamin C. Cod liver oil, a preventive treatment for rickets, is an excellent source of vitamin D. The mineral water prescribed by Sydenham supplied iron for his patients suffering from chlorosis, a form of iron-deficiency anemia.

Vitamin C, vitamin D, and iron are a few examples of micronutrients—nutrients that yield no energy and are required in small amounts (milligrams or micrograms). However slight its requirement, each micronutrient is essential for one or more functions in the body (Fig. 8-1). In Chapter 8, let's get started with an overview of the micronutrients. You will gain general knowledge about the micronutrients and begin to see how the vitamins and minerals work together to perform various physiological functions. Later, in Chapters 9 through 12, the functional roles of these micronutrients will be examined in greater detail.

Refresh Your Memory

As you begin your study of vitamins and minerals, you may want to review:

- Application of the Dietary Reference Intakes and implications of the Dietary Supplement Health and Education Act (DSHEA) in Chapter 2.
- The digestion and absorption of nutrients in Chapter 3.
- The digestion, absorption, and metabolism of dietary lipids in Chapter 5.

8.1 Vitamins: Vital Dietary Components

By definition, **vitamins** are essential organic (carbon-containing) substances needed in small amounts in the diet for normal function, growth, and maintenance of the body. In general, humans require a total of about 1 ounce (28 grams) of vitamins for

Can my food choices now affect my future risk of osteoporosis? What can I do to correct anemia? Will a megadose of zinc protect me from catching a cold? How can I get the most nutrition out of my food? Do I need to take supplements? Chapter 8 provides some answers.

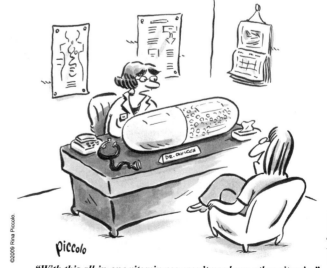

"With this all-in-one vitamin you won't need any other vitamin."

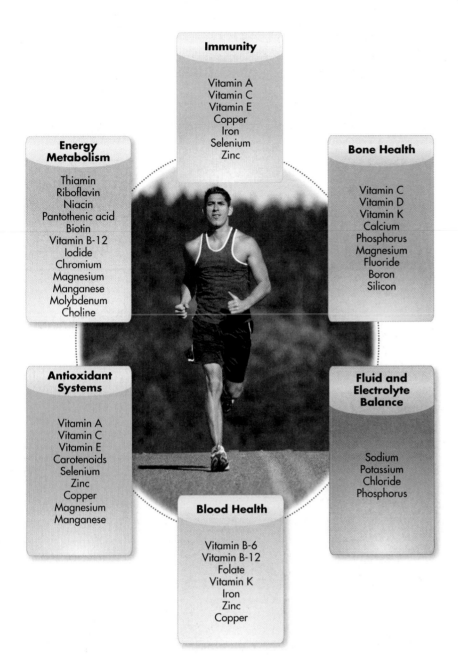

Immunity

Vitamin A
Vitamin C
Vitamin E
Copper
Iron
Selenium
Zinc

Energy Metabolism

Thiamin
Riboflavin
Niacin
Pantothenic acid
Biotin
Vitamin B-12
Iodide
Chromium
Magnesium
Manganese
Molybdenum
Choline

Bone Health

Vitamin C
Vitamin D
Vitamin K
Calcium
Phosphorus
Magnesium
Fluoride
Boron
Silicon

Antioxidant Systems

Vitamin A
Vitamin C
Vitamin E
Carotenoids
Selenium
Zinc
Copper
Magnesium
Manganese

Fluid and Electrolyte Balance

Sodium
Potassium
Chloride
Phosphorus

Blood Health

Vitamin B-6
Vitamin B-12
Folate
Vitamin K
Iron
Zinc
Copper

FIGURE 8-1 ▶ Micronutrients contribute to many functions in the body.

every 150 pounds (70 kilograms) of food consumed. Vitamins can be divided into two broad classes based on solubility. Vitamins A, D, E, and K are **fat-soluble vitamins** (Table 8-1). whereas the B vitamins and vitamin C are **water-soluble vitamins** (Table 8-2). The B vitamins include thiamin, riboflavin, niacin, pantothenic acid, biotin, vitamin B-6, folate, and vitamin B-12. Choline is a related nutrient but is not classified as a vitamin.

Vitamins are generally essential in human diets because they cannot be synthesized in the human body or because their synthesis can be decreased by environmental factors. Notable exceptions to having a strict dietary need for a vitamin are vitamin A, which we can synthesize from certain pigments in plants; vitamin D, synthesized in the body if the skin is exposed to adequate sunlight; niacin, synthesized from the amino acid tryptophan; and vitamin K and biotin, synthesized to some extent by bacteria in the intestinal tract.

To be classified as a vitamin, a compound must meet the following criteria: (1) the body is unable to synthesize enough of the compound to maintain health; and (2) absence of the compound from the diet for a defined period produces deficiency

fat-soluble vitamins Vitamins that dissolve in fat and such substances as ether and benzene but not readily in water. These vitamins are A, D, E, and K.

water-soluble vitamins Vitamins that dissolve in water. These vitamins are the B vitamins and vitamin C.

TABLE 8-1 Summary of the Fat-Soluble Vitamins

Vitamin	Major Functions	RDA or Adequate Intake	Dietary Sources	Deficiency Symptoms	Toxicity Symptoms
Vitamin A (preformed vitamin A and provitamin A)	• Promote vision: night and color • Promote growth • Prevent drying of skin and eyes • Promote resistance to bacterial infection and overall immune system function	Females: 700 micrograms RAE Males: 900 micrograms RAE 2300–3000 IU if as preformed (vitamin A)	Preformed vitamin A: • Liver • Fortified milk • Fortified breakfast cereals Provitamin A: • Sweet potatoes • Spinach • Greens • Carrots • Cantaloupe • Apricots • Broccoli	• Night blindness • Xerophthalmia • Poor growth • Dry skin	• Fetal malformations • Hair loss • Skin changes • Bone pain • Fractures Upper Level is 3000 micrograms of preformed vitamin A (10,000 IU) based on the risk of birth defects and liver toxicity.
Vitamin D	• Increase absorption of calcium and phosphorus • Maintain optimal blood calcium and calcification of bone • Regulation of cell development	15 micrograms (600 IU)	• Vitamin D fortified milk • Fortified breakfast cereals • Fish oils • Sardines • Salmon	• Rickets in children • Osteomalacia in adults	• Growth retardation • Kidney damage • Calcium deposits in soft tissue Upper Level is 100 micrograms (4000 IU) based on the risk of elevated blood calcium.
Vitamin E	• Antioxidant; prevents breakdown of vitamin A and unsaturated fatty acids	15 milligrams alpha-tocopherol 22 IU natural form, 33 IU (synthetic form)	• Plant oils • Products made from plant oils • Some greens • Some fruits • Nuts and seeds • Fortified breakfast cereals	• Hemolysis of red blood cells • Nerve degeneration	• Muscle weakness • Headaches • Nausea • Inhibition of vitamin K metabolism Upper Level is 1000 milligrams (1100 IU synthetic form, 1500 IU natural form) based on the risk of hemorrhage.
Vitamin K	• Activation of blood-clotting factors • Activation of proteins involved in bone metabolism	Females: 90 micrograms Males: 120 micrograms	• Green vegetables • Liver • Some plant oils • Some calcium supplements	• Hemorrhage • Fractures	No Upper Level has been set.

Abbreviations: RAE = retinol activity equivalents; IU = international units.

TABLE 8-2 Summary of the Water-Soluble Vitamins and Choline

Vitamin	Major Functions	RDA or Adequate Intake	Dietary Sources*	Deficiency Symptoms	Toxicity Symptoms
Thiamin	• Coenzyme of carbohydrate metabolism • Nerve function	1.1–1.2 milligrams	• Sunflower seeds • Pork • Whole and enriched grains • Dried beans • Peas	*Beriberi* • Nervous tingling • Poor coordination • Edema • Heart changes • Weakness	None
Riboflavin†	• Coenzyme of carbohydrate metabolism	1.1–1.3 milligrams	• Milk • Mushrooms • Spinach • Liver • Enriched grains	• Inflammation of the mouth and tongue • Cracks at the corners of the mouth • Eye disorders	None
Niacin	• Coenzyme of energy metabolism • Coenzyme of fat synthesis	14–16 milligrams (niacin equivalents)	• Mushrooms • Bran • Tuna • Salmon • Chicken • Beef • Liver • Peanuts • Enriched grains	*Pellagra* • Diarrhea • Dermatitis • Dementia • Death	Upper Level is 35 milligrams from supplements, based on flushing of skin.
Pantothenic acid	• Coenzyme of energy metabolism • Coenzyme of fat synthesis	5 milligrams	• Mushrooms • Liver • Broccoli • Eggs *Most foods have some*	• No natural deficiency disease or symptoms	None
Biotin	• Coenzyme of glucose production • Coenzyme of fat synthesis	30 micrograms	• Cheese • Egg yolks • Cauliflower • Peanut butter • Liver	• Dermatitis • Tongue soreness • Anemia • Depression	Unknown
Vitamin B-6†	• Coenzyme of energy metabolism, especially protein • Neurotransmitter synthesis • Red blood cell synthesis *Many other functions*	1.3–1.7 milligrams	• Animal protein foods • Spinach • Broccoli • Bananas • Salmon • Sunflower seeds	• Headache • Anemia • Convulsions • Nausea • Vomiting • Flaky skin • Sore tongue	Upper Level is 100 milligrams, based on nerve destruction.
Folate (folic acid)†	• Coenzyme involved in DNA synthesis *Many other functions*	400 micrograms (dietary folate equivalents)	• Green leafy vegetables • Orange juice • Organ meats • Sprouts • Sunflower seeds	• Megaloblastic anemia • Inflammation of tongue • Diarrhea • Poor growth • Depression	None likely Upper Level for adults is set at 1000 micrograms for synthetic folic acid (exclusive of food folate), based on masking of B-12 deficiency.

(continued)

(concluded)

Vitamin	Major Functions	RDA or Adequate Intake	Dietary Sources*	Deficiency Symptoms	Toxicity Symptoms
Vitamin B-12†	• Coenzyme of folate metabolism • Nerve function *Many other functions*	2.4 micrograms *Older adults and vegans should use fortified foods or supplements.*	• Animal foods (not natural in plants) • Organ meats • Oysters • Clams • Fortified, ready-to-eat breakfast cereals	• Macrocytic anemia • Poor nerve function	None
Vitamin C	• Connective tissue synthesis • Hormone synthesis • Neurotransmitter synthesis • Possible antioxidant activity	75–90 milligrams *Smokers should add 35 milligrams.*	• Citrus fruits • Strawberries • Broccoli • Greens	• Scurvy • Poor wound healing • Pinpoint hemorrhages • Bleeding gums	Upper Level is 2 grams, based on development of diarrhea. Can also alter some diagnostic tests
Choline†	• Neurotransmitter synthesis • Phospholipid synthesis	425–550 milligrams	Widely distributed in foods and synthesized by the body	No natural deficiency	Upper Level is 3.5 grams per day, based on development of fishy body odor and reduced blood pressure.

*Fortified ready-to-eat breakfast cereals are good sources for most of these vitamins and a common source of B vitamins for many of us.

†These nutrients also participate in homocysteine metabolism, which in turn may reduce the risk of developing cardiovascular disease.

megadose Intake of a nutrient beyond estimates of needs to prevent a deficiency or what would be found in a balanced diet; 2 to 10 times human needs is a starting point for such a dosage.

symptoms that, if caught in time, are quickly cured when the compound is resupplied. A compound does not qualify as a vitamin merely because the body cannot make it. Evidence must suggest that health declines when the substance is not consumed.

As scientists began to identify various vitamins, related deficiency diseases such as scurvy and rickets were dramatically cured. For the most part, as the vitamins were discovered, they were named alphabetically: A, B, C, D, E, and so on. Later, many substances originally classified as vitamins were found not to be essential for humans and were dropped from the list. Other vitamins, thought at first to be only one chemical, turned out to be several chemicals, so the alphabetical names had to be broken down by numbers (B-6, B-12, and so on).

In addition to their use in correcting deficiency diseases, a few vitamins have also proved useful in treating several nondeficiency diseases. These medical applications require administration of **megadoses**, well above typical human needs for the vitamins. For example, megadoses of a form of niacin can be used as part of blood cholesterol-lowering treatment for certain individuals. Still, any claimed benefits from use of vitamin supplements, especially intakes in excess of the Upper Level (if set), should be viewed critically because unproved claims are common. Remember, whenever you take a supplement at high doses, you are taking it at a pharmacological dose—that of a drug. Expect side effects as you would from any drug.

Vitamins isolated from foods or synthesized in the laboratory are the same chemical compounds and work equally well in the body. Contrary to claims in the health-food literature, "natural" vitamins isolated from foods are, for the most part, no more healthful than those synthesized in a laboratory, but there are exceptions. Vitamin E is much more potent in its natural form. In contrast, synthetic folic acid, the form of the vitamin added to ready-to-eat breakfast cereals and flour, is 1.7 times more potent than the natural vitamin form (see Further Reading 3).

Absorption and Storage of Vitamins in the Body

The fat-soluble vitamins A, D, E, and K are absorbed along with dietary fat. These vitamins then travel with dietary fats as part of chylomicrons through the bloodstream to reach body cells. Special carriers in the bloodstream help distribute some of these vitamins. Fat-soluble vitamins are stored mostly in the liver and fatty tissues.

When fat absorption is efficient, about 40% to 90% of the fat-soluble vitamins are absorbed. Anything that interferes with normal digestion and absorption of fats, however, also interferes with fat-soluble vitamin absorption. For example, people with cystic fibrosis, a disease that often hampers fat absorption, may develop deficiencies of fat-soluble vitamins. Some medications, such as the weight-loss drug orlistat (Alli), discussed in Chapter 7, also interfere with fat absorption. Unabsorbed fat carries these vitamins to the large intestine, where they are excreted in the feces. People with such conditions are especially susceptible to vitamin K deficiency because body stores of vitamin K are lower than those of the other fat-soluble vitamins. Vitamin supplements, taken under a physician's guidance, are part of the treatment for preventing a vitamin deficiency associated with fat malabsorption. Finally, people who use mineral oil as a laxative at mealtimes risk fat-soluble vitamin deficiencies. The intestine does not absorb mineral oil, but the mineral oil absorbs the vitamins. So, fat-soluble vitamins are eliminated with the mineral oil in the feces.

Water-soluble vitamins are handled much differently than fat-soluble vitamins. After being ingested, the B vitamins are first broken down from their active coenzyme forms into free vitamins in the stomach and small intestine. The vitamins are then absorbed, primarily in the small intestine. Typically, about 50% to 90% of the B vitamins in the diet are absorbed, which means they have relatively high **bioavailability**. Water-soluble vitamins are transported to the liver via the portal vein and are distributed to body tissues. Once inside cells, the active coenzyme forms are resynthesized. Note that some supplement manufacturers sell vitamins in their coenzyme forms, There is no benefit of consuming the coenzyme forms, as these are broken down during digestion and activated inside cells when needed.

Excretion of vitamins varies primarily on their solubility. Except for vitamin K, fat-soluble vitamins are not readily excreted from the body. Hence, toxicity can be an issue. Water-soluble vitamins are excreted based on **tissue saturation,** the degree to which the tissue vitamin stores are full. Tissue storage capacity is limited. As the tissues become saturated, the rate of excretion via the kidney increases sharply, preventing potential toxicity. This is also why we need to replenish the vitamins daily. Notable exceptions are water-soluble B-6 and B-12, as they are stored in the liver and not easily excreted in the urine.

The limited tissue saturation of many vitamins dictates that they should be consumed in the diet daily, although an occasional lapse in the intake of even water-soluble vitamins causes no harm. Symptoms of a vitamin deficiency occur only when that vitamin is lacking in the diet and the body stores are essentially exhausted. For example, for an average person, the diet must be devoid of thiamin for 10 days or lacking in vitamin C for 20 to 40 days before developing the first symptoms of deficiency of these vitamins.

bioavailability The degree to which an ingested nutrient is digested and absorbed and thus is available to the body.

tissue saturation The limited storage capacity of water-soluble vitamins in the tissues.

Vitamin Toxicity

Intakes in excess of daily needs for most water-soluble vitamins are rapidly lost from the body because the kidneys efficiently filter the excess from the blood and excrete these compounds in urine. Notable exceptions are vitamin B-6 and vitamin B-12, which are stored in the liver. Although they are water-soluble, these two B vitamins may accumulate to toxic levels.

In contrast to the water-soluble vitamins, fat-soluble vitamins are not readily excreted, so some can easily accumulate in the body and cause toxic effects. Although a toxic effect from an excessive intake of any vitamin is theoretically possible, toxicity of the fat-soluble vitamin A is the most frequently observed. Vitamin A causes toxicity at intakes as little as two times human need. Vitamin E and the water-soluble vitamins niacin, vitamin B-6, and vitamin C can also cause toxic effects but only when consumed in very large amounts (15 to 100 times human needs or more). Vitamins are unlikely to cause toxic effects unless taken in supplement (pill) form.

Some people believe that consuming vitamins far in excess of their needs provides them with extra energy, protection from disease, and prolonged youth. They seem to think that if a little is good, then more must be better. A "one-a-day" type of multivitamin and mineral supplement usually contains less than two times the Daily Values of its components, so daily use of these products is unlikely to cause toxic effects in men and nonpregnant women. However, consuming many vitamin pills, especially potent sources of vitamin A, can cause problems.

Preservation of Vitamins in Foods

Good sources of vitamins can be found in all food groups, especially fruits and vegetables (Fig. 8-2). However, storage time and several environmental factors can affect vitamin content of foods. Substantial amounts of vitamins can be lost from the time a fruit or vegetable is picked until it is eaten. The water-soluble vitamins, particularly thiamin, vitamin C, and folate, can be destroyed with improper storage and excessive cooking. Heat, light, exposure to the air, cooking in water, and alkalinity are factors that can destroy vitamins. The riper the food, the more vitamins it will contain. The sooner a food is eaten after harvest, the less chance of nutrient loss.

There are several steps you can take to preserve the vitamin content of fruits and vegetables (Table 8-3). Purchasing, storing, and preparing foods are points at which you can be cognizant of preserving nutrients. Frozen vegetables and fruits are often as nutrient-rich as freshly picked ones because fruits and vegetables are typically frozen immediately after harvesting. As part of the freezing process, vegetables are quickly blanched in boiling water. Blanching destroys the enzymes that would otherwise degrade the vitamins. If a food is not to be eaten within a few days, freezing is the best preservation method to retain nutrients.

FIGURE 8-2 ▶ Certain food groups on MyPlate are especially rich sources of various vitamins and choline. This is true for those listed. Each may be also found in other MyPlate groups, but in lower amounts. In addition to those vitamins listed here, pantothenic acid is present in moderate amounts in many groups and vitamin E is abundant in plant oils.

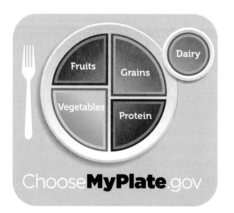

**MyPlate:
Sources of Vitamins
and Choline**

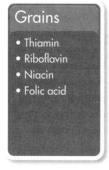
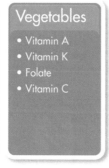
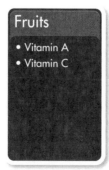
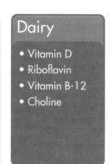
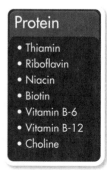

Grains
• Thiamin
• Riboflavin
• Niacin
• Folic acid

Vegetables
• Vitamin A
• Vitamin K
• Folate
• Vitamin C

Fruits
• Vitamin A
• Vitamin C

Dairy
• Vitamin D
• Riboflavin
• Vitamin B-12
• Choline

Protein
• Thiamin
• Riboflavin
• Niacin
• Biotin
• Vitamin B-6
• Vitamin B-12
• Choline

TABLE 8-3 Tips for Preserving Vitamins in Fruits and Vegetables

Preservation Methods	Why?
Keep fruits and vegetables cool until eaten.	Enzymes in fruits and vegetables begin to degrade vitamins once they are harvested. Chilling limits this process.
Refrigerate fruits and vegetables (except bananas, onions, potatoes, and tomatoes) in moisture-proof, airtight containers or in the vegetables drawer.	Nutrients keep best at temperatures near freezing, at high humidity, and away from air.
Trim, peel, and cut fruits and vegetables minimally—just enough to remove inedible parts.	Oxygen breaks down vitamins faster when more of the food surface is exposed. Whenever possible, cook fruits and vegetables in their skins.
Microwave, steam, or stir-fry vegetables.	More nutrients are retained when there is less contact with water and shorter cooking time.
Minimize cooking time.	Prolonged cooking (slow simmering) and reheating reduce vitamin content.
Avoid adding fats to vegetables during cooking if you plan to discard the liquid.	Fat-soluble vitamins will be lost in discarded fat. if you want to add fats, do so after vegetables are fully cooked and drained.
Do not add baking soda to vegetables to enhance the green color.	Alkalinity destroys vitamin D, thiamin, and other vitamins.
Store canned and frozen fruits and vegetables carefully.	To protect canned foods, store them in a cool, dry location. To protect frozen foods, store them at 0° F (−32°C) or colder. Eat within 12 months.

CONCEPT CHECK

Vitamins are organic compounds required in small amounts by the body for proper function growth, and maintenance. They cannot be synthesized in adequate quantities by the body to maintain health and are therefore essential in the diet. Prolonged absence of a vitamin from the diet leads to deficiency symptoms. Vitamins A, D, E, and K are fat soluble; whereas the B vitamins, vitamin C, and choline (a related nutrient) are water soluble. Toxicities of fat-soluble vitamins are most common because these vitamins are stored in body tissues and not easily excreted. Food-handling practices, such as cooking methods, can lead to vitamin losses from foods. Vitamin bioavailability varies based on the body's ability to digest and absorb the vitamin.

8.2 Minerals: Essential Elements For Health

Whereas vitamins are compounds consisting of many elements (e.g., carbon, oxygen, and hydrogen), **minerals** are individual chemical elements. They cannot be broken down further. The mineral content of foods is sometimes called "ash" because it is all that remains after the whole food has been destroyed by high temperatures or chemical degradation. In humans, minerals make up about 4% of adult body weight (Fig. 8-3). A mineral is essential for humans if a dietary inadequacy results in a physiological or structural abnormality, and its addition to the diet prevents such

mineral Element used in the body to promote chemical reactions and to form body structures.

FIGURE 8-3 ▶ Approximate amounts of various minerals present in the average human body. Other trace minerals of nutritional importance not listed include chromium, fluoride, molybdenum, selenium, and zinc.

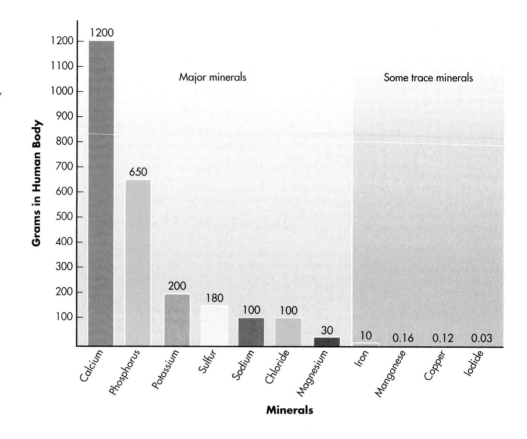

major mineral Vital to health, a mineral required in the diet in amounts greater than 100 milligrams per day.

trace mineral Vital to health, a mineral required in the diet in amounts less than 100 milligrams per day.

ultratrace mineral A mineral present in the human diet in trace amounts but that has not been shown to be essential to human health.

illness or reinstates normal health. Sixteen minerals are known to be essential in the diet.

Minerals are categorized based on the amount we need per day. Recall from Chapter 1 that if we require greater than 100 milligrams (1/50 of a teaspoon) of a mineral per day, it is considered a **major mineral** (Table 8-4). These include calcium, phosphorus, magnesium, sulfur, sodium, potassium, and chloride. **Trace minerals** are required at levels less than 100 milligrams per day (Table 8-5). Nine essential trace minerals (iron, zinc, copper, iodine, selenium, molybdenum, fluoride, manganese, and chromium) have been identified for humans.

Information about trace minerals is perhaps the most rapidly expanding area of knowledge in nutrition. With the exceptions of iron and iodide, the importance of trace minerals to humans has been recognized only within the last 50 years or so. Although we need 100 milligrams or less of each trace mineral daily, they are as essential to good health as are major minerals.

In some cases, discovering the importance of a trace mineral reads like a detective story, and the evidence is still unfolding. In 1961, researchers linked dwarfism in Middle Eastern villagers to a zinc deficiency. Other scientists recognized that a rare form of heart disease in an isolated area of China was linked to a selenium deficiency. In North America, some trace mineral deficiencies were first observed in the late 1960s and early 1970s when the minerals were not added to synthetic formulas used for intravenous feeding.

It is difficult to define precisely our trace mineral needs because we need only minute amounts. Highly sophisticated technology is required to measure such small amounts in both food and body tissues.

There are several additional trace minerals (sometimes called **ultratrace minerals**) found in the human body, but many of them have no known requirements. These include arsenic, boron, nickel, silicon, and vanadium.

TABLE 8-4 Summary of the Major Minerals

Mineral	Major Functions	RDA, or Adequate Intake	Dietary Sources	Deficiency Symptoms	Toxicity Symptoms
Sodium	• Major positive ion of the extracellular fluid • Aids nerve impulse transmission • Water balance	*Age 19–50 years:* 1500 milligrams *Age 51–70 years:* 1300 milligrams *Age > 70 years* 1200 milligrams	• Table salt • Processed foods • Condiments • Sauces • Soups • Chips	• Muscle cramps	• Contributes to hypertension in susceptible individuals • Increases calcium loss in urine • Upper Level is 2300 milligrams.
Potassium	• Major positive ion of intracellular fluid • Aids nerve impulse transmission • Water balance	4700 milligrams	• Spinach • Squash • Bananas • Orange juice • Milk • Meat • Legumes • Whole grains	• Irregular heartbeat • Loss of appetite • Muscle cramps	• Slowing of the heartbeat, as seen in kidney failure
Chloride	• Major negative ion of extracellular fluid • Participates in acid production in stomach • Aids nerve impulse transmission • Water balance	2300 milligrams	• Table salt • Some vegetables • Processed foods	• Convulsions in infants	• Linked to hypertension in susceptible people when combined with sodium • Upper Level is 3600 milligrams.
Calcium	• Bone and tooth structure • Blood clotting • Aids in nerve impulse transmission • Muscle contractions • Other cell functions	*Age 9–18 years:* 1300 milligrams *Age > 18 years:* 1000–1200 milligrams	• Dairy products • Canned fish • Leafy vegetables • Tofu • Fortified orange juice (and other fortified foods)	• Increased risk of osteoporosis	• May cause kidney stones and other problems in susceptible people • Upper Level is 2500 milligrams.
Phosphorus	• Major negative ion of intracellular fluid • Bone and tooth strength • Part of various metabolic compounds • Acid-base balance	*Age 9–18 years:* 1250 milligrams *Age > 18 years:* 700 milligrams	• Dairy products • Processed foods • Fish • Soft drinks • Bakery products • Meats	• Possibility of poor bone maintenance	• Impairs bone health in people with kidney failure • Poor bone mineralization if calcium intakes are low • Upper Level is 3 to 4 grams.
Magnesium	• Bone formation • Aids enzyme function • Aids nerve and heart function	*Men:* 400–420 milligrams *Women:* 310–320 milligrams	• Wheat bran • Green vegetables • Nuts • Chocolate • Legumes	• Weakness • Muscle pain • Poor heart function	• Causes diarrhea and weakness in people with kidney failure • Upper Level is 350 milligrams but refers to nonfood sources (e.g., supplements) only.
Sulfur	• Part of vitamins and amino acids • Aids in drug detoxification • Acid-base balance	None	• Protein foods	• None observed	• None likely

TABLE 8-5 Summary of Key Trace Minerals

Mineral	Major Functions	RDA, or Adequate Intake	Dietary Sources	Deficiency Symptoms	Toxicity Symptoms
Iron	• Component of hemoglobin and other key compounds used in respiration • Immune function • Cognitive development	*Men:* 8 milligrams *Premenopausal Women:* 18 milligrams	• Meats • Seafood • Broccoli • Peas • Bran • Enriched breads	• Fatigue • Anemia • Low blood hemoglobin values	• Liver and heart damage (extreme cases) • GI upset • Upper Level is 45 milligrams.
Zinc	• Required for nearly 200 enzymes • Growth • Immunity • Alcohol metabolism • Sexual development • Reproduction • Antioxidant protection	*Men:* 11 milligrams *Women:* 8 milligrams	• Seafood • Meats • Greens • Whole grains	• Skin rash • Diarrhea • Decreased appetite and sense of taste • Hair loss • Poor growth and development • Poor wound healing	• Reduced copper absorption • Diarrhea • Cramps • Depressed immune function • Upper Level is 40 milligrams.
Selenium	• Part of an antioxidant system	55 micrograms	• Meats • Eggs • Fish • Seafood • Whole grains	• Muscle pain • Weakness • Form of heart disease	• Nausea • Vomiting • Hair loss • Weakness • Liver disease • Upper Level is 400 micrograms.
Iodide	• Component of thyroid hormones	150 micrograms	• Iodized salt • White bread • Saltwater fish • Dairy products	• Goiter • Mental retardation • Poor growth in infancy when mother is iodide deficient during pregnancy	• Inhibition of thyroid gland function • Upper Level is 1.1 milligrams.
Copper	• Aids in iron metabolism • Works with many antioxidant enzymes • Involved with enzymes of protein metabolism and hormone synthesis	900 micrograms	• Liver • Cocoa • Beans • Nuts • Whole grains • Dried fruits	• Anemia • Low white blood cell count • Poor growth	• Vomiting • Nervous system disorders • Upper Level is 8–10 milligrams.
Fluoride	• Increases resistance of tooth enamel to dental caries	*Men:* 3.8 milligrams *Women:* 3.1 milligrams	• Fluoridated water • Toothpaste • Tea • Seaweed • Dental treatments	• Increased risk of dental caries	• Stomach upset • Mottling (staining) of teeth during development • Bone pain • Upper Level is 10 milligrams for adults.
Chromium	• Enhances insulin action	25–35 micrograms	• Egg yolks • Whole grains • Pork • Nuts • Mushrooms • Beer	• High blood glucose after eating	Caused by industrial contamination, not dietary excesses, so no Upper Level has been set.
Manganese	• Cofactor of some enzymes, such as those involved in carbohydrate metabolism • Works with some antioxidant systems	1.8–2.3 milligrams	• Nuts • Oats • Beans • Tea	None observed in humans	• Nervous system disorders • Upper Level is 11 milligrams.
Molybdenum	• Aids in action of some enzymes	45 micrograms	• Beans • Grains • Nuts	None observed in healthy humans	• Poor growth in laboratory animals • Upper Level is 2 milligrams.

Absorption and Storage of Minerals in the Body

Foods offer us a plentiful supply of many minerals, but the ability of our bodies to absorb and use them varies. The bioavailability of minerals depends on many factors, including many nonmineral components of foods. Age, gender, genetic variables, nutritional status, and diet will affect mineral absorption and bioavailability. Numerous prescription drugs also adversely affect mineral absorption. The mineral content listed in a food composition table is a starting point for estimating the contribution the food will make to our mineral needs.

Components of fiber, such as **phytic acid (phytate)** and **oxalic acid (oxalate),** can limit absorption of some minerals by binding to them. Spinach, for example, contains plenty of calcium, but only about 5% (compared to the average 25% bioavailability of calcium from foods) of it can be absorbed because of the vegetable's high concentration of oxalic acid, which binds calcium. High-fiber diets—particularly those in excess of current recommendations of 25 (adult women) to 38 grams (adult men) of fiber per day—can decrease the absorption of iron, zinc, and possibly other minerals.

Many minerals, such as magnesium, calcium, iron, and copper, are of similar sizes and electrical charges (+2 charge). Having similar sizes and the same electrical charge causes these minerals to compete with each other for absorption; therefore, they affect each other's bioavailabilty. An excess of one mineral decreases the absorption and metabolism of other minerals. For example, a large intake of zinc decreases copper absorption. Therefore, people should avoid taking individual mineral supplements unless a dietary deficiency or medical condition specifically warrants it. Food sources, however, pose little risk for these mineral interactions, giving us another reason to emphasize foods in meeting nutrient needs.

Several beneficial vitamin-mineral interactions occur during nutrient absorption and metabolism. When consumed in conjunction with vitamin C, absorption of certain forms of iron—such as that in plant products—improves. The active form of vitamin D hormone improves calcium absorption. Many vitamins require specific minerals to act as components in their structure and as cofactors for their function. For example, without magnesium or manganese, the thiamin coenzyme cannot function efficiently.

The average North American diet derives minerals from both plant and animal sources. Overall, minerals from animal products are better absorbed than those from plants because binders such as fiber are not present to hinder absorption. The mineral content of plants greatly depends on mineral concentrations of the soil in which they are grown. Vegans must be aware of the potentially poor mineral content of some plant foods and choose some concentrated sources of minerals. Soil conditions have less of an influence on the mineral content of animal products because livestock usually consume a variety of plant products grown from soils of differing mineral contents.

Like vitamins, the majority of the minerals are absorbed in the small intestine. Minor amounts may be absorbed in the stomach, and some sodium and potassium are absorbed in the large intestine. After minerals are absorbed, some travel freely in the bloodstream, but many are carried by specific transport proteins to their sites of action or storage. Calcium is one example of a mineral that can travel as an ion in the blood or bound to a blood protein called albumin. Iron, on the other hand, has damaging effects in its unbound form, so it is transported bound to proteins, such as transferrin. Minerals are stored in various tissues throughout the body. Some minerals must remain in the bloodstream to maintain fluid balance and supply body functions. Others, such as calcium, phosphorus, magnesium, and fluoride, are stored mainly in bones. Iron, copper, zinc, and many trace minerals are stored in the liver. Still others are stored in muscle tissue, organs, or glands.

Mineral Toxicities

Excessive mineral intake, especially of trace minerals such as iron and copper, can have toxic results. For many trace minerals, the gap between just enough and too much is small. Taking minerals as supplements poses the biggest threat for mineral

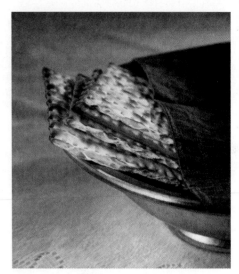

▲ If grains are leavened with yeast, as they are in bread making, enzymes produced by the yeast can break some of the bonds between phytic acid and minerals. This increases mineral absorption. The zinc deficiencies found among some Middle Eastern populations are attributed partly to their consumption of unleavened breads, such as matzo, resulting in low bioavailability of dietary zinc.

phytic acid (phytate) A constituent of plant fibers that binds positive ions to its multiple phosphate groups.

oxalic acid (oxalate) An organic acid found in spinach, rhubarb, and sweet potatoes that can depress the absorption of certain minerals present in the food, such as calcium.

CRITICAL THINKING

Gwen follows a vegetarian diet. What factors in plant food may limit the bioavailability of minerals, such as calcium and zinc, in her diet?

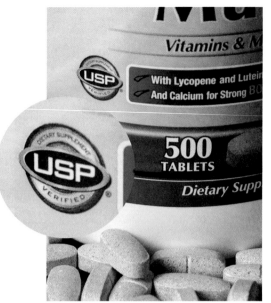

▲ Look for the USP symbol on your vitamin or mineral supplement.

toxicity, whereas food sources are unlikely culprits. Mineral supplements exceeding current standards for mineral needs—especially those that supply more than 100% of the Daily Values on supplement labels—should be taken only under a physician's supervision. The Daily Values are for the most part higher than our current standards (e.g., Recommended Dietary Allowances [RDA]) for mineral needs. Without close monitoring, doses of minerals should not exceed any Upper Level set on a long-term basis.

The potential for toxicity is not the only reason to carefully consider the use of mineral supplements. Harmful interactions with other nutrients are possible. Also, contamination of mineral supplements—with lead, for example—is a possibility. Use of brands approved by the United States Pharmacopeia (USP) lessens this risk. Even with the best intentions, people can harm themselves using mineral supplements.

Preservation of Minerals in Foods

Minerals are found in plant and animal foods (Fig. 8-4), but as you previously read, the bioavailability of minerals varies widely. Minerals are not typically lost from animal sources during processing, storage, or cooking; but for plant sources, significant amounts may be lost during food processing. When grains are refined, the final products have lost the majority of their vitamin E, many B vitamins, and trace minerals. The more refined a plant food, as in the case of white flour, the lower its mineral content. During the enrichment of refined grain products, iron is the only mineral added, whereas the selenium, zinc, copper, and other minerals lost during refinement are not replaced. Following the recommendation of the 2010 Dietary Guidelines for Americans to "make half your grains whole" will effectively preserve the mineral content of foods.

FIGURE 8-4 ▶ Certain groups of MyPlate are especially rich sources of various minerals. This is true for the minerals listed. Each mineral may also be found in other groups but in lower amounts. Other trace minerals are also present in moderate amounts in many groups. With regard to the grains group, whole-grain varieties are the richest sources of most trace minerals listed.

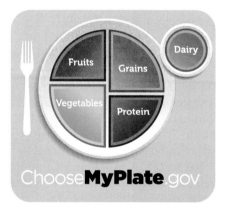

MyPlate:
Sources of Minerals

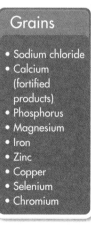

Grains

- Sodium chloride
- Calcium (fortified products)
- Phosphorus
- Magnesium
- Iron
- Zinc
- Copper
- Selenium
- Chromium

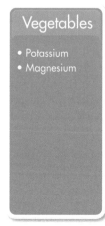

Vegetables

- Potassium
- Magnesium

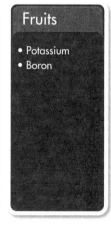

Fruits

- Potassium
- Boron

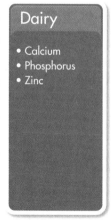

Dairy

- Calcium
- Phosphorus
- Zinc

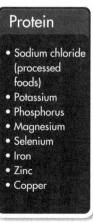

Protein

- Sodium chloride (processed foods)
- Potassium
- Phosphorus
- Magnesium
- Selenium
- Iron
- Zinc
- Copper

8.3 The Functional Roles of Micronutrients

The next four chapters will explore the vitamins and minerals from a functional perspective. The micronutrients will be grouped and discussed as they apply to various metabolic roles in the body. Keep in mind that each vitamin and mineral has multiple roles in metabolism. For example, calcium, best known for its role in bone formation, is also crucial for the transmission of nerve impulses through the body and plays a role in blood clotting. Vitamin C contributes to cellular antioxidant function, bone health, and metabolism of proteins. At all levels—cellular, tissue, organ, and whole body—vitamins and minerals clearly play important and interrelated roles in maintaining healthy body functions.

Enzymes, Coenzymes, and Cofactors

Before moving ahead in your study of the functional roles of vitamins and minerals, it is important to understand how enzymes work. **Enzymes** are catalysts for biochemical reactions in living organisms. A catalyst is a compound that speeds the rate of a reaction but is not altered by the reaction. Most of the chemical reactions in the body would not occur (or would occur only at very slow rates) in the absence of catalysts. As you will learn in Chapter 10, enzymes are crucial players in antioxidant reactions, which neutralize free radicals in the body. In Chapter 12, you will see that enzymes allow for the breakdown of carbohydrates, lipids, and proteins to generate energy. They also catalyze synthetic reactions, such as the assembly of triglycerides for storage in adipose tissue. These are the roles of just a few of the enzymes in the human body—thousands of other enzymes have been identified and studied.

Typically, enzymes are made of proteins, but many such proteins require the aid of another compound—a **cofactor**—for biological activity (Fig. 8-5). Frequently, the assisting compounds are one or more vitamins or minerals. A cofactor is a general term referring to any organic or inorganic substance that binds to an enzyme to aid enzyme activity. A **coenzyme** is one type of cofactor that is organic. In our discussion of vitamins and minerals, vitamins (organic molecules) are called coenzymes and minerals (inorganic molecules) are called cofactors.

Requirements for an enzyme and its cofactors are specific, with little or no enzymatic activity observed if another cofactor is substituted for the required one. The B vitamins function as coenzymes in many chemical reactions of energy metabolism. For example, thiamin is part of the coenzyme thiamin pyrophosphate, which catalyzes several reactions in carbohydrate and protein metabolism. Minerals are required as cofactors for activation of about 30% of all known enzymes. Selenium's role in the function of glutathione peroxidase, one of the body's antioxidant enzyme systems, is one example.

enzyme A compound that speeds the rate of a chemical reaction but is not altered by the reaction. Almost all enzymes are proteins (some are made of genetic material).

cofactor A substance (e.g., mineral) that binds to a specific region on a protein, such as an enzyme, and is necessary for the protein's function.

coenzyme A compound (e.g., water-soluble vitamin) that combines with an inactive enzyme to form a catalytically active form. In this manner, coenzymes aid in enzyme function.

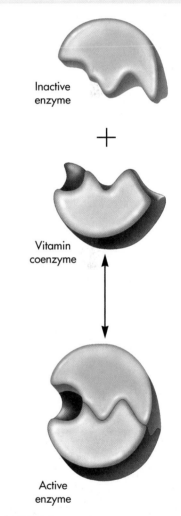

FIGURE 8-5 ► Coenzymes, such as those formed from B vitamins, aid in the function of various enzymes. Without the coenzyme, the enzyme cannot function, and deficiency symptoms associated with the missing vitamin eventually appear. Health-food stores sell the coenzyme forms of some vitamins. These more expensive forms of vitamins are unnecessary. The body makes all the coenzymes it needs from vitamin precursors.

NEWSWORTHY NUTRITION Multivitamin use linked to lower heart attack risk

A study of more than 30,000 Swedish women revealed an association between multivitamin use and approximately 25% reduced risk of heart attacks. The data came from a survey regarding diet, supplement use, and lifestyle that was part of a 10-year prospective cohort study. Possible explanations for a link between multivitamin use and heart attack risk include antioxidant effects, the homocysteine-lowering ability of certain B vitamins, or heart-protecting effects of some minerals, such as potassium and magnesium. These data are promising but need to be confirmed by randomized, controlled trials. In an epidemiological study, many lifestyle and genetic factors could influence heart attack risk. For example, dietary supplements are generally used by individuals who have other health-promoting habits. It is possible that multivitamin use is simply a marker of a healthy lifestyle (see also Further Reading 2).

Source: Rautiainen S and others: Multivitamin use and the risk of myocardial infarction: A population-based cohort of Swedish women. *American Journal of Clinical Nutrition* 92:1251, 2010.

connect | NUTRITION **Check out the Connect site** www.mcgrawhillconnect.com **to further explore research for and against regular use of multivitamins.**

Fluid and Electrolyte Balance

Chapter 9 focuses on the roles of the micronutrients in fluid and electrolyte balance. Water balance requires sodium, potassium, chloride, and phosphorus. Levels of these minerals in the blood are tightly regulated by the body, and imbalances can have dire consequences. In addition to maintaining the delicate balance between intracellular and extracellular water, these minerals participate in the transmission of nerve impulses and acid-base balance, which will be discussed briefly in Chapter 9.

Antioxidant Systems

Chapter 10 will enhance your understanding of the body's antioxidant systems and how various vitamins and minerals take part in protecting tissues from oxidative damage. Some vitamins and minerals, as already discussed, aid in antioxidant function as components of antioxidant enzymes, such as glutathione peroxidase. In other cases, the vitamin itself can function as an antioxidant. Vitamin E, vitamin C, vitamin A and its precursor carotenoids, and selenium are discussed in Chapter 10. In addition, the roles of beneficial plant chemicals in protection of human health will be explored.

Building Bones

In Chapter 11, you will learn how micronutrients are vital to bone health. When we think of bone, we often imagine the hard, lifeless architecture of a skeleton hanging in the back of our high school science classroom. However, bone is a living and dynamic tissue that supports growth, houses nerves and blood vessels, produces blood cells, and helps regulate blood levels of certain minerals. Chapter 11 explores the roles of vitamin D, vitamin K, calcium, phosphorus, magnesium, and fluoride in bone health.

MAKING DECISIONS

Sulfur is a Major Mineral With No Known Requirement

Sulfur is found in many important compounds in the body, such as some amino acids (e.g., methionine) and vitamins (e.g., biotin and thiamin). Sulfur helps in the balance of acids and bases in the body and is an important part of the liver's drug-detoxifying pathways. Proteins supply the sulfur we need, so it is not an essential nutrient *per se*. Sulfur is naturally a part of a healthy diet. Sulfur compounds (e.g., sulfites) are also used to preserve foods (see Chapter 16).

Energy Metabolism

Chapter 12 delves into the roles of vitamins and minerals in energy metabolism. Although vitamins and minerals yield no energy to the body, they often participate as cofactors or coenzymes in energy-yielding reactions, as introduced previously. The B vitamins are integrally involved in metabolism of the macronutrients.

Immune Function

Recall from Chapter 3 that the immune system is the body's defense against pathogens. Skin, intestinal cells, and white blood cells operate together to fend off infections. Adequate protein and essential fatty acids support the immune system. As for micronutrients, optimal immune function relies on vitamin A, some B vitamins, vitamin C, vitamin D, vitamin E, chromium, copper, selenium, iron, and zinc. Each of these nutrients has multiple functional roles, which will be detailed in other sections of the book; but the roles of micronutrients in immunity are summarized in Chapter 12.

Blood Health

Chapter 12 also presents the roles of micronutrients in the maintenance of blood health. Blood health encompasses clotting ability and the transport of oxygen, nutrients, and waste products. Vitamin K and calcium participate in blood clotting. The health of blood cells is influenced by iron, copper, folate, vitamin B-6, and vitamin B-12.

Micronutrients Are Multitaskers

Micronutrients are vital to every aspect of human health. Although requirements for vitamins and minerals are small, depriving the body of any one of these important dietary factors can be debilitating or deadly. Although dietary supplements may be useful under some circumstances, foods are safe, effective, and enjoyable sources of vitamins and minerals for most healthy children and adults. As you study the next four chapters, prepare to be amazed by the intricate interplay of micronutrients and human health.

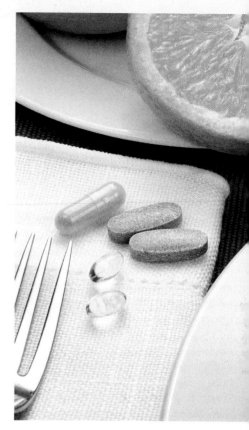

▲ It is better to get nutrients from foods or dietary supplements?

CONCEPT CHECK

Vitamins and minerals play important and interrelated roles in the body. In some cases, one micronutrient serves multiple functions. Fluid balance depends on sodium, potassium, chloride, and phosphorus. Vitamin E, vitamin C, vitamin A, carotenoids, and selenium function in the body's antioxidant systems. Calcium, phosphorus, vitamin D, magnesium, and fluoride work together to support bone health. Use of macronutrients for fuel relies on B vitamins and several trace minerals as coenzymes or cofactors in reactions of energy metabolism. Also important for energy metabolism, iodide is essential for synthesis of thyroid hormones and chromium is involved in glucose metabolism. Iron, zinc, copper, vitamin K, vitamin B-6, vitamin B-12, and folate are implicated in blood health. Immune function requires vitamin A, some B vitamins, vitamin C, vitamin D, vitamin E, chromium, copper, selenium, iron, and zinc.

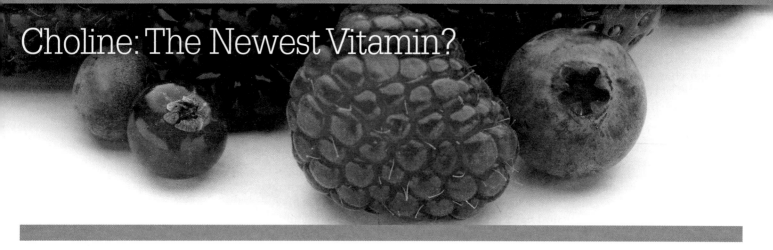

Choline: The Newest Vitamin?

Our knowledge of micronutrients is a relatively recent innovation that continues to evolve. Although certain components of foods have been linked to prevention of diseases since ancient times, the first vitamin was not isolated until 1913—a mere century ago. Over the next 25 years, all the vitamins we know to be essential in the human diet—from A to E—were identified. For choline, a water-soluble compound that is important for many aspects of human health, the story is still unfolding.

In 1998, the Institute of Medicine recognized choline as an essential nutrient. Dietary Reference Intakes were released in 2000. At the time of the DRI report, only limited research on the dietary requirements for choline existed. One study of male volunteers showed decreased choline stores and liver damage when they were fed choline-deficient total parenteral (intravenous) nutrition solutions. Based on this human study, plus laboratory animal studies, choline has been deemed essential, but it is not yet classified as a vitamin.

Functions of Choline

Despite its lack of vitamin status, choline is needed by all cells and plays several important roles in the body.

Cell Membrane Structure

Choline is a precursor for several phospholipids. **Phosphatidylcholine** (also known as **lecithin**) accounts for about half of the phospholipids in cell membranes. Recall from Chapter 5 that phospholipids contribute to the flexibility of cell membranes and also allow for the presence of both water- and fat-soluble compounds in cell membranes. With its role in cell membrane structure, choline is important for the health of every cell and particularly for the health of brain tissue, where it is present in high levels.

Single-Carbon Metabolism

Choline is a precursor for **betaine,** a compound that participates in many chemical reactions that involve the transfer of single-carbon groups in human metabolism. Important examples of metabolic pathways that involve the transfer of single-carbon groups include the synthesis of neurotransmitters, modifications of DNA during embryonic development, and the metabolism of homocysteine. As you will learn in Chapter 12, high levels of homocysteine in the blood are related to increased risk of heart disease. Betaine and the B vitamin folate both donate single-carbon groups to convert homocysteine to another compound, thus reducing levels of homocysteine in the blood. The role of choline in single-carbon metabolism has broad implications, from embryonic development through old age.

Nerve Function and Brain Development

Choline is part of acetylcholine, a neurotransmitter associated with attention, learning, memory, muscle control, and many other functions. Sphingomyelin, a choline-containing phospholipid, is part of the myelin sheath that insulates nerve cells. As already mentioned, brain tissue is particularly high in choline. During pregnancy, the concentration of choline in amniotic fluid is high, supplying choline to the developing brain of the fetus.

Animal studies demonstrate that choline deficiencies during pregnancy lead to poor brain development, learning ability, and memory. The AI for choline is increased during pregnancy and breastfeeding to assist in proper brain development.

Lipid Transport

As part of phospholipids, choline is a component of lipoproteins, which carry lipids through the blood. Choline deficiencies in animals and humans lead to development of fatty liver because lipid transport

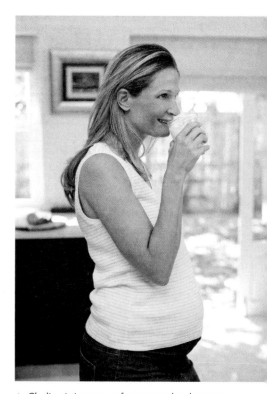

▲ Choline is important for proper development of the fetal brain. Milk and other dairy products supply some choline.

is impaired. Indeed, choline deficiency can lead to high levels of very-low-density lipoproteins and triglycerides in the blood. Compounding its role in homocysteine metabolism, choline deficiency may also contribute to cardiovascular disease due to this negative impact on blood lipids.

Sources of Choline

Choline is widely distributed in foods (Fig. 8-6). Soybeans, egg yolks, beef, cauliflower, almonds, and peanuts are good sources. In addition to natural food sources, lecithin is often added to food products as an emulsifier during processing, so many other foods are sources of choline.

Choline can exist in foods as free choline or as part of other compounds, such as phospholipids. Pancreatic enzymes break down some of the phospholipid forms prior to absorption. Free choline is water soluble and can be absorbed from the small intestine into portal circulation for transport to the liver. Choline that is part of phospholipids, on the other hand, is fat soluble and gets absorbed into the lymphatic system.

To some extent, choline also can be synthesized in the body by a process that involves other nutrients, such as folate and the amino acid methionine. If the body must synthesize choline to meet its needs, functional deficiencies of folate could result.

Eggs (with yolks) are by far the most nutrient-dense source of choline. One whole egg supplies about ¼ of the daily choline needs in a 70-kcal package. However, dietary advice to limit saturated fat and cholesterol discourages frequent intake of egg yolks. Choline researchers suggest that an average of one egg per day would assist in achieving the AI for choline while still supplying less than the 300-milligram-per-day limit for cholesterol.

Dietary Requirements for Choline

The AI for choline for adults is 425 milligrams per day for women or 550 milligrams per day for men (see Further Reading 5). It is unknown whether a dietary supply is essential for infants or children. As already noted, some choline can be synthesized in the body, but recent research indicates that synthesis by the body is not sufficient to meet the body's needs for choline. Nutrition surveys indicate that fewer than 10% of Americans meet the AI for choline. In addition, the AIs do not reflect wide genetic variation in individual choline requirements. Research indicates that at least half the population

Food Sources of Choline

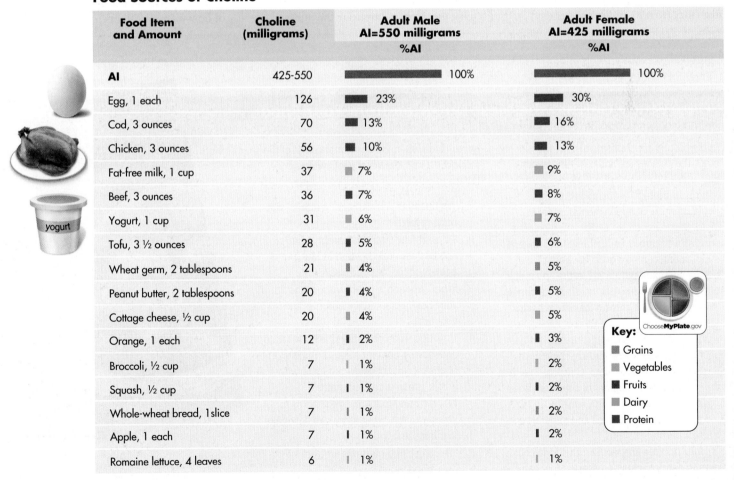

Food Item and Amount	Choline (milligrams)	Adult Male AI=550 milligrams %AI	Adult Female AI=425 milligrams %AI
AI	425-550	100%	100%
Egg, 1 each	126	23%	30%
Cod, 3 ounces	70	13%	16%
Chicken, 3 ounces	56	10%	13%
Fat-free milk, 1 cup	37	7%	9%
Beef, 3 ounces	36	7%	8%
Yogurt, 1 cup	31	6%	7%
Tofu, 3 ½ ounces	28	5%	6%
Wheat germ, 2 tablespoons	21	4%	5%
Peanut butter, 2 tablespoons	20	4%	5%
Cottage cheese, ½ cup	20	4%	5%
Orange, 1 each	12	2%	3%
Broccoli, ½ cup	7	1%	2%
Squash, ½ cup	7	1%	2%
Whole-wheat bread, 1 slice	7	1%	2%
Apple, 1 each	7	1%	2%
Romaine lettuce, 4 leaves	6	1%	1%

Key:
■ Grains
■ Vegetables
■ Fruits
■ Dairy
■ Protein

FIGURE 8-6 ▶ Food sources of choline compared to the AI for adult males and females.

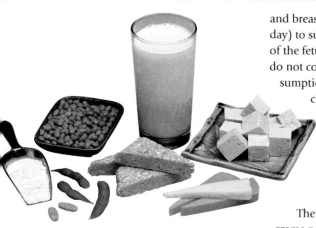

▲ Soy, almonds, and peanuts are natural sources of choline.

has genetic variations that increase dietary requirements for nutrients that serve in single-carbon metabolism, including choline and folate. Thus, even meeting the AI may not provide enough choline to support the body's needs for some people.

The AI for choline increases during pregnancy (to 450 milligrams per day) and breastfeeding (to 550 milligrams per day) to support the brain development of the fetus or infant. Prenatal vitamins do not contain choline. Therefore, consumption of rich dietary sources of choline, such as eggs, is important for pregnant and breastfeeding women.

Upper Level for Choline

The UL for adults is set at 3.5 grams per day. Routinely exceeding the UL will result in a fishy body odor and low blood pressure.

Possible Health Benefits

There are many proposed health benefits for adequate choline intake (see Further Reading 6). For certain, achieving adequate choline intake helps to avoid development of fatty liver. The roles of choline in lipid transport and homocysteine metabolism implicate the nutrient in prevention of cardiovascular disease, as well. Choline also may be useful for preventing or treating cancer or neurological disorders, such as Alzheimer's disease.

Recent research points to a role of adequate choline for the prevention of birth defects. Choline's purported role in prevention of birth defects is similar to that of folate. Both folate and choline are involved in formation of DNA during embryonic development. As you will read in Chapters 12 and 17, problems with DNA formation lead to birth defects. Indeed, animal studies show that maternal choline supplementation during critical stages of embryonic development can improve learning and memory in the offspring. In humans, as well, studies show that babies born to women with low choline intakes have four times higher rates of birth defects as babies born to women with high choline intakes.

Nutrition science is exciting, dynamic, and so immediately applicable to each of our lives. Emerging knowledge on the importance of choline is just one example of how there is still much left to discover.

Case Study Getting the Most Nutrition from Your Food

In the dietary supplements aisle of the grocery store, the choices are endless—and expensive. Julie, a college sophomore, just read the American Dietetic Association's position paper on nutrient supplementation for her class. She learned that dietary supplements, such as a balanced multivitamin and mineral supplement, can be a good back-up plan to ensure adequate nutrition, but the jury is still out when it comes to demonstrating a benefit of dietary supplements for long-term health and longevity. About one-third of Americans regularly take nutrient supplements, but it is usually the people who already consume a healthy diet who take them. Getting more than the recommended amount of a nutrient does not confer additional health benefits. In fact, too much of some vitamins and minerals can lead to toxicity.

Julie decides she would rather focus on getting her nutrients from foods. How can she get the most vitamins and minerals out of the foods she eats? Answer the following questions and check your responses in Appendix A.

1. What factors can damage or reduce vitamins in food?
2. To maximize vitamin content, what should Julie keep in mind as she selects fresh produce for purchase?
3. When produce is out of season, should Julie buy frozen or canned fruits and vegetables?
4. How does food processing affect vitamin and mineral content? Does it make a difference if Julie chooses products with whole grains or refined grains?
5. When storing fruits and vegetables in her apartment, what steps can Julie take to minimize nutrient losses?
6. Which cooking methods are best for preserving vitamin content?

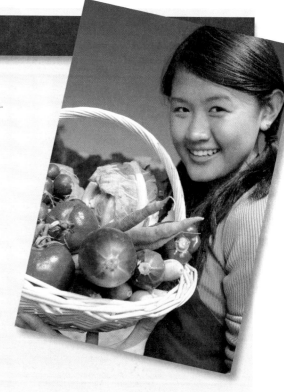

Summary (Numbers refer to numbered sections in the chapter.)

8.1 Vitamins are organic substances required in small amounts in the diet for growth, function, and body maintenance. These can be categorized as fat soluble (vitamins A, D, E, and K) or water soluble (B vitamins and vitamin C). Vitamins cannot be synthesized by the body in adequate amounts to support health, and absence of a vitamin from the diet leads to development of a deficiency disease. Fat-soluble vitamins require dietary fat for absorption and are carried by lipoproteins in the blood. Vitamin toxicity is most likely to occur from megadoses of fat-soluble vitamins because they are readily stored in the body. Intakes of water-soluble vitamins that exceed the storage ability of tissues are typically excreted in urine. Some vitamins are susceptible to destruction by light, heat, air, or alkalinity or may be lost from foods in cooking water or fats.

8.2 Minerals are inorganic elements, some of which are required for human health. Major minerals are required in amounts of 100 milligrams or more per day. These include calcium, phosphorus, magnesium, sulfur, sodium, potassium, and chloride. Trace minerals are required in amounts less than 100 milligrams per day and include iron, zinc, copper, iodine, selenium, molybdenum, fluoride, manganese, and chromium. Other minerals that are present in small amounts in the diet but have no known requirements are called ultratrace minerals. Mineral bioavailability is affected by age, gender, heredity, nutritional status, and other components of the diet. Any toxicities are likely to result from dietary supplementation, not food sources. Refinement greatly reduces mineral content of grain products.

8.3 Vitamins and minerals serve multiple roles in the body but can be grouped by their common functions. The B vitamins, iodide, chromium, magnesium, manganese, molybdenum, and choline are involved in energy metabolism. Immune function depends on vitamins A, C, and E; copper; iron; selenium; and zinc. Bone health relies on vitamins C, D, and K; calcium; phosphorus; magnesium; fluoride, boron, and silicon. Fluid and electrolyte balance is regulated by sodium, potassium, chloride, and phosphorus. The health of blood cells requires vitamins B-6, B-12, and K; folate; iron; copper; and zinc. Vitamins A (and carotenoids), C, and E; selenium; zinc; copper; magnesium; and manganese function in the body's antioxidant systems.

N&YH Choline is an essential nutrient, but has not yet been classified as a vitamin. As a component of phospholipids, it contributes to cell membrane structure, the myelin sheath that surrounds nerves, and functions in lipid transport. Like folate, choline plays a role in single-carbon metabolism, which has implications for prevention of birth defects, cancer, and heart disease. Egg yolks, meats, dairy products, soybeans, and nuts are good food sources of choline.

Check Your Knowledge (Answers to the following questions are below.)

1. An organic compound needed in small amounts by the body for normal growth, function, and maintenance is a
   a. vitamin.
   b. major mineral.
   c. trace mineral.
   d. phytochemical.

2. An inorganic element used by the body in chemical reactions and to form body structures is a
   a. vitamin.
   b. mineral.
   c. coenzyme.
   d. phytochemical.

3. Which of the following is a water-soluble vitamin?
   a. vitamin A
   b. vitamin K
   c. thiamin
   d. choline

4. Which of the following is a trace mineral?
   a. selenium
   b. phosphorus
   c. calcium
   d. silicon

5. Fat-soluble vitamins are absorbed into
   a. plasma.
   b. serum.
   c. lymph.
   d. urine.

6. A megadose of which of the following micronutrients is most likely to lead to toxicity?
   a. vitamin A
   b. niacin
   c. vitamin K
   d. magnesium

7. Certain compounds in plant foods, such as phytic acid, can limit the bioavailability of
   a. vitamins.
   b. minerals.
   c. phytochemicals.
   d. choline.

8. Which of the following cooking methods is best for preservation of vitamins in foods?
   a. boiling
   b. deep-frying
   c. stir-frying
   d. pressure cooking

9. Vitamin A participates in
   a. antioxidant systems.
   b. fluid and electrolyte balance.
   c. bone health.
   d. All of the above.

10. Choline is important for
    a. nerve transmission.
    b. prevention of birth defects.
    c. learning and memory.
    d. All of the above.

Answer Key: 1. a (LO 8.1), 2. b (LO 8.1), 3. c (LO 8.2), 4. a (LO 8.3), 5. c (LO 8.4), 6. a (LO 8.4), 7. b (LO 8.5), 8. c (LO 8.5), 9. a (LO 8.6), 10. d (LO 8.7)

Study Questions (Numbers refer to Learning Outcomes)

1. Compare and contrast vitamins and minerals. (**LO 8.1**)

2. What are two defining characteristics of vitamins? (**LO 8.1**)

3. List two examples of fat-soluble vitamins and two examples of water-soluble vitamins. (**LO 8.2**)

4. Provide two examples of major minerals and two examples of trace minerals. (**LO 8.3**)

5. What are ultratrace minerals? (**LO 8.3**)

6. Explain why fat-soluble vitamins are more likely to cause toxicity than water-soluble vitamins. (**LO 8.4**)

7. List two components of plant foods that limit mineral bioavailability. (**LO 8.5**)

8. Contrast the micronutrient content of whole versus refined grains by

listing three examples of differences in vitamin or mineral content. (**LO 8.5**)

9. Provide one example of a micronutrient that has more than one functional role in the body. List its multiple functional roles. (**LO 8.6**)

10. List three functions of choline in the body. (**LO 8.7**)

What Would You Choose Recommendations

The B-complex supplements shown at the beginning of the chapter all provide vitamins in excess of the Daily Value for most nutrients listed. Were you surprised to see that one of these supplements provided 10,000% of the Daily Value for one vitamin? When it comes to micronutrients, more is not always better. For some vitamins and minerals, such as vitamin A, there is a fairly narrow range between not enough and too much. Excess intakes of the fat-soluble vitamins and some minerals, especially, can lead to toxicity. For these water-soluble B vitamins, however, the excesses will be excreted in the urine.

Supplement C contains the B vitamins in their coenzyme forms "for enhanced absorption." B vitamins are present in free and coenzyme forms in the foods you eat, but the coenzyme forms are broken down by digestive enzymes prior to absorption. The coenzymes will be reformed as needed in the cells. Thus, there is no advantage of consuming the coenzyme forms of vitamins.

Though the megadoses shown here are not likely to harm your health, they are unnecessary and might just harm your bank account. Supplement A costs $7.99 for 100 capsules, Supplement B costs $17.99 for 100 capsules, and Supplement C costs $19.99 for 60 capsules. That is kind of pricey for vitamin-fortified urine!

In the absence of a specific medical need, it is not necessary to supplement with more than 100% of the Daily Value for any nutrient. In fact, for the most part, typical American diets provide ample B vitamins. Grain products are enriched with thiamin, niacin, riboflavin, and folate. Fortified breakfast cereals are especially rich sources of B vitamins and many other micronutrients (see the Rate Your Plate activity at the end of this chapter). Consuming a diet that adheres to the 2010 Dietary Guidelines for Americans and MyPlate will provide enough B vitamins to meet daily needs. If you feel that a supplement would be a good back-up plan for days when your dietary intake is less than

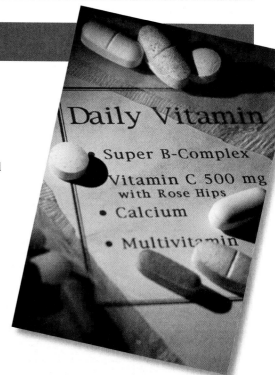

adequate, a balanced multivitamin-mineral supplement providing no more than 100% of the DV for nutrients is a prudent idea (see Further Readings 1 and 4).

Supplement A		
	Amount Per Serving	% DV
Thiamin (as thiamin mononitrate)	50 mg	3333%
Riboflavin	50 mg	2941%
Niacin (as niacinamide)	50 mg	250%
Vitamin B-6 (as pyridoxine hydrochloride)	50 mg	2500%
Folic acid	400 mcg	100%
Vitamin B-12 (as cyanocobalamin)	50 mcg	833%
Biotin	50 mcg	17%
Pantothenic acid (as calcium d-pantothenate)	50 mg	500%

Supplement B		
	Amount Per Serving	% DV
Thiamin (as thiamin mononitrate)	150 mg	10,000%
Riboflavin	150 mg	8824%
Niacin (as niacinamide)	150 mg	750%
Vitamin B-6 (as pyridoxine hydrochloride)	150 mg	7500%
Folic acid	400 mcg	100%
Vitamin B-12 (as cyanocobalamin)	150 mcg	2500%
Biotin	150 mcg	50%
Pantothenic acid (as calcium d-pantothenate)	150 mg	1500%

Supplement C with coenzyme forms of B vitamins		
	Amount Per Serving	% DV
Thiamin (as thiamin HCl, thiamin cocarboxylase)	50 mg	3333%
Riboflavin (as riboflavin 5' phosphate)	50 mg	2941%
Niacin (as inositol hexaniacinate)	100 mg	500%
Vitamin B-6 (as pyridoxine HCl, pyridoxal 5'phosphate)	80 mg	4000%
Folic acid	800 mcg	200%
Vitamin B-12 (as dibencozide methylcobalamin)	500 mcg	8333%
d-Biotin	200 mcg	67%
Pantothenic acid (as pantethine, d-calcium pantothenate)	50 mg	500%

Further Readings

1. ADA Reports: Position of the American Dietetic Association: Nutrient supplementation. *Journal of the American Dietetic Association* 109:2073, 2009.

   The best nutrition-based strategy for promoting optimal health and reducing the risk of chronic disease is to choose a wide variety of nutrient-dense foods. Additional nutrients from supplements can help some people meet their nutritional needs as set by science-based nutrition standards (e.g., the Dietary Reference Intakes).

2. Don't jump to conclusions on multivitamin heart-attack protection. *Tufts University Health & Nutrition Letter* 28:1, 2011.

   Results of a recent study linked multivitamin use with lower risk of heart attacks, but experts caution consumers that other factors besides multivitamin use are likely involved. In epidemiological studies, it can be difficult to discern the effects of confounding variables. For example, use of multivitamins may be a marker for an overall healthy lifestyle that includes healthy foods, physical activity, and avoidance of tobacco.

3. Fulgoni VL 3rd and others: Foods, fortificants, and supplements: Where do Americans get their nutrients? *Journal of Nutrition* 141:1847, 2011.

   Estimating the actual nutrient intakes of Americans is complicated by the consumption of many fortified and enriched foods and dietary supplements. The researchers used data collected from the National Health and Nutrition Examination Survey from 2003 to 2006 to determine usual nutrient intakes compared to the DRIs. Results indicate that most Americans achieve adequate intakes (from the combination of foods, fortified foods, and supplements) of B vitamins and the minerals zinc, phosphorus, iron, copper, and selenium. Micronutrients of concern include all the fat-soluble vitamins; vitamin C; and the minerals calcium, magnesium, and potassium. Fortification/enrichment of foods and use of dietary supplements make a significant contribution to micronutrient intake for Americans, with little evidence of micronutrient excess.

4. NIH State-of-the-Science Conference Statement on Multivitamin/Mineral Supplements and Chronic Disease Prevention. *NIH Consensus State-of-the-Science Statements* 23(2):1, 2006.

   Use of multivitamins/minerals (MVMs) has grown rapidly over the past several decades. Due in part to the fortification of foods, there is still insufficient knowledge about the actual amount of total nutrients that Americans consume from diet and supplements. The cumulative effects of supplementation and fortification have raised safety concerns about exceeding upper levels. Most studies do not provide strong evidence for beneficial health-related effects of supplements taken singly, in pairs, or in combinations of three or more. Although there is encouraging evidence of increased bone mineral density and decreased fractures in postmenopausal women who use calcium and vitamin D supplements, several other studies provide disturbing evidence of risk, such as increased lung cancer risk with beta-carotene use among smokers. The present evidence is insufficient to recommend either for or against the use of MVMs by the American public to prevent chronic disease.

5. Webb D: Choline—rethinking the dietary requirement. *Today's Dietitian* 13:38, 2011.

   Although still not considered a vitamin, choline was recognized as an essential nutrient in 1998, and useful databases of choline content of food have been available since 2004. This article reviews the functions, dietary requirements, and dietary sources of choline and examines the consequences of choline deficiency and toxicity.

6. Zeisel SH and da Costa K: Choline: An essential nutrient for public health. *Nutrition Reviews* 67:615, 2009.

   The essentiality of choline for human health is well documented, but recent research indicates Americans are not consuming enough of this nutrient. Health professionals must educate themselves about the importance of choline, especially during critical times of pregnancy and breastfeeding, and encourage individuals to consume adequate food sources of choline.

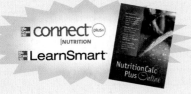

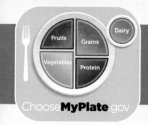

RATE YOUR PLATE

Throughout the chapters on vitamins and minerals, you will see breakfast cereals described as enriched, fortified, cold, or ready to eat. What do these terms mean? The cereal you pour out of the box, add milk to, and enjoy is called ready-to-eat or cold cereal. All cereals have a standard enrichment (or fortification) with iron, niacin, riboflavin, thiamin, and folic acid. Others are enriched at a higher level or with more nutrients. In this section, when you read "enriched" or "fortified" cereals, it is this latter group that we are referring to. The way you can tell is by reading the label. See for yourself in the following table.

Cereal A has the traditional supplementation in the range of 25% to 35%. Iron is a bit higher. Cereal B, the enriched or fortified choice, contains 100% of the DV for select vitamins and minerals, especially the B vitamins and iron. Manufacturers vary which nutrients and which cereals they wish to enrich.

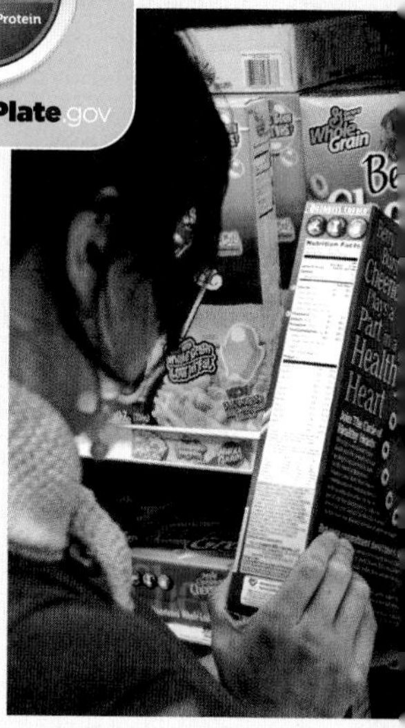

Nutrient	Cereal A (1 ounce) % DV	Cereal B (1 ounce) % DV	Your Favorite Cereal % DV	One Cup of Milk % DV
Vitamin A	25	15		
Vitamin C	25	100		
Calcium	0	0		
Iron	50	100		
Vitamin D	10	10		
Vitamin E	25	100		
Thiamin	25	100		
Riboflavin	25	100		
Niacin	25	100		
Vitamin B-6	25	100		
Folic acid	25	100		
Pantothenic acid	—*	100		
Phosphorus	4	4		
Magnesium	—*	4		
Zinc	—*	100		

*Information not provided on label.

Locate a nutrition facts panel for one of your favorite breakfast cereals. In the blank spaces in the table, record the % DV for each nutrient provided by one serving. If some data are missing, fill in the blanks with an asterisk. Based on your observations, answer the following questions.

1. Is your favorite cereal fortified? How can you tell?

   _____

   _____

   _____

2. Examine the calorie, fat, and sugar content listed on your Nutrition Facts panel. How does the cereal compare to the recommendations of the Dietary Guidelines for Americans and other health authorities to limit calories, fat, and added sugars?

   _____

   _____

   _____

3. Now locate the Nutrition Facts panel of your favorite type of milk and record its % DV for one cup in the blank spaces in the table. For which nutrients does the addition of milk further enhance the nutritional value?

   _____

   _____

   _____

4. Which special population groups can especially benefit from daily use of a fortified breakfast cereal?

   _____

   _____

   _____

5. What could you eat with your breakfast cereal to build a meal that meets MyPlate standards?

   _____

   _____

   _____

Chapter 9 Nutrients Involved in Fluid and Electrolyte Balance

Student Learning Outcomes

Chapter 9 is designed to allow you to:

9.1 List and explain the functions of water in the body.

9.2 List the four minerals that function as electrolytes.

9.3 Describe how electrolytes control fluid balance, acid-base balance, and nerve impulse transmission.

9.4 Describe the control mechanisms that regulate water intake and output.

9.5 Identify recommended intakes and sources of water.

9.6 Describe the health consequences of dehydration.

9.7 List dietary sources of the electrolyte minerals.

9.8 Describe factors that can contribute to the development of hypertension.

What Would You Choose?

Water is the best choice for everyday hydration—it quenches thirst without calories. There are currently many "water" choices available. Do you need water that contains vitamins and minerals? What is the difference between spring water and mineral water? Is bottled water safer to drink than tap water? As you peruse the convenience store shelves, which is the healthiest choice to take along to the student recreation center for your workout?

a 20-ounce reusable bottle filled with tap water

b 16.9-ounce bottle of Aquafina® Pure Water

c 16.9-ounce bottle of San Pellegrino Mineral Water

d 20-ounce bottle of vitaminwater®

 Think about your choice as you read Chapter 9, then see our recommendations at the end of the chapter. To learn more about the costs and benefits of bottled water, check out the Connect site: www.mcgrawhillconnect.com

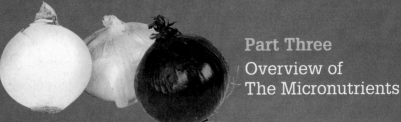

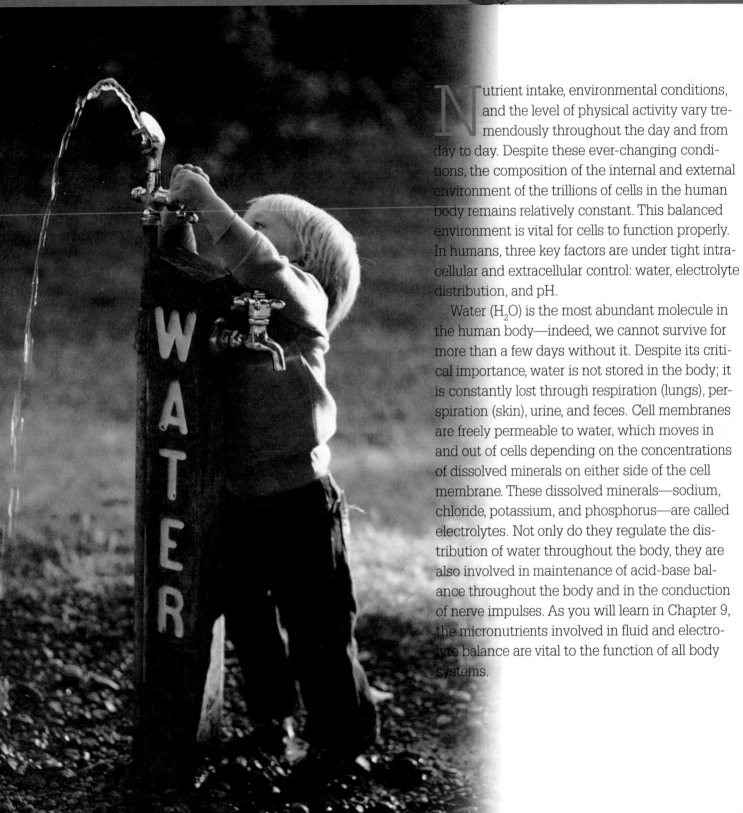

Nutrient intake, environmental conditions, and the level of physical activity vary tremendously throughout the day and from day to day. Despite these ever-changing conditions, the composition of the internal and external environment of the trillions of cells in the human body remains relatively constant. This balanced environment is vital for cells to function properly. In humans, three key factors are under tight intracellular and extracellular control: water, electrolyte distribution, and pH.

Water (H_2O) is the most abundant molecule in the human body—indeed, we cannot survive for more than a few days without it. Despite its critical importance, water is not stored in the body; it is constantly lost through respiration (lungs), perspiration (skin), urine, and feces. Cell membranes are freely permeable to water, which moves in and out of cells depending on the concentrations of dissolved minerals on either side of the cell membrane. These dissolved minerals—sodium, chloride, potassium, and phosphorus—are called electrolytes. Not only do they regulate the distribution of water throughout the body, they are also involved in maintenance of acid-base balance throughout the body and in the conduction of nerve impulses. As you will learn in Chapter 9, the micronutrients involved in fluid and electrolyte balance are vital to the function of all body systems.

Refresh Your Memory

As you begin the study of water and other nutrients involved in fluid balance in Chapter 9, you may want to review:

- Cell structure and function, digestion and absorption of nutrients, cardiovascular function, immunity, and endocrine function in Chapter 3.
- The functions of phosphorus related to bone health in Chapter 11.

9.1 Intracellular and Extracellular Fluid Distribution—A Delicate Balance Between Water and Electrolytes

electrolytes Minerals that separate into positively or negatively charged ions in water. They are able to transmit an electrical current.

intracellular fluid Fluid contained within a cell; it represents about two-thirds of body fluid.

ion A positively or negatively charged atom.

extracellular fluid Fluid found outside the cells; it represents about one-third of all body fluid.

osmosis The passage of water through a membrane from a less concentrated compartment to a more concentrated compartment.

Each cell of the body is surrounded by a membrane. This membrane allows water to pass freely through it. Water found inside the cell membrane is part of the **intracellular fluid.** Intracellular fluid accounts for 63% of fluid in the body. The remaining body fluid is found outside of cells in one of two extracellular spaces: (1) the fluid portion of blood (plasma) and lymph, accounting for 7% of body fluid; or (2) the fluid between cells (interstitial), making up 30% of the body fluid (Fig. 9-1).

Although water can freely travel into and out of cells across the cell membrane, the body controls the amount of water in the intracellular and extracellular compartments mainly by controlling ion concentrations. **Ions** are minerals that dissolve in water and are either positively (+) or negatively (−) charged. These charged ions allow the transfer of electrical current so they are called **electrolytes.** Four electrolytes predominate: sodium (Na^+) and chloride (Cl^-) are primarily found in the **extracellular fluid,** and potassium (K^+) and phosphate (PO_4^-) are the principal electrolytes in the intracellular fluid (Fig. 9-2).

The term **osmosis** is used to describe the passage of water through a membrane from an area of lower electrolyte concentration to an area of higher electrolyte concentration. Where ions move, water follows passively. Under normal conditions, the flow of electrolytes is controlled in such a way that water movement into and out of

FRANK & ERNEST by Bob Thaves

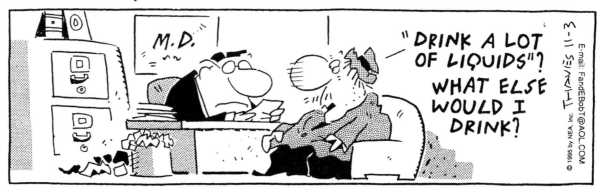

Replacing fluids—water as part of foods, beverages, and water itself—is an important daily task. Why is this so critical for maintaining health? Why are infants, athletes, and older adults particularly at risk for dehydration? Are you at risk? How does water interact with some of the minerals used by the body? Chapter 9 provides some answers.

FRANK & ERNEST © Reprinted by permission of Newspaper Enterprise Association, Inc.

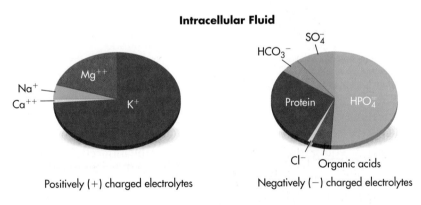

FIGURE 9-1 ▶ Fluid compartments in the body. Total fluid volume is about 40 liters (about 165 cups).

Fluid compartments

3 Liters
Blood plasma

14 Liters
Fluid between cells
Lymph
Gastrointestinal fluid
Spinal column fluid
Fluid in eyes
Tears
Synovial fluid (in joints)

25 Liters
Fluid found inside every type of cell (e.g., blood, bone, muscle, adipose)

Extracellular fluid (37%)

Intracellular fluid (63%)

Total fluid (40 liters)

Liters

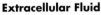

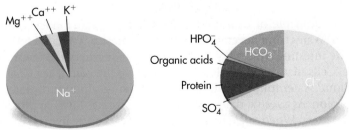

Intracellular Fluid

Na$^+$
Ca^{++}
Mg^{++}
K$^+$

Positively (+) charged electrolytes

SO$_4^-$
HCO$_3^-$
Protein
HPO$_4^=$
Cl$^-$
Organic acids

Negatively (−) charged electrolytes

Extracellular Fluid

Mg^{++}
Ca^{++}
K$^+$
Na$^+$

Positively (+) charged electrolytes

HPO$_4^-$
Organic acids
Protein
SO$_4^-$
HCO$_3^-$
Cl$^-$

Negatively (−) charged electrolytes

FIGURE 9-2 ▶ Intracellular and extracellular percent distribution of electrolytes. Each figure shows the percent distribution of electrolytes inside and outside cells. The total concentration of positively and negatively charged electrolytes is equal in the intracellular and extracellular fluid.

FIGURE 9-3 ▶ Effects of various ion concentrations in a fluid on plant and human cells. This shows the process of osmosis. Fluid is shifting into and out of the cells in response to changing ion concentrations in the fluid surrounding the cells.

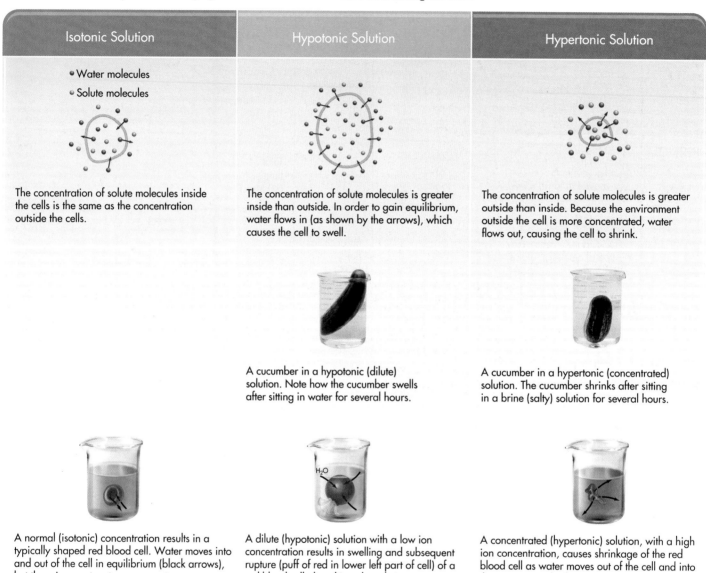

Isotonic Solution	Hypotonic Solution	Hypertonic Solution
• Water molecules • Solute molecules		
The concentration of solute molecules inside the cells is the same as the concentration outside the cells.	The concentration of solute molecules is greater inside than outside. In order to gain equilibrium, water flows in (as shown by the arrows), which causes the cell to swell.	The concentration of solute molecules is greater outside than inside. Because the environment outside the cell is more concentrated, water flows out, causing the cell to shrink.
	A cucumber in a hypotonic (dilute) solution. Note how the cucumber swells after sitting in water for several hours.	A cucumber in a hypertonic (concentrated) solution. The cucumber shrinks after sitting in a brine (salty) solution for several hours.
A normal (isotonic) concentration results in a typically shaped red blood cell. Water moves into and out of the cell in equilibrium (black arrows), but there is no net water movement.	A dilute (hypotonic) solution with a low ion concentration results in swelling and subsequent rupture (puff of red in lower left part of cell) of a red blood cell placed into the solution.	A concentrated (hypertonic) solution, with a high ion concentration, causes shrinkage of the red blood cell as water moves out of the cell and into the concentrated solution.

the cell is in equilibrium (Fig. 9-3). However, if the intracellular concentration of electrolytes is greater than the extracellular concentration, water will freely flow into the cell. If too much water flows in, the cell can burst—similar to filling a balloon with too much air. The opposite can also occur, where the intracellular concentration of electrolytes is relatively low compared to the extracellular environment and water will exit the cell, leading to cell shrinkage.

The principle of osmosis is used by the digestive tract to absorb water from the colon. Water from beverages, foods, and intestinal tract secretions make the contents of the intestinal tract very high in water as it enters the colon from the small intestine. Cells that line the colon lumen (inside the colon, see Chapter 2) actively absorb sodium. Water follows sodium, causing a large amount of water to be absorbed from the colon. As a result, daily water loss from feces is low—approximately 150 milliliters, or 5 ounces. When taken to the extreme, or especially in cases of very vulnerable people (infants, very old), osmosis can lead to life-threatening medical conditions in response to long bouts of diarrhea and vomiting. The large loss of fluid from the intestinal tract causes a loss of water from the extracellular space, resulting in a high concentration of electrolytes in the extracellular space. Intracellular water exits the cells in an attempt to balance the water loss from the extracellular space. There is then an imbalance in fluid and electrolyte concentration across the cell membrane. This imbalance can lead to a decreased ability of cells to function normally. In the heart, this imbalance can lead to a decreased ability of the heart to pump blood and, ultimately, to cardiac failure.

9.2 Electrolytes—Essential for Nerve Function and Acid-Base Balance

Sodium, potassium, chloride, and phosphate ions are found in very different concentrations on either side of the cell membrane, as shown in Figure 9-2. These ions are charged, so there is an electrochemical gradient across the cell membrane. Let's investigate this a little further.

All membranes contain an energy-dependent pump that can transfer sodium from inside to outside the cell. When Na^+ is actively pumped out of the cell, K^+ enters the cell in an attempt to balance the loss of the positively charged sodium ions. The inside of the cell becomes slightly negatively charged relative to the outside. This difference in electrical charge allows transmission of nerve impulses (Fig. 9-4).

Nerve impulses are transmitted along a cell by the following process. In response to stimulation, positively charged sodium ions rush into the cell, causing the cell to become less negatively charged. The change in electrical charge is transmitted from one cell to the next (like dominoes falling), which leads to the electrical signal being transmitted from one nerve cell to the next. Immediately after the change in electrolyte balance, sodium is actively pumped out of the cell to reestablish the normal electrolyte balance.

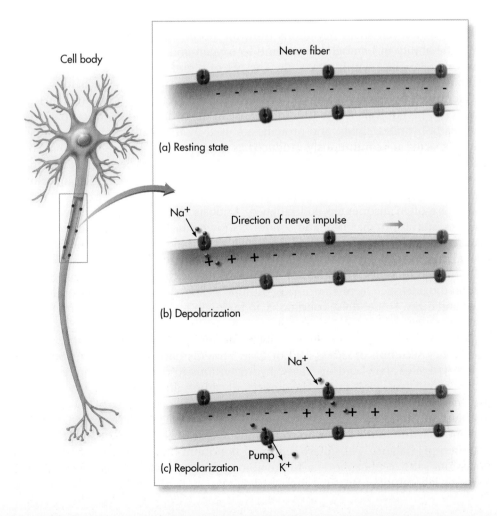

FIGURE 9-4 ▶ Electrolytes control the conduction of a nerve impulse. (a) Under resting conditions, the intracellular fluid has slightly more electrolytes with a negative charge. (b) Nervous stimulation causes the influx of sodium into the interior of the cell. The intracellular charge changes from slightly negative to slightly positive (depolarization). This results in an electrical signal (action potential) transmitted along the surface of the membrane. (c) The pumping of positive ions from intracellular to extracellular space allows the membrane to return to the resting state. This process is called repolarization.

FIGURE 9-5 ▶ pH scale. The diagonal line indicates the proportionate number of hydrogen ions to hydroxide ions. Any pH value above 7 is basic, and any pH value below 7 is acidic.

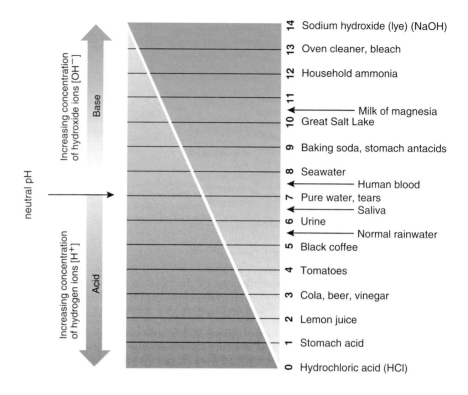

pH	Substance
14	Sodium hydroxide (lye) (NaOH)
13	Oven cleaner, bleach
12	Household ammonia
11	Milk of magnesia
10	Great Salt Lake
9	Baking soda, stomach antacids
8	Seawater
	Human blood
7	Pure water, tears
	Saliva
6	Urine
	Normal rainwater
5	Black coffee
4	Tomatoes
3	Cola, beer, vinegar
2	Lemon juice
1	Stomach acid
0	Hydrochloric acid (HCl)

Acid-Base Balance

Electrolytes provide another critical function by maintaining fluid **pH** in a very narrow range. Even small deviations from the normal range of pH will negatively affect the ability of hemoglobin to bind to oxygen and the rate at which chemical reactions take place within the body. The pH of blood, foods, and other common substances is shown in Figure 9-5. The pH scale is logarithmic. The pH of a fluid is determined by the concentration of hydrogen ions (H^+). A change of 1 pH unit (e.g., 8 to 7) is equivalent to a 10-fold increase in the hydrogen-ion concentration.

As carbohydrates, lipids, and proteins are used by the body to provide energy to the cells, acids are continuously produced as a by-product of these reactions. These acids must be neutralized; otherwise, the pH of the body would become acidic. Under normal conditions, the body is easily able to maintain a pH of 7.4 in the extracellular fluids. A large production of acids results in acidosis, in which blood pH is 7.0 to 7.3. People are often disoriented and fatigued. Acidosis can occur in poorly controlled diabetes, starvation, diarrhea, and conditions in which there is excessive production of carbon dioxide for an extended time such as emphysema. Less often, though as critical, alkalosis may occur (blood pH 7.5 to 5.8). Here, the body loses too much acid through diuretics, vomiting, or conditions in which you breathe off too much carbon dioxide, such as pneumonia or altitude sickness. With alkalosis, you feel agitated and dizzy. Under these conditions, to maintain normal pH, the control systems may be inadequate.

Regulation of pH is complex, involving **buffer** systems, the respiratory system, and kidney secretion of excess acid or base. Proteins have a critical function in the buffer system as they bind or release hydrogen ions to control pH. The respiratory system can increase or decrease the amount of carbon dioxide exhaled when breathing. Increased production and release of carbon dioxide can lower pH because CO_2 dissolves in blood or water, creating an acidic compound. Electrolytes, especially sodium, function in the kidney to control the release of acid and base in the urine to maintain pH balance. Phosphate is also an important buffering agent. Sodium and potassium salts of phosphoric acid are among the most widely used buffers in the scientific laboratory.

pH A measure of the concentration of hydrogen ions. A pH below 7.0 is acidic.

buffer Compound that functions to take up or release hydrogen ions, thereby causing a fluid to resist changes in pH.

9.3 Water

Water provides a number of vital functions essential for life. Water is the perfect medium for body processes because it is the universal **solvent.** Carbohydrates, proteins, minerals, water-soluble vitamins, and many enzymes and hormones dissolve in water. The primary component of blood is water, making it an excellent transportation medium. Lipids do not mix or dissolve in water, so the ability to transport lipids in the blood could be a serious problem. To solve this problem, lipids are coated with a layer of water-soluble protein allowing them to be dispersed throughout the body via the blood. Recall from Chapter 5, these lipid transport vehicles are called lipoproteins.

In addition to its function as a solvent, water has a number of other critical functions in the body (Fig. 9-6). These functions include:

- Providing a medium in which chemical reactions take place
- Actively participating in many chemical reactions
- Distributing nutrients to cells in the body
- Removing waste products from cells for elimination
- Acting as a lubricant for joints
- Moistening the respiratory, gastrointestinal, and urogenital tracts, as well as the eyes and skin
- Maintaining body temperature
- Maintaining blood volume as the major component of blood

A Closer Look at the Functions of Water

Water Contributes to Body Temperature Regulation. Water temperature changes slowly because it has a great ability to hold heat. It takes much more energy to heat water than it does to heat air. Water molecules are polar (charged) so they are attracted to each other. This attractive force is strong and requires energy to separate the water

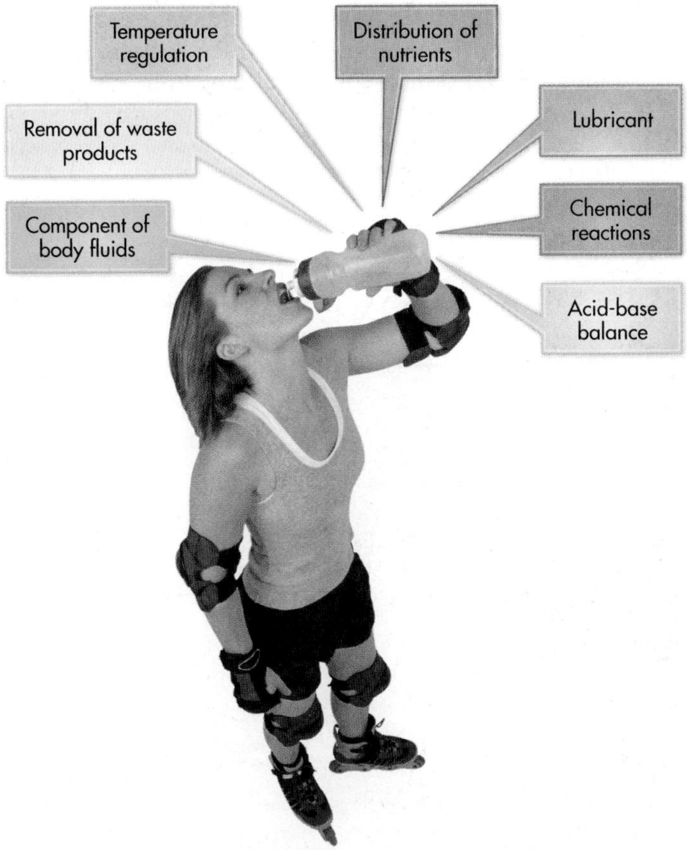

solvent A liquid substance in which other substances dissolve.

FIGURE 9-6 ▶ Water has many essential functions in the body.

FIGURE 9-7 ▶ Although the percentages vary for men and women, the main constituent of the body is water.

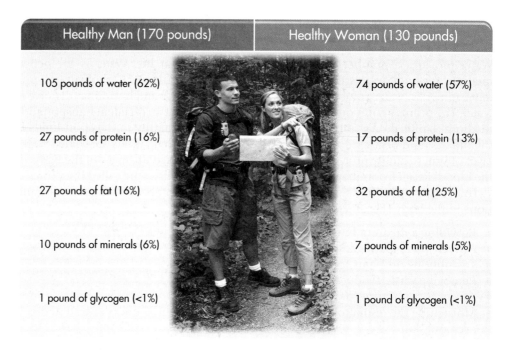

Healthy Man (170 pounds)	Healthy Woman (130 pounds)
105 pounds of water (62%)	74 pounds of water (57%)
27 pounds of protein (16%)	17 pounds of protein (13%)
27 pounds of fat (16%)	32 pounds of fat (25%)
10 pounds of minerals (6%)	7 pounds of minerals (5%)
1 pound of glycogen (<1%)	1 pound of glycogen (<1%)

molecules. Because the human body is 50% to 70% water (Fig. 9-7) it takes a lot of energy to change body temperature.

When overheated, the body secretes fluids in the form of perspiration, which evaporates through skin pores. As water evaporates from the skin, heat energy is released. So, as perspiration evaporates, heat energy is removed from the skin, cooling the body in the process (Fig. 9-8). In response to an increased body temperature, blood vessels in the skin become larger, allowing greater water loss through perspiration. Each quart (approximately 1 liter or 2 pounds) of perspiration evaporated represents approximately 600 kilocalories of energy lost from the skin and surrounding tissues.

So, should you feed a fever? Fever is an increase in body temperature caused by an infection. When you have a fever, you do need more energy. For every increase of 1°F (0.5°C) in internal temperature above normal, your basal metabolic rate (BMR)

FIGURE 9-8 ▶ Body temperature is reduced when heat is transported from the body through the bloodstream to the surface of the skin. The water evaporates from the surface of the skin and heat is removed with it. This cools the blood, which circulates back to the body, reducing body temperature.

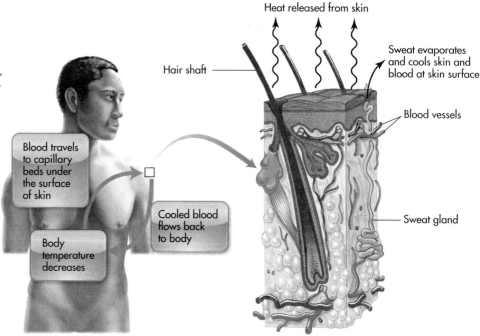

Heat released from skin

Hair shaft

Sweat evaporates and cools skin and blood at skin surface

Blood vessels

Sweat gland

Blood travels to capillary beds under the surface of skin

Cooled blood flows back to body

Body temperature decreases

increases by 7%. Do not go overboard with this information, though. Take into account that you are not moving around much with a 101°F temperature, so your physical activity factor will be quite low.

When carbohydrate, lipid, and protein are used by cells in the body, energy is released in the form of heat. About 60% of the chemical energy in food is turned into body heat; the other 40% is converted to forms of energy that cells can use (principally ATP). Almost all of that energy eventually leaves the body in the form of heat. If this heat could not be dissipated, the body temperature would rise enough to prevent enzyme systems from functioning efficiently, ultimately leading to death. Perspiration is the primary way to prevent this rise in body temperature.

Water Dissolves and Transports Substances Throughout the Body. Besides transporting and distributing body heat, water transports nutrients to the cells and removes waste products. The majority of the nutrients consumed are water soluble; therefore, they can be dissolved in blood and moved into the water-based environment within and around cells and tissues. Most unusable substances or waste products in the body can dissolve in water and so exit the body through the urine.

When carbohydrates and lipids are used as energy sources, water and carbon dioxide are produced. Protein breakdown also produces water and carbon dioxide; however, the nitrogen portion of amino acids cannot be used for energy production. The liver converts the nitrogen by-product into urea. The more protein consumed in excess of needs, the more nitrogen must be excreted in the form of urea in the urine. Likewise, the more sodium we consume, the more sodium we excrete in the urine. As a result, the amount of urine a person needs to produce is determined primarily by excess protein and salt intake. Strict attention to protein and sodium intake is also used to treat some diseases that hamper the kidneys' ability to produce urine.

Typical urine volume is about 1 liter per day, depending mostly on the intake of fluid, protein, and sodium. A somewhat greater urine output than that is fine, but less—especially less than 500 milliliters (2 cups)—forces the kidneys to form concentrated urine.

Heavy ion concentration, in turn, increases the risk of kidney stone formation in susceptible people (generally men). Kidney stones form from minerals and other substances that have precipitated out of the urine and accumulate in the kidney. The simplest way to determine if water intake is adequate is to observe the urine color (Fig. 9-9). Urine should be clear or pale yellow (like pale lemonade or the color of straw) with adequate hydration; concentrated urine is dark yellow (like apple juice). Urine color can be influenced by consuming supplements (especially some B vitamins), medications, and food. Lots of carrot juice, pumpkin, or winter squash can tint your urine orange. Too many fava beans or too much rhubarb will turn it dark brown. A reddish or pinkish urine results from eating too many beets or blackberries. In the spring, too much asparagus not only makes your urine smell funny but can also turn it a bit green.

Water Functions as an Important Lubricant. The body secretes many fluids that are primarily water. Water-based solutions are produced by the digestive tract, respiratory tract, urogenital tract, eyes, and skin. Saliva acts as a lubricant, allowing food to pass through the esophagus to the stomach. Mucus provides a protective fluid coating throughout the digestive tract. The lungs are coated with a layer of mucus that provides an important immunologic function. Water helps form the lubricant found in knees and other joints of the body. The spinal cord and brain are cushioned in cerebral spinal fluid. Water is also the basis of amniotic fluid, which functions as a shock absorber surrounding the growing fetus in the mother's womb. Without adequate availability of water, the ability of the body to produce these critical secretions will be limited.

Water Balance

Every cell, tissue, and organ contains water, although the percentage of water varies tremendously between tissues. For example, muscle is 73% water, adipose tissue is 10% to 20% water, and bone contains approximately 20% water. Overall, the

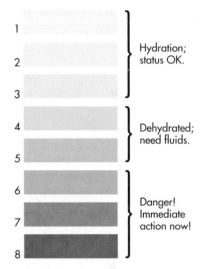

1
2 } Hydration; status OK.
3

4 } Dehydrated; need fluids.
5

6
7 } Danger! Immediate action now!
8

FIGURE 9-9 ▶ Monitoring the color of urine is a good gauge of hydration.

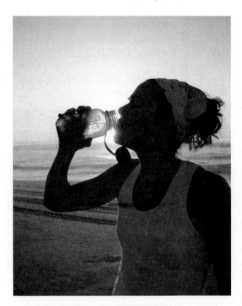

▲ Regular intake of water and water-rich fluids is essential to replace daily fluid losses. One trend in North America is to carry bottles of water.

human body contains 50% to 70% water (see Fig. 9-7). As the fat content of the body increases, the percentage of lean decreases and subsequently the total body water content decreases. When body composition measurements are performed on extremely lean athletes, the percentage body water will be around 70%.

If you do not drink enough water, your body eventually lets you know by signaling thirst. Your brain is communicating the need to drink. This thirst mechanism can lag behind actual water loss during prolonged exercise and illness, as well as in older adults. Sick children, especially those with fever, vomiting, diarrhea, and increased perspiration, and older persons often need to be reminded to drink plenty of fluids because their thirst mechanism may be duller.

Athletes should monitor fluid status. They should weigh themselves before and after training sessions to determine their rate of water loss and, thus, their water needs. The old saying, "A pint's a pound the world around" does not apply here. True, 1 pound of water is 1 pint (2 cups) of water. However, the body can absorb only about 60% of the water consumed. So athletes should drink about 50% more than what they lose through sweat in a workout. Their goal is to consume 2 to 3 cups of fluid for every pound lost.

Once the body registers a shortage of available water, it increases fluid conservation. Two hormones that participate in this process are **antidiuretic hormone (ADH)** and **aldosterone.** The pituitary gland, located in the brain, releases ADH to force the kidneys to conserve water. The kidneys respond by reducing urine production and output. As fluid volume decreases in the bloodstream, blood pressure decreases. ADH also causes blood vessel constriction, which acts to raise blood pressure. Low blood pressure triggers the release of the hormone aldosterone, which signals the kidneys to retain more sodium and, in turn, more water via osmosis.

Despite mechanisms that work to conserve water, fluid continues to be lost via the feces, skin, and lungs. Those losses must be replaced. In addition, there is a limit to how concentrated urine can become. Eventually, if fluid is not consumed, the body becomes dehydrated and suffers ill effects.

By the time a person loses 1% to 2% of body weight in fluids, he or she will be thirsty (Fig. 9-10). Even this small water deficit can cause one to feel tired and dizzy and to experience headaches. At a 4% loss of body weight, muscles lose significant strength and endurance and central nervous system function is negatively affected (e.g., memory and reaction time are compromised and one becomes impatient). By the time the body weight is reduced by 10%, heat tolerance is decreased and weakness results. Ultimately, **dehydration** will lead to kidney failure, coma, and death. Dehydration is a contributing factor to the development of the very serious condition, heatstroke. Performing strenuous physical activity in hot, humid conditions can lead to dehydration and the inability to control body temperature. In addition to an elevated body temperature and dehydration, heart rate is increased and the skin becomes dry. Unassisted, the individual will become unconscious and die. Adequate fluid intake and cessation of physical activity in hot, humid conditions are the best recommendations to prevent heat illness.

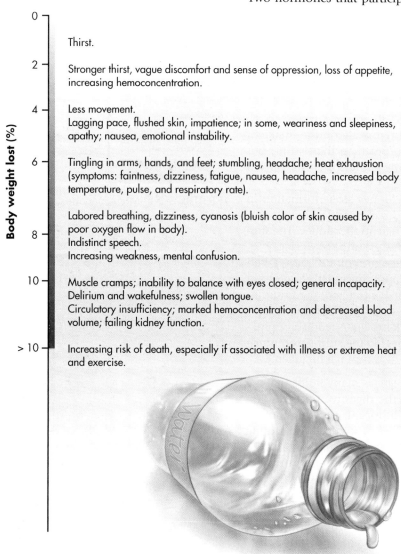

Body weight lost (%)

0 — Thirst.

2 — Stronger thirst, vague discomfort and sense of oppression, loss of appetite, increasing hemoconcentration.

4 — Less movement.
Lagging pace, flushed skin, impatience; in some, weariness and sleepiness, apathy; nausea, emotional instability.

6 — Tingling in arms, hands, and feet; stumbling, headache; heat exhaustion (symptoms: faintness, dizziness, fatigue, nausea, headache, increased body temperature, pulse, and respiratory rate).

Labored breathing, dizziness, cyanosis (bluish color of skin caused by poor oxygen flow in body).
8 — Indistinct speech.
Increasing weakness, mental confusion.

10 — Muscle cramps; inability to balance with eyes closed; general incapacity. Delirium and wakefulness; swollen tongue.
Circulatory insufficiency; marked hemoconcentration and decreased blood volume; failing kidney function.

> 10 — Increasing risk of death, especially if associated with illness or extreme heat and exercise.

FIGURE 9-10 ▶ The effects of dehydration can range from thirst to death, depending on the extent of water weight lost.

Water Intake and Output

The Adequate Intake (AI) for total water intake is 2.7 liters (11 cups) for adult women and 3.7 liters (15 cups) for adult men. This amount is based primarily on average water intake from fluids and foods. For fluid alone, this corresponds to about 2.2 liters (9 cups) for women and about 3 liters (13 cups) for men.

Drinking water is not the only way we consume water. We also consume water in fruit juice, coffee, tea, soft drinks, and milk. Nearly all foods contain water. Many fruits and vegetables are more than 80% water, and many meats contain at least 50% water (Fig. 9-11). The body produces 250 to 350 milliliters (1 to 1½ cups) of water each day as a result of the chemical reactions used to metabolize energy. The amount of **metabolic water** produced can double in physically active people.

Usually, urinary excretion of water accounts for the greatest source of output. Average urinary water loss per day is approximately 1650 milliliters (7½ cups). The daily amount of urine produced depends very strongly on water intake. To remove the waste products generated each day, the minimum daily urine excretion is about 500 milliliters (2 cups). Urine output consistently below this level is often a sign of chronic dehydration due to low fluid intake.

Water is also lost through the skin in the form of perspiration and from the lungs. On days of low physical activity, these losses amount to about 1 liter. Under hot, humid conditions or with strenuous physical activity, losses can be much greater than 1 liter per day. A relatively small amount of water is lost daily in the feces. When we consider the large amount of water used to lubricate the digestive tract, the loss of only 100 milliliters (½ cup) of water each day through the feces is remarkable. About 8000 milliliters (35 cups) of water enters the digestive tract daily through secretions from the mouth, stomach, intestine, pancreas, and other organs. The diet supplies another 500 to 1000 milliliters (2 to 4 cups). The small intestine reabsorbs most of this water, while the colon takes up a lesser but still important amount. The kidneys also greatly conserve water. They can reabsorb as much as 97% of the water filtered each day.

The volumes of water intake and output shown in Figure 9-12 are estimates. Altitude, caffeine and alcohol intake, ambient temperature, humidity, and physical activity will influence water loss.

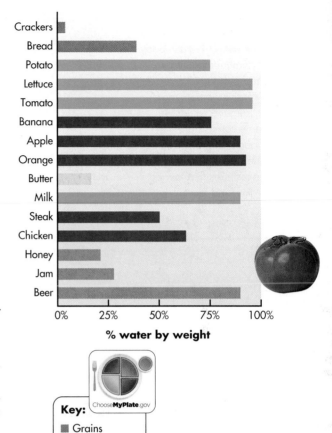

FIGURE 9-11 ▶ Water content of foods by weight. In addition to the MyPlate food groups, pink is used for substances that do not fit easily into food groups (e.g., honey, candy, coffee, alcohol, and table salt.

MAKING DECISIONS

Can a Person Consume Too Much Water?

Even though the kidneys of a healthy person can process up to 15 liters per day, it is possible to drink too much water. As water intake increases above what is needed, kidneys process the excess fluid and excrete dilute urine. If water intake far exceeds the kidneys' processing ability, overhydration and sodium dilution in the blood result. This condition is **hyponatremia**. Endurance athletes exercising for prolonged times, drinking large volumes of water to replace sweat losses, are especially at risk. Using sport drinks (see Chapter 13) will help replace the sodium lost in sweat. **Water intoxication** can happen to healthy people when they drink a great deal of water in a very short period of time. Severe hyponatremia results along with extreme and rapid blood dilution, causing tissue swelling, just as shown in the example with red blood cells in Figure 9-3. Heartbeat becomes irregular, allowing fluid to enter the lungs; brain and nerves swell causing severe headaches, confusion, seizure, and coma. Unless water is restricted and a concentrated salt solution administered under close medical monitoring, the person will die.

metabolic water Water formed as a by-product of carbohydrate, lipid, and protein metabolism.

hyponatremia Dangerously low blood sodium level.

water intoxication Potentially fatal condition that occurs with a high intake of water, which results in a severe dilution of the blood and other fluid compartments.

FIGURE 9-12 ▶ Estimate of water balance—intake versus output—in a woman. We primarily maintain body fluids at an optimum amount by adjusting water output to intake. As you can see for this woman, most water comes from the liquids we consume. Some comes from the moisture in foods, and the remainder is manufactured during metabolism. Water output includes that lost via lungs, urine, skin, and feces.

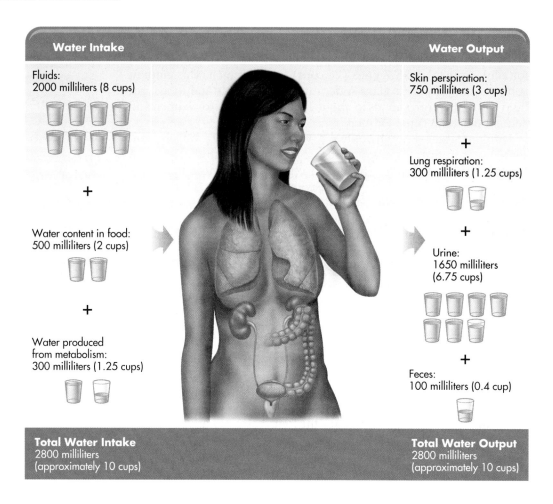

hard water Water that contains high levels of calcium and magnesium.

soft water Water that contains a high level of sodium.

hypertension High blood pressure. The pressure inside the blood vessels exceeds 140/90 millimeters of mercury.

Water Sources

Water consumed each day comes from one of the following sources: well, spring, public water supply, or bottled water. The water source and how it is processed will influence the composition of the water. Water can be classified as either hard or soft. In North America, 89% of homes have hard water. Naturally soft water is found in the Pacific North and Northwest, New England, South-Atlantic gulf, and Hawaii. **Hard water** contains relatively large levels of the minerals calcium and magnesium. It is easy to determine if your water is hard or soft. When washing with hard water, it is difficult to work up lather, and a pronounced ring is left around the bathtub or sink. **Soft water** does a better job of cleaning clothes and feels much better when bathing. Naturally occurring soft water can be high in sodium. Hard water can be converted into soft water through the use of a commercial water softener. As water travels through the water softener, calcium and magnesium exchange with sodium found in the water softener device. The water that exits the softener has a low calcium and magnesium content; however, the sodium content is high. The water filtered through your refrigerator is charcoal activated, removing off flavors but not removing fluoride, a mineral essential to help fight tooth decay. The additional intake of sodium from soft water is undesirable for people restricting sodium intake due to **hypertension**. The additional intake of calcium and magnesium afforded by consuming hard water would be more beneficial than increasing sodium intake through the use of softened water.

Bottled water is a popular alternative to consuming tap water. Rather than using chlorine to disinfect water, most bottled water is treated with ozone, which does not impart a flavor in the water. The Environmental Protection Agency regulates and monitors public water supplies, whereas the Food and Drug Administration regulates bottled water. The standards for quality and contaminants are identical for both regulatory agencies, so the perception that bottled water is safer is unfounded. Much of the bottled water produced in the United States is processed municipal tap water. Very few bottled water manufacturers add the cavity preventive mineral fluoride to the water. The large amount of plastic used to package the over 8.5 billion gallons of bottled water consumed by Americans each year creates a huge energy, recycling, and solid waste disposal concern. People who drink primarily bottled water must be careful to include regular tap water throughout the day in order to receive the benefits of fluoride. Trips to the drinking fountain or making coffee or tea with tap water should suffice.

Have you ever asked yourself these questions? Should I buy bottled water? Can I reuse the bottles? Does it matter what material is used to make the bottle? Is there more to drinking water from plastic bottles than just the recycling issue?

Drinking water from a freshly washed or newly opened bottle is fine. But plastic, like the food we eat, has a shelf life. Over time, the chemicals that make up plastic break down and can leach into the liquid inside the container. Temperature, age of the bottle, acidity of the contents, and type of plastic (recycling code), all make a difference. Age of the consumer makes a difference, too, as babies and young children are more susceptible to problems than adults. Here are some guidelines for the use of water bottles:

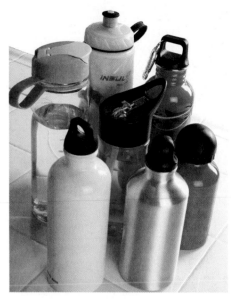

▲ So many ways to hydrate. How to choose?

1. Stainless steel bottles are best for the long run if you are going to use your bottles over and over.
2. If you choose plastic, look for recycling codes 2 and 4 (see Further Reading 4). These are the best for plastics and when they break down, they are the least harmful. You can also use recycling code 7 as long as it also has "BPA free" molded into the bottom of the bottle next to the recycle code.
3. Avoid recycle codes 3 and 7 without "BPA free" embedded in the plastic. These hard plastics may contain BPA (bisphenyl A). Since the 1930s, this organic compound has been used to make clear bottles. When such a bottle is cleaned with harsh detergents (laboratory) or used to hold acidic or high-temperature liquids, BPA can leach into its contents. Exposure can occur through air and skin in addition to diet. BPA is considered an endocrine disrupter. At low doses, it can mimic the body's own hormones. Thus, there is concern about chronic exposure for infants and young children. BPA has been banned for use in Canada and many European countries. In the United States, the Food and Drug Administration recommends limiting infants' exposure to BPA. The major baby bottle manufacturers have stopped using BPA in their products. Many reusable water bottles are switching to "BPA free." If the bottom of your water bottle does not have it molded near the recycling symbol, your bottle contains BPA. Be careful to avoid putting acidic (lemonade, juices, etc.) or hot beverages in your bottle (see Further Reading 3).
4. Choose a reusable bottle with a wide mouth so you can easily clean it.
5. When your plastic bottle becomes scratched or cracked, throw it away. Bacteria can get inside.
6. Do not store your cartons of water in a hot garage or in the back of your hot car. The heat quickly breaks down the plastic. If a bottle has been open and exposed to heat, do not drink it. Pitch the water and recycle the bottle. If it is your reusable bottle, wash and soak it in a sanitizer, such as ¼ teaspoon (4 milliliters) bleach in 1 quart (1 liter) water.

CONCEPT CHECK

Water dissolves substances, serves as a medium for chemical reactions and as a lubricant, and aids in temperature regulation. Water is the most abundant molecule in the body; however, we cannot store water. Daily water intake is balanced with output. Water accounts for 50% to 70% of body weight and distributes itself throughout the body in intracellular and extracellular fluids. The distribution of water between cellular compartments is tightly regulated. The AI for total water intake is 2.7 liters (11 cups) for women and 3.7 liters (15 cups) for men. This level includes beverages as well as the water naturally in food. Thirst is the body's first sign of dehydration. If the thirst mechanism is faulty, as it may be during vigorous exercise, illness, or as a natural part of aging, hormonal mechanisms also help to conserve water by reducing urine output. Excess fluid intake can be dangerous, even fatal.

9.4 Sodium (Na)

Table salt (sodium chloride) is the primary dietary source of sodium. (The chemical symbol Na represents the Latin term *natrium.*) Table salt is 40% sodium by weight, and 1 teaspoon of table salt contains 2400 milligrams of sodium. This mineral is an essential constituent of our diets, adds flavor to our food, and has been used as a preservative for many generations. There is concern that high intakes of sodium may have harmful health effects.

Functions of Sodium

The digestive tract absorbs nearly all consumed sodium. When sodium chloride (NaCl) is dissolved in water, the chemical bond holding the two atoms together breaks and the charged ions Na^+ and Cl^- are released. These electrolytes, as well as others, attract water. The concentration of intracellular and extracellular water is controlled by the concentration of the electrolytes. Fluid balance is maintained by moving or actively pumping sodium ions where more water is needed. Sodium ions also function in nerve impulse conduction and absorption of some nutrients (e.g., glucose).

Unless purposely controlled for health reasons, sodium consumption varies tremendously from day to day, even meal to meal. Yet, our blood levels vary only slightly. Kidneys function as a filter. If blood sodium is low, as blood flows through the kidney, sodium is secreted back into the blood, resulting in a decreased urine output. Conversely, if our blood sodium levels are too high, the sodium is filtered out by the kidneys and excreted into the urine. When this excess sodium is removed, water follows, resulting in greater urine output. Without drinking extra water, dehydration can result. Fortunately, high-sodium (salty) foods make us thirsty and drive us to drink more fluids.

A diet low in sodium, coupled with excessive perspiration and persistent vomiting or diarrhea, has the ability to deplete the body of sodium. This state can lead to muscle cramps, nausea, vomiting, dizziness, and later shock and coma. The likelihood of this occurring is low because the kidney is very efficient at conserving sodium under conditions of low-sodium status.

When weight loss from perspiration exceeds 2% to 3% of total body weight (or about 5 to 6 pounds), sodium losses should raise concern. Even then, merely salting food, or selecting some salty foods such as soup or crackers, is sufficient to restore body sodium for most people. Athletes who perspire for hours during endurance activities need to consume electrolyte-replacement drinks during competition to avoid depletion of sodium, which can lead to hyponatremia. Perspiration contains about two-thirds the sodium concentration found in blood or about 1 gram of sodium per liter.

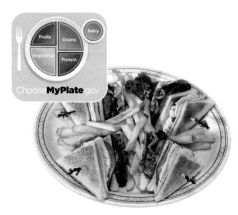

▲ How does this meal of a turkey club sandwich and French fries compare to MyPlate? How could you reduce the sodium content of this meal?

Sodium Sources and Needs

About 80% of the sodium we consume is added in the form of salt during food manufacturing and food preparation at restaurants. Sodium added while cooking or at the table at home provides about 10% of our intake, and naturally occurring sodium in foods provides the remaining 10% (Fig. 9-13). Most unprocessed foods are relatively low in sodium; milk is one exception (about 120 milligrams per cup).

The more processed and restaurant food consumed, the higher one's sodium intake. Conversely, the more home-cooked meals prepared, the more control a person has over sodium in the diet. Major contributors of sodium in the adult diet are white bread and rolls; hot dogs and lunch meat; cheese; soups; and foods with tomato sauce—partly because these foods are consumed so often. Other foods that can be major contributors to sodium intake include salted snack foods, French fries, potato chips, sauces, and gravies.

If we ate only unprocessed foods and added no salt, we would consume about 500 milligrams of sodium per day. The AI for sodium is 1500 milligrams for adults less than age 51, 1300 milligrams for people ages 51 through 70, and 1200 milligrams for those over 70. If we compare 500 milligrams of sodium from a diet of unprocessed foods with the 2300 to 4700 milligrams or more typically consumed by adults, it is clear that food processing, dining out, and salt added while cooking are the major contributors to sodium intake. When dietary sodium must be restricted, attention to food labels is valuable to monitor sodium intake. The Daily Value (DV) on food labels is 2400 milligrams.

Most people can adapt to wide variations in dietary sodium intakes—today's sodium intake is found in tomorrow's urine. However, approximately 10% to 15% of adults are *sodium sensitive*; that is, sodium intake has a direct effect on their blood pressure. As their sodium intake increases, so does their blood pressure. Among these people, lower-sodium diets (about 2000 milligrams daily) often decrease blood pressure. Groups that appear to be especially affected are African-Americans, Asian-Americans, and people who have diabetes and/or are overweight (see Newsworthy Nutrition in the margin and the Nutrition and Your Health section on minerals and hypertension at the end of the chapter). Lifestyle factors such as being overweight and inactive are the major contributors to the development of hypertension.

The medical community suggests that adults should reduce salt and sodium consumption to limit the risk of developing hypertension later in life (see Further Reading 2). It is also a good idea to have your blood pressure checked regularly. If you are diagnosed with hypertension, you should reduce sodium intake as you follow a comprehensive plan to treat this disease. Reducing sodium intake may also help maintain a healthy calcium status, as sodium intake greater than about 2000 milligrams per day may increase urinary calcium loss along with the sodium excreted. The effect of this increased urinary calcium loss on bone health is controversial.

Adopting a reduced-salt diet is a significant lifestyle change for most people because many typical food choices will have to be limited (Fig. 9-14). At first, foods may taste bland, but eventually you will perceive more flavor as the taste receptors in the tongue become more sensitive to the salt content of foods. It takes 6 to 8 weeks to retrain your taste buds to sense sodium at a lower level. Slowly reducing sodium intake by substituting lemon juice, herbs, and spices will allow you to become accustomed to a diet that contains minimal amounts of salt. Many cookbooks and online sources offer excellent recipes for flavorful dishes.

Upper Level for Sodium

The Upper Level (UL) for sodium for adults is 2300 milligrams (2.3 grams), approximately 1 teaspoon. Intakes exceeding this amount typically increase blood pressure. About 95% of North American adults have sodium intakes that exceed that UL. It must be noted that the Daily Value (DV) of 2400 milligrams exceeds the UL for sodium. A healthier goal is to aim for the AI of 1500 milligrams.

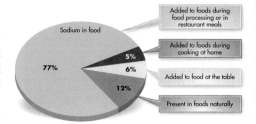

FIGURE 9-13 ▶ Salt arrives in the American diet largely as a result of food processing.

The 2010 Dietary Guidelines for Americans recommend less than 2300 milligrams of sodium (approximately 1 teaspoon of salt) per day for the general population. African-Americans; middle-aged or older adults; and individuals with hypertension, diabetes, or chronic kidney disease should consume no more than 1500 milligrams of sodium per day. The American Heart Association takes a stronger position, advising no more than 1500 milligrams of sodium per day for all Americans.

NEWSWORTHY NUTRITION

Lower sodium and higher potassium intakes reduce risk of cardiovascular disease

Increasing potassium intakes appears effective in lowering blood pressure and is most effective at reducing risk of cardiovascular disease when combined with lower intakes of sodium. The sodium-to-potassium ratio in urine is a good predictor of cardiovascular disease.

Source: Cook NR and others: Joint effects of sodium and potassium intake on subsequent cardiovascular disease. *Archives of Internal Medicine* 169:32, 2009.

connect NUTRITION **Check out the Connect site www.mcgrawhillconnect.com to further explore the roles of sodium and potassium in cardiovascular health.**

FIGURE 9-14 ▶ Food sources of sodium compared to the Adequate Intake.

Food Sources of Sodium

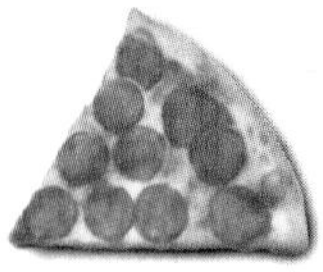

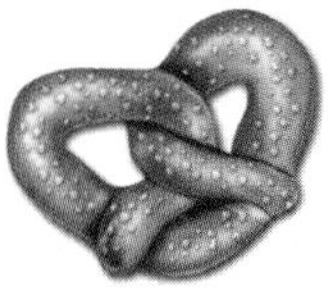

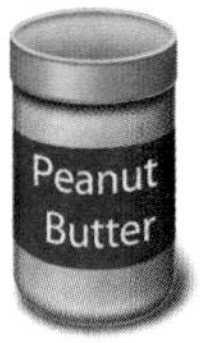

Food Item and Amount	Sodium Content (milligrams)	Adult Male and Female AI = 1500 milligrams
		Daily Value = 2400 milligrams %AI
AI*	1500	100%
Pepperoni pizza, 2 slices	2045	136%
Ham, sliced, 1 ounce	1215	81%
Chicken noodle soup, canned, 1 cup	1106	74%
V8 vegetable juice, 8 ounces	620	41%
Macaroni salad, ½ cup	561	37%
Hard pretzels, 1 ounce	486	32%
Hamburger with bun, 1 each	474	32%
Green beans, canned, ½ cup	390	26%
Saltine crackers, 6 each	234	16%
Cheddar cheese, 1 ounce	176	12%
Peanut butter, 2 tablespoons	156	10%
Nonfat milk, 1 cup	127	8%
Seven-grain bread, 1 slice	126	8%
Animal crackers, 1 ounce	112	7%
Grape juice, 1 cup	10	1%

Key:
- Grains
- Vegetables
- Fruits
- Dairy
- Protein

ChooseMyPlate.gov

* For adults; see the DRI table in the back of this book for age-specific recommendations.

CONCEPT CHECK

Sodium is the major positive ion in the extracellular fluid. It is important for maintaining fluid balance and conducting nerve impulses. Sodium depletion is unlikely, because the typical diet has abundant sources of sodium. Compared to dining out or buying commercially prepared foods, preparation of foods in the home allows greater control over sodium intake. The AI for sodium for adults is 1500 milligrams per day. The average adult consumes 2300 to 4700 milligrams or more daily. Some adults are sensitive to sodium intake, and blood pressure will increase as sodium intake increases. Sodium in the North American diet is provided in the form of salt, predominantly through processed and restaurant foods.

9.5 Potassium (K)

Potassium performs many of the same functions as sodium, such as water balance and nerve impulse transmission. (The chemical symbol K represents the Latin term *Kalium.*) It is the principal positively charged ion inside cells. Intracellular fluids contain 95% of the potassium in the body. Higher potassium intake is associated with lower rather than higher blood pressure values. Approximately 90% of the potassium consumed is absorbed.

Low blood potassium from chronic diarrhea, vomiting, or laxative abuse is a life-threatening problem. Symptoms often include a loss of appetite, muscle cramps, confusion, and constipation. Eventually, the heart beats irregularly, decreasing its capacity to pump blood.

Potassium Sources and Needs

Unprocessed foods are rich sources of potassium, including fruits, vegetables, milk, whole grains, dried beans, and meats (Fig. 9-15). Here is an easy guide: the more processed your food, the higher it is in sodium and the lower it is in potassium. Major contributors of potassium to the adult diet include milk, potatoes, beef, coffee, tomatoes, and orange juice (Fig. 9-16).

The Adequate Intake for potassium for adults is 4700 milligrams (4.7 grams) per day. The DV used on food and supplement labels is 3500 milligrams. Typically, North Americans consume 2000 to 3000 milligrams per day. Thus, many of us need to increase potassium intake, preferably by increasing fruit and vegetable intake.

Diets are more likely to be lower in potassium than sodium because we add salt to our food, not potassium. Some **diuretics** used to treat high blood pressure also deplete the body's potassium. Thus, people who take potassium-wasting diuretics need

▲ Vegetables in general are a rich source of potassium, as are fruits.

diuretic A substance that increases urinary fluid excretion.

FIGURE 9-15 ▶ Food sources of potassium compared to the Adequate Intake.

Food Sources of Potassium

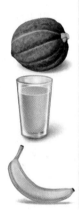

Food Item and Amount	Potassium (milligrams)	Adult Male and Female AI = 4700 milligrams
		Daily Value = 3500 milligrams %AI
AI*	4700	100%
Kidney beans, 1 cup	715	15%
Winter squash, ¾ cup	670	14%
Plain yogurt, 1 cup	570	12%
Orange juice, 1 cup	495	11%
Cantaloupe, 1 cup	495	11%
Lima beans, ½ cup	480	10%
Banana, 1 medium	470	10%
Zucchini, 1 cup	450	10%
Soybeans, ½ cup	440	9%
Artichoke, 1 medium	425	9%
Tomato juice, ¾ cup	400	9%
Pinto beans, ½ cup	400	9%
Baked potato, 1 small	385	8%
Buttermilk, 1 cup	370	8%
Sirloin steak, 3 ounces	345	7%

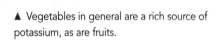

Key:
■ Grains
■ Vegetables
■ Fruits
■ Dairy
■ Protein

* For adults; see the DRI table in the back of this book for age-specific recommendations.

FIGURE 9-16 ▶ Sources of potassium from MyPlate. The fill of the background color (none, 1/3, 2/3, or completely covered) within each group on the plate indicates the average nutrient density for potassium in that group. Overall, the vegetables group and the fruits group contain many foods that are nutrient-dense sources of potassium, with the dairy group and protein group following close behind. With regard to physical activity, potassium is especially needed for cardiovascular function.

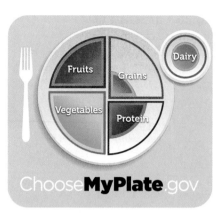

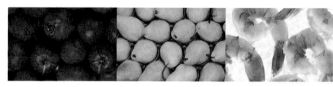

MyPlate: Sources of Potassium

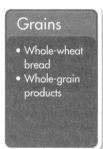 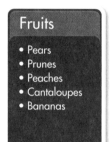 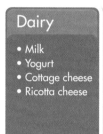 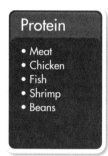

Grains	Vegetables	Fruits	Dairy	Protein
• Whole-wheat bread • Whole-grain products	• Avocados • Spinach • Squash • Potatoes • Tomatoes • Lettuce • Lima beans	• Pears • Prunes • Peaches • Cantaloupes • Bananas	• Milk • Yogurt • Cottage cheese • Ricotta cheese	• Meat • Chicken • Fish • Shrimp • Beans

to monitor their potassium intake carefully. For these people, high-potassium foods are good additions to the diet, as are potassium chloride supplements prescribed by a physician.

A continually deficient food intake, as may be the case in alcoholism, can result in a potassium deficiency and low blood potassium levels called hypokalemia. People with certain eating disorders whose diets are poor and whose bodies can be depleted of nutrients because of vomiting and diarrhea are also at risk for potassium deficiency (see Chapter 14). Other populations especially at risk for potassium deficiency include people on very low-calorie diets and athletes who exercise for prolonged periods. These people should compensate for potentially low body potassium by consuming potassium-rich foods.

Upper Level of Potassium

If the kidneys function normally, typical food intakes will not lead to potassium toxicity. Thus, no Upper Level for potassium has been set. When the kidneys function poorly, potassium builds in the blood, inhibiting heart function and leading to a slowed heartbeat. If left untreated, the heart eventually stops beating, resulting in a cardiac arrest and death. Therefore, in cases of kidney failure or kidney disease, close monitoring of blood levels of potassium and potassium intake becomes critical.

9.6 Chloride (Cl)

Chloride is a negative ion found primarily in the extracellular fluid. Chlorine (Cl_2) is a poisonous gas used to disinfect municipal water supplies. Chloride ions are a component of the acid produced in the stomach (hydrochloric acid) and are used during immune responses as white blood cells attack foreign cells. In addition, nerve function relies on the presence of chloride. Like sodium, nearly all the chloride consumed is efficiently absorbed and the principal route of excretion is the kidneys; some is lost in perspiration. Chloride has been linked to the blood-pressure-raising ability of sodium

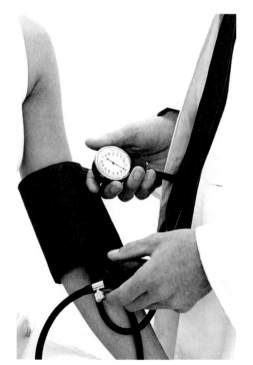

▲ Chloride is likely part of the blood-pressure-raising property of sodium chloride (salt).

chloride. Prolonged vomiting, as can occur in bulimia or severe cases of the flu, can lead to a disturbance of the body's acid-base balance due to the large loss of stomach acid.

A chloride deficiency is unlikely because our dietary salt intake is so high. Frequent and lengthy bouts of vomiting, if coupled with a nutrient-poor diet, can contribute to a deficiency because stomach secretions contain a lot of chloride.

Chloride Sources and Needs

A few fruits and some vegetables are naturally good sources of chloride. Chlorinated water is also a source. Most chloride is consumed as salt added to foods. Knowing a food's salt content allows for a close prediction of its chloride content. Salt is 60% chloride by weight.

The Adequate Intake for chloride for adults is 2300 milligrams per day. This value is based on the 40:60 ratio of sodium to chloride in salt (1500 milligrams of sodium: 2300 milligrams of chloride). The DV used on food and supplement labels is 3400 milligrams. If the average adult consumes about 9 grams of salt daily, that yields 5.4 grams (5400 milligrams) of chloride. Because chloride has a role in raising blood pressure, it is important that aging adults consciously control salt intake to decrease risk of developing hypertension. Learning at a young age to select lower-salt foods is the best way to start.

Upper Level of Chloride

The UL of chloride is 3600 milligrams. Thus, the average adult typically consumes an excess of this ion.

CONCEPT CHECK

Potassium performs functions similar to those of sodium, except that it is the main positive ion found inside cells. Potassium is vital to fluid balance and nerve transmission. A potassium deficiency—caused by an inadequate intake of potassium, persistent vomiting, or use of some diuretics—can lead to loss of appetite, muscle cramps, confusion, and heartbeat irregularities. Fruits and vegetables are good sources of potassium. Potassium intake can be toxic if a person's kidneys do not function properly. Chloride is the major negative ion found in the extracellular fluid. Chloride also functions in digestion as part of hydrochloric acid and in immune and nervous system responses. Deficiencies of chloride are highly unlikely because we eat so much salt.

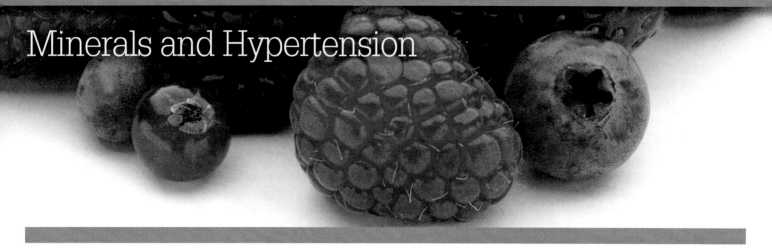

Minerals and Hypertension

Among North Americans, an estimated one in five adults has hypertension. Over the age of 65, the number rises to one in every two adults. Only about half of cases are being treated. Blood pressure is expressed by two numbers. The higher number represents systolic blood pressure, the pressure in the arteries when the heart muscle is contracting and pumping blood into the arteries. Optimal systolic blood pressure is 120 millimeters of mercury (mm Hg) or less. The second value is diastolic blood pressure, the artery pressure when the heart is relaxed. Optimal diastolic blood pressure is 80 mm Hg or less. Elevations in both systolic and diastolic blood pressure are strong predictors of disease (Fig. 9-17).

How High Is High?

If your systolic and diastolic pressures fall into different categories, your risk depends on the higher category

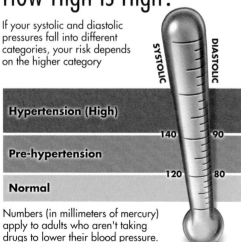

Numbers (in millimeters of mercury) apply to adults who aren't taking drugs to lower their blood pressure.

FIGURE 9-17 ▶ The cutoff for hypertension is 140/90 mm Hg, but the risk of heart attacks and stroke precedes the rise in blood pressure.

Hypertension is defined as sustained systolic pressure exceeding 139 mm Hg or diastolic blood pressure exceeding 89 mm Hg. Most cases of hypertension (about 95%) have no clear-cut cause. Such cases are classified as primary or essential hypertension. Kidney disease, sleep-disordered breathing (sleep apnea), and other causes often lead to the other 5% of cases, classified as secondary hypertension. African-Americans and Asian-Americans are more likely than Caucasians to develop hypertension and to do so earlier in life.

Unless blood pressure is periodically measured, the development of hypertension is easily overlooked. Thus, it is described as a silent disorder, because it usually does not cause symptoms.

Why Control Blood Pressure?

Blood pressure needs to be controlled mainly to prevent cardiovascular disease, kidney disease, strokes and related declines in brain function, poor blood circulation in the legs, problems with vision, and sudden death. These conditions are much more likely to be found in individuals with hypertension than in people with normal blood pressure. Smoking and elevated blood lipoproteins make these diseases even more likely. Individuals with hypertension need to be diagnosed and treated as soon as possible, as the condition generally progresses to a more serious stage over time and even resists therapy if it persists for years.

Contributors to Hypertension

Because we do not know the cause of 95% of the cases of hypertension, we can identify only risk factors that contribute to its development (see Further Reading 1). A family history of hypertension is a risk factor, especially if both parents have (or had) the problem. In addition, blood pressure can increase as a person ages. Some increase is caused by atherosclerosis. As plaque builds up in the arteries, the arteries become less flexible and cannot expand. When vessels remain rigid, blood pressure remains high. Eventually, the plaque begins to decrease the blood supply to the kidneys, decreasing their ability to control blood volume and, in turn, blood pressure.

Overweight people have six times greater risk of having hypertension than lean people. Overall, obesity is considered the number one lifestyle factor related to hypertension. This is especially the case in minority populations.

How High Is High?

Additional blood vessels develop to support excess tissue in overweight and obese individuals, and these extra miles of associated blood vessels increase work by the heart and also blood pressure. Hypertension is linked to obesity if elevated blood insulin levels result from insulin-resistant adipose cells. This increased insulin level augments sodium retention in the body and accelerates atherosclerosis. In such cases, a weight loss of as little as 10 to 15 pounds often can help treat hypertension.

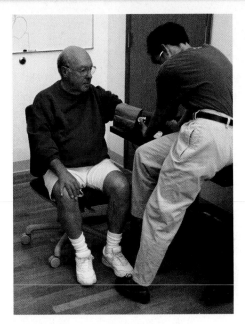

▲ Older adults are particularly at risk of hypertension.

Inactivity is considered the number two lifestyle factor related to hypertension. If an obese person can engage in regular physical activity (at least 5 days per week for 30 to 60 minutes) and lose weight, blood pressure often returns to normal.

Third, excess alcohol intake is responsible for about 10% of all cases of hypertension, especially in middle-aged males and among African-Americans in general. When hypertension is caused by excessive alcohol intake, it is usually reversible. A sensible alcohol intake for people with hypertension is two or fewer drinks per day for men and one or no drinks per day for women and all older adults. Did you recognize that this is the same recommendation given in the 2010 Dietary Guidelines for Americans? Some studies suggest that such a minimal alcohol intake may reduce the risk of ischemic stroke. These data, however, should not be used to encourage alcohol use.

In some people, particularly African-Americans and older overweight persons, blood pressure is especially sensitive to sodium. In these people, excess salt leads to fluid retention by the kidney and a corresponding increase in blood volume, resulting in increased blood pressure. It is not clear whether sodium or chloride is more responsible for the effect. Still, as reviewed in this chapter, if one reduces sodium intake, chloride intake naturally falls; the opposite is also true. For the most part, a recommendation to consume less sodium is equivalent to a call for less salt in the diet. Only some North Americans are susceptible to increases in blood pressure from salt intake, so it is only the number four lifestyle factor related to hypertension. It is unfortunate that salt intake receives the major portion of public attention with regard to hypertension. Efforts to prevent hypertension should also focus on obesity, inactivity, and excessive consumption of alcohol.

Other Minerals and Blood Pressure

Minerals such as calcium, potassium, and magnesium also deserve attention when it comes to prevention and treatment of hypertension. Studies show that a diet rich in these minerals and low in salt can decrease blood pressure within days of beginning this type of diet, especially among African-Americans. The response is even similar to that seen with commonly used medications. The diet is called the Dietary Approaches to Stop Hypertension (DASH) diet (Table 9-1). The diet is rich in calcium, phosphorus, and magnesium and low in salt. It takes a standard MyPlate Daily Food Plan; adds one to two extra vegetables and fruits servings; and emphasizes consumption of nuts, seeds, or legumes (beans) 4 to 5 days of the week. In DASH studies, participants also consumed no more than 3 grams of sodium and no more than one to two alcoholic drinks

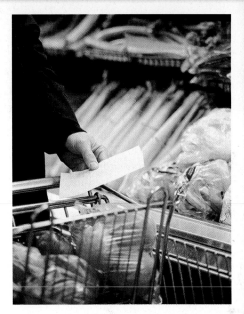

▲ Opting for the fruits, vegetables, and other foods recommended by the DASH diet is good nutrition advice regardless of hypertension.

per day. A DASH 2 diet trial tested three daily sodium intakes (3300 milligrams, 2400 milligrams, and 1500 milligrams). People showed a steady decline in blood pressure on the DASH diet as sodium intake declined. Overall, the DASH diet is seen as a total dietary approach to treating hypertension. It is not clear which of the many healthful practices of this diet are responsible for the fall in blood pressure.

Other studies also show a reduction in stroke risk among people who consume a diet rich in fruits, vegetables, and vitamin C (recall that fruits and vegetables are rich in vitamin C). Overall, a diet low in salt and rich in low-fat and fat-free

TABLE 9-1 What Is the DASH Diet?
The DASH diet is characterized as low in fat and sodium and rich in fruits, vegetables, and low-fat dairy products. Here is the breakdown:

Per Day	Per Week
6–8 servings of grains and grain products	4–5 servings of nuts, seeds, or legumes
4–5 servings of fruit	5 servings of sweets and added sugars
4–5 servings of vegetables	
2–3 servings of low-fat or fat-free dairy products	
2 or less servings of meats, poultry, and fish	
2–3 servings of fats/oils	

dairy products, fruits, vegetables, whole grains, and some nuts can substantially reduce hypertension and stroke risk in many people, especially those with hypertension (see Further Reading 7).

Medications to Treat Hypertension

Diuretic medications are one class of drugs used to treat hypertension. These "water pills" work to reduce blood volume (and therefore blood pressure) by increasing fluid output in the urine. Other medications act by slowing heart rate or by causing relaxation of the small muscles lining the blood vessels. A combination of two or more medications is commonly required to treat hypertension that does not respond to diet and lifestyle therapy.

Prevention of Hypertension

Many of the risk factors for hypertension and stroke are controllable, and appropriate lifestyle changes can reduce a person's risk (Fig. 9-18), depending on the severity of the hypertension. Experts also recommend that those with hypertension lower blood pressure through diet and lifestyle changes before resorting to blood pressure medications.

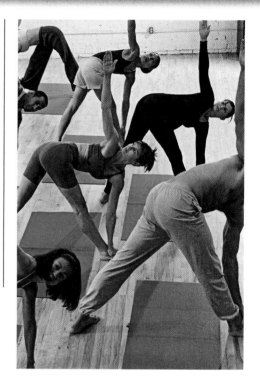

▲ Regular, moderate physical activity contributes to better blood pressure control.

FIGURE 9-18 ▶ What works? If your blood pressure is high, here's how much lifestyle changes should lower it.

Advice	Details	Drop in Systolic Blood Pressure
Lose excess weight	For every 20 pounds you lose (if BMI > 25)	5 to 20 points
Follow a DASH diet	Eat a lower-fat diet rich in vegetables, fruits, and low-fat dairy foods	8 to 14 points
Exercise daily	Get 30 minutes a day of aerobic activity (such as brisk walking)	4 to 9 points
Limit sodium	Eat no more than 2400 mg per day (1500 mg per day is better)	2 to 8 points
Limit alcohol	Have no more than 2 drinks per day for men, 1 drink per day for women (1 drink = 12 oz beer, 5 oz wine, or 1.5 oz 80-proof whiskey)	2 to 4 points

Source: *The Seventh Report of the Joint National Committee on Prevention, Detection, Evaluation, and Treatment of High Blood Pressure* (www.nhlbi.nih.gov/guidelines/hypertension).

Case Study Let's Focus on the Positive

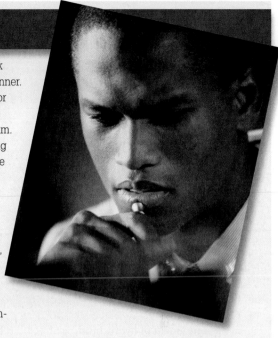

Jerome enjoys listening to his nutrition professor's experiences with successes and failures in advising people on diet change. The instructor says that when people focus on doing something positive in their diet, they automatically start to do less of the negative—like substituting one behavior with another. While at the pharmacy the other day, Jerome stopped at the station to check his blood pressure. He did not like the results. He went to the student health center for a recheck, as advised by the American Heart Association. He was diagnosed as prehypertensive, with a blood pressure of 129/85. Jerome was sad but not shocked. He is African-American and has a family history of hypertension. He exercises four times/week, controls stress through playing piano, is close to his family, enjoys friends, and does not drink or smoke. Jerome lives in an apartment with three friends. His mom taught him to cook, which he does three nights per week. Jerome does not skip meals (eats breakfast) and packs a lunch to eat on campus. However, too often

dinner is late and he grabs packaged snack foods to ward off hunger until he can fix dinner.

Jerome talks with his nutrition professor about his dilemma. She wants him to stay positive and asks him to focus on potassium. She tells him that if he focuses on including high-potassium foods, he will receive some added benefits.

Answer the following questions about Jerome's situation and check your responses in Appendix A.

1. Since Jerome is an African-American, why is it prudent for him to do something about his blood pressure right now?
2. In what other nutrients are potassium-rich foods high?
3. How might these foods be beneficial for Jerome in his desire to control his blood pressure?
4. What are some potassium-rich foods that Jerome could have readily available at

home to help him ward off hunger until he is ready to eat his dinner? Can he pack any of these for a quick snack?

Summary (Numbers refer to numbered sections in the chapter.)

9.1 The body contains about 40 liters of water. Intracellular fluid is fluid contained within cells, accounting for about two-thirds of total fluid. Extracellular fluid (e.g., plasma, lymph, gastrointestinal secretions, synovial fluid) makes up the remaining one-third of body fluid. Water moves freely across cell membranes by osmosis. The distribution of water in various body compartments is strictly regulated by the concentrations of electrolytes, including sodium, potassium, chloride, and phosphate. Intakes of sodium, potassium, and chloride are related to the development of hypertension.

9.2 Electrolyes are involved in transmission of nerve impulses. At rest, the inside of the nerve cell membrane has a slightly negative charge. Stimulation of the nerve cell leads to depolarization of the cell membrane: sodium ions flow into the cell, leading to a slightly positive charge within the cell membrane. Depolarization of one part of the nerve cell membrane triggers

depolarization of an adjacent area, so an electrical signal can be transmitted along the cell. After nervous stimulation, sodium ions are pumped back into the cell and the membrane is repolarized.

The pH is a measure of the concentration of hydrogen ions in a solution. A pH of 7 is neutral, >7 is basic, and <7 is acidic. The pH of the blood is maintained close to 7.4. Sodium, potassium, and phosphate function in the pH regulation of body fluids.

9.3 Water constitutes 50% to 70% of the human body. Its unique chemical properties enable it to dissolve substances as well as serve as a medium for chemical reactions, temperature regulation, and lubrication. Water also helps regulate the acid-base balance in the body. For adults, daily water needs from the combination of food and drink are estimated at 11 cups (women) and 15 cups (men) per day.

9.4 Sodium, the major positive ion found outside cells, is vital in fluid balance and

nerve impulse transmission. The North American diet provides abundant sodium through processed foods and table salt. About 10% to 15% of the adult population is sensitive to sodium intake. Overweight people and African-Americans are especially at risk for developing hypertension from consuming excessive sodium.

9.5 Potassium, the major positive ion found inside cells, has a similar function to sodium. Fruits, vegetables, and dairy are good sources.

9.6 Chloride is the major negative ion found outside cells. It is important in digestion as part of stomach acid and in immune and nerve functions. Table salt supplies most of the chloride in our diets.

N&YH Maintaining a healthy weight; limiting alcohol intake; exercising regularly; decreasing salt intake; and ensuring adequate potassium, magnesium, and calcium in the diet all can play a part in controlling high blood pressure.

Check Your Knowledge (Answers to the following questions are below.)

1. Which of the following is a function of water in the body?
   a. temperature regulation
   b. acid-base balance
   c. nerve impulse transmission
   d. All of the above

2. Minerals involved in fluid balance are
   a. calcium and magnesium.
   b. copper and iron.
   c. calcium and phosphorus.
   d. sodium and potassium.

3. The primary function of sodium is to maintain
   a. bone mineral content.
   b. hemoglobin concentration.
   c. immune function.
   d. fluid distribution.

4. Chloride is
   a. a component of hydrochloric acid.
   b. an intracellular fluid ion.

   c. a positively charged ion.
   d. converted to chlorine in the intestinal tract.

5. Hypertension is defined as a blood pressure greater than
   a. 110/60.
   b. 120/65.
   c. 140/90.
   d. 190/80.

6. Fatigue, headaches, dizziness and muscle weakness are signs of
   a. hypertension.
   b. dehydration.
   c. kidney stones.
   d. low blood potassium.

7. A hormone that causes the kidneys to conserve sodium is called
   a. glucagon.
   b. parathyroid hormone.

   c. antidiuretic hormone.
   d. aldosterone.

8. Total water needs are about _____ cups per day for women and about _____ cups per day for men.
   a. 8, 10
   b. 9, 13
   c. 11, 15
   d. 15, 18

9. The major intracellular positive ion is
   a. sodium.
   b. potassium.
   c. chloride.
   d. calcium.

10. Food sources of potassium include
    a. milk.
    b. kidney beans.
    c. orange juice.
    d. All of the above.

Answer Key: 1. a (LO 9.1), 2. d (LO 9.3), 3. d (LO 9.3), 4. a (LO 9.2), 5. c (LO 9.8), 6. b (LO 9.6), 7. d (LO 9.4), 8. c (LO 9.5), 9. b (LO 9.2), 10. d (LO 9.7)

Study Questions (Numbers refer to Learning Outcomes)

1. List five functions of water in the body. **(LO 9.1)**

2. What are two similarities and differences between sodium and potassium? Sodium and chloride? **(LO 9.2)**

3. What is the relationship between sodium and water balance, and how is that relationship monitored as well as maintained in the body? **(LO 9.3)**

4. How do sodium and potassium participate in nerve impulse transmission? **(LO 9.3)**

5. What metabolic processes affect the pH of body fluids? Why is it important for pH to be maintained within a narrow range? **(LO 9.3)**

6. Describe the effects of antidiuretic hormone (ADH) and aldosterone on body water. **(LO 9.4)**

7. Approximately how much water do you need each day to stay healthy? Identify at least two situations that increase the need for water. Then list three sources of water in the average person's diet. **(LO 9.5)**

8. Name three consequences of mild (1% to 2% loss of body weight) dehydration. List three consequences of severe dehydration. **(LO 9.6)**

9. Of the micronutrients discussed in this chapter, which are typically consumed in excess? Which of the micronutrients in this chapter are typically lacking in North American diets? **(LO 9.7)**

10. List three dietary strategies to lower blood pressure. **(LO 9.8)**

What Would You Choose Recommendations

Bottled water has become very popular. In 2009, each American consumed almost 28 gallons of bottled water, adding up to about 8.5 billion gallons for the nation. The public perception that bottled water is safer and healthier than tap water has stimulated the current bottle-toting habit. The truth is that bottled and tap water are both regulated: bottled water by the FDA and tap water by the Environmental Protection Agency (EPA). The FDA requirements for bottled water mimic those of the EPA for water quality, but neither has to be contaminant-free.

"Pure" is an advertising term and means nothing about the quality of the water. Recent controversy over misleading advertising by major companies such as Pepsico and Coca-Cola that use public source water in their respective products, Aquafina and Dasani, has led to the printing of "Public Source Water" or "PSW" on labels.

Mineral water must contain consistent levels of natural elements from an underground source; no minerals may be added to the water. The precise mineral content varies by source; but some common minerals found in water include calcium, magnesium, potassium, sodium, sulfur, iron, fluoride, zinc, and some ultratrace minerals. The minerals impart some taste to the water but are typically a minor contributor to overall mineral intake.

There is no legal definition for "vitamin water." Manufacturers of vitamin water (i.e., soft-drink companies) usually use filtered or distilled water and add sweeteners (e.g., high-fructose corn syrup) and citric

acid as flavoring agents, plus several vitamins (mostly vitamin C and an assortment of B vitamins). In 2010, the Coca-Cola Bottling Company was sued by the Center for Science in the Public Interest for false marketing of its popular vitaminwater® brand as "nutritious." These products are marketed as healthy because they contain added vitamins, but most of them also supply a surprising amount of sugar. Recall that the American Heart Association recommends that men and women get no more than 150 or 100 kcal per day, respectively, from added sugars. A 20-ounce bottle of vitaminwater® has 33 grams of sugar, providing 132 kcal from added sugar. This is about half the sugar in a regular soft drink, but you can see how this can add up to excess. Furthermore, most North Americans consume adequate amounts of vitamin C and the B vitamins without the aid of these beverages.

Consumers should also be aware of the FDA definitions for other types of bottled water.

- Artesian water must come from a confined aquifer.
- Springwater must flow naturally to the surface.
- Purified water is produced through an approved process such as distillation or reverse osmosis.

Relying on bottled water is an expensive habit, personally and environmentally. If you use bottled water to meet your recommended fluid needs, you will spend close

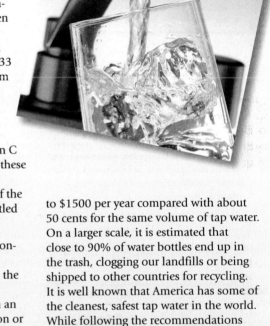

to $1500 per year compared with about 50 cents for the same volume of tap water. On a larger scale, it is estimated that close to 90% of water bottles end up in the trash, clogging our landfills or being shipped to other countries for recycling. It is well known that America has some of the cleanest, safest tap water in the world. While following the recommendations to drink more water, hydrate with tap or home-filtered water in a reusable container (see Further Reading 5).

Further Readings

1. American Society of Hypertension: Reference list in clinical hypertension. *The American Society of Hypertension:* 2007. Available at: www.ash-us.org/pub/curriculum.htm.

This reference list outlines research articles and reviews of many topics that contribute to hypertension. If interested in a contributor to hypertension, this 56-page document lists many articles that will provide information for further study on the topic.

2. Appel LJ and others: The importance of population-wide sodium reduction as a means to prevent cardiovascular disease and stroke: A call to action from the American Heart Association. *Circulation* 123:1138, 2011.

High blood pressure is the second leading cause of preventable death in the United States, contributing to cardiovascular disease, stroke, and kidney disease. This statement of the American Heart Association summarizes the abundant evidence linking excessive sodium intake with hypertension and damage to the heart, kidneys, and blood vessels. The AHA calls for individuals, their healthcare providers, government, and the food manufacturing and restaurant industry to work together to decrease sodium intake among all Americans.

3. Food and Drug Administration. U.S. Department of Health and Human Services: Update on bisphenol A for use in food contact applications: January 2010. Available at: www.fda.gov/NewsEvents/PublicHealth Focus/ucm197739.htm#interim.

This update gives an historical perspective on the use of bisphenol A (BPA) in the United States and the current status of legislation on its use. Controversy exists regarding its use in water bottles and other hard plastics.

4. Howard BC: What do recycling symbols on plastics mean? *The Daily Green:* March 2008 Available at: www.thedailygreen.com/green-homes/latest/recycling-symbols-plastics-460321.

This slideshow provides the recycling code on plastic items (1–7) as well as pictures of these items, what they may be recycled into, and possible issues with their chemical makeup. Because this is a "green" site, it contains comments.

5. Palmer S: Busting bottled water. *Today's Dietitian* 9(12):60, 2007.

This article highlights several reasons why consumers have been wrong in assuming that bottled water is always better than tap water. It addresses the ecological, environmental, and economic problems with relying on bottled water for our fluid needs. The laws regulating bottled and tap water are also compared, suggesting that bottled water is generally not safer and healthier than tap water. The author recommends that we drink more water but do it from the tap.

6. Popkin BM and others: A new proposed guidance system for beverage consumption in the United States. *American Journal of Clinical Nutrition* 83:529, 2006.

Water is recommended as the preferred beverage to fulfill water needs, with tea, coffee, and low-fat and skim milk also ranked high. The Beverage Guidance Panel suggests that beverages with no or few calories should be consumed more often than calorie-containing beverages. An intake of 98 fluid ounces is recommended daily for a person consuming 2200 calories.

7. Savica V and others: The effect of nutrition on blood pressure. *Annual Review of Nutrition* 30:365, 2010.

The most important predictors of development of hypertension are excess energy intake and obesity. Excessive intakes of sodium and alcohol are also factors. Well-studied dietary components that can lower blood pressure include potassium and polyunsaturated fatty acids (e.g., fish oil). Other compounds of interest for blood pressure reduction are certain amino acids, vitamin D, green coffee bean extract, dark chocolate, and tea. The DASH low-sodium diet is effective at lowering blood pressure and preventing development of hypertension, but efforts are needed to improve long-term compliance with such dietary interventions.

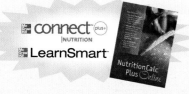

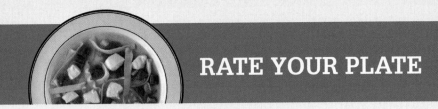

RATE YOUR PLATE

I. How High Is Your Sodium Intake?

Complete this questionnaire to evaluate your sodium habits with respect to typically rich sources.

How Often Do You . . .	Rarely	Occasionally	Often	Regularly (Daily)
1. Eat cured or processed meats, such as ham, bacon, sausage, frankfurters, and other luncheon meats?				
2. Choose canned or frozen vegetables with sauce?				
3. Use commercially prepared meals, main dishes, or canned or dehydrated soups?				
4. Eat cheese, especially processed cheese?				
5. Eat salted nuts, popcorn, pretzels, corn chips, or potato chips?				
6. Add salt to cooking water for vegetables, rice, or pasta?				
7. Add salt, seasoning mixes, salad dressings, or condiments—such as soy sauce, steak sauce, catsup, and mustard—to foods during preparation or at the table?				
8. Salt your food before tasting it?				
9. Ignore labels for sodium content when buying foods?				
10. When dining out, choose obviously salty sauces or foods?				

The more checks you put in the "often" or "regularly" columns, the higher your dietary sodium intake. However, not all the habits in the table contribute the same amount of sodium. For example, many natural cheeses such as cheddar are relatively moderate in sodium, whereas processed cheeses and cottage cheese are much higher. To moderate sodium intake, choose lower-sodium foods from each food group more often and balance high-sodium food choices with low-sodium ones.

Adapted from *USDA Home and Garden Bulletin* No. 232-6, April 1986.

II. Rate Your Beverage Choices

Water is the key component in the beverage-consumption guidelines that have been recently developed (Table 9-2). These recommendations give guidance on the health and nutritional benefits as well as the risks of various beverage categories. The basis of the Beverage Guidance System is that fluids should not provide a significant amount of the energy nutrients in a healthy diet. More specifically, the system recommends that beverages provide less than 10% of total calories consumed for a 2200 kcal diet (see Further Reading 6).

TABLE 9-2 The Beverage Guidance System

Level	Category *	Recommended Servings per Day
1	Water	50 fluid ounces (1.7 liters)
2	Tea or coffee, unsweetened	0 to 40 fluid ounces (0 to 1.4 liters)
3	Low-fat and skim milk and soy beverages	0 to 16 fluid ounces (0 to 0.5 liter)
4	Noncalorically sweetened beverages (diet drinks)	0 to 32 fluid ounces (0 to 1 liter)
5	Calorie beverages with some nutrients (100% fruit juices, alcoholic beverages, whole milk, sports drinks)	0 to 8 fluid ounces 100% fruit juices (0 to 0.25 liter) 0 to 1 alcoholic drink for women 0 to 2 alcoholic drinks for men
6	Calorically sweetened beverages (regular soft drinks)	0 to 8 fluid ounces (0 to 0.25 liter)

*Categories established based on their possible health benefits or risks.

Adapted from Popkin and others: *American Journal of Clinical Nutrition* 83:529, 2006.

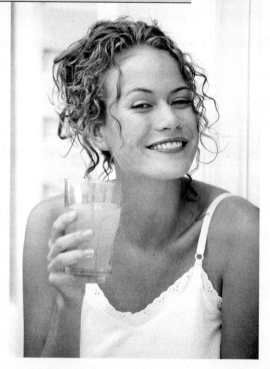

1. Think of all the beverages you drank yesterday, from the time you woke up to the time you went to bed. Do your best to recall the types and amounts of your fluid intake in the space below.

    _____

    _____

    _____

    _____

2. Next to each beverage choice you listed for question 1, indicate its category from the Beverage Guidance System.

3. Did you come close to the recommendation to consume 50 fluid ounces (1.7 liters) of fluid in the form of water yesterday?

    _____

    _____

4. How many fluid ounces of your beverages fit into categories 2, 3, 4, or 5? Did you exceed the recommended servings per day for these categories?

    _____

    _____

5. What changes could you make in your beverage choices to follow the Beverage Guidance System more closely? How does following the Beverage Guidance System contribute to good health?

    _____

    _____

Chapter 10 Nutrients That Function as Antioxidants

Student Learning Outcomes

Chapter 10 is designed to allow you to:

10.1 Define the terms *oxidation*, *reduction*, and *free radical* and understand how free radicals can alter normal cell function.

10.2 Describe how antioxidants function to neutralize free radicals.

10.3 Summarize the functions of important micronutrients shown to have antioxidant properties and describe their deficiency and toxicity symptoms.

10.4 List major food sources of the antioxidants.

10.5 Describe the relationship between consumption of foods that are rich sources of antioxidants and a decreased risk for disease.

10.6 Define *functional foods* and *phytochemicals*.

10.7 Understand appropriate uses of dietary supplements.

What Would You Choose?

To make a few extra bucks, you have been working as a hot-dog vendor in the football stadium on campus. At the end of your shift, your supervisors allow the vendors to take home any extras to eat or share with friends. You have heard that eating a lot of processed meats, like hot dogs, increases the risk of cancer. Which of the following nutrients is added to processed meats to reduce their cancer-causing potential?

 a Vitamin E

 b Vitamin C

 c Vitamin A

 d Selenium

 Think about your choice as you read Chapter 10, then see our recommendations at the end of the chapter. To learn more about the link between red or processed meats and cancer, check out the Connect site: www.mcgrawhill connect.com

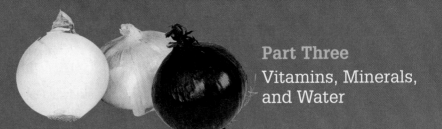

Some vitamins, minerals, and plant compounds can function as antioxidants. They protect our cells from the damaging effects of compounds called free radicals. Free radicals are produced naturally in energy metabolism but may also be overproduced with an immune reaction or exposure to adverse environmental conditions, such as air pollution or tobacco smoke. Nutrients that act as antioxidants may help prevent diseases of aging, such as macular degeneration, cataracts, and some cancers.

In order for nutrients to carry out this free-radical neutralizing role, they must be consumed in adequate amounts and optimally in their natural forms. Researchers are learning more and more about how nutrients help in disease prevention, and their role as antioxidants is a major one. This chapter will describe how free radicals are produced and the damage they can cause. Then we will describe how specific vitamins, minerals, and plant compounds can act as a defense against them.

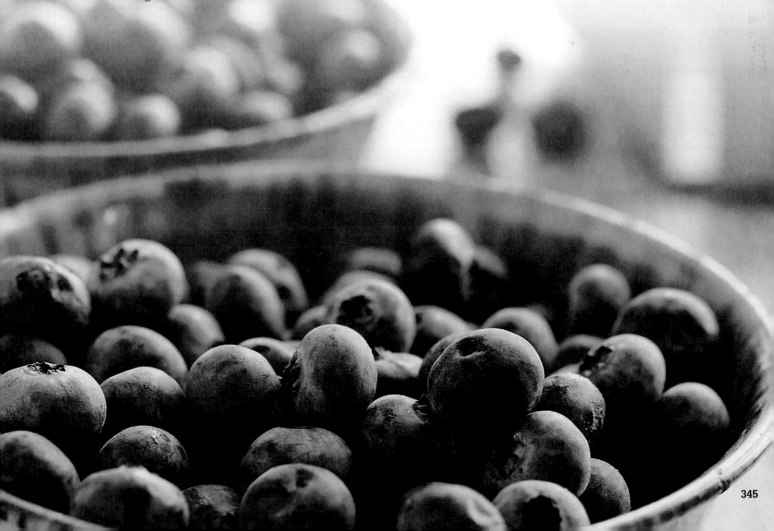

Refresh Your Memory

As you begin the study in Chapter 10 of nutrients that have **antioxidant** functions, you might want to review:

- Implications of the Dietary Supplement Health and Education Act (DSHEA) in Chapter 1.
- Cell structure and function, digestion and absorption of nutrients, and immunity in Chapter 3.

Oxidation
Electrons from molecule A are transferred to molecule B. Molecule A has been oxidized.

Reduction
Electrons are added to molecule B from molecule A. Molecule B has been reduced.

FIGURE 10-1 ▶ Electrons are transferred between molecules in oxidation-reduction reactions.

reduction The process of gaining an electron during a chemical reaction.

oxidation The process of losing an electron during a chemical reaction.

10.1 Oxidation and Reduction

To have an understanding of how antioxidants function, a brief review of the anatomy of an atom is necessary. Atoms contain protons and neutrons found in the nucleus. Electrons circle the nucleus and are found in pairs. The nucleus is positively $(+)$ charged and the electrons are negatively $(-)$ charged. The positive and negative charges are balanced so there is no overall charge to the atom.

Atoms join together (or bond) to form molecules. For example, hydrogen (H) and oxygen (O) are individual atoms; they bond to form a molecule of water (H_2O). Carbohydrates, lipids, and protein are examples of molecules. Approximately half of all enzymatic (chemical) reactions in the body involve the exchange of electrons between atoms and molecules. The gain of a negatively charged electron is called **reduction,** and the loss of an electron is termed **oxidation** (Fig. 10-1).

Within the human body, millions of metabolic processes occur all the time. Many of these processes require oxygen. The key to human life is respiration, in which we inhale oxygen (O_2) and exhale carbon dioxide (CO_2). That inspired O_2 reacts with atoms and molecules in food to produce the CO_2 we exhale, energy we derive from food, and water as a waste product. This reaction occurs within the cell, in its respiratory center (mitochondria). The energy we derive from food is in the form of ATP and other high-energy compounds. This energy allows us to do work (Fig. 10-2).

Normally, bonds between atoms or molecules are strong; sharing electrons in the outer shell makes the bond strong. Oxidation of these bonds usually produces stable compounds. However, sometimes bonds between atoms or molecules may be weak. When these bonds split, a molecule or atom may be left with an unpaired electron in its outer shell.

Rhymes with Orange

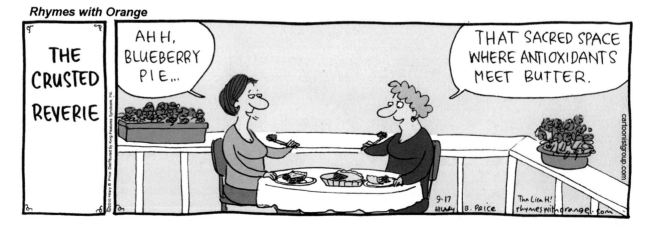

Can antioxidants prevent disease? What foods are the best sources of antioxidants? Is it better to get antioxidants from food or supplements? What role do phytochemicals play in disease prevention? Can I rationalize eating a lot of chocolate or blueberry pie if it contains phytochemicals? Chapter 10 provides some answers.

The presence of the free electron results in a situation in which the number of positive charges contributed by the nucleus of the atom is no longer equal to the number of negative charges in the electrons surrounding the nucleus. These chemically unstable atoms are classified as **free radicals.** Free radicals are chemically reactive and sometimes aggressive. To reestablish a balance between positive and negative charges, the free radical pilfers an electron from an adjacent stable atom or molecule. Once this process starts, it leads to a chain reaction. With the loss of an electron, that nearby molecule now becomes an unstable free radical. In order to reestablish neutrality, it looks to acquire an electron from another adjacent molecule. The body's natural defenses and repair systems try to control the destruction caused by free radicals, but these systems are not 100% effective.

The production of free radicals is a normal consequence of cellular respiration and metabolism. To a degree, free radicals are purposefully produced to protect our health. For example, white blood cells produce highly reactive free radicals that assist in the destruction of bacteria, viruses, and fungi. The production of free radicals has also been shown to be an important component of the mechanism by which the body destroys altered cells, which could potentially proceed to cancerous growth (see Further Reading 12).

On the other hand, overproduction of free radicals can be deleterious to healthy cells. The damage can happen at two levels: at the cell membrane or inside the cell, disrupting cell function and growth. Remember, the cell membrane is a lipid bilayer. Phospholipids primarily compose these layers. The hydrophilic (attracted to water) heads of phospholipid molecules are aligned to the inside (cytoplasm) or outside (extracellular fluid) of the cell. The tails, which are fatty acids, are hydrophobic (or lipophilic—attracted to fat) and are aligned toward each other in the interior of the cell membrane. When free radicals pilfer electrons from the heads of the phospholipids,

free radical An unstable atom with an unpaired electron in its outermost shell.

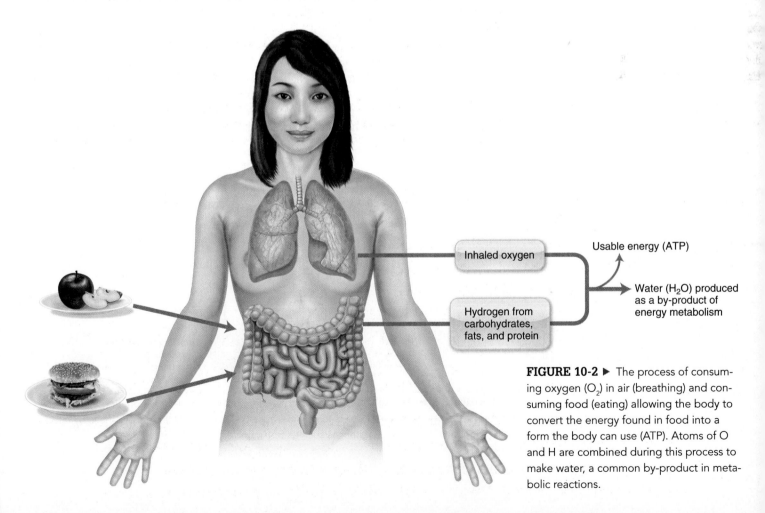

Inhaled oxygen

Hydrogen from carbohydrates, fats, and protein

Usable energy (ATP)

Water (H_2O) produced as a by-product of energy metabolism

FIGURE 10-2 ▶ The process of consuming oxygen (O_2) in air (breathing) and consuming food (eating) allowing the body to convert the energy found in food into a form the body can use (ATP). Atoms of O and H are combined during this process to make water, a common by-product in metabolic reactions.

the cell membrane loses its integrity. The chain of lipid heads is "broken," and so is the cell's ability to regulate the flow of water and nutrients in and out of it. Eventually, with enough breakage, the cell will collapse.

Specific structures and molecules within the cells can be damaged by free-radical overproduction. Damage to LDL proteins (low-density lipoproteins) can contribute to plaque formation and atherosclerosis (see Further Readings 4, 5, 8, 9 and 10). Alteration of DNA, as in the case of some skin cancer, results in altered protein synthesis. The chemical damage produced by free radicals has been linked to numerous diseases including:

cancer   kidney disease
atherosclerosis   Alzheimer's disease
arthritis   Parkinson's disease
diabetes   cataracts
emphysema

Several environmental substances have been shown to accelerate the formation of free radicals. Examples are excessive sunlight, water and air pollution, radiation, asbestos, ozone, and toxic chemicals.

10.2 Defense Against Free Radicals

antioxidant A substance that has the ability to prevent or repair the damage caused by oxidation.

vitamin Compound needed in small amounts to help regulate and support chemical reactions and processes in the body.

phytochemical A chemical Found in Plants. Some phytochemicals may contribute to a reduced risk of cancer or cardiovascular disease in people who consume them regularly.

The body has two principal defense mechanisms to limit or defend against the adverse effects of free radicals: enzyme systems and **antioxidant** chemicals. Enzyme systems have a close relationship with nutrition in that enzyme activity requires the presence of such minerals as selenium, manganese, zinc, iron, and copper. These enzyme systems detoxify free radicals or related compounds at specific locations within cells.

Antioxidant chemicals are derived from food. They include **vitamins,** a vitamin precursor, and **phytochemicals.** These antioxidants principally function by donating an electron or hydrogen atom to reactive molecules to stabilize the molecule's structure (Fig. 10-3). The antioxidants then become chemically unstable; but because of their unique structure, they are not reactive molecules prone to induce cellular damage. The enzyme systems and dietary antioxidants work in concert to limit free radical

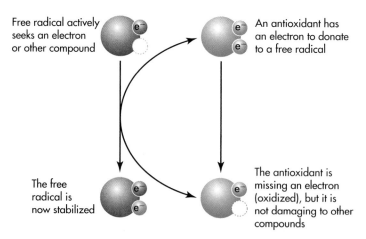

FIGURE 10-3 ▶ Antioxidants (in blue) stabilize free radicals (in red) by donating electrons to them. Free radicals are dangerous to cells because they seek to fill their outer shells by removing electrons from other substances such as DNA, proteins, and lipids.

formation, destroy free radicals, and assist in repairing oxidative damage induced by reactive molecules. Dietary recommendations, including those found in the 2010 Dietary Guidelines for Americans, MyPlate, and the Fruits & Veggies: More Matters© campaign, are based on the premise that increased consumption of fruits and vegetables will increase intake of fiber, antioxidant vitamins, minerals, and phytochemicals. These latter chemicals help detoxify reactive molecules, including free radicals.

10.3 Nutrients That Provide an Antioxidant Role

Antioxidant minerals, vitamins, and phytochemicals may help prevent or postpone diseases that have oxidation as a component to their development. These nutrients must be consumed in the diet as the body cannot synthesize them. The principal antioxidant vitamins are E and C. Vitamin A and its precursor, the **carotenoids**, are discussed in this chapter as they also have antioxidant properties. The antioxidant function of phytochemicals and selenium are examined in this chapter (see Further Reading 6). Iron, zinc, manganese, and copper also participate to some extent in antioxidant enzyme systems, but these minerals will be discussed in Chapters 11 and 12.

carotenoids Pigment materials that range in color from yellow to orange to red; three of the carotenoids are converted into vitamin A. Many are antioxidants.

CONCEPT CHECK

As cells in the body metabolize the molecules found in foods, atoms gain pairs of electrons (reduction) and lose pairs of electrons (oxidation). Free radicals are formed when atoms contain an unpaired electron and form naturally in metabolic reactions, and a number of environmental factors (e.g., pollution, radiation) increase their formation. Free radicals are chemically destructive, aggressive, and play a role in the development of numerous diseases. Nutrients with antioxidant roles in the body include vitamins A, C and E; selenium; and some phytochemicals. Antioxidant chemicals and enzyme system stabilize or detoxify free radicals, thereby reducing the cellular damage they can induce.

10.4 Vitamin E (Tocopherol)

Functions of Vitamin E

In the 1920s, a fat-soluble compound was found to be essential for fertility in rats. This compound was named tocopherol from the Greek words *tokos*, meaning birth, and *phero*, meaning to bring forth. Later, this essential nutrient was named vitamin E. Vitamin E is a family of four tocopherols and four tocotrienols called alpha, beta, gamma, and delta. They differ in that tocopherols have a saturated side chain whereas the tocotrienols have an unsaturated side chain. Tocotrienols have not been as extensively studied as tocopherols, but recent research explores their potential roles in prevention of cancer, diabetes, and cardiovascular diseases. Of the four tocopherols, alpha (α)-tocopherol is the most biologically active and the most potent.

Vitamin E is unique in that in many animal species it has an essential function in fertility, whereas it does not appear to have this function in humans. It is, however, important for the formation of muscles and the central nervous system in early human development.

The principal function of vitamin E in humans is as an antioxidant. Vitamin E is a fat-soluble vitamin found primarily in adipose tissue and in the lipid bilayers of cell membranes (Fig. 10.4). Many of the lipids within these membranes are polyunsaturated fatty acids (PUFA). The unsaturated double bond is not as stable as a saturated single bond in saturated fatty acids. PUFAs are particularly susceptible to oxidative

FIGURE 10-4 ▶ Fat-soluble vitamin E can insert itself into cell membranes, where it helps stop free-radical chain reactions. If not interrupted, these reactions cause extensive oxidative damage to cells and ultimately cell death.

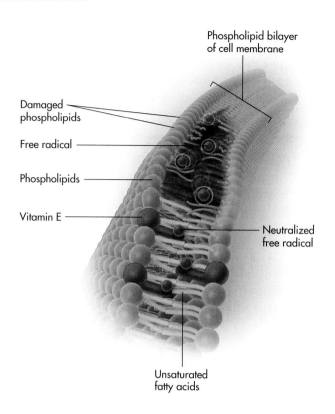

megadose Intake of a nutrient beyond estimates of needs to prevent a deficiency or what would be found in a balanced diet; 2 to 10 times human needs is a starting point for such a dosage.

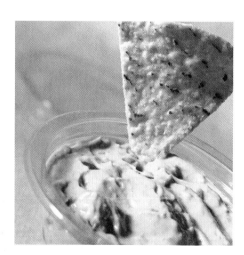

▲ The avacado in guacarnole and the oil in the tortilla chip are good sources of vitamin E.

attack by free radicals. The formation of free radicals may destabilize the cell membrane, which may ultimately alter the ability of the cell to function properly. Vitamin E can donate electrons or hydrogen to free radicals found in membranes, thereby making them more stable. The antioxidant function of vitamin E appears to be critical in cells continually exposed to high levels of oxygen, particularly red blood cells and the cells lining the lungs.

Increasing vitamin E intake has also been suggested as a way to prevent several chronic diseases that are linked to oxidative damage. For example, oxidized LDL cholesterol is a major component of the plaque that develops in arteries, which leads to atherosclerosis. Vitamin E is thought to attenuate the development of atherogenic plaque due to its ability to prevent or reduce the formation of oxidized LDL cholesterol (see Further Reading 2). Also, oxidative damage to proteins in the eye leads to the development of cataracts. Oxidized proteins combine and precipitate in the lens, causing cloudiness and decreasing visual acuity. Low intakes of foods that are good sources of antioxidants have been shown to be related to an increased incidence of these diseases.

Experts do not know whether supplementation with **megadoses** of vitamin E can confer any significant protection against diseases linked to oxidative damage. The consensus among the scientific community is that the established benefits of lifestyle choices have a far greater effect than any proposed benefits of antioxidant supplementation. The position of scientific research groups (e.g., American Heart Association, U.S. Preventive Services Task Force) is that it is premature to recommend vitamin E supplements to the general population, based on current knowledge and the failure of large clinical trials to show any consistent benefit. This conclusion is in agreement with the latest report on vitamin E by the Food and Nutrition Board of the National Academy of Sciences. In addition, the Food and Drug Administration has denied the request of the dietary supplement industry to make a health claim that vitamin E supplements reduce the risk of cardiovascular disease and cancer.

Vitamin E has been shown to improve vitamin A absorption if the dietary intake of vitamin A is low. Vitamin E also functions in the metabolism of iron within cells, and it helps maintain nervous tissue and immune function.

Vitamin E Sources and Needs

Because vitamin E is only synthesized by plants, plant products (especially the oils) are the best sources. In the North American diet, nearly two-thirds of vitamin E is supplied by salad oils, margarines, spreads (low-fat margarine), and shortening (Fig. 10-5). Breakfast cereals fortified with vitamin E are good sources, but other than wheat germ, few other grain products provide much vitamin E. Milling of grains removes the germ, which contains the oils, mostly PUFAs and vitamin E. By removing the germ, the resulting grain product has less chance of spoiling (i.e., rancidity of the PUFAs), and thus a longer shelf life. Other good sources of vitamin E are nuts and seeds.

Because plant oils are made up of mainly unsaturated fatty acids, the relatively high amount of vitamin E in plant oils naturally protects these unsaturated lipids from oxidation. Animal products (meat, dairy, eggs) and fish oils, on the other hand, contain almost no vitamin E (Fig. 10-6). Vitamin E is susceptible to destruction by oxygen, metals, light, and especially repeated use in deep-fat frying; thus, the vitamin E content of a food depends on how it is harvested, processed, stored, and cooked.

The RDA of vitamin E for adults is 15 milligrams per day of alpha-tocopherol, the most active, natural form of vitamin E (d isomer). This amount equals 22.4 milligrams of the less active, synthetic source (dl isomer). Typically, North American adults consume about two-thirds of the RDA for vitamin E from food sources. The Daily Value used on food and supplement labels is 30 milligrams.

Specific population groups are especially susceptible to developing marginal vitamin E status. Preterm infants tend to have low vitamin E stores because this vitamin is transferred from mother to baby during the late stages of pregnancy. Hence,

Food Sources of Vitamin E

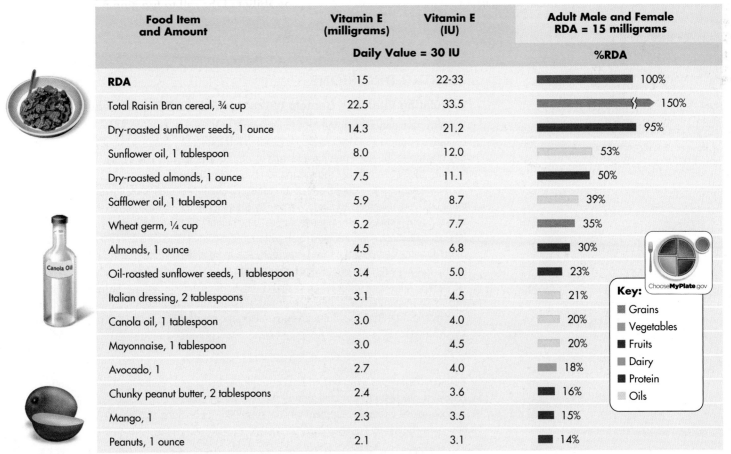

Food Item and Amount	Vitamin E (milligrams)	Vitamin E (IU)	Adult Male and Female RDA = 15 milligrams
	Daily Value = 30 IU		%RDA
RDA	15	22-33	100%
Total Raisin Bran cereal, ¾ cup	22.5	33.5	150%
Dry-roasted sunflower seeds, 1 ounce	14.3	21.2	95%
Sunflower oil, 1 tablespoon	8.0	12.0	53%
Dry-roasted almonds, 1 ounce	7.5	11.1	50%
Safflower oil, 1 tablespoon	5.9	8.7	39%
Wheat germ, ¼ cup	5.2	7.7	35%
Almonds, 1 ounce	4.5	6.8	30%
Oil-roasted sunflower seeds, 1 tablespoon	3.4	5.0	23%
Italian dressing, 2 tablespoons	3.1	4.5	21%
Canola oil, 1 tablespoon	3.0	4.0	20%
Mayonnaise, 1 tablespoon	3.0	4.5	20%
Avocado, 1	2.7	4.0	18%
Chunky peanut butter, 2 tablespoons	2.4	3.6	16%
Mango, 1	2.3	3.5	15%
Peanuts, 1 ounce	2.1	3.1	14%

Key:
- Grains
- Vegetables
- Fruits
- Dairy
- Protein
- Oils

ChooseMyPlate.gov

FIGURE 10-5 ▶ Food sources of vitamin E compared to the RDA for adults.

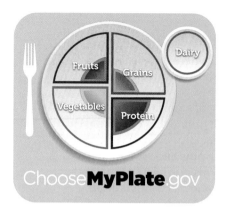

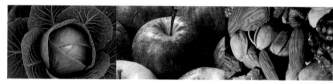

MyPlate:
Sources of Vitamin E

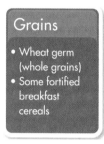

Grains
- Wheat germ (whole grains)
- Some fortified breakfast cereals

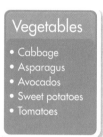

Vegetables
- Cabbage
- Asparagus
- Avocados
- Sweet potatoes
- Tomatoes

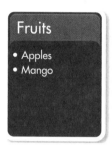

Fruits
- Apples
- Mango

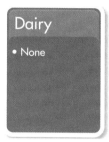

Dairy
- None

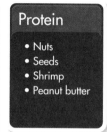

Protein
- Nuts
- Seeds
- Shrimp
- Peanut butter

FIGURE 10-6 ▶ Sources of vitamin E from MyPlate. The fill of the background color (none, 1/3, 2/3, or completely covered) within each group on the plate indicates the average nutrient density for vitamin E in that group. Overall, plant oils are the richest source, followed by nuts and seeds in the protein group. With regard to physical activity, vitamin E has no primary role in the related energy metabolism per se but likely limits some oxidative damage during such endeavors.

MAKING DECISIONS

Calculating Vitamin E Content of Dietary Vitamin E Supplements

You may have noticed that the RDA for vitamin E is given in milligrams, whereas the vitamin E content on Supplement Facts labels is given in international units (IU). Legally, supplement manufacturers still must provide amounts of vitamin E in IU, which is a measure of the biological activity of a nutrient rather than its absolute quantity.

Supplements may contain any of the variety of chemical forms and stereoisomers of vitamin E you have learned about. Typical synthetic preparations of vitamin E contain a mixture of equal parts of d and l stereoisomers, only half of which are biologically active. Therefore, a supplement containing synthetic vitamin E has lower biological activity (i.e., lower IU) than the same quantity of natural vitamin E. The more expensive natural vitamin E supplements contain only the biologically active d-form.

To find milligrams of *natural* vitamin E (d-alpha-tocopherol), multiply IU by 0.67. Conversely, to calculate IU from milligrams, multiply milligrams by 1.49.

Example: The RDA for vitamin E is 15 milligrams per day. This is equal to how many IU of natural vitamin E?

$$15 \text{ mg} \times 1.49 \text{ IU/mg} = 22.35 \text{ IU}$$

To find milligrams of *synthetic* vitamin E (dl-alpha-tocopherol), multiply IU by 0.45. Conversely, to calculate IU from milligrams, multiply milligrams by 2.22.

Example: A vitamin E supplement contains 400 IU of dl-alpha-tocopherol. This is equal to how many milligrams of vitamin E?

$$400 \text{ IU} \times 0.45 \text{ mg/IU} = 180 \text{ mg}$$

the potential for oxidative damage, which could cause the cell membranes of red blood cells to break (hemolysis), is of particular concern for preterm infants. The rapid growth of preterm infants, coupled with the high oxygen needs of their immature lungs, greatly increases the stress on red blood cells. Special vitamin-E-fortified formulas and supplements designed for preterm infants compensate for lack of vitamin E. Smokers are another group at high risk for vitamin E deficiency, as smoking readily destroys vitamin E in the lungs. One study showed that megadosing will not correct this vitamin E destruction by smokers. Others at risk of vitamin E deficiency include adults on very low-fat diets (< 15% total fat) or those with fat malabsorption.

Upper Level for Vitamin E

Unlike other fat-soluble vitamins, vitamin E is not stored in the liver. It is stored in adipose tissue throughout the body. The Upper Level for vitamin E is 1000 milligrams per day of supplemental alpha-tocopherol. Excessive intake of vitamin E can interfere with vitamin K's role in the clotting mechanism, leading to hemorrhage. The risk of insufficient blood clotting is especially high if vitamin E is taken in conjunction with anticoagulant medications (e.g., Coumadin or heavy aspirin use).

Caution should always be taken with supplementation. In addition to the significant risk of drug interference and prolonged bleeding, vitamin E supplements can produce nausea, gastrointestinal distress, and diarrhea.

CONCEPT CHECK

By providing electrons to free radicals, vitamin E helps prevent oxidative damage, especially of cell membranes. Dietary sources of vitamin E include plant oils and fortified foods, such as breakfast cereal. Preterm infants are particularly susceptible to oxidative breakdown of their red blood cell membranes (hemolysis) because of their poor vitamin E status. Among adults, overt deficiency is rare. People who smoke or experience long-term fat malabsorption run the biggest risk of vitamin E deficiency. There is controversy about the utility of megadose vitamin E supplementation for chronic disease prevention; research is ongoing. Toxicity of vitamin E reduces blood clotting, possibly leading to a hemorrhage.

10.5 Vitamin C (Ascorbic Acid)

On long sea voyages, half or more of sailing crews died due to scurvy, the vitamin C deficiency disease. In 1740, the Englishman Dr. James Lind first showed that citrus fruits—two oranges and one lemon a day—could prevent the development of scurvy. Fifty years after Lind's discovery, daily rations for British sailors included limes (thus their nickname, limeys). Even after this discovery, scurvy continued to affect many people as thousands died during the American Civil War due to inadequate intake of vitamin C.

Functions of Vitamin C

Vitamin C (also known as ascorbic acid or ascorbate) has a specific function in the synthesis of numerous compounds in the body, including collagen; carnitine; and two neurotransmitters, serotonin and norepinephrine. Vitamin C is required for the synthesis of carnitine, a compound that transports fatty acids into the mitochondria. The best understood function of vitamin C is its role in the synthesis of collagen. This protein is highly concentrated in connective tissue, bone, teeth, tendons, and blood vessels. The important function of vitamin C in the formation of connective tissue is exemplified in the early

▲ Citrus fruits are good sources of vitamin C.

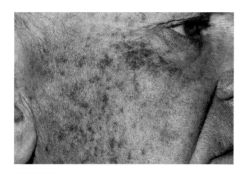

FIGURE 10-7 ▶ Pinpoint hemorrhages of the skin—an early symptom of scurvy. The spots on the skin are caused by slight bleeding. The person may experience poor wound healing. These are signs of defective collagen synthesis.

symptoms of a deficiency: pinpoint hemorrhages under the skin (Fig. 10-7), bleeding gums, and joint pain. Vitamin C is very important for wound healing; it increases the cross-connections between amino acids found in collagen, greatly strengthening the structural tissues it helps form. Without adequate vitamin C, wounds will not heal.

Vitamin C also has a more general function acting as antioxidant because it can readily accept and denote electrons. These antioxidant properties have been postulated to reduce the formation of cancer-causing nitrosamines in the stomach (see What Would You Choose Recommendations). Vitamin C also aids in the reactivation of vitamin E after it has donated an electron to a free radical. Population studies suggest that the antioxidant properties of vitamin C may be effective in the prevention of certain cancers (esophagus, mouth, and stomach) and cataracts. The extent to which vitamin C functions in the reduction of diseases is debatable based on the scientific studies to this point.

Vitamin C enhances iron absorption by keeping iron in its most absorbable form, especially as the mineral travels through the alkaline environment of the small intestine. Consuming 75 milligrams or more of vitamin C at a meal significantly increases absorption of the iron consumed at that meal. Increasing intake of vitamin-C-rich foods is beneficial for those with poor iron status or for those who choose to limit iron-rich food sources. Iron-deficiency anemia is common in the United States and is the number one nutritional deficiency worldwide.

Vitamin C is vital for the function of the immune system, especially for the activity of certain cells (leukocytes) in the immune system. Thus, diseases and infections can increase the need for vitamin C. It is unknown if this increased need is greater than the RDA. Partly on the basis of this observation of promoting resistance to infection, Nobel laureate Dr. Linus Pauling claimed that supplementation with large doses of vitamin C could combat the common cold. In the 1970s, he advocated the consumption of at least 1000 milligrams of vitamin C daily. As a result of the popularity of his books and the respectability of his scientific credentials, millions of North Americans supplement their diets with vitamin C.

MAKING DECISIONS

Vitamin C and the Common Cold

Does vitamin C reliably and effectively lower the likelihood of developing an upper respiratory infection? Numerous well-designed, double-blind studies have failed to show that vitamin C prevents colds. Nevertheless, vitamin C does appear to reduce the duration of symptoms by a day or so and to lessen the severity of the symptoms. The key to success is to start the supplement or added fruit juice as soon as symptoms start. Once the cold has taken hold, it is too late! The effect of vitamin C on cold symptoms may be due to a general role in stimulating immune function and the ability to increase the breakdown of histamine. The reaction of vitamin C with the oxidized products formed in upper respiratory infection minimizes the inflammatory effects of these oxidized products and therefore may reduce the severity of these infections.

Vitamin C Sources and Needs

Major sources of vitamin C are citrus fruits, strawberries, green peppers, cauliflower, broccoli, cabbage, papayas, and romaine lettuce (Fig. 10-8). The brighter the fruit or vegetable, the higher it tends to be in vitamin C. Look at Figure 10-8 and compare red peppers to green peppers, and oranges to pineapple chunks, in terms of brightness. Just picked, most ripe fruits and vegetables will be loaded with vitamin C. Allowing them to "ripen" further in the grocery store or on your countertop at home will not increase vitamin C and actually can decrease it.

Food Sources of Vitamin C

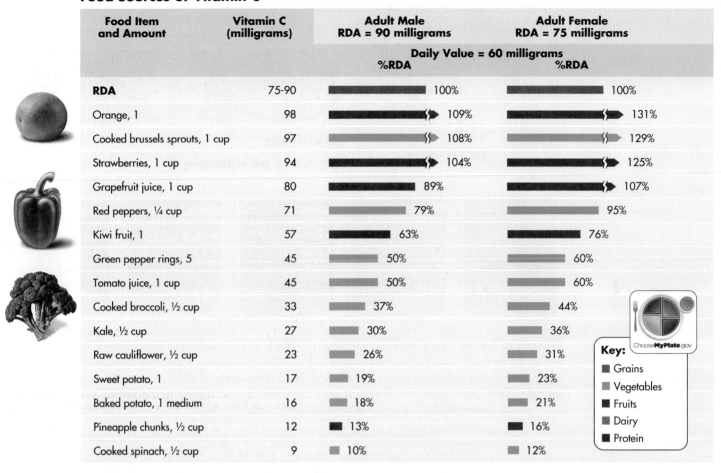

Food Item and Amount	Vitamin C (milligrams)	Adult Male RDA = 90 milligrams %RDA	Adult Female RDA = 75 milligrams %RDA
RDA	75-90	100%	100%
Orange, 1	98	109%	131%
Cooked brussels sprouts, 1 cup	97	108%	129%
Strawberries, 1 cup	94	104%	125%
Grapefruit juice, 1 cup	80	89%	107%
Red peppers, ¼ cup	71	79%	95%
Kiwi fruit, 1	57	63%	76%
Green pepper rings, 5	45	50%	60%
Tomato juice, 1 cup	45	50%	60%
Cooked broccoli, ½ cup	33	37%	44%
Kale, ½ cup	27	30%	36%
Raw cauliflower, ½ cup	23	26%	31%
Sweet potato, 1	17	19%	23%
Baked potato, 1 medium	16	18%	21%
Pineapple chunks, ½ cup	12	13%	16%
Cooked spinach, ½ cup	9	10%	12%

Daily Value = 60 milligrams

Key:
- Grains
- Vegetables
- Fruits
- Dairy
- Protein

FIGURE 10-8 ▶ Food sources of vitamin C compared to the RDA for adult males and females.

Ready-to-eat breakfast cereals, potatoes, and fortified fruit drinks are also good sources of vitamin C (Fig. 10-9). The five to nine servings of fruit and vegetables suggested by MyPlate's Daily Food Plan can easily provide enough vitamin C. Vitamin C is rapidly lost in processing and cooking as it is unstable in the presence of heat, iron, copper, or oxygen and is water soluble. When fruits and vegetables are boiled for an extended time, much of the vitamin C is destroyed or leached out of the food and found in the often discarded water.

The adult RDA of vitamin C is 75 milligrams for women and 90 milligrams for men per day. The Daily Value used on food and supplement labels is 60 milligrams. Tobacco users need to add an extra 35 milligrams per day to the RDA. The toxic by-products of cigarette smoke and the oxidizing agents found in tobacco products increase the need for the antioxidant action of vitamin C. Average daily consumption of vitamin C in the United States is 70 to 100 milligrams, reflecting our poor intake of fruits and vegetables. Absorption efficiency is about 80% to 90% for moderate intakes (i.e., 60 to 100 milligrams per day).

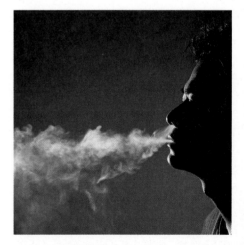

▲ If you smoke or chew tobacco, you need more vitamin C—at least 33% more.

Upper Level for Vitamin C

The Upper Level (UL) of vitamin C is 2000 milligrams. Note that when vitamin C is consumed in large doses, the amount in excess of daily needs mostly ends up in the feces or urine. The kidneys start rapidly excreting vitamin C when intakes exceed 100 milligrams per day. As the amount ingested increases, absorption efficiency decreases precipitously—to approximately 50% with intake of 1000 milligrams per day and to 20% with intakes of 6000 milligrams daily. Regular consumption of more

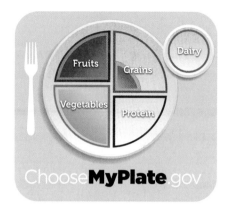

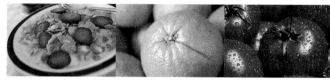

**MyPlate:
Sources of Vitamin C**

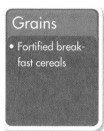

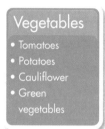

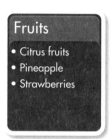

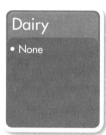

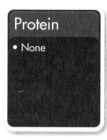

Grains
• Fortified break-
  fast cereals

Vegetables
• Tomatoes
• Potatoes
• Cauliflower
• Green
  vegetables

Fruits
• Citrus fruits
• Pineapple
• Strawberries

Dairy
• None

Protein
• None

FIGURE 10-9 ▶ Sources of vitamin C from MyPlate. The fill of the background color (none, 1/3, 2/3, or completely covered) within each group on the plate indicates the average nutrient density for vitamin C in the group. Overall, the vegetables group and the fruits group contain many foods that are nutrient-dense sources of vitamin C. With regard to physical activity, vitamin C has no primary role in the related energy metabolism per se but likely limits some oxidative damage during such endeavors.

than 2000 milligrams per day may cause stomach inflammation and diarrhea. Even 1000 mg supplement pills can cause some nausea and GI distress. Ingesting large amounts of vitamin C supplements is discouraged in people predisposed to kidney stones and those who overabsorb iron or have excessive iron stores. High doses of vitamin C may interfere with medical tests for diabetes or blood in the feces. If you take vitamin C supplements at any dose, be sure to inform your doctor. Physicians may misdiagnose conditions when large doses of vitamin C are consumed without their knowledge.

CONCEPT CHECK

Vitamin C functions as an antioxidant by donating electrons that chemically stabilize free radicals. Vitamin C also regenerates vitamin E after vitamin E has stabilized free radicals. In addition, vitamin C is required for the synthesis of collagen, carnitine, and neurotransmitters. A vitamin C deficiency causes scurvy, marked by many changes in the skin and gums, because of reduced collagen synthesis. Vitamin C also modestly improves iron absorption. Many fruits and vegetables are good sources of vitamin C. Fresh or lightly cooked foods are the best sources because vitamin C is easily lost during storage and cooling.

10.6 Vitamin A (Retinoids)

Vitamin A was the first fat-soluble vitamin to be recognized as an important component of food essential for human health. Almost all (90%) of vitamin A is stored in the liver; the remaining 10% is in adipose tissue, kidneys, and lung. Either a deficiency or toxicity can cause severe problems; there is a narrow range of optimal intakes between these two states. Vitamin A has many important functions in the body. The best known and most clearly understood involves vision. A more well-known role to teens is vitamin A's role in acne control. In this role, vitamin A is functioning in cellular reproduction. Vitamin A may have antioxidant functions in the body; recent research indicates a stronger role in this area. **Carotenoids,** which are precursors of vitamin A, have profound antioxidant properties. Vitamin A and carotenoids are discussed in this chapter.

Vitamin A is in a group of compounds known as **retinoids.** There are three active forms of vitamin A: **retinol** (an alcohol), **retinal** (an aldehyde), and **retinoic acid** (an acid). These are often called preformed vitamin A. They exist only in animal products. When retinol is stored, it is esterified (joined to a fatty acid) and becomes **retinyl.** In supplements, you will often find vitamin A listed as retinyl acetate, a stored form of retinol. Plants contain carotenoids, a group of compounds that humans can convert to vitamin A to some extent. Beta carotene (β-carotene) is the only carotenoid that can be sufficiently absorbed and converted to retinol to play a significant role as a source of vitamin A and as a powerful antioxidant.

Functions of Vitamin A

Vision. The link between vitamin A and night vision has been known since ancient Egyptian times when juice extracted from liver was used to cure **night blindness.** Vitamin A performs important functions in light-dark vision and, to a lesser extent, color vision. Light entering the back of the eye reaches a lining called the **retina.** The retina consists of rods, cones, and nerve cells. Rods detect black and white and are responsible for night vision. Cones are responsible for color vision. Rods and cones require vitamin A for normal function. One form of vitamin A (retinal) allows certain cells in the eye to adjust from dim light (such as after seeing the headlights of an oncoming car) (Fig. 10-10). Without sufficient dietary vitamin A, the cells in the eye cannot quickly readjust to dim light, causing night blindness.

carotenoids Precursors of vitamin A found in plant foods.

retinoids Chemical forms of preformed vitamin A; one source is animal foods.

retinol Alcohol form of vitamin A.

retinal Aldehyde form of vitamin A.

retinoic acid Acid form of vitamin A.

retinyl Storage form of vitamin A.

night blindness A vitamin A-deficiency disorder that results in loss of the ability to see under low-light conditions.

retina A light-sensitive lining in the back of the eye. It contains retinal.

xerophthalmia Hardening of the cornea and drying of the surface of the eye, which can result in blindness.

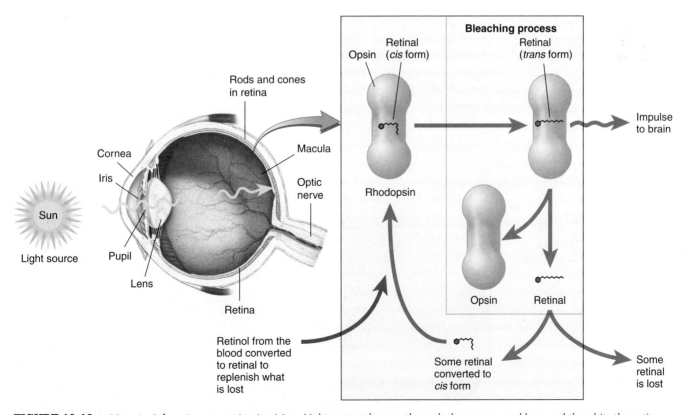

FIGURE 10-10 ▶ Vitamin A functions to maintain vision. Light enters the eye through the cornea and lens and then hits the retina. The light reacts with vitamin-A-containing rhodopsin, which is stored in the rod cells of the retina. Rod cells allow us to see black-and-white images. When light reacts with rhodopsin, retinal is cleaved from rhodopsin (bleaching), a process that stimulates an electrical impulse to the brain. A new molecule of vitamin A then combines with opsin to regenerate rhodopsin.

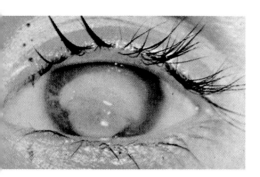

FIGURE 10-11 ▶ Vitamin A deficiency that eventually led to blindness. Note the severe effects on this eye. This problem is commonly seen today in Southeast Asia.

If vitamin A deficiency progresses, the cells that line the cornea of the eye (the clear window of the eye) lose the ability to produce mucus. The eye then becomes dry. Eventually, dirt particles scratch the dry surface of the eye, leading to blindness. This disease is called **xerophthalmia**, which means dry eye. Xerophthalmia can progress to the stage where there is an accumulation of dead cells and secretions on the surface of the eye. This condition is called Bitot's spots (Fig. 10-11).

Vitamin A deficiency is the leading cause of blindness worldwide (Fig. 10-12). North Americans are at little risk because typical American diets contain plentiful sources of preformed vitamin A, such as fortified milk and eggs. However, poor vitamin A intakes, low fat intakes that do not allow for sufficient vitamin A absorption, and low stores of vitamin A lessen the ability of children to meet high needs during rapid childhood growth. Hundreds of thousands of children in developing nations, especially Southeast Asia and Africa, become blind each year because of vitamin A deficiency. Some of these children ultimately die from infections. Worldwide, attempts to reduce this problem have included giving large doses of vitamin A twice yearly and fortifying sugar, margarine, and monosodium glutamate with vitamin A. These food vehicles are used because they are commonly consumed by the populations of less-developed nations. This effort has proven effective in some countries.

Another effort is to treat maternal night blindness in these same areas of the world. Among pregnant women, night blindness is a marker of vitamin A deficiency that will likely lead to pregnancy-related deaths, malnutrition, anemia, and infant mortality. Screening and supplementing populations of pregnant women can be effective in treating and preventing this public health problem.

Health of Epithelial Cells and Immune Function. Vitamin A maintains the health of epithelial cells, which line internal and external surfaces of the lungs, intestines, stomach, vagina, urinary tract, and bladder, as well as those of the eyes and skin. Retinoic acid is required for immature epithelial cells to develop into mature, functional epithelial cells. Without vitamin A, mucus-forming cells, such as those in the intestines and lungs, deteriorate and lose function. As just noted for the eye, this can lead to blindness. Hyperkeratosis, also a result of vitamin A deficiency, is a condition in which skin cells produce too much keratin, blocking the hair follicles and causing "gooseflesh" or "toadskin" appearance. The excessive keratin in these skin cells causes the skin to be hard and dry.

For many years, vitamin A has been dubbed the "anti-infection" vitamin. The epithelial tissues described above serve as important barriers to infection. Vitamin A also supports the activity of certain immune system cells, specifically, the T-lymphocytes,

FIGURE 10-12 ▶ Areas of the world where vitamin A represents a major malnutrition problem. Every year, 250,000 to 500,000 children become blind due to vitamin A deficiency.

Source: WHO

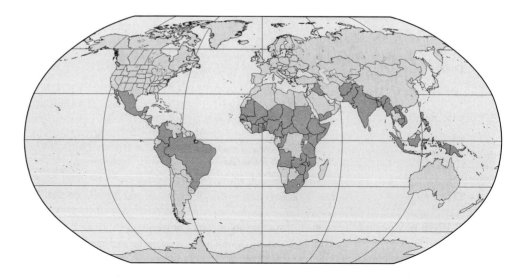

or T-cells. Together, these effects leave the vitamin A-deficient person at great risk for infections. Vitamin-A-deficient animals and humans have an increased infection rate, but when they are supplemented with vitamin A, the immune response improves.

Growth, Development, and Reproduction. Vitamin A participates in the processes of growth, development, and reproduction in several ways. At the genetic level, vitamin A binds to receptors on DNA to increase synthesis of a variety of proteins. Some of these proteins are required for growth, such as bone growth. During early fetal growth, vitamin A functions in the differentiation and maturation of cells, ultimately forming tissues and organs. Vitamin-A-deficient children experience stunted growth. For bone to grow and elongate, old bone must be remodeled (broken down) so that new bone can be formed. Vitamin A assists with breakdown and formation of healthy bone tissue. Adequate intake of vitamin A is needed for reproduction; it aids in sperm production (associated with its epithelial role) and in a normal reproductive cycle for women.

Possible Cancer Prevention. Vitamin A has potential benefits but also potential dangers where cancer prevention is concerned. Vitamin A plays a role in cellular differentiation and embryonic development. Numerous studies have found that diets rich in **provitamin A** carotenoids are associated with a lower risk of skin, lung, bladder, and breast cancers. Still, because of the potential for toxicity, unsupervised use of megadose vitamin A supplements to reduce cancer risk is not advised and can be potentially dangerous. More about the effects of carotenoids on the incidence of cancer is covered later in this chapter.

provitamin A A substance that can be converted into vitamin A.

Vitamin A Analogs for Acne. Taking vitamin A supplements or making a paste from supplements and applying it to your skin will have no effect on acne. It is the analog form of vitamin A in medication that works. Tretinoin (Retin-A), a topical treatment (applied to the skin) for acne, appears to work by altering cell activity in the skin (gene-expression role discussed earlier). Another derivative of vitamin A, 13-*cis* retinoic acid (Accutane), is an oral drug used to treat serious acne. Taking high doses of vitamin A would not be safe. Even Accutane, a less potentially toxic form, can induce toxic symptoms, as well as birth defects in the offspring of women using it during pregnancy. A pregnancy test is required before Accutane is prescribed to women.

Vitamin A Sources and Needs

Preformed vitamin A (e.g., retinol, retinal, and retinoic acid) is found in liver, fish, fish oils, fortified milk, butter, yogurt, and eggs (Figs. 10-13 and 10-14). Margarine and spreads are also fortified with vitamin A. About 65% of the vitamin A in the typical North American diet comes from preformed vitamin A sources, whereas provitamin A (carotenoids) dominates in the diet among poor people in other parts of the world.

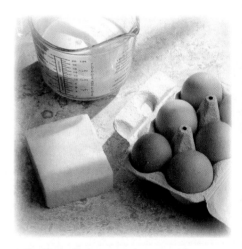

▲ Fortified milk, butter, and eggs are dietary sources of preformed vitamin A.

The RDA for vitamin A is 700 micrograms for women and 900 micrograms for men of retinol activity equivalents (RAE). These RAE units take into account the activity of both preformed vitamin A and the three carotenoids that are synthesized into vitamin A in humans. The total RAE value for a food is calculated by adding the concentration of preformed vitamin A to the amount of provitamin A carotenoids in the food that will be converted to vitamin A. The Daily Value used on food and supplement labels is 1000 micrograms (5000 IU). As with vitamin E, vitamin A legally must be expressed as IU on supplement labels.

The diets of North American adults typically contain adequate vitamin A from both preformed retinoids and carotenoids. Many supplements contain both forms, too. Most adults in North America have liver reserves of vitamin A three to five times

Food Sources of Vitamin A

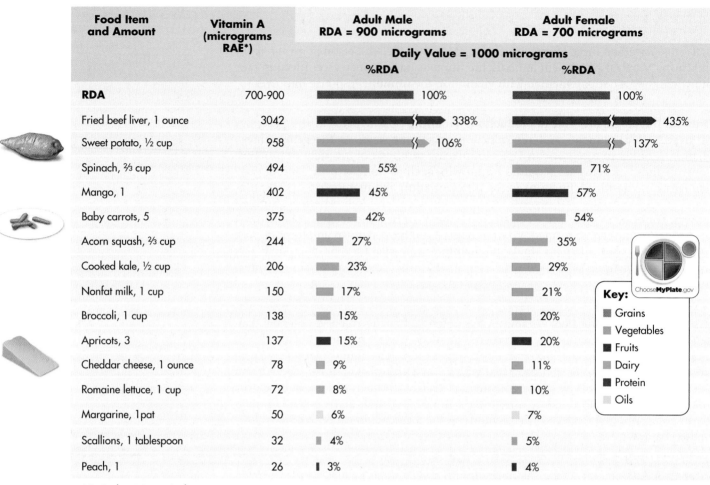

Food Item and Amount	Vitamin A (micrograms RAE*)	Adult Male RDA = 900 micrograms	Adult Female RDA = 700 micrograms
		Daily Value = 1000 micrograms	
		%RDA	%RDA
RDA	700-900	100%	100%
Fried beef liver, 1 ounce	3042	338%	435%
Sweet potato, ½ cup	958	106%	137%
Spinach, ⅔ cup	494	55%	71%
Mango, 1	402	45%	57%
Baby carrots, 5	375	42%	54%
Acorn squash, ⅔ cup	244	27%	35%
Cooked kale, ½ cup	206	23%	29%
Nonfat milk, 1 cup	150	17%	21%
Broccoli, 1 cup	138	15%	20%
Apricots, 3	137	15%	20%
Cheddar cheese, 1 ounce	78	9%	11%
Romaine lettuce, 1 cup	72	8%	10%
Margarine, 1 pat	50	6%	7%
Scallions, 1 tablespoon	32	4%	5%
Peach, 1	26	3%	4%

Key:
- Grains
- Vegetables
- Fruits
- Dairy
- Protein
- Oils

* Retinol activity equivalents.

FIGURE 10-13 ▶ Food sources of vitamin A compared to the RDA for adult males and females.

MAKING DECISIONS

Calculating RAE and IU for vitamin A

Supplements legally must report vitamin A content in international units (IU), an antiquated, less-accurate method than the RAE (retinol activity equivalent) used today. All preformed vitamin A is grouped as retinol, whereas the carotenoids are grouped based on the ability to be synthesized into vitamin A. Following are the retinol activity equivalents:

1 RAE =

- 1 microgram of retinol (or retinal or retinoic acid—all the same)
- 12 micrograms of β-carotene from food or a supplement
- 24 micrograms of other carotenoids from food

How do you convert to RAE (or micrograms) when the supplement label is still in IU?

- IU ÷ 3.3 if the supplement is preformed vitamin A (such as retinyl acetate)
- IU ÷ 6.6 if the supplement is carotenoids (usually β-carotene)

Example: A supplement contains 2500 IU of vitamin A (as retinyl acetate and 40% β-carotene) which is 50% of the Daily Value. How would you express this as RAE or micrograms?

- First calculate carotene: 2500 IU × 40% = 2500 × .40 = 1000 IU from β-carotene
  - 1000 IU ÷ 6.6 = 151 RAE or micrograms of vitamin A
- Retinyl acetate: 2500 IU − 1000 IU (from β-carotene) = 1500 IU
  - 1500 IU ÷ 3.3 = 455 RAE or micrograms of vitamin A
- Total: 151 + 455 = 606 RAE or micrograms of vitamin A

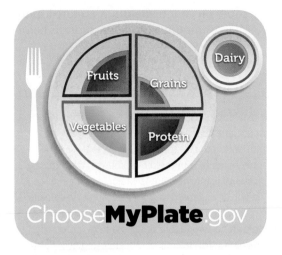

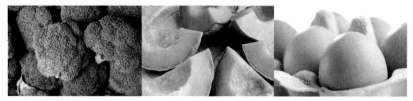

MyPlate:
Sources of Vitamin A

Grains
- Fortified break-fast cereals
- Fortified meal replacement bars

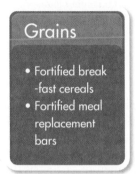

Vegetables
- Carrots
- Broccoli
- Spinach
- Squash
- Sweet potatoes

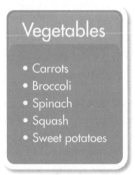

Fruits
- Peaches
- Apricots
- Cantaloupes
- Mangoes
- Papayas

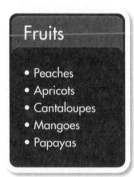

Dairy
- Fortified milk
- Fortified yogurt
- Cheese

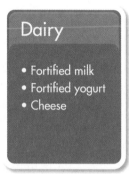

Protein
- Liver
- Eggs
- Fish

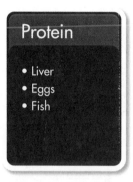

FIGURE 10-14 ▶ Sources of vitamin A from MyPlate. The fill of the background color (none, 1/3, 2/3, or completely covered) within each group on the plate indicates the average nutrient density for vitamin A in that group. Overall richest sources are found in the vegetables group, fruits group, and certain choices in the protein group. The grains group contains some foods that are nutrient dense because they are vitamin A fortified. With regard to physical activity, vitamin A plays no specific role *per se*.

higher than needed to provide good health. Thus, the use of vitamin A supplements by most people is unnecessary. Deficient vitamin A status in North America may be seen in preschool children who do not eat enough vegetables. The urban poor, older adults, and people with alcoholism or liver disease (which limits vitamin A storage) can show diminished vitamin A status, especially with respect to stores. Finally, children and adults with severe fat malabsorption may also experience vitamin A deficiency.

Upper Level for Vitamin A

The UL for vitamin A intake is established at 3000 micrograms of preformed vitamin A (3000 RAE or 10,000 IU) per day for adult men and women. This level is based on the increases in birth defects and liver toxicity that accompany intakes in excess of 3000 micrograms of vitamin A per day. Above the Upper Level, other possible side effects include an increased risk of hip fracture and poor pregnancy outcomes.

During the early months of pregnancy, a high intake of preformed vitamin A is especially dangerous because it may cause fetal malformations and spontaneous abortions. This is because vitamin A binds to DNA and thus influences cell development. The Food and Drug Administration (FDA) recommends that women of childbearing age limit their overall intake in diet plus supplements of preformed vitamin A to a total of about 100% of the Daily Value (1000 micrograms or 5000 IU). It is also important to limit consumption of rich food sources, such as liver. These precautions

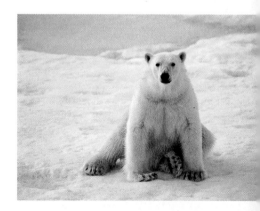

▲ Inuits long knew and explorers soon learned to avoid eating the liver of polar bears. Just 4 ounces (120 grams) of polar bear liver will deliver a toxic dose of 1.36 million RAE of vitamin A. That's 136 times the UL!

also apply to women who may possibly become pregnant; vitamin A is stored in the body for long periods, so women who ingest large amounts during the months before pregnancy place their fetus at risk.

CONCEPT CHECK

Vitamin A has diverse functions. The binding of a form of vitamin A to DNA can influence cell growth and differentiation. Vitamin A is important for maintaining vision and epithelial tissues, reproduction, growth, and ensuring proper function of the immune system. The role of vitamin A as an antioxidant is under study. Vitamin A in the diet comes in two forms: retinoids (preformed vitamin A) and certain carotenoids (provitamin A). Major food sources of vitamin A include carrots, eggs, mangoes, milk, butter, and many vegetables. North Americans most at risk for poor vitamin A status are preschool children and alcoholics. Large doses of retinoids can be toxic, even at chronic dosages only about two to four times the RDA, especially during early pregnancy. Outcomes of toxicity include birth defects, poor vision, and liver damage. Deficiency symptoms include poor growth, increased infection rates, and night blindness.

10.7 Carotenoids

Plants contain pigments called carotenoids. Carotenoids are phytochemicals, that is, chemicals within plants that have health-promoting properties for humans. Because carotenoids can be turned into vitamin A, they are termed provitamin A. Only three of the more than 600 identified carotenoids are currently known to serve as provitamin A in humans. Beta-carotene (β-carotene), the orange-yellow pigment in carrots, is the most potent form of provitamin A. The other two carotenoids that can be converted into vitamin A, though not very effectively, are alpha-carotene and beta-cryptoxanthin. Other carotenoids that may play a role in human health but are not vitamin A precursors include lycopene, zeaxanthin, and lutein. Beta-carotene is split in half by cells in the body to form two molecules of retinal. Neither the conversion of the provitamin A carotenoids into vitamin A nor the absorption of carotenoids is an efficient process. See Making Decisions on page 360 for an example.

Functions of the Carotenoids

Vision. Age-related macular degeneration is a leading cause of legal blindness among North American adults over age 65 (Fig. 10-15). The disease is associated with changes in the macular area of the retina, which provides the most detailed vision. Age, smoking, and genetics are risk factors. The macula contains the carotenoids lutein and zeaxanthin in high enough concentrations to impart a yellow color. In one study of older adults, the higher the total number of carotenoids (beta-carotene, lutein, and zeaxanthin) consumed in the diet, the lower was the risk for age-related macular degeneration.

These carotenoids may also decrease the risk of cataracts in the eyes. Research studies point toward the actual fruit and vegetables with their high carotenoid content as contributing to reduced risk for eye disorders. Consuming just carotenoids as supplements for this purpose is not recommended. Multivitamin and mineral supplements formulated for older adults (e.g., Centrum Silver™) are being marketed as a source of lutein. Consumers must be aware that studies on carotenoids are generally conducted with food rather than supplements.

Cardiovascular Disease Prevention. Carotenoids may play a role in preventing cardiovascular disease in persons at high risk (see Further Reading 13). This role may be linked to carotenoids' ability to inhibit the oxidation of low-density lipoproteins

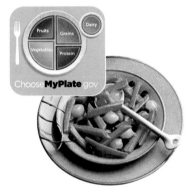

▲ Provitamin A carotenoids are the safest way to meet vitamin A needs. A serving of these carrots would be an excellent addition to the vegetable section of MyPlate. Cooking food sources of carotenoids actually makes them more bioavailable.

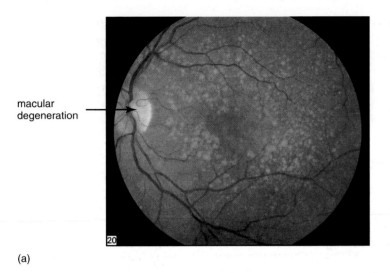

macular
degeneration

(a)

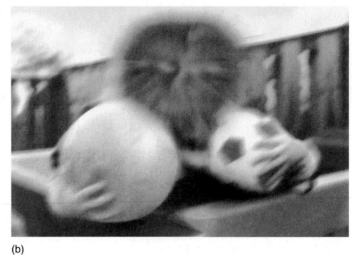

(b)

FIGURE 10-15 ▶ (a) Age-related degeneration of the macular region as noted by the black arrow. (b) The blurry center of the image simulates the vision of a person with macular degeneration.

(LDLs). Until definitive studies are complete, many scientists recommend that we consume a total of at least five servings of a combination of fruits and vegetables per day as part of an overall effort to reduce the risk of cardiovascular disease. Other phytochemicals, including flavonoids, phenolic acids, and phytoestrogens, may have a more positive effect in cardiovascular disease prevention than carotenoids.

Cancer Prevention. Carotenoids by themselves may play a role in preventing cancer, as a by-product of their antioxidant activity. Population studies show that regular consumption of foods rich in carotenoids decreases the risk of lung and oral cancers. The carotenoid lycopene may decrease skin cancer risk. In contrast, recall from Chapter 1 that studies from the United States and Finland failed to show a reduction in lung cancer in male smokers and nonsmokers given supplements of the carotenoid β-carotene for 5 or more years. In fact, β-carotene use in male smokers increased the number of lung cancer cases compared with control groups. No comparable studies have been conducted with women. Although further research continues, most researchers are convinced that β-carotene supplementation offers no protection against cancer. Again, the best advice is to rely on food sources for this or any other carotenoid.

Cancer of the **prostate gland** is one of the most common cancers among North American men. The dietary carotenoid lycopene (the red pigment found in tomatoes, watermelon, pink grapefruit, and guava) seems to protect against this type of cancer. The proposed biological role of lycopene again appears to be that of an antioxidant. Some food companies (e.g., Campbell Soup Company) have even marketed their products as important sources of lycopene.

Carotenoid Sources and Needs

The provitamin A carotenoids are mainly found in dark green and yellow-orange vegetables and some fruits (see Further Reading 11). Carrots, spinach and other greens, winter squash, sweet potatoes, broccoli, mangoes, cantaloupe, peaches, and apricots are examples of such sources. Beta-carotene accounts for some of the orange color of carrots. In vegetables such as broccoli, this yellow-orange color is masked by dark-green chlorophyll pigments. Still, green vegetables contain provitamin A. Green,

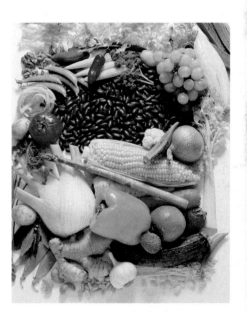

▲ More research is needed to understand the relationship of carotenoids and cancer prevention.

prostate gland A solid, chestnut-shaped organ surrounding the first part of the urinary tract in the male. The prostate gland secretes substances into the semen.

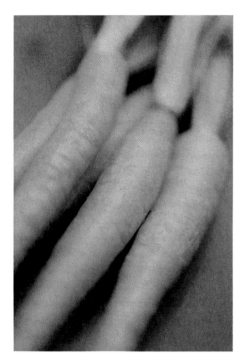

▲ As little as four to five large carrots daily can produce hypercarotenemia. Taking a break from carrots, squash, and pumpkins will turn the skin back to normal.

leafy vegetables, such as spinach and kale, have high concentrations of lutein and zeaxanthin. Tomato juice and other tomato products, such as pizza or spaghetti sauce, contain significant amounts of lycopene. In contrast to many other nutrients, cooking food improves the bioavailability of carotenoids. In raw fruits and vegetables, carotenoids are bound to proteins. Cooking disrupts this protein bond and frees up the carotenoid for better absorption. There is no separate DRI for beta-carotene or any of the other provitamin A carotenoids.

Upper Level for Carotenoids

Ingesting large amounts of vitamin-A-yielding carotenoids does not cause toxic effects. A high carotenoid concentration in the blood (called hypercarotenemia) can occur if someone routinely consumes large amounts of carrots or takes pills containing beta-carotene (more than 30 milligrams daily), or if infants eat a great deal of squash. The skin turns yellow-orange, particularly the palms of the hands and soles of the feet. It differs from jaundice, a sign of liver failure. In jaundice, the yellow discoloration extends to the sclera (whites) of the eye, whereas in hypercarotenemia it does not. Hypercarotenemia does not appear to cause harm and disappears when carotenoid intake decreases. Dietary carotenoids do not produce toxic effects because (1) their rate of conversion into vitamin A is relatively slow and regulated and (2) the efficiency of carotenoid absorption from the small intestine decreases markedly as oral intake increases.

CONCEPT CHECK

The carotenoids are a chemically similar group of over 600 compounds found in plants. Three provitamin A carotenoids can be converted into vitamin A by the body. Carotenoids act as antioxidants and have been shown to have beneficial effects in the prevention of oxidative damage and subsequent development of macular degeneration, cardiovascular disease, and cancer. Many fruits and vegetables are good sources of the carotenoids. No toxicity or deficiency symptoms have been reported.

10.8 Other Phytochemicals

functional foods Foods that have health benefits beyond basic nutrition.

zoochemicals Chemicals found in animal products that have health-protective actions.

In addition to the approximately 45 essential nutrients, there are thousands of other substances in food. For many years, a great deal of nutrition research concentrated on gaining knowledge about carbohydrates, lipids, proteins, vitamins, and minerals. Now, there is growing interest about the potential health benefits of other substances found in food (see Further Reading 1). Foods that are sources of the chemicals that provide health benefits beyond being essential dietary nutrients are termed **functional foods**. These chemicals are placed into one of two categories: **zoochemicals**, health-promoting compounds found in animal food; and phytochemicals, health-promoting compounds found in plant food. Phytochemicals are responsible for the colors observed in plants and their unique flavors. Improved health has been linked to consuming diets high in plant foods, so most of the nutrition research on functional foods has focused on phytochemicals. In addition to the carotenoids discussed in the previous section, some of the phytochemicals being studied include allicin, dithiolthione, ellagic acid, flavonoids, glucarates, indoles, isothiocyanates, lignans, phthalides, phytoestrogens, polyacetylenes, saponins, stanols, and terpenes. Examples of foods that are rich sources of phytochemicals include apples, celery, citrus fruit, cruciferous vegetables, garlic, green tea, soybeans, tomatoes, whole grains, and a number of herbs and spices. Individual foods may contain hundreds of different phytochemicals.

Functions of Phytochemicals

Over 600 carotenoids are found in plants, and the full extent of their health benefits has yet to be determined. See Table 1-4 on page 14 to review foodsources of a variety of phytochemicals. Phytochemicals are not essential nutrients because a deficiency disease is not observed when they are removed from the diet. Phytochemicals cannot be synthesized in the body; therefore, we must ingest them from food. Although the study of the metabolic actions of phytochemicals is relatively new, numerous functions of phytochemicals have been elucidated. Phytochemicals have the following functions:

- Act as antioxidants
- Inhibit the initiation and proliferation of cancer and stimulate spontaneous cell death (see Further Reading 3)
- Alter the absorption, production, and metabolism of cholesterol
- Mimic or inhibit hormones and enzymes
- Decrease the formation of blood clots
- Reduce inflammation, affecting immune-related diseases

A number of phytochemicals are strong antioxidants. As mentioned in the previous section, beta-carotene has been shown to exert powerful antioxidant properties. Lycopene, a red carotenoid found in tomatoes and pink grapefruit, appears to have even stronger antioxidant properties than beta-carotene. Flavonoids function as antioxidants by inhibiting the oxidation of cholesterol, an initial step in the development of atherogenic plaques. Rich sources of flavonoids include blueberries, chocolate, citrus fruit, and raspberries. Other commonly eaten carotenoids that have antioxidant properties include alpha-carotene, beta-cryptoxanthin, lutein, and zeaxanthin.

There are no specific dietary recommendations for the amount of phytochemicals that should be consumed, except that they should be consumed as food. Building meals that resemble MyPlate will provide a diet rich in phytochemicals (at least five servings of fruits and vegetables). In the United States, average consumption of fruits and vegetables falls far short of these recommendations.

Many phytochemicals are available as single and combined supplements on grocery, pharmacy, health-food, and department store shelves. At present, we know that phytochemicals have protective functions with minimal side effects when consumed naturally in a variety of foods. What we do not know is their effect if we take them in large doses, consistently, from the same source. Will the phytochemical still have a protective role? Will there be side effects?

10.9 Selenium (Se)

It was only in the late 1970s that an RDA was established for selenium. Until that time, toxicity symptoms had been observed but not deficiency. Because selenium is found in both plant and animal foodstuffs, both are strongly directly dependent upon soil selenium content. Worldwide, only one region, the Keshan province in China, has such low soil levels that selenium deficiencies result. Such deficiencies were first reported by Chinese scientists in 1979. Of note, communication and relations between the West and China were closed from 1949 until 1972. In the mid and late 1970s, medical dialogue opened significantly.

Selenium is a trace mineral that exists in many readily absorbed chemical forms. Selenium's best-understood role is aiding the activity of one of the body's natural antioxidant enzymes—glutathione peroxidase. Glutathione peroxidase chemically converts potentially damaging peroxides (hydrogen peroxide, for example) into water. In functioning as part of our natural antioxidant enzyme system, selenium spares vitamin E and indirectly helps maintain cell-membrane integrity. Selenium also functions by activating thyroid hormone and in immune function.

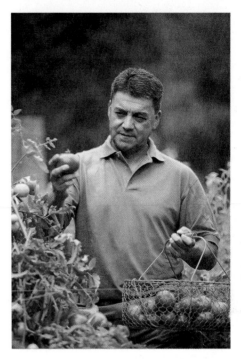

▲ Not all phytochemicals are beneficial to human health. As a form of self-defense, some plants do produce chemicals that act as toxins. These tomatoes are a source of lycopene, a cancer-fighting phytochemical. However, the leaves of a tomato plant contain harmful toxins.

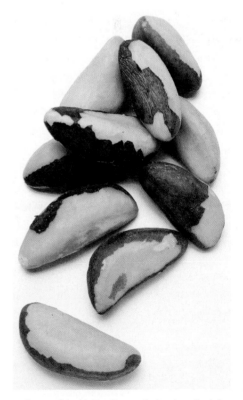

▲ Be careful with Brazil nuts. Eating just six daily exceeds the Upper Limit for selenium.

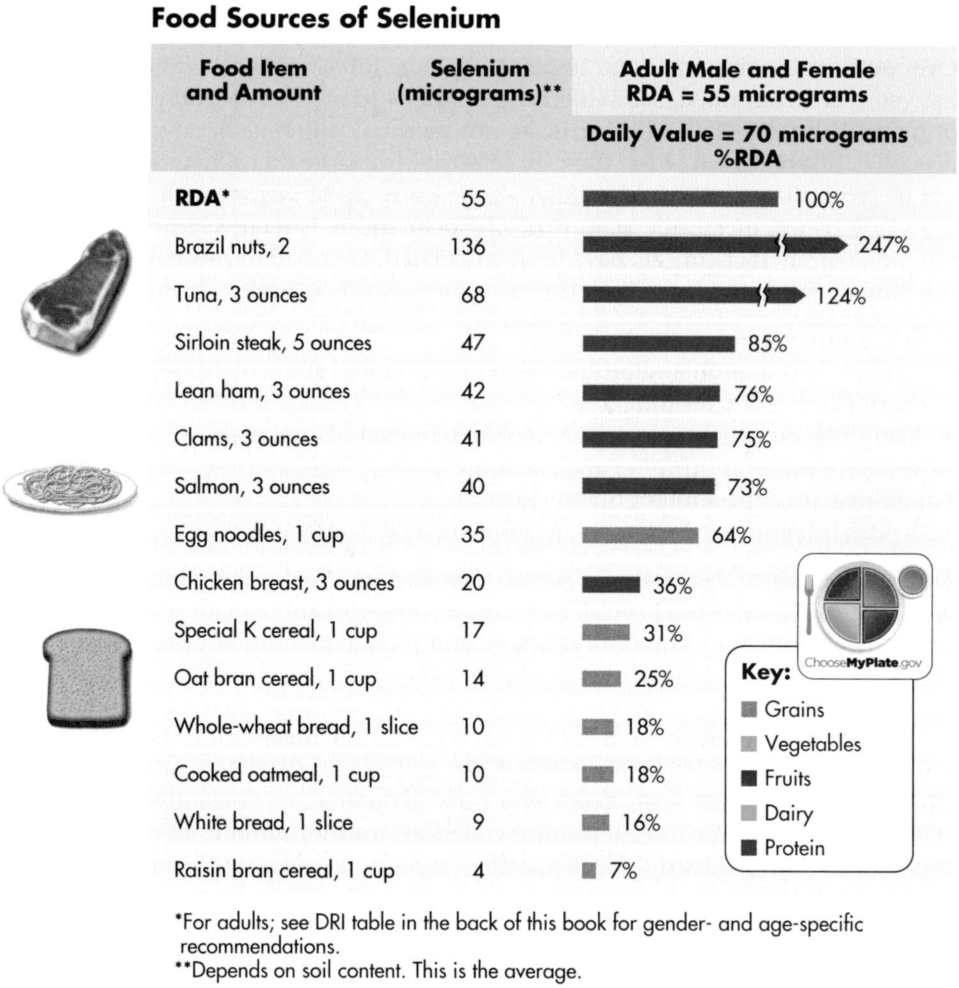

FIGURE 10-16 ▶ Food sources of selenium compared to the RDA.

Food Sources of Selenium

Food Item and Amount	Selenium (micrograms)**	Adult Male and Female RDA = 55 micrograms
		Daily Value = 70 micrograms %RDA
RDA*	55	100%
Brazil nuts, 2	136	247%
Tuna, 3 ounces	68	124%
Sirloin steak, 5 ounces	47	85%
Lean ham, 3 ounces	42	76%
Clams, 3 ounces	41	75%
Salmon, 3 ounces	40	73%
Egg noodles, 1 cup	35	64%
Chicken breast, 3 ounces	20	36%
Special K cereal, 1 cup	17	31%
Oat bran cereal, 1 cup	14	25%
Whole-wheat bread, 1 slice	10	18%
Cooked oatmeal, 1 cup	10	18%
White bread, 1 slice	9	16%
Raisin bran cereal, 1 cup	4	7%

Key:
- Grains
- Vegetables
- Fruits
- Dairy
- Protein

ChooseMyPlate.gov

*For adults; see DRI table in the back of this book for gender- and age-specific recommendations.
**Depends on soil content. This is the average.

Low blood levels of selenium have been linked with an increased incidence of some forms of cancer, specifically prostate cancer. Although selenium could prove to have a role in prevention of cancers in those with low or marginal selenium stores, it is premature to recommend selenium supplementation for this purpose. Animal studies in this area are conflicting. Current studies address the interaction of selenium and vitamin E on gene expression in some cancers.

Selenium deficiency symptoms in humans include muscle pain and wasting and a certain form of heart damage. In China's Keshan province, unless they are supplemented, children and adults develop characteristic muscle and heart disorders associated with inadequate selenium intake.

Selenium Sources and Needs

Brazil nuts, fish, meat (especially organ meats), shellfish, and eggs are good animal sources of selenium (Fig. 10-16). Grains and seeds grown in soils containing selenium are good plant sources. Major selenium contributors to the adult diet are animal and grain products. Some geographic regions identified with low-selenium soil in North America include the Northeast, Pacific, Southwest, and coastal plain of the Southeast in the United States; and the north central and eastern regions in Canada. We eat a varied diet of foods supplied from many geographic areas, so it is unlikely that local areas with low soil selenium will mean inadequate selenium in our diets.

The RDA for selenium is 55 micrograms per day for adults. This intake maximizes the activity of selenium-dependent enzymes. The Daily Value used on food and supplement labels is 70 micrograms. Adults meet the RDA, consuming on average 105 micrograms each day.

Upper Level for Selenium

Selenium toxicity has not been reported from eating food. Excessive supplementation for an extended period has been shown to be toxic. The UL for selenium is 400 micrograms per day for adults. This is based on overt signs of selenium toxicity, such as hair loss, weakness, nausea, vomiting, and cirrhosis. Because Brazil nuts are such a concentrated source of selenium, it is recommended to avoid consuming them daily, thus preventing an inadvertent overload.

CONCEPT CHECK

Selenium activates an enzyme (glutathione peroxidase) that helps change electron-seeking free-radical (oxidizing) compounds into less toxic compounds so these do not attack and break down cell membranes. Selenium also functions in the maintenance of the immune system and production of thyroid hormones. A selenium deficiency results in muscle and heart disorders. Animal products and grains are good selenium sources; however, the selenium content in plants depends on the selenium concentration in the soil. The misuse of selenium supplements can readily lead to toxicity. Toxicity symptoms include brittle hair and nails, vomiting, and liver damage.

NEWSWORTHY NUTRITION   Selenium and vitamin E supplements offer no benefit for cancer prevention

In the late 1990s and early 2000s, secondary results of two large trials of nutrient supplementation in cancer prevention hinted at possible roles for micronutrients in the prevention of prostate cancer. As a result, the 12-year Selenium and Vitamin E Cancer Prevention Trial (SELECT) was designed to further explore the roles of selenium and vitamin E for the prevention of prostate cancer. After just 7 years, the trial was stopped due to lack of evidence of any beneficial effect of the supplements on endpoints related to cancer. This trial demonstrated that neither selenium (200 micrograms per day of selenomethionine) nor vitamin E (400 IU per day of dl-alpha-tocopherol), either alone or in combination, reduced risk for prostate cancer. This is an example of why replication of research results is so important. The results of one study are not sufficient to inform clinical practice.

Source: Lippman SM and others: Effect of selenium and vitamin E on risk of prostate cancer and other cancers: The Selenium and Vitamin E Cancer Prevention Trial (SELECT). *JAMA* 301:39, 2009.

connect NUTRITION   **Check out the Connect site** www.mcgrawhillconnect.com **to futher explore nutrition research on cancer prevention.**

Dietary Supplements— Who Needs Them?

The phrase *multivitamin and mineral supplement* has been mentioned many times so far in this textbook. Often, these and other supplements are marketed as cures for anything and everything. This cure-all approach is promoted by the supplement industry and countless health-food stores, pharmacies, and supermarkets.

According to the Dietary Supplement Health and Education Act of 1994 (discussed in Chapter 1), a supplement in the United States is a product intended to supplement the diet that bears or contains one or more of the following ingredients:

- A vitamin
- A mineral
- An herb or another botanical
- An amino acid
- A dietary substance to supplement the diet, which could be an extract or a combination of the first four ingredients in this list

The definition is broad and covers a wide variety of nutritional substances. The use of dietary supplements is a common practice among North Americans and generates about $28–29 billion annually for the industry in the United States (Fig. 10-17). Supplements can be sold without proof that they are safe and effective. Unless the FDA has evidence that a supplement is inherently dangerous or marketed with an illegal claim, it will not regulate such products closely. (The vitamin folate is an exception.) The FDA has limited resources to police supplement manufacturers and has to act against these manufacturers one at a time. Thus, we cannot rely on the FDA to protect us from vitamin and mineral supplement overuse and misuse. We bear that responsibility ourselves, with the help of professional advice from a physician or registered dietitian.

The supplement makers can make broad claims about their products under the "structure or function" provision of the law. The products, however, cannot claim to prevent, treat, or cure a disease. Menopause in women and aging are not diseases *per se*, so products alleging to treat symptoms of these conditions can be marketed without FDA approval. For example, a product that claims to treat hot flashes arising during menopause can be sold without any evidence to prove that the product works, but a product that claims to decrease the risk of cardiovascular disease by reducing blood cholesterol must have results from scientific studies that justify the claim.

Why do people take supplements? Frequently given reasons include to:
- Reduce susceptibility to health problems (e.g., colds)
- Prevent heart attacks
- Prevent cancer
- Reduce stress
- Increase "energy"

FIGURE 10-17 ▶ The dietary supplement industry is a growing multibillion dollar business.

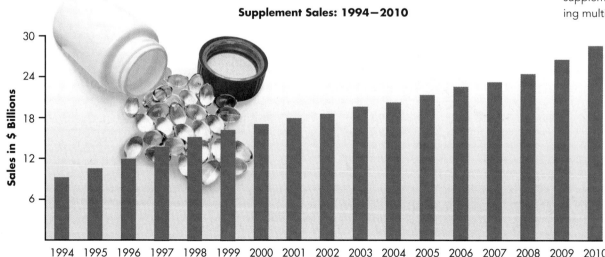

Supplement Sales: 1994—2010

Should You Take a Supplement?

The choice to take a supplement is up to you. Opinions vary about the wisdom and safety of supplement use even among knowledgeable scientists. Typically, nutrition scientists have recommended that supplement use is needed only by a few groups. The National Institutes of Health came to the same conclusion, noting there is insufficient evidence to support the recommendation of use of a multivitamin and mineral supplement by the general population (see Further Reading 7). The experts found that only a few studies of vitamins and minerals demonstrate beneficial effects for the prevention of chronic disease, including increased bone mineral density and decreased fractures in postmenopausal women who use calcium and vitamin D supplements. (See the next section in this feature for more specific examples.) In contrast, several other studies provide disturbing evidence of risk, such as increased lung cancer risk with beta-carotene use among smokers. The NIH State-of-the Science report concludes that the present evidence is insufficient to recommend either for or against the use of multivitamin/mineral supplements by Americans to prevent chronic disease.

The rationale for widespread use of a multivitamin and mineral supplement is primarily because many North Americans have been unwilling to change their food habits to include the recommended servings of fruits, vegetables, and whole grains. As for individual vitamins, there are specific cases in which supplements are advised. As discussed in Chapter 12, adequate folate status when a woman becomes pregnant helps reduce the risk of certain birth defects in her offspring (400 micrograms per day of synthetic folic acid is recommended). Folate also limits homocysteine in the blood, a likely risk factor for cardiovascular disease that can affect all of us. In addition, the committee appointed by the Food and Nutrition Board that set current nutrient standards for vitamin B-12 suggested that adults over age 50 consume vitamin B-12 in a synthetic form, such as that added to ready-to-eat breakfast cereals or present in supplements. Synthetic vitamin B-12 is more easily absorbed than that found in food; this helps compensate for the fall in vitamin B-12 absorption often seen in one's older years.

Whether experts support use of a multivitamin and mineral supplement or not, they all emphasize that many of the health-promoting effects of foods cannot be found in a bottle. Recall the discussions of phytochemicals in Chapter 2 and the benefits of fiber in Chapter 4. Few or no phytochemicals and no fiber are present in most supplements. Multivitamin and mineral supplements also contain little calcium to keep the pill size small; and the oxide forms of magnesium, zinc, and copper used in many supplements are not as well absorbed as forms found in foods.

Overall, supplement use cannot fix a poor diet in all respects. Uninformed megadose supplement use also can lead to harm—most cases of nutrient toxicity are a result of supplement use. Thus, we are advised to first take a good look at our dietary habits and then improve them, as outlined in Chapter 2 (Fig. 10-18). Then we should find out which nutrient gaps remain and identify food sources that can help. Such a source could be ready-to-eat breakfast cereals to increase vitamin E, folic acid, and vitamin B-6 intake, and as well provide highly absorbable forms of vitamin B-12. Calcium-fortified orange juice could be used to increase calcium intake, or milk and yogurt to increase vitamin D and calcium intake. You need to be careful of highly fortified foods, however, as these products may provide the appropriate amount of nutrients in one serving, but the typical consumer may eat more than one serving. This can lead to an excessive intake of some nutrients, such as vitamin A, iron, and synthetic folic acid.

If supplement use is desired, you should discuss this practice with a physician or registered dietitian, as some supplements can interfere with certain medicines. For example, high intakes of vitamin K or vitamin E alter the action of anticlotting medications. Vitamin B-6 can offset the action of L-dopa (used in treating Parkinson's disease). Large doses of vitamin C can interfere with certain cancer therapy regimens. Excessive zinc intake can inhibit copper absorption. Large amounts of folate can mask signs and symptoms of a vitamin B-12

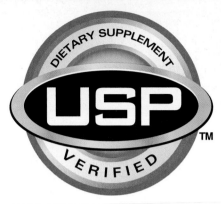

▲ The USP (United States Pharmacopeia) label indicates the product meets USP standards.

▶ Because research on a variety of nutrient supplements has revealed a lack of product quality, FDA now requires supplement makers to test the purity, strength, and composition of all their products. The USP (United States Pharmacopeia) designation, which has been extended to an increasing number of nutrient supplements, establishes professionally accepted standards for these products and can be used to evaluate supplements. The USP standards designate strength, quality, purity, packaging, labeling, speed of dissolution, and acceptable length of storage of ingredients for drugs.

Top Five Dietary Supplements in 2010

1. Fish oil
2. Multivitamins
3. Vitamin D
4. Calcium
5. Coenzyme Q

Source: Consumerlab.com

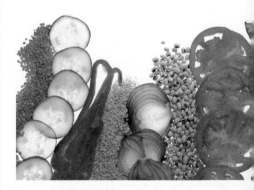

▲ Focus first on foods that meet nutrient needs.

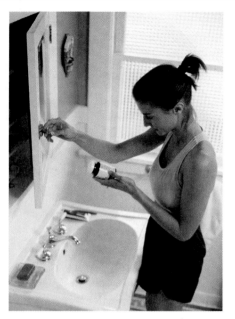

▲ Long-term intake of just three times the Daily Value for some fat-soluble vitamins—particularly preformed vitamin A—can cause toxic effects. Know what you are taking if you use supplements.

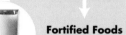

Healthy Diet Rich in Vitamins and Minerals

↓

Fortified Foods

↓

Possible Multivitamin and Mineral Supplement Use

↓

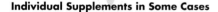

Individual Supplements in Some Cases

FIGURE 10-18 ▶ Supplement savvy—an approach to the use of nutrient supplements. Emphasizing a healthy diet rich in vitamins and minerals is always the first option.

CRITICAL THINKING

Believing that supplements provide the nutrition her body needs, Janice regularly takes numerous supplements while paying relatively little attention to daily food choices. How would you explain to her that this practice may lead to health problems?

deficiency see Chapter 12. Remember, you *can* get too much of a good thing.

People Most Likely to Need Supplements

As you might guess, generally the people who take supplements in our society are already healthy. Various medical and health-related organizations suggest that the following vitamin and mineral supplements can be important for certain groups of healthy people:

- Women of childbearing age may need extra synthetic folic acid if their dietary patterns do not supply the recommended amount (400 micrograms).
- Women with excessive bleeding during menstruation may need extra iron.
- Women who are pregnant or breastfeeding may need extra iron, folate, and calcium.
- People with low calorie intakes (less than about 1200 kcal per day) may need a range of vitamins and minerals. This is true of some women and many older people.
- Strict vegans may need extra calcium, iron, zinc, and vitamin B-12.
- Newborns need a single dose of vitamin K, as directed by a physician.
- Some older infants may need fluoride supplements, as directed by a dentist.
- People with limited milk intake and sunlight exposure may need extra vitamin D. This includes all infants, many African-Americans, and older people.
- People with lactose maldigestion or lactose intolerance, and those with allergies to dairy products, may need extra calcium.
- Adults over age 50 may need a synthetic source of vitamin B-12.
- People on low-fat diets or diets low in plant oils and nuts may need some extra vitamin E.
- People who consume a large part of their diet as refined foods rather than as fruits, vegetables, or whole grains may need a range of vitamins and minerals. Individuals with certain medical conditions (e.g., vitamin-resistant diseases

deficiency see Chapter 12. Remember, you *can* get too much of a good thing.

long-standing fat malabsorption) and those who use certain medications also may require supplementation with specific vitamins and minerals. Children who are "picky eaters" may require supplementation as well (see Chapter 18). Finally, smokers and alcohol abusers may benefit from supplementation, but cessation of these two activities is far more beneficial than any supplementation.

Which Supplement Should You Choose?

If you decide to take a multivitamin and mineral supplement, which one should you choose? As a start, choose a nationally recognized brand (from a supermarket or pharmacy) that contains about 100% of the Daily Values for the nutrients present. A multivitamin and mineral supplement should generally be taken with or just after meals to maximize absorption. Make sure also that intake from the total of this supplement, any other supplements used, and highly fortified foods (such as ready-to-eat breakfast cereals) provides no more than the Upper Level for each vitamin and mineral. (See the inside cover of this text book for Upper Levels.) This is especially important with regard to preformed vitamin A intake. Two exceptions are: (1) both men and older women should make sure any product used is low in iron or iron-free to avoid possible iron overload (see Chapter 12 for details), and (2) somewhat exceeding the Upper Level for vitamin D is likely a safe practice for adults. One should read the labels carefully to be sure of what is being taken (Fig. 10-19).

Another consideration in choosing a supplement is avoiding superfluous ingredients, such as para-aminobenzoic acid (PABA), hesperidin complex, inositol, bee pollen, and lecithins. These are not needed in our diets. They are especially common in expensive supplements sold in health-food stores and by mail. In addition, use of l-tryptophan and high doses of beta-carotene or fish oils is discouraged.

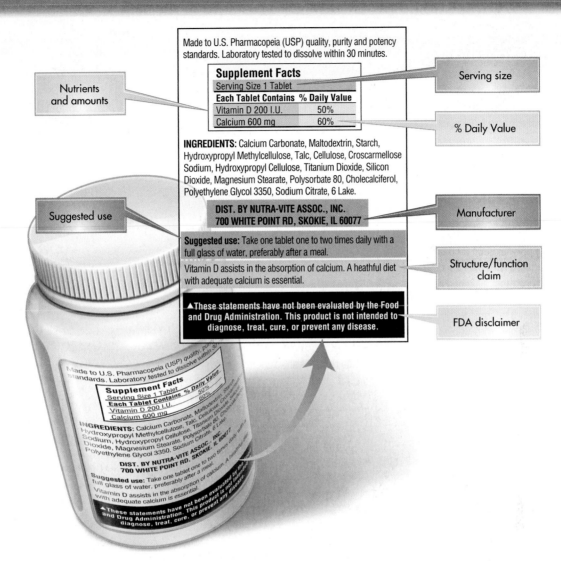

Made to U.S. Pharmacopeia (USP) quality, purity and potency standards. Laboratory tested to dissolve within 30 minutes.

Supplement Facts

Serving Size 1 Tablet

Each Tablet Contains	% Daily Value
Vitamin D 200 I.U.	50%
Calcium 600 mg	60%

INGREDIENTS: Calcium Carbonate, Maltodextrin, Starch, Hydroxypropyl Methylcellulose, Talc, Cellulose, Croscarmellose Sodium, Hydroxypropyl Cellulose, Titanium Dioxide, Silicon Dioxide, Magnesium Stearate, Polysorbate 80, Cholecalciferol, Polyethylene Glycol 3350, Sodium Citrate, 6 Lake.

**DIST. BY NUTRA-VITE ASSOC., INC.
700 WHITE POINT RD, SKOKIE, IL 60077**

Suggested use: Take one tablet one to two times daily with a full glass of water, preferably after a meal.

Vitamin D assists in the absorption of calcium. A heathful diet with adequate calcium is essential.

▲These statements have not been evaluated by the Food and Drug Administration. This product is not intended to diagnose, treat, cure, or prevent any disease.

Nutrients and amounts

Suggested use

Serving size

% Daily Value

Manufacturer

Structure/function claim

FDA disclaimer

FIGURE 10-19 ▶ Nutrient supplements display a nutrition label different from that of foods. This Supplement Facts label must list the ingredient(s), amount(s) per serving, serving size, suggested use, and % Daily Value if one has been established. This label also includes structure/function claims. Thus, it also must include the FDA warning that these claims have not been evaluated by the agency.

▶ The regular use of individual nutrient supplements could lead to health risks. These should be used with caution.

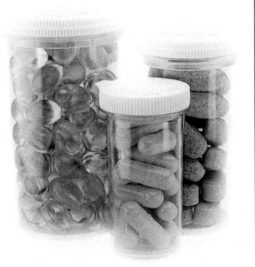

A Few websites to help you evaluate ongoing claims and evaluate safety of supplements are:

www.acsh.org
www.quackwatch.com
www.ncahf.org
http://ods.od.nih.gov
www.eatright.org
www.usp.org/USPVerified/
  dietarySupplements/

These sites are maintained by groups or individuals committed to providing reasoned and authoritative nutrition and health advice to consumers.

Case Study Choosing a Dietary Supplement

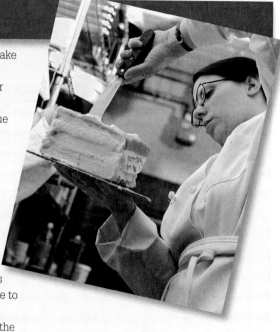

Amy works the predawn shift as a baker at a popular bistro. Amy is also a full-time student, and the combination of taking a full course load at college and working early hours while her friends are sleeping has created a lot of stress for her. Amy's many commitments also make it important that she not become ill. Recently, one of her coworkers suggested that she take Nutramega supplements to help prevent colds, flu, and other illnesses. The product's label suggests that Nutramega helps prevent such problems, especially those associated with the changing of seasons. The label recommends taking two to three tablets daily for health maintenance and two to three tablets every 3 hours at the first sign of feeling ill. Amy looks at the Supplement Facts label on the bottle and finds that each tablet contains (as percent of the DV): 33% for vitamin A (three-quarters is preformed vitamin A), 700% for vitamin C, 50% for zinc, and 10% for selenium. A month's supply costs about $50.

Answer the following questions and check your responses in Appendix A.

1. Are there any health risks associated with taking the "maintenance" dose of two to three tablets per day? How does this dose compare with the Tolerable Upper Intake Levels for the four nutrients?
2. How many tablets would be taken per day if Amy was feeling ill?
   a. For vitamin A, use the % Daily Value to calculate the micrograms RAE that would be in this larger dose. How does this compare to the UL for vitamin A?
   b. Use the % Daily Value to calculate the milligrams of vitamin C in this larger dose. How does this compare to the UL for vitamin C?
   c. Use the % Daily Value to calculate the milligrams of zinc in this larger dose. How does this compare to the UL for zinc?
   d. Use the % Daily Value to calculate the micrograms of selenium in this larger dose. How does this compare to the UL for selenium?
   e. Does the recommended dosage of any of these nutrients pose any health risks?
3. Does the cost of this supplement seem reasonable? How does it compare to the cost of a typical multivitamin/mineral supplement available at your local drug store?
4. Should Amy be concerned about meeting her nutrient needs? Does the type of stress she is under increase her nutrient needs?
5. After studying Chapter 10, what diet and supplement advice would you offer to Amy?

Summary (Numbers refer to numbered sections in the chapter.)

10.1 Many chemical reactions involve the transfer of electrons between molecules. A molecule is oxidized when it loses an electron; a molecule is reduced when it gains an electron. Typically, all these electrons are paired, but when such reactions result in an unpaired electron, the molecule is called a free radical. Production of free radicals is a normal consequence of metabolism, but an overabundance of free radicals can cause damage to cells, especially cell membranes and DNA. This damage can lead to many diseases, including cancer and atherosclerosis.

10.2 The body has natural defenses against damage by free radicals. Antioxidant enzyme systems detoxify free radicals, often with the aid of mineral cofactors. Antioxidant chemicals can donate electrons to free radicals without becoming reactive themselves, a process that halts cellular damage.

10.3 Vitamins that function as antioxidant chemicals include vitamin C, vitamin E, vitamin A, and some carotenoids. Minerals that function as cofactors in antioxidant enzyme systems include selenium, manganese, zinc, iron, and copper. Some phytochemicals also possess antioxidant activity.

10.4 Vitamin E functions primarily as an antioxidant and is found in plant oils. By donating electrons to electron-seeking free-radical (oxidizing) compounds, it neutralizes them. This effect shields cell membranes and red blood cells from breakdown. Claims are made about the curative powers of vitamin E, but more information is needed before megadose vitamin E recommendations for healthy adults can be made with certainty. The Upper Level is set at about 50 times adult needs.

10.5 Vitamin C is a potent antioxidant and also functions to synthesize collagen, carnitine, and neurotransmitters. A vitamin C deficiency results in scurvy, evidenced by pinpoint hemorrhages in the skin, bleeding gums, and joint pain. Vitamin C also modestly enhances iron absorption. Fresh fruits and vegetables, especially citrus fruits, are good sources. A great amount of vitamin C is lost in storage and cooking; therefore, the diet should emphasize fresh or minimally cooked vegetables. Deficiencies can occur in people with alcoholism and those whose diets lack sufficient fruit and vegetable intake. Smoking increases the possibility of vitamin C deficiency. The Upper Level is set at about 20 times adult needs.

10.6 Vitamin A is a family of compounds that includes several forms of preformed vitamin A (retinoids): retinol, retinal, and retinoic acid. Vitamin A contributes to vision, immune function, cell development, and possibly antioxidant activity. Precursors to vitamin A—carotenoids—have profound antioxidant activity. Preformed vitamin A is found in liver and fish oils. Vitamin A can be toxic, especially during pregnancy, even when taken at doses just three times the RDA for preformed vitamin A.

10.7 Carotenoids are phytochemicals that can be converted to vitamin A in the body. Three forms of carotenoids can yield vitamin A in humans: beta-carotene, alpha-carotene, and beta-cryptoxanthin. Although carotenoids are not essential nutrients, some have health-promoting qualities for humans. In addition to their contribution to vitamin A intake, carotenoids are powerful antioxidants. The antioxidant abilities of several carotenoids are linked to prevention of macular degeneration, cataracts, cardiovascular disease, and cancer. Carotenoids are plentiful in dark-green and orange vegetables.

10.8 In addition to carotenoids, other phytochemicals have health benefits related to their effects in antioxidant activity, DNA expression, cholesterol metabolism, and the inflammatory process, among others. Notable health-promoting phytochemicals include lycopene (in tomatoes, watermelon, and pink grapefruit) and flavonoids (in blueberries, raspberries, citrus fruit, and chocolate).

10.9 Selenium is a cofactor in the glutathione peroxidase system, which detoxifies free radicals. It acts along with vitamin E to provide antioxidant protection. Muscle pain, wasting, and a form of heart damage may result from a selenium deficiency. Meats, eggs, fish, and shellfish are good animal sources of selenium. Good plant sources include grains and seeds.

Check Your Knowledge (Answers to the following questions are below.)

1. Free radicals can
   a. damage DNA
   b. disrupt cell membranes.
   c. destroy pathogens.
   d. All of the above.

2. A deficiency of vitamin A can lead to the disease called
   a. xerophthalmia.
   b. osteomalacia.
   c. scurvy.
   d. pellagra.

3. A high intake of vitamin E can
   a. inhibit vitamin K metabolism.
   b. result in lead poisoning.
   c. inhibit copper absorption.
   d. cause baldness.

4. Vitamin C is necessary for the production of
   a. stomach acid.
   b. collagen.
   c. hormones.
   d. clotting factors.

5. Damage caused by free radicals is thought to contribute to
   a. atherosclerosis.
   b. diabetes.
   c. Alzheimer's disease.
   d. All of the above.

6. Good food sources of vitamin E include
   a. meats.
   b. white bread.
   c. nuts.
   d. All of the above.

7. Which of the following micronutrients is *not* involved in immune function?
   a. vitamin A
   b. vitamin C
   c. vitamin E
   d. None of the above.

8. Supplementation with certain vitamin or mineral supplements is most likely to be useful for
   a. college students studying for finals.

   b. older adults with low stomach acid production.
   c. curing cancer.
   d. preventing AIDS.

9. Phytochemicals are
   a. a new type of vitamin.
   b. plant chemicals that protect health.
   c. plant pigments that may be converted into vitamin A.
   d. animal chemicals that protect health.

10. Selenium is an antioxidant micronutrient because it
    a. donates electrons to free radicals.
    b. accepts electrons from free radicals.
    c. aids glutathione peroxidase activity.
    d. enhances the absorption of vitamin E.

Answer key: 1. d (LO 10.1), 2. a (LO 10.3), 3. a (LO 10.3), 4. b (LO 10.3), 5. d (LO 10.5), 6. c (LO 10.4), 7. d (LO 10.3), 8. b (LO 10.7), 9. b (LO 10.6), 10. c (LO 10.2)

Study Questions (Numbers refer to Learning Outcomes)

1. What is the difference between reduction and oxidation? How do free radicals arise? (LO 10.1)

2. Identify two beneficial roles of free radicals in the body. (LO 10.1)

3. Describe the process by which an antioxidant can prevent a free radical from damaging cells. (LO 10.2)

4. Name three micronutrients that act as antioxidants by donating electrons or hydrogen atoms to unstable free radicals. (LO 10.3)

5. Describe the varied functions of vitamin A. (LO 10.3)

6. Describe three functions of vitamin C. **(LO 10.3)**

7. How would you determine which fruits and vegetables displayed in the produce section of your supermarket are likely to provide plenty of carotenoids? **(LO 10.4)**

8. What is the role of vitamin E in the prevention of cardiovascular disease? Should people at risk for cardiovascular disease take vitamin E supplements? **(LO 10.5)**

9. Define the terms *phytochemicals* and *functional foods.* How do carotenoids fit into these definitions? **(LO 10.6)**

10. What is the contribution of dietary supplements to human health? Do nutrient intakes well above the DV have any consequences? **(LO 10.7)**

What Would You Choose Recommendations

Most cured meats contain sodium nitrite. This food additive has many useful purposes. It inhibits the growth of the botulinum toxin; staves off rancidity and off-flavors during storage; adds color to meats; and develops and preserves the flavor of cured meats, such as deli meats, bologna, hot dogs, sausage, and bacon.

A downside of sodium nitrite is that it can combine with amines (i.e., protein) to form nitrosamines when exposed to high heat (e.g., grilling of meats) or acid (e.g., stomach acid). Nitrosamines are carcinogenic, and because nitrosamines are ingested, they are associated with cancers of the digestive tract.

The conversion of nitrites to nitrosamine compounds involves oxidation-reduction reactions. As an antioxidant, vitamin C can inhibit the formation of nitrosamines from nitrites or convert nitrosamines into less harmful chemicals. For about the last 40 years, vitamin C or related compounds have been a required addition to cured meats to reduce the formation of nitrosamines. In addition to

vitamin C, some manufacturers of cured meats also add vitamin E to products to further reduce nitrosamine formation.

Although the addition of vitamin C and vitamin E to cured meats has decreased exposure to nitrosamines among Americans, such foods are still not altogether healthy choices. Many cured meats, such as sausage, bacon, and some types of hot dogs, are high in calories, total fat, saturated fat, and cholesterol. Excesses of these nutrients contribute to obesity, cancer, heart disease, stroke, and diabetes. Also, cured meats are high in sodium. One hot dog, for example, contains about 500 milligrams of sodium. As you learned in Chapter 9, most Americans need to reduce their intake of sodium to combat hypertension.

Recall from Chapter 2 that variety, balance, and moderation are important concepts to keep in mind when planning a healthy diet. Reasonable portions of cured or processed meats can be an occasional inclusion in a healthy diet, especially if you choose reduced-fat and

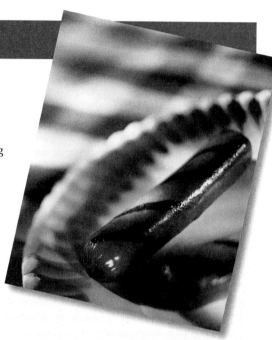

reduced-sodium varieties. Balancing occasional intakes of less nutrient-dense foods, such as hot dogs, with ample intake of whole grains, fruits, and vegetables will lead to an overall diet that meets micronutrient needs without supplying too many calories and too much fat.

Further Readings

1. Basu A and others: Berries: Emerging impact on cardiovascular health. *Nutrition Reviews* 68:168, 2010.

   Consumption of berries or their extracts is linked to improved cardiovascular health parameters. Berries are good sources of polyphenols, several vitamins and minerals involved in cardiovascular health, and fiber. In addition to the antioxidant effects of nutrients and phytochemicals, berries also may influence heart health by modulating expression of genes that lead to inflammation and formation of plaques

   in blood vessels. Freeze drying or heat-treatment of berries reduces their nutrient content, so consuming fresh or frozen berries is preferable to consuming processed versions of the fruit.

2. Cordero Z and others: Vitamin E and risk of cardiovascular diseases: A review of epidemiologic and clinical trial studies. *Critical Reviews in Food Science and Nutrition* 50:420, 2010.

   Although epidemiological studies suggest an association between vitamin E intake and reduced risk of cardiovascular diseases, most

   randomized controlled trials do not provide evidence of a benefit of vitamin E supplementation for prevention of cardiovascular diseases. Studies of the relationships between vitamin E intake and cardiovascular disease risk are complicated by the presence of other dietary components, including other chemical forms of vitamin E, as well as inaccuracies of data-collection methods. Current evidence does not support the use of vitamin E supplements to prevent cardiovascular diseases, but research is ongoing. Most research has focused on alpha-tocopherol, but the contributions of other forms of vitamin E warrant further exploration.

3. Johnson IT: Phytochemicals and cancer. *Proceedings of the Nutrition Society* 66:207, 2007.

   The author reviews current evidence on the roles of phytochemicals in the prevention of cancer, including a discussion of possible mechanisms of action. An important research need is to conduct in vivo *studies, as* in vitro *studies may overestimate the bioavailability and overlook metabolism of phytochemicals.*

4. Kaliora AC and others: Dietary antioxidants in preventing atherogenesis. *Atherosclerosis* 187:1, 2006.

   The role of oxidation in the development of cardiovascular disease is well accepted. This article reviews the evidence for antioxidant nutrients, including vitamin C, vitamin E, phytochemicals, and coenzyme Q10, in prevention of LDL oxidation and plaque formation. The authors highlight the anticipated importance of nutrigenomics in the prevention of cardiovascular disease.

5. Martini LA and others: Role of vitamins and minerals in prevention and management of type 2 diabetes mellitus. *Nutrition Reviews* 68:341, 2010.

   Guidelines for the dietary management of diabetes mellitus outline optimal macronutrient intakes but steer clear of recommending supplements of any micronutrients. Theoretical uses of vitamins and minerals for people with diabetes abound: B vitamins are associated with energy metabolism and antioxidant nutrients are involved in amelioration of oxidative stress associated with diabetes. Current research does not support a specific role for supplementation of any micronutrients for people with diabetes. Rather, meeting micronutrient needs from food sources, including fruits, vegetables, whole grains, and low-fat dairy products, is the safest plan of action.

6. National Institutes of Health, Office of Dietary Supplements: Dietary supplement fact sheet: Vitamin E. Updated 12/15/2009. Available at: http://ods.od.nih.gov/factsheets/vitaminE.asp; Vitamin A and carotenoids. Updated 4/23/2006. http://ods.od.nih.gov/factsheets/vitamina.asp; and, Vitamin C. Updated 11/12/2009. http://ods.od.nih.gov/factsheets/vitaminc.asp.

   These reader-friendly fact sheets provide the most recent information on supplements. Food sources, deficiencies, at-risk groups, and nutrient-drug interactions are highlighted. Current research and controversial areas are discussed.

7. NIH State-of-the-Science Panel: National Institutes of Health State-of-the-Science Conference Statement: Multivitamin/mineral supplements and chronic disease prevention. *Annals of Internal Medicine* 145(5):364, 2006.

   This report is the result of a thorough assessment of current medical knowledge of multivitamin/mineral supplements (MVMs). The effectiveness and safety of MVMs in relation to chronic disease prevention was systemically evaluated. The panel found few rigorous studies on which to base conclusions and recommendations. Only a few trials of vitamins and minerals demonstrate beneficial effects for the prevention of chronic disease, including increased bone mineral density and decreased fractures in postmenopausal women who use calcium and vitamin D supplements. In contrast, several other studies provide disturbing evidence of risk, such as increased lung cancer with beta-carotene use among smokers. The report concludes that the present evidence is insufficient to recommend either for or against the use of MVMs by the American public to prevent chronic disease. This conclusion is important to remember because manufacturers of these products are not required to report adverse events, and the FDA has no regulatory authority to require labeling or to help inform the public of these issues and concerns.

8. Park Y and others: Intakes of vitamins A, C, and E and use of multiple vitamin supplements and risk of colon cancer: A pooled analysis of prospective cohort studies. *Cancer Causes and Control* 21:1745, 2010.

   An analysis of many studies showed that intakes of vitamins A, C, and E from the diet were not related to reduced risk for colon cancer. However, total intakes (including food and supplemental sources) of vitamins C and E were associated with decreased risk of colon cancer. The authors suggest that because diets high in vitamins C and E are also usually high in folate, intake of folate may actually be responsible for the reduced risk of colon cancer observed in research studies.

9. Ramesh BN and others: Neuronutrition and Alzheimer's disease. *Journal of Alzheimer's Disease* 19:1123, 2010.

   Alzheimer's disease is characterized by the appearance of plaques in the brain. Oxidative stress contributes to plaque formation. Therefore, nutritional strategies to decrease oxidative stress are hypothesized to prevent or delay the development of Alzheimer's disease. For prevention of Alzheimer's disease, research supports maintaining high levels of physical activity, keeping the brain active, avoiding excessive intakes of calories and saturated fat, and consuming a diet high in antioxidants and omega-3 fatty acids.

10. Sesso HD and others: Vitamins E and C in the prevention of cardiovascular disease in men. The Physicians' Health Study II Randomized Controlled Trial. *Journal of American Medical Association* 300:2123, 2008.

    Men enrolled in the Physician's Health Study II were placed into four groups, which were given vitamin C and a placebo, vitamin E and a placebo, C and E together, and placebo only. Neither C nor E had an effect on major cardiovascular events, which include heart attacks, stroke, or death. The results suggest that when you pull a nutrient out of the whole diet, you don't see the same effects.

11. Stimpson JP and others: Acculturation in the United States is associated with lower serum carotenoid levels: Third National Health and Nutrition Examination Survey. *Journal of the American Dietetic Association* 107:1218, 2007.

    Despite public health campaigns promoting fruit and vegetable consumption, intakes of fruits and vegetables remain below recommendations for the majority of Americans. This study showed that for Mexican-Americans, acculturation is associated with declines in fruit and vegetable intake, as reflected by declines in serum carotenoid levels. Among immigrant populations, targeted public health messages should focus on maintenance of existing positive dietary habits.

12. Valko M and others: Free radicals and antioxidants in normal physiological functions and human disease. *International Journal of Biochemistry and Cell Biology* 39:44, 2007.

    Clearly, overproduction of free radicals has deleterious effects. However, free radicals do play important roles in normal human physiology. For example, free radicals are involved in cellular signaling pathways that protect the body against pathogens or identify and destroy tumors. This article reviews the roles of free radicals—good and bad—in human health.

13. Voutilainen S and others: Carotenoids and cardiovascular health. *American Journal of Clinical Nutrition* 83:1265, 2006.

    This report reviews the role of carotenoids in the prevention of heart disease. Although fruits and vegetables are recognized as having protective effects against cardiovascular disease, the role of a single group of compounds such as carotenoids cannot be ascertained. Therefore, the consumption of carotenoids in supplemental forms cannot be recommended.

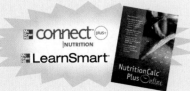

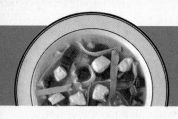

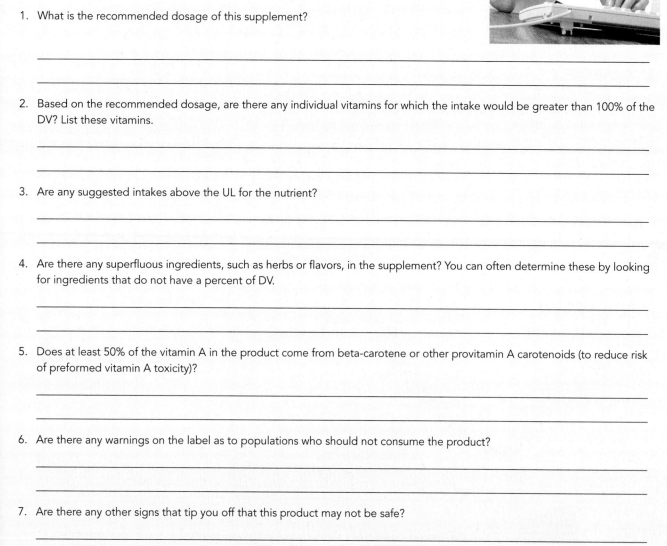

RATE YOUR PLATE

I. Spotting Fraudulent Claims on the Internet

Search for vitamins and vitaminlike substances sold over the Internet. Then write a report concerning any fraudulent or misleading claims made on behalf of these products. Are the websites selling vitamins, or are they a cover for selling something else? Compare the price of the vitamins from these sites with the price you would pay at the local supermarket or drugstore. Do any of these sites display any disclaimers or warnings about the products?

II. A Closer Look at Supplement Use

With the popularity of vitamin and mineral supplements, it is important to understand how to evaluate a supplement. Study the label of a supplement you use or one readily available from a friend or the supermarket. Then answer the following questions.

1. What is the recommended dosage of this supplement?

_____

_____

2. Based on the recommended dosage, are there any individual vitamins for which the intake would be greater than 100% of the DV? List these vitamins.

_____

_____

3. Are any suggested intakes above the UL for the nutrient?

_____

_____

4. Are there any superfluous ingredients, such as herbs or flavors, in the supplement? You can often determine these by looking for ingredients that do not have a percent of DV.

_____

_____

5. Does at least 50% of the vitamin A in the product come from beta-carotene or other provitamin A carotenoids (to reduce risk of preformed vitamin A toxicity)?

_____

_____

6. Are there any warnings on the label as to populations who should not consume the product?

_____

_____

7. Are there any other signs that tip you off that this product may not be safe?

_____

_____

Chapter 11 Nutrients Involved in Bone Health

Student Learning Outcomes

Chapter 11 is designed to allow you to:

11.1 Classify bone as either cortical or trabecular.

11.2 Describe the process by which bone cells synthesize and degrade bone.

11.3 List hormonal, lifestyle, and nutritional factors that influence bone health.

11.4 List key functions of the vitamins and minerals involved in bone health.

11.5 Describe current methods used to assess bone health.

11.6 List three important sources for each vitamin and mineral involved in bone health.

11.7 Identify deficiency and toxicity symptoms associated with vitamins and minerals involved in bone health.

What Would You Choose?

Vitamin D has been in the news a lot lately—it has been linked to prevention of several diseases, and the dietary reference intakes for vitamin D have recently changed. You know the "sunshine vitamin" is an important nutrient for bone health. Which type of milk contains the most vitamin D?

a Fat-free (skim) milk

b Reduced-fat (2%) milk

c Whole milk

d All contain the same amount of vitamin D.

 Think about your choice as you read Chapter 11, then see our recommendations at the end of the chapter. To learn more about vitamin D, check out the Connect site: www.mcgrawhillconnect.com

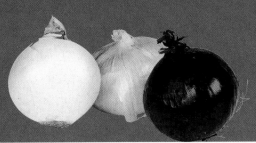
The human skeletal system can be thought of as the bricks and mortar that provide the structural support for the body. One major difference, however, is that bone is a vibrant, living tissue that flexes and undergoes constant breakdown and resynthesis. It is estimated that in the middle-aged adult, 9% of bone is removed and replaced by new bone every year. In addition to providing architectural framework, bone contains nerves and cartilage and is the source of red and white blood cells and platelets. Numerous minerals and vitamins are essential to synthesize and maintain bone. This chapter will explore how these nutrients function together to achieve optimal bone health.

Maintenance of healthy bone is critical for an active, productive life. The human body contains 206 bones, infiltrated by blood vessels that supply nutrients and hormones to the cells found in bone. The interactions among genes, hormones, body weight, physical activity, nutrition, and other lifestyle factors will ultimately determine bone health.

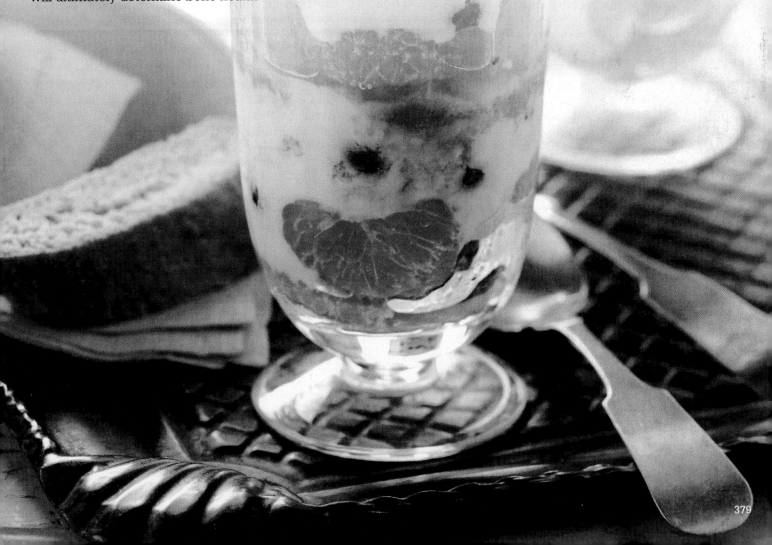

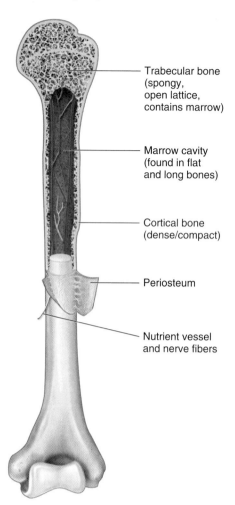

Trabecular bone (spongy, open lattice, contains marrow)

Marrow cavity (found in flat and long bones)

Cortical bone (dense/compact)

Periosteum

Nutrient vessel and nerve fibers

FIGURE 11-1 ▶ There are two types of bone: cortical and trabecular. Cortical bone forms the shafts of bones and the outer mineral covering. Trabecular bone supports the outer shell of cortical bone in various bones of the body.

 Refresh Your Memory

As you begin the study of nutritional factors that influence bone health in Chapter 11, you may want to review:

- Implications of the Dietary Supplement Health and Education Act (DSHEA) in Chapter 1.
- Cell structure, function, digestion, and absorption of nutrients in Chapter 3.
- The importance of adequate protein for bone development in Chapter 6.
- The role of vitamin C in collagen synthesis in Chapter 10.

11.1 Bone Structure

Think of bone as having three major components, each with a specific function (Fig. 11-1):

1. **Periosteum:** This thick, fibrous vascular membrane covers most of the (cortical) bone surface. Muscles, tendons, and ligaments connect to it. The periosteum does not cover the ends of long bones, as you need cartilage there for joint articulation.

2. **Bone, cortical and trabecular:**
   Cortical bone is sometimes called dense or compact bone. It comprises 80% of adult bone mass. The outer portion of nearly all bones is composed of dense, strong cortical bone. The principal function of cortical bone is to provide strength and stability. Microscopic openings in cortical bone allow blood vessels and nerves to pass through, providing nutrients and hormones to bone cells.

   Where cortical bone provides strength and stability, trabecular bone provides more. It, too, provides structural stability, but because it is not so rigid, it acts more like a shock absorber. It also lightens bones. The latticelike matrix of trabecular bone has small cavities that can be filled with marrow or connective tissue. Trabecular bone is predominant in the ends of long bones, vertebrae, rib cage, and flat bones of the pelvis. About 20% of adult bone mass is trabecular.

Rhymes with Orange

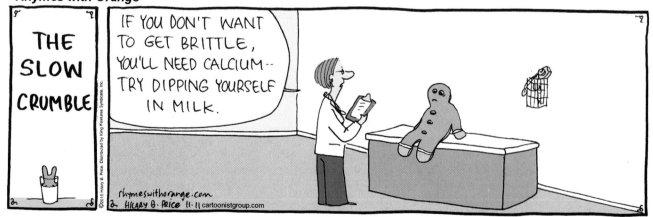

What are the new RDAs for calcium and vitamin D? Are supplements as good as food sources when it comes to getting proper nutrition for bone health? What if I am allergic to milk—can I still get enough bone-building nutrients? How can I find out if I am at risk for osteoporosis? Chapter 11 provides some answers.

3. **Bone marrow:** Marrow is a spongy tissue that contains stem cells. These cells are of two types: **hemopoietic,** meaning they are capable of developing into blood cells (see Chapter 12); or **stromal,** cells that can produce fat, cartilage, and bone. In infancy, all marrow is red in color due to the high number of blood-producing cells. With age, more and more marrow becomes yellow, reflecting a higher number of fat cells. By adulthood, only 50% of marrow is red. Bone marrow is primarily located in flat bones (hip, breast, rib, shoulder blade, and vertebrae) and in the shafts of long bones. You will find it in the head of the femur (ball joint at hip) and humerus (forearm at elbow). As noted earlier, marrow is located in pockets of trabecular bone.

Are teeth bone? Teeth have the same properties as bone plus a hard protective outer covering called enamel, not infiltrated by vessels or nerves.

11.2 Bone Growth and Remodeling

The growth, maintenance, and repair of bone involve a complex relationship between the synthesis of new bone by the **osteoblasts** and the breakdown of bone by **osteoclasts.** The degradation and resynthesis of bone is termed **bone remodeling** (Fig. 11-2). When you remodel a room, you tear down first and then you rebuild or you add on. The same principle applies to bone. Osteoclasts produced from stem cell bone marrow bring about **resorption,** that is, they break down or degrade small

periosteum A specialized connective tissue covering all bones and having bone-forming potential.

cortical bone The compact or dense bone found on the outer surfaces of bone.

trabecular bone The less dense, more open structure bone found in the inner layer of bones.

bone marrow The spongy tissue in flat bones and trabecular bone that contains stem cells.

osteoblast Bone cells that initiate the synthesis of new bone.

osteoclast Bone cells that break down bone and subsequently release bone minerals into the blood.

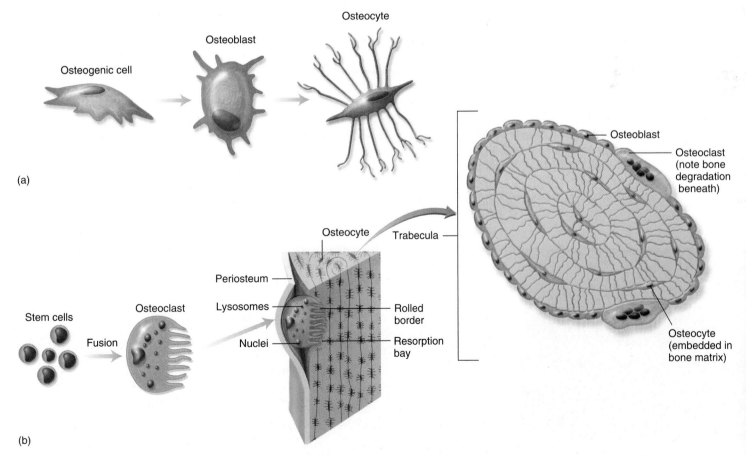

FIGURE 11-2 ▶ Bone remodeling. (a) Osteogenic cells (new bone cells produced in bone marrow) produce osteoblasts that develop into osteocytes. (b) Stem cells (from bone marrow) fuse together and form osteoclasts. These cells dissolve bone via the lysosomes and acids they contain. The osteoclasts degrade the bone (resorption) so that osteoblasts can embed and add more minerals and connective tissue (resynthesis).

bone remodeling The chemical process by which bone is broken down and replaced by new bone.

resorption The process of losing substance. Bone resorption is part of the initial process for remodeling and growth.

osteocyte Osteoblast embedded into the bone matrix.

hydroxyapatite Crystalline compound containing calcium, phosphorus, and sometimes fluoride, also known as bone mineral.

amounts of bone. In doing so, minerals embedded in bone matrix, including calcium, phosphorus, and magnesium, are freed and released into the blood. The resynthesis of new bone is then accomplished by the activity of osteoblasts from bone marrow. These osteoblasts embed within the dissolved "resorption bay" (Fig. 11-2) provided by the osteoclasts. The osteoblasts take up free calcium and phosphorus and, along with collagen, form a complex mixture called **hydroxyapatite.** This mixture adds strength and structure to the bone. Some osteoblasts become embedded within the bone matrix and become osteocytes. Figure 11-2 shows the relationship of these three cells in the bone. Synthesis of bone, for repair or growth, is a function of the osteoblast.

Bone growth occurs in length and width during the first two decades of life. The rate of bone formation exceeds the rate of bone breakdown during infancy, childhood, and young adulthood. The majority of bone growth occurs before adulthood, although in both males and females, peak bone mass is usually achieved a few years before age 30. Genetics as well as nutrient intake, drugs, hormones, physical activity, and lifestyle choices will influence the age at which peak bone mass is achieved. People with a larger frame size and body weight will have a greater bone mass due to the additional stress on the bone associated with the extra weight.

The optimal situation throughout adulthood would be to maintain peak bone mass through an equal amount of bone resorption and resynthesis. However, after 30 years of age, bone resorption occurs at a faster rate than synthesis, resulting in a loss of bone mass and a decrease in bone mineral density. Bone mineral density is the concentration of minerals found in the bone and is used as an indicator of bone health. Bone is composed of approximately 65% minerals and 35% connective tissue. Minerals provide the strength and rigidity, whereas the connective tissue provides flexibility.

11.3 Factors That Influence Bone Health

The rate of bone remodeling is different between trabecular and cortical bone. The breakdown and resynthesis of trabecular bone occur at a faster rate when compared to cortical bone. This subsequently makes the trabecular bone more responsive to factors that influence bone remodeling. Biological and lifestyle factors have a large role in the growth, maintenance, and overall health of bone.

Biological factors (Table 11-1) are predetermined by genetics; an individual has little or no ability to change these factors. People with larger frames tend to have higher peak bone mass than do people with smaller frames, and women have lower peak bone mass than men. The greater the bone mineral density, the stronger the bone. Individuals need to focus on meeting calcium, vitamin D, protein, and other nutrient needs to provide the building blocks to synthesize bone.

The hormone estrogen, produced by the ovaries in females and by adipose tissue in both men and women, is a major contributor to bone maintenance because estrogen has been shown to stimulate osteoblast activity (bone formation). Therefore, any sign of menstrual irregularities (defined as no menstrual period for 3 consecutive months or more, unless medically supervised) is reason to see a physician. Nonmenstruating

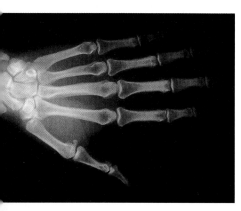

▲ Ninety-nine percent of calcium in the body is in bones.

TABLE 11-1 Biological Factors Associated with Bone Status

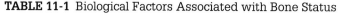

Biological Factors	Effect on Bone Status
Sex	Women have lower bone mass and density than men.
Age	Bone loss occurs after age 30.
Ethnicity	Individuals of Caucasian or Asian heritage are at greater risk for poor bone health than individuals of African descent.
Frame size	People with "small bones" have a lower bone mass.

female athletes and other women with irregular menstrual cycles (e.g., women with eating disorders) typically exhibit low bone mineral density. Physical activity alone cannot prevent bone loss associated with irregular menstruation. Even though female athletes may perform an extensive amount of weight-bearing physical activity, high levels of physical activity not balanced with adequate energy intake result in "low energy availability" to support reproductive function. The hormone estrogen also plays an important role in the decline of bone mass and bone mineral density in later life. When a woman reaches menopause and the ovaries stop producing estrogen, bone loss accelerates.

In contrast to the biological factors already described, we have the ability to influence bone health through various lifestyle choices (Table 11-2). An active lifestyle that includes weight-bearing physical activity is an important factor in bone health. The increased muscle mass that stems from weight-bearing physical activity is associated with greater bone mineral density. Muscle keeps tension on bone and the hormonal changes that occur with the stress associated with exercise cause bones to retain and possibly gain density (Fig. 11-3). Upper-body strength training is especially encouraged, as this area can be easily overlooked. Older adults especially need to stay physically active—including some weight-bearing and resistance activities.

At any age, smoking and excessive alcohol intake decrease bone mass. Smoking lowers the estrogen concentration in the blood in women, increasing bone loss. Smoking one pack of cigarettes per day throughout your adult life could result in a 5% to 10% acceleration of bone loss. Alcohol is toxic to bone cells for both men and

TABLE 11-2 Modifiable Lifestyle Factors Associated with Bone Status

Lifestyle Factors	Call to Action
Adequate diet containing an appropriate amount of nutrients	• Follow MyPlate with special emphasis on adequate amounts of fruits, vegetables, and low-fat and fat-free dairy products. • Consider use of fortified foods (or supplements) to make up for specific nutrient shortfalls, such as vitamin D and calcium.
Healthy body weight	• Maintain a healthy body weight (BMI of 18.5–24.9) to support bone health.
Normal menses	• During childbearing years, seek medical advice if menses cease (such as in cases of anorexia nervosa or extreme athletic training). • Women at menopause and beyond should consider use of current medical therapies to reduce bone loss linked to the fall in estrogen output.
Weight-bearing physical activity	• Perform weight-bearing activity as this contributes to bone maintenance, whereas bed rest and a sedentary lifestyle lead to bone loss. Strength training, especially upper body, is helpful to bone maintenance.
Smoking	• Smoking lowers estrogen synthesis in women. Cessation is advised. Passive exposure is a risk.
Medications	• Some medications (e.g., thyroid hormone, cortisol, diuretics) stimulate urinary calcium excretion. • Some medications (e.g., alcohol, diuretics, cancer medications) stimulate urinary excretion of magnesium.
Excessive intake of protein, phosphorus, sodium, caffeine, wheat bran, or alcohol	• Moderate intake of these dietary constituents is recommended. Problems primarily arise when excessive intakes of these nutrients are combined with inadequate calcium consumption. • Excessive soft drink consumption is especially discouraged.
Inadequate UV-B exposure	• If sunlight exposure is limited (< 10–15 minutes per day without sunscreen), focus on food or supplements to meet current RDA for vitamin D.

FIGURE 11-3 ▶ The stress of muscles pulling on bone during exercise increases bone mineral density.

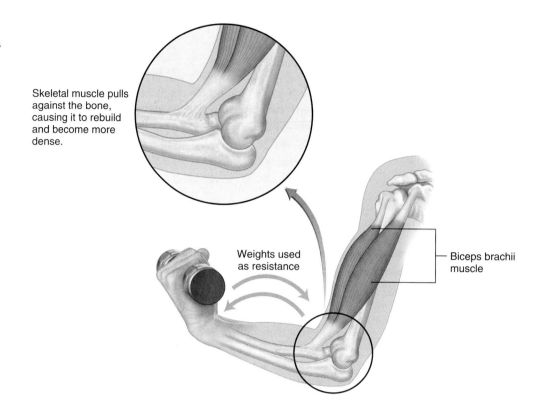

Skeletal muscle pulls against the bone, causing it to rebuild and become more dense.

Weights used as resistance

Biceps brachii muscle

women, and alcoholism is probably a major undiagnosed and unrecognized cause of low bone mineral density. Excessive intakes of phosphorus, caffeine, and sodium also adversely affect bone health but only if calcium intake is low or marginal.

11.4 Osteoporosis

osteoporosis The presence of a stress-induced fracture or a T-score of −2.5 or lower. The bones are porous and fragile due to low mineral density.

Healthy People 2020 identified the prevention of bone disease, or **osteoporosis,** as one of its major focus areas. About 10 million Americans over the age of 50 currently have osteoporosis. Of these, about 8 million are women. An additional 34 million Americans have low bone density, placing them at risk for developing osteoporosis. By 2020, these numbers are expected to increase to 10.5 million women and 3.3 million men with osteoporosis, and another 48 million with low bone mass. Consistently, osteoporosis has led to approximately 2 million bone fractures per year in the United States, including nearly 300,000 broken hips. The health care costs associated with these fractures was about $19 billion in 2005. These costs are projected to reach more than $25 billion by the year 2025, with the most rapid increases among minority populations (see Fig. 11-4 and Further Reading 3).

The personal cost with a hip fracture surpasses any financial cost. Hip fractures are regarded as devastating. They result in loss of mobility and need for long-term care. The average age for hip fracture is 82 years. Thus, long-term care may be for life. Only 40% of people with hip fractures regain their earlier level of independence. Hip fracture is associated with significant mortality. Results from the national Fracture Intervention Trial showed a six times greater risk of mortality associated with a hip fracture among postmenopausal women with low bone mass. Other types of fractures or even fear of fracture due to osteoporosis can affect quality of life. Vertebral fractures, especially if there are several of them, cause significant pain, reduced lung function, loss of height, and a curved spine. Movement can be restricted and gait altered, increasing the risk and fear of falls and/or more fractures.

Women tend to lose 1% to 3% of their bone mass each year after menopause. Men also lose bone mass as they age, but the loss is more gradual. When the

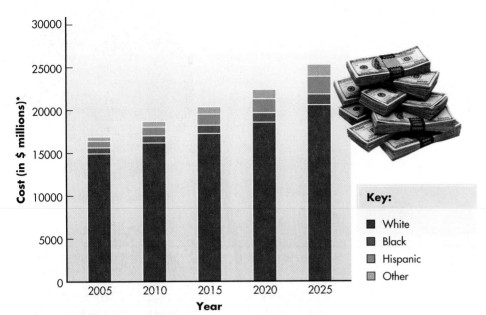

* Projected costs are not adjusted for inflation.

FIGURE 11-4 ▶ Projected economic burden of osteoporosis by race/ethnicity, 2005–2025.

Source: Burge R and others: 2007 (see Further Reading 3).

bone-demineralization activities of osteoclasts exceed the bone-building activities of osteoblasts, bone mass declines. This is a normal part of aging and does not always lead to unhealthy bones. However, if bone mass is low when this process begins, even moderate bone demineralization can lead to a condition called **osteopenia.** As more bone is lost, the entire matrix of the bone tissue also begins to break down. When this occurs, osteoporosis is likely to result. About 25% of women older than age 50 develop or have osteoporosis. Among people older than age 80, osteoporosis becomes the rule, not the exception. To young adults, it may sound benign to have osteoporosis. To older adults, the diagnosis presents the reality of life permanently changed.

osteopenia A bone disease defined by low mineral density.

type 1 osteoporosis Porous trabecular bone characterized by rapid bone demineralization following menopause.

type 2 osteoporosis Porous trabecular and cortical bone observed in men and women after the age of 60.

Type 1 and Type 2 Osteoporosis

There are two types of osteoporosis. **Type 1 osteoporosis,** also called postmenopausal osteoporosis, typically occurs in women between 50 and 60 years of age. This type of osteoporosis is directly linked to decreased estrogen concentrations that occur at menopause. Type 1 osteoporosis most dramatically affects trabecular bone, as this type of bone undergoes faster remodeling than cortical bone (Fig. 11-5). A woman can lose 20% to 30% of trabecular bone and 5% to 10% of cortical bone between ages 50 and 60, unless intervention occurs (Fig. 11-6).

Trabecular bone has a much higher density of osteoblast and osteoclast cells than cortical bone. The osteoblast cells require estrogen for maximal activity. After menopause, osteoblast activity decreases; however, osteoclast activity remains high. The result is greater bone resorption than resynthesis. Minerals are released but not reincorporated into bone, so the locations where the osteoclasts left reserves or pockets for osteoblasts to rebuild the collagen mineral matrix will now become holes. The trabecular-rich bones of the pelvis, vertebrae, and portions of long bones are at greatest risk for fracture in people with osteoporosis (Fig. 11-7).

Type 2 osteoporosis occurs in both men and women and tends to be diagnosed later in life (70 to 75 years of age). Type 2 osteoporosis is a result of breakdown of both cortical and trabecular bone. It is due to a combination of dietary and age-related factors; low dietary intake of bone-building nutrients compounds the problems associated with decreased ability to absorb or metabolize nutrients.

People with either form of osteoporosis can lose significant height and experience severe pain, especially in the vertebrae. A woman may lose an inch or more in height as the bone is demineralized (Fig. 11-8). Both men and women can develop a curvature

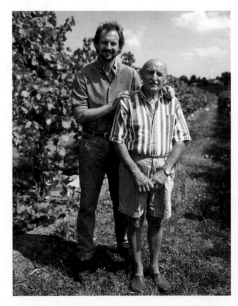

▲ Men are at risk for osteoporosis when they reach their 70s. As with women, it can be prevented.

FIGURE 11-5 ▶ Cortical and trabecular bone. Cortical bone forms the shafts of bones and their outer mineral covering. Trabecular bone supports the outer shell of cortical bone in various bones of the body. Note how the osteoporotic bone has much less trabecular bone. This leads to a more fragile bone and is not reversible to any major extent with current therapies.

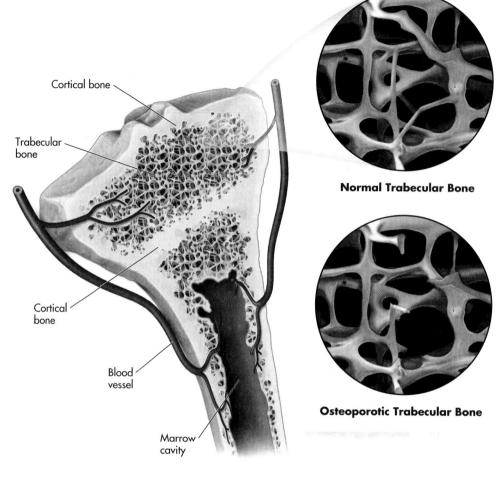

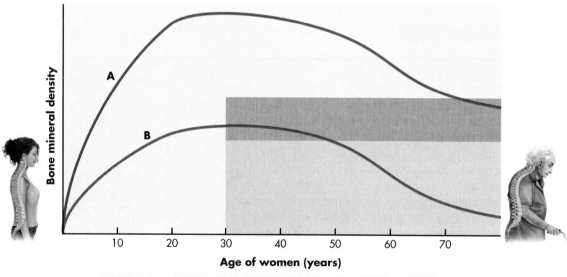

☐ Healthy bone mineral density ☐ Low bone mineral density ☐ Osteoporosis

FIGURE 11-6 ▶ The relationship between peak bone mass and the ultimate risk of developing osteoporosis and related bone fractures.
• **Woman A** had developed a high peak bone mass by age 30. Her bone loss was slow and steady between ages 30 and 50 and sped up somewhat after age 50 because of the effects of menopause. At age 75, the woman had a healthy bone mineral density value and did not show evidence of osteoporosis.
• **Woman B** with low peak bone mass experienced the same rate of bone loss as Woman A. By age 50, she already had low bone mineral density and by age 70, kyphosis and spinal fractures had occurred.
Given the low calcium intakes common among young women today, line B is a sobering reality. Following a diet and lifestyle pattern that contributes to maximal bone mineral density can help women follow line A and significantly reduce their risk of developing osteoporosis.

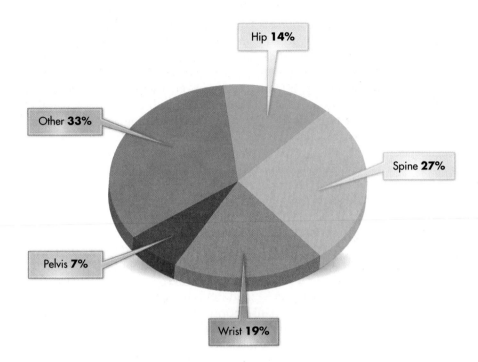

FIGURE 11-7 ▶ Sites of osteoporotic fractures.

Source: Burge R and others: 2007 (see Further Reading 3).

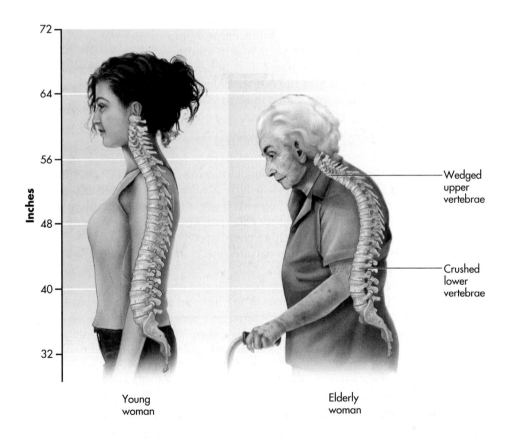

FIGURE 11-8 ▶ Normal and osteoporotic woman. Osteoporotic bones have less substance, so osteoporosis generally leads to loss of height, distorted body shape, fractures, and possibly loss of teeth. Monitoring changes in adult height is one way to detect early evidence of osteoporosis.

in the upper spine called **kyphosis** or dowager's hump (Fig. 11-9). Kyphosis is a major concern because the bending of the spine may decrease the volume of the chest cavity, resulting in difficulty breathing, abdominal pain, decreased appetite, and premature satiety. Osteoporotic bone is also more susceptible to fracture following a fall. Bone fractures often result in hospitalization and loss of the ability to live independently, so preventing osteoporosis means enhanced health and well-being as we age.

kyphosis Abnormally increased bending of the spine.

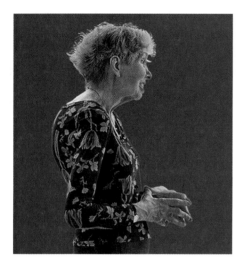

FIGURE 11-9 ▲ Kyphosis, or curvature of the upper spine, results from demineralization of the vertebrae. This can lead to both physical and emotional pain. Kyphosis occurs in both men and women.

According to the National Osteoporosis Foundation 2010 guidelines (see Further Reading 9), all men and women diagnosed with osteoporosis should first be counseled on risk factor reduction. Daily habits of calcium and vitamin D consumption as well as exercise should be stressed. Clear guidelines are provided to physicians for patients to be considered for pharmacological (drug) intervention. These drugs are indicated for postmenopausal women and men over 50 who meet specific standards for level of risk of future fracture as well as medical history (see Further Reading 7). Current medication options for men and women are bisphosphonates (Fosamax, Boniva, Actonel, and Reclast) and parathyroid hormone (Forteo), and, for women only, calcitonin (Miacalcin or Fortical) and hormone therapy (estrogens or Raloxifene).

Bisphosphonates are antiresorptive drugs; they inhibit bone breakdown by limiting osteoclast activity. Though commonly prescribed for low bone mass or osteoporosis, they are not easy to tolerate. Problems swallowing, esophageal inflammation, and gastric ulcers have been reported with their use.

Estrogen/hormone therapy is used to prevent osteoporosis and to relieve the symptoms of menopause. It is not used to treat low bone mass or osteoporosis. Raloxifene, on the other hand, is used for both prevention and treatment of osteoporosis. The types of therapy, mode (pill, cream, patch), and duration are chosen by the woman and her health care professional. Menopause hormone therapy can carry some risk: vaginal bleeding, increased risk for some cancers (cervical, breast, ovarian, uterine), and increased risk of cardiovascular disease, depending on family history.

The incidence of osteoporosis increases as a person ages. Its importance as a personal and public health problem is intensifying as the U.S. population ages. It appears, however, that a large percentage of the cases of osteoporosis can be prevented. The key to prevention is to build dense bones during the first 30 years of life and then limit the amount of bone loss in adulthood. People with higher peak bone mass have more calcium to lose before bones become weak and fracture easily. A higher peak bone mass is also the reason males experience osteoporosis less often than females do; they have more bone mass to lose.

11.5 Bone Health Assessment

Until the 1990s, there were no convenient clinical measurement devices health care professionals could use to assess bone health. A routine X-ray could detect osteoporosis, but not until 30% or more of bone mass was already lost. A hairline fracture of the vertebrae also was used to diagnose osteoporosis. Both of these tools diagnosed the presence of osteoporosis, but neither could predict risk. Today, we have tools that can quantitate bone mass and bone density, and, subsequently, the likelihood of a person's developing bone disease.

The most accurate test for assessing bone density is the central **dual energy X-ray absorptiometry (DEXA)** measurement of the hip and spine. The central DEXA procedure is simple, painless, safe, noninvasive and generally takes less than 15 minutes. The hip and spine are measured because these sites are commonly affected by osteoporosis and are likely to result in more serious injuries. The ability of the bone to block the path of a low-level X-ray is used as a measure of bone mineral density. A very low dose of radiation is used for the DEXA—about one-tenth of the exposure from a chest X-ray.

From the DEXA measurement of bone density, a T-score is generated, which compares the observed bone density to that of a person at peak bone mass (e.g., age 30). The T-score is interpreted as follows:

0 to −1	Normal
−1 to −2.4	Low bone mineral density
−2.5 or lower	Osteoporosis

bisphosphonates Drugs that bind minerals and prevent osteoclast breakdown of bone. Examples are alendronate (Fosamax) and risedronate (Actonel).

dual energy X-ray absorptiometry (DEXA) A scientific tool used to measure bone mineral density.

The National Osteoporosis Foundation 2010 recommendations call for DEXA testing for the following groups of people.

- All women age 65 and older and men age 70 and older
- Younger postmenopausal women and men (ages 50 to 69) who have risk factors
- Women going through perimenopause (transitioning into menopause) who have low body weight, have prior low-trauma fracture, or take high-risk medications, such as steroids
- Adults with fracture after age 50
- Adults with a health condition for which they take steroids for a prolonged period (e.g., rheumatoid arthritis, Crohn's disease, asthma)
- Anyone being considered for medication for osteoporosis or receiving therapy for osteoporosis

When DEXA measurements of the hip and spine are not feasible due to portability or expense, several peripheral measurements of bone density can be used as screening methods at various sites on the body. Peripheral DEXA uses the same technology as central DEXA but scans only the ankle or wrist. Peripheral quantitative computed tomography (pQCT) generates a three-dimensional scan of the radius in the arm or the tibia in the lower leg. It measures bone mineral density and can provide information on cortical and trabecular bone density, area, and thickness, as well as some measurements of bone strength. The quantitative ultrasound (QUS) technique uses sound waves to measure the density of bone in the heel, shin, and kneecap. These peripheral tests are sometimes used at health fairs, medical offices, and research settings. Although they cannot be used to diagnose osteoporosis, they can inform the health care provider if additional testing (i.e., central DEXA) is warranted.

The incidence of osteoporosis is far less in many other countries than in the United States. In reviewing Tables 11-1 and 11-2, you can see that the contributions for the greater incidence in the United States are mainly related to diet and other lifestyle behaviors. That means that osteoporosis can largely be prevented.

To synthesize, maintain, and repair bone requires several vitamins, minerals, and hormones. The key nutrients include vitamin D and the minerals calcium, phosphorus, magnesium, and fluoride. Other nutrients that support bone health include vitamin C, vitamin K, boron, and silicon. In addition, adequate protein must be consumed, especially in the elderly, to reduce bone loss.

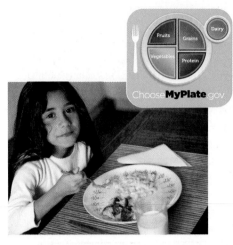

▲ Macaroni and cheese, broccoli, and milk provide calcium. How does this young girl's meal compare to MyPlate?

11.6 Critical Nutrients Required for Bone Growth, Maintenance, and Repair

Calcium (Ca)

All cells require calcium to function; however, more than 99% of the calcium in the body is used to strengthen bones and teeth. Calcium represents 40% of all the minerals present in the body and equals about 2.5 pounds (1200 grams) in the average person. Less than 1% of calcium is found in blood, but this circulating calcium is critical to supply the needs of cells other than bone cells (e.g., muscle, nerve).

Bone growth, development, and maintenance require an adequate calcium intake. Calcium requires an acidic environment in the gastrointestinal tract to be absorbed efficiently. Absorption occurs primarily in the upper part of the small intestine. This area tends to remain somewhat acidic because it receives the acidic stomach contents. After the first loop of the small intestine, secretions from the pancreas enter the small intestine and the pH becomes neutral to slightly basic. Calcium absorption decreases. Efficient calcium absorption in the upper small intestine depends on the presence of the active form of vitamin D.

parathyroid hormone (PTH) A hormone made by the parathyroid gland that increases synthesis of the active form of vitamin D. This hormone works with vitamin D to increase blood levels of calcium.

phytic acid (phytate) A constituent of plant fiber that chemically binds minerals and prevents their absorption. Phytic acid can depress calcium absorption from other foods present in the GI tract.

oxalic acid (oxalate) An organic acid found in spinach, rhubarb, beet greens, chard, and sweet potatoes. It can depress the absorption of certain minerals, such as calcium, but only in the food itself.

cellular differentiation The process of a less-specialized cell becoming a more specialized type. Think of stem cells in the bone marrow becoming red and white blood cells.

Adults absorb about 30% of the calcium in the foods eaten, but during times when the body needs extra calcium, such as in infancy and pregnancy, absorption increases to as high as 60%. Young people tend to absorb calcium better than do older people, especially those older than 70.

Many factors *enhance* calcium absorption, including:

- High need (e.g., during growth, pregnancy, lactation)
- Blood levels of **parathyroid hormone** and vitamin D
- The presence of lactose in the diet
- The flow rate (motility) of digestive contents through the intestine
- Acidic environment of the stomach

Many factors *inhibit* calcium absorption, including:

- Large amounts of **phytic acid** and fiber from grains (if fiber intake >30 grams/day)
- **Oxalates** found in specific foods—only inhibit calcium in those foods.
- Great excess of phosphorus, magnesium, sodium, and zinc in the diet (only if calcium intake is very low)
- Tannins (polyphenols) in tea and some legumes (e.g., soy)
- A vitamin D deficiency
- Diarrhea (as a result of chronic or acute health conditions or induced by laxatives)
- Old age
- Some medications (anticonvulsants, cortisone, antacids)

The body tightly regulates a constant blood calcium concentration, regardless of dietary intake. If dietary calcium intake is inadequate and blood calcium concentration begins to decrease, three hormonally controlled actions are stimulated to reestablish calcium blood levels. Bones release calcium, intestines absorb more calcium, and the kidneys retain more calcium in the blood. The skeleton provides the framework of the body, and it functions as a bank from which calcium can be added or withdrawn. Only about 1% of the calcium in bone is available at any time for this purpose. Even so, bone loss due to inadequate calcium intake and/or absorption may occur, though slowly. Clinical symptoms show after many years. By not meeting calcium needs, some people, especially women, are most likely setting the stage for osteoporosis and future bone fractures.

NEWSWORTHY NUTRITION | Calcium supplements and cardiovascular health

Two recent analyses revealed a small but statistically significant increase in the rate of heart attacks among older adults taking calcium supplements with or without vitamin D. Meeting daily needs for calcium and vitamin D is recommended for prevention of osteoporosis. Although achieving the RDAs for calcium and vitamin D through dietary modifications is associated with improved bone mineral density and reduced rate of fractures, use of supplements to meet RDAs may actually impair skeletal health and worsen cardiovascular health. Although the observed relationships between calcium supplements and heart attack risk are small, the regular use of calcium supplements by so many older adults could translate into a large public health problem. Obtaining adequate calcium and vitamin D through dietary sources, if possible, appears to be the safest means to prevent osteoporosis without jeopardizing heart health.

Sources: Bolland MJ and others: Effect of calcium supplements on risk of myocardial infarction and cardiovascular events: meta-analysis. *British Medical Journal* 341:c3691, 2010.

Bolland MJ and others: Calcium supplements with or without vitamin D and risk of cardiovascular events: Reanalysis of the Women's Health Initiative limited access dataset and meta-analysis. *British Medical Journal* 342:d2040, 2011.

connect **Check out the Connect site www.mcgrawhillconnect .com to further explore calcium and heart health.**

Additional Functions of Calcium. Forming and maintaining bone are calcium's major roles in the body. However, calcium is critical for many other processes. Calcium is essential for formation of a blood clot. Muscle contraction is activated by calcium release and the flow of calcium along the surface of the muscle cell. If blood calcium falls below a critical point, muscles cannot relax after contraction; the body stiffens and shows involuntary twitching, called tetany. In nerve transmission, calcium assists in the release of neurotransmitters and permits the flow of ions in and out of nerve cells. Without sufficient calcium, nerve function fails, opening another path to tetany. Calcium helps regulate cellular metabolism by influencing the activities of various enzymes and hormonal responses. Calcium also functions in the maintenance of cell membrane integrity, normal blood pressure, regulation of glucose concentration, and **cellular differentiation.** It is the tight regulation of the concentration of calcium in the blood that keeps these processes going, even if a person fails to consume enough dietary calcium from day to day.

Other Possible Health Benefits of Calcium. Researchers have been examining links between calcium intake and risks for a wide array of diseases. An adequate calcium intake can reduce the risk of colon cancer, especially in people who consume a high-fat diet (see Further Reading 13). A decreased risk of some forms of kidney stones and reduced lead absorption are other possible benefits when calcium is part of a meal. Calcium intakes of 800 to 1200 milligrams per day can also decrease blood pressure, compared with intakes of 400 milligrams per day or less. Calcium intakes of 1200 milligrams per day in combination with a low-fat, low-cholesterol diet can help people with elevated LDL improve their blood lipid profiles. For women, an adequate calcium intake might also reduce the risk of premenstrual syndrome and high blood pressure that can develop during pregnancy. Overall, the benefits of a diet providing adequate calcium extend beyond bone health.

Calcium Sources and Needs. Calcium is found in both plant and animal foods, although the best sources are dairy products. Milk is also a source of vitamin D and lactose, two nutrients that enhance calcium absorption. Dairy products, such as milk and cheese, provide about 75% of the calcium in North American diets. An exception is cottage cheese, because most calcium is bound and unavailable for absorption.

Bread, rolls, crackers, and foods made with milk products are secondary contributors. Other calcium sources are leafy greens (such as kale), almonds, some legumes, sardines, and canned salmon. Overall, fat-free milk is the most nutrient-dense (milligrams per kcal) source of calcium because of its relatively high **bioavailability** and low calorie content, with some vegetable sources following close behind (Fig. 11-10). Calcium-fortified foods such as orange juice, breakfast cereals, breakfast bars, waffles, and soy products provide considerable amounts of calcium. High-calcium mineral

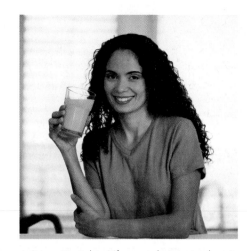

▲ It is not just dairy! If you are lactose intolerant or just do not like dairy, you can still find calcium in foods. Soy and rice milks as well as some types of orange juice are fortified with calcium. Almonds are a natural source of calcium. One ounce contains 80 milligrams.

bioavailability The degree to which a consumed nutrient is absorbed and used by the body.

Food Sources of Calcium

Food Item and Amount	Calcium (milligrams)	Adult Male and Female RDA = 1000 milligrams	
		Daily Value = 1000 milligrams %RDA	
RDA*	1000		100%
Plain yogurt, 1 cup	450		45%
Parmesan cheese, 1 ounce	390		39%
Fortified orange juice, 1 cup	350		35%
Romano cheese, 1 ounce	300		30%
Skim milk, 1 cup	300		30%
Swiss cheese, 1 ounce	275		28%
Salmon (with bones), 3 ounces	210		21%
Cheddar cheese, 1 ounce	200		20%
Soy milk, fortified with calcium, 1 cup	200		20%
Total Raisin Bran cereal, ¾ cup	180		18%
Sardines (with bones), 2 ounces	170		17%
Chocolate pudding, ½ cup	160		16%
Tofu, ½ cup	140		14%

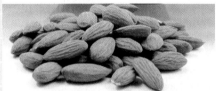

Key:
- Grains
- Vegetables
- Fruits
- Dairy
- Protein

*For adults; see the DRI table in the back of this book for age-specific recommendations.

FIGURE 11-10 ▶ Food sources of calcium compared to the Recommended Dietary Allowance.

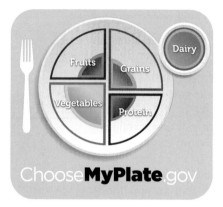

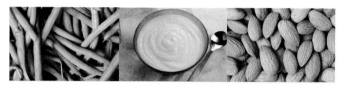

**MyPlate:
Sources of Calcium**

Grains	Vegetables	Fruits	Dairy	Protein
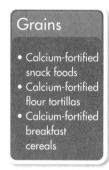 • Calcium-fortified snack foods • Calcium-fortified flour tortillas • Calcium-fortified breakfast cereals	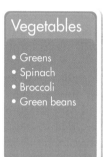 • Greens • Spinach • Broccoli • Green beans	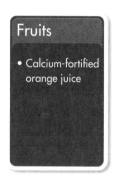 • Calcium-fortified orange juice	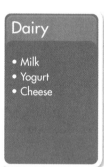 • Milk • Yogurt • Cheese	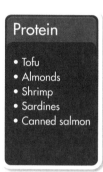 • Tofu • Almonds • Shrimp • Sardines • Canned salmon

FIGURE 11-11 ▶ Sources of calcium from MyPlate. The fill of the background color (none, 1/3, 2/3, or completely covered) within each group on the plate indicates the average nutrient density for calcium in that group. Overall, foods from the dairy group and many fortified foods are nutrient-dense and bioavailable sources of calcium. More calcium-fortified foods appear in stores each year and thus add to the food sources listed for various groups. With regard to physical activity, calcium is especially important for related muscle contraction and to maintain a strong skeleton to support the body.

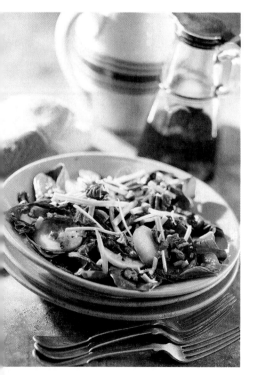

▲ Spinach may be loaded with vitamin A, but the calcium (and iron) in it are largely unavailable. Oxalic acid in spinach binds these minerals, making them less bioavailable.

waters also appear to provide useful quantities of bioavailable calcium (see Further Reading 4). Through the production of more products fortified with calcium, food and beverage companies are responding to consumers' desire to increase consumption of calcium (Fig. 11-11).

A serving of some calcium-fortified foods may exceed the amount of calcium contained in a cup of milk. An 8-ounce glass of calcium-fortified orange juice can provide up to 350 milligrams of calcium, whereas 8 ounces of milk has 300. Another source of calcium is soybean curd (tofu) if it is made with calcium carbonate (check the label). It is easy to assess the calcium content of foods because it is among those nutrients that are required to be listed on the Nutrition Facts panel on food labels. The Daily Value (DV) for calcium used for food and supplement labels is 1000 milligrams. To determine the amount of calcium in a food, use this trick. If a food label states a serving supplies 30% of the DV for calcium, convert this to milligrams by adding a 0, so 30% is the same as 300 milligrams. See Making Decisions at the end of this section for further discussion.

Many factors can influence the bioavailability of calcium. Calcium absorption can be reduced by the presence of oxalates, tannins, and phytic acid. These compounds chelate (chemically bind) calcium in the digestive tract. Oxalates are found in sweet potatoes, collard greens, spinach, and rhubarb. It is estimated that a person would have to consume over eight servings (8 cups) of spinach to absorb the same amount of calcium present in one serving (1 cup) of milk. Oxalates bind only the calcium in the food they are in; oxalate-containing foods do not affect the calcium availability from other foods. This does not hold true for phytates or tannins. Tea and some legumes are rich sources of tannins. Phytates are found in whole grains, raw beans, and nuts. Diets high in dietary fiber reduce mineral absorption. Age also influences the bio-availabilty of calcium; calcium absorption decreases in the fifth decade of life due to decreased acid secretion in the stomach and lower synthesis, absorption, and activation of vitamin D, which makes it more difficult for older people to meet their need for calcium.

The Recommended Dietary Allowance for calcium is 1000 milligrams/day for adults up through 50 years of age. For women older than age 50, and both men and women over age 70, the RDA increases to 1200 milligrams per day. The RDA is based on the amount of calcium needed each day to offset calcium losses in urine, feces, and other routes. The RDA for young people includes an additional amount to allow for increases in bone mass during growth and development. Most older children and adolescents in the United States do not consume the recommended amount of calcium.

In the United States, average daily calcium intakes are approximately 800 milligrams for women and 1000 milligrams for men. Approximately half of adult women in the United States consume less than 60% of the recommended intake of calcium (Fig. 11-12). Many women have low calcium intake for several reasons. Dairy products are perceived to be high in calories. The food industry has responded to this concern through the introduction of many reduced-fat dairy products. Many adults report losing a taste for milk as they age. In addition, lactose intolerance becomes more prevalent as people age. Thus, dietary intakes of calcium by many women, especially young women, are below the RDA, whereas intakes by most men are roughly equivalent to the RDA. It is also important for vegans to focus on eating good plant sources of calcium, as well as on the total amount of calcium ingested.

MAKING DECISIONS

To estimate your calcium intake, use the rule of 300s. Count 300 milligrams for the calcium provided by foods scattered throughout the diet. Add to that another 300 milligrams for every cup of milk or yogurt or 1.5 ounces of cheese. If you eat a lot of tofu, almonds, or sardines or drink calcium-fortified beverages, use Figure 11-10 or diet-analysis software to get a more accurate calculation of calcium intake.

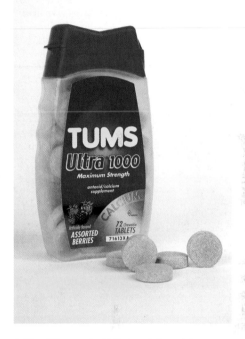

▲ Tums® is an antacid that contains calcium carbonate. It can be used as a relatively inexpensive calcium supplement.

FIGURE 11-12 ▶ The gap between recommended daily intake of calcium and daily consumption of calcium in males and females in the United States.

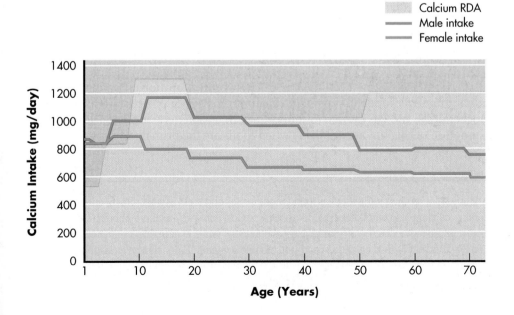

Legend:
- Calcium RDA
- Male intake
- Female intake

TABLE 11-3 Calcium Supplement Comparisons

Supplement form	% Calcium*	Comments
Calcium carbonate • tablets • chewable tablets • soft chews	40% calcium	• Most common form. • Least expensive. • Needs acid environment in stomach, so take with acid food or take with meals.
Calcium citrate • pills • liquid	21% calcium	• Best absorbed. • Most expensive. • *Does not* need acid environment to be absorbed. • Pills can be quite large. • Liquid (colloidal) form sometimes easier to tolerate.

*By weight.

Calcium Supplements. People who have a milk allergy, do not like milk, are ovo vegetarian, vegan, lactose intolerant, or who cannot incorporate enough calcium-containing foods into their diets can increase calcium intake through the use of calcium supplements (see Further Reading 11). Always look for a supplement with added vitamin D, as it enhances calcium uptake. This additional vitamin D routinely does not add to the cost of the supplement. Table 11-3 compares the two most common forms of calcium supplements. Calcium citrate is indicated for people who cannot remember to take calcium carbonate with meals, and for those who have low-acid stomach conditions, such as people who have ulcers, have gastric reflux, or have had surgery for obesity reduction. Calcium supplements do have side effects including gas, bloating, or constipation. Distributing small-dose supplements throughout the day, taking it with meals, or even changing the brand of supplement may alleviate some problems. Intake of calcium from supplements and/or food above 500 milligrams at any one time significantly reduces the percent absorbed. High intake of calcium at one time may also inhibit absorption of other minerals.

With calcium supplements, interactions with other minerals are a concern. There is evidence that calcium supplements may decrease zinc, iron, and other mineral absorption. An effect of calcium supplementation on iron absorption is possible; however, this appears to be small over the long term. To be safe, people using a calcium supplement on a regular basis should notify their physician of the practice. Calcium supplements can also interfere with the body's ability to absorb certain antibiotics. If your doctor prescribes antibiotics, especially tetracycline, be sure to talk with your pharmacist about timing of your supplement, medication, and meals.

In 1981, the FDA cautioned the public on calcium supplements from bone meal or dolomite due to their unhealthy level of contaminants. Concern was also expressed about oyster shell calcium supplements. Today, measures have been taken to clearly label such products as clear of contaminants. Tablet or liquid calcium supplements with the United States Pharmacopeia (USP) symbol are considered the safest. If you purchase calcium supplements from dolomite, bone meal, or oyster shell, look for those marked "purified."

Upper Level for Calcium The Upper Level (UL) for calcium intake is 2500 milligrams per day for young adults, based on the observation that greater intakes increase the risk for some forms of kidney stones. Excessive calcium intakes by some people can also cause high blood and urinary calcium concentrations, irritability, headache, kidney failure, soft tissue calcification, and decreased absorption of other minerals, as noted previously.

So which is better: calcium from food or supplements? Taking 1000 milligrams of calcium carbonate or calcium citrate daily in divided doses (about 500 milligrams per tablet) is probably safe in many instances. However, people often have difficulty adhering to a supplement regimen. Plus, the GI side effects may be a bit unpleasant. Modification of eating habits to include foods that are good sources of calcium is a better plan of action (see Further Reading 5 and Newsworthy Nutrition). In addition to this important mineral, foods that contain calcium also supply other vitamins, minerals, phytochemicals, and fats needed to support health. Problems associated with excessive consumption of calcium are not likely when foods are the primary sources of calcium.

CONCEPT CHECK

About 99% of calcium in the body is found in the bones and teeth. Aside from its critical role in bone, calcium also functions in blood clotting, muscle contraction, nerve-impulse transmission, and cell metabolism. Calcium requires the active vitamin D hormone for efficient absorption. Factors that reduce calcium absorption include a vitamin D deficiency; ingestion of large amounts of fiber, oxalate, or phytate; and old age. Blood calcium is regulated primarily by hormones and does not closely reflect daily intake.

Phosphorus (P)

Functions of Phosphorus. Phosphorus is the second most abundant mineral in the body. Approximately 85% of phosphorus is found as a component of hydroxyapatite crystals that provide the functional component of bone and teeth. The remaining 15% of phosphorus is in the soft tissues, blood, and extracellular fluid (see Chapter 9). Phosphorus is part of DNA and RNA, the genetic material present in every cell. Therefore, phosphorus is critical for cellular replication and growth because DNA and RNA are responsible for mitosis and protein synthesis. Phosphorus is also a primary component of adenosine triphosphate (ATP), the energy molecule that fuels body functions. Phosphorus is essential for the activation and deactivation of many enzymes. Many enzymes and the B vitamins are functional only when a phosphate group is attached.

A major class of lipids contains phosphorus (phospholipids). Phospholipids are the principal structural component of cell membranes, making up approximately 60% of membranes. These phospholipid membranes regulate the transport of nutrients and waste products into and out of cells. Phosphorus also functions to maintain blood pH and fluid balance because phosphates can accept and donate charged hydrogen atoms.

Phosphorus Sources and Needs. In contrast to calcium, phosphorus is naturally abundant in many foods. Milk, cheese, meat, and bread provide most of the phosphorus in the adult diet. Nuts, fish, breakfast cereals, bran, and eggs are also good sources (Fig. 11-13). About 20% to 30% of dietary phosphorus comes from food additives, especially in baked goods, cheeses, processed meats, and many soft drinks (about 75 milligrams per 12 ounces). As a food additive, phosphorus is considered a GRAS (generally recognized as safe) substance, and its function is to increase water binding and taste. Phosphoric acid, which gives a tangy, sour taste, will also significantly lower the pH of a food or beverage (pH of a soft drink is less than 3). Absorption of phosphorus is high, ranging from 55% to 80%, yet the phosphorus absorption from grains is reduced because of the high phytic acid content. Vitamin D enhances phosphorus absorption. Average daily adult consumption is about 1000 to 1600 milligrams. As a general rule, deficiencies of phosphorus are unlikely in healthy adults, especially because it is so efficiently absorbed.

Marginal phosphorus status can be found in preterm infants, vegans, people with alcoholism, older people on nutrient-poor diets, and people with long-term bouts of diarrhea. A 2004 review of older women undergoing osteoporosis treatment identified a small but significant group at high risk for phosphorus deficiency. These women, estimated to comprise 10% to 15% of all women ages 60 years and older, tend to live alone and eat a poor-quality diet, including below 70% of the RDA for phosphorus. To control their osteoporosis, these women are taking calcium supplements as well as antiresorptive medications to inhibit further bone loss. To maintain bone hydroxyapatite, both calcium and phosphorus must be available. High calcium carbonate or citrate supplements can bind the low food phosphorus in the intestine, thus inhibiting its absorption. These women are at high risk for phosphorus deficiency, as their intake is low and their absorption is inhibited. Attempts must be made to enhance dietary intake or calcium supplements should be switched to calcium phosphate, all under close medical supervision.

Upper Level for Phosphorus. The UL for phosphorus intake is 3 to 4 grams per day. Intakes greater than this can result in mineralization of soft tissues. Phosphorus levels in the blood are regulated primarily by the kidneys and these organs are particularly sensitive to phosphorus toxicity. High intakes can lead to serious problems in people with certain kidney diseases. In addition, chronic imbalance in the calcium-to-phosphorus ratio in the diet, resulting from a high phosphorus intake coupled with a low calcium intake, also can contribute to bone loss. This situation most likely arises when the RDA for calcium is not met, as can occur in adolescents and adults who regularly substitute soft drinks for milk or otherwise underconsume calcium.

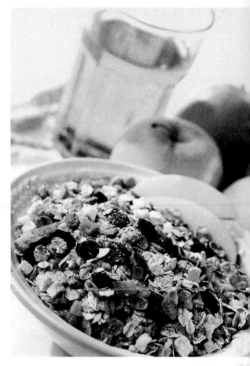

▲ Muesli (with milk), granola, and trail mix are rich in phosphorus.

FIGURE 11-13 ▶ Food sources of phosphorus compared to the RDA.

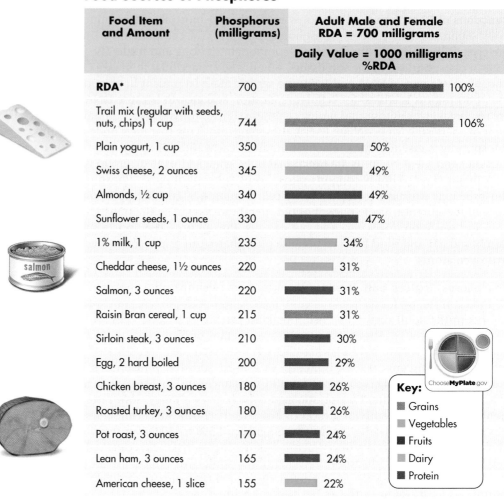

Food Sources of Phosphorus

Food Item and Amount	Phosphorus (milligrams)	Adult Male and Female RDA = 700 milligrams Daily Value = 1000 milligrams %RDA
RDA*	700	100%
Trail mix (regular with seeds, nuts, chips) 1 cup	744	106%
Plain yogurt, 1 cup	350	50%
Swiss cheese, 2 ounces	345	49%
Almonds, ½ cup	340	49%
Sunflower seeds, 1 ounce	330	47%
1% milk, 1 cup	235	34%
Cheddar cheese, 1½ ounces	220	31%
Salmon, 3 ounces	220	31%
Raisin Bran cereal, 1 cup	215	31%
Sirloin steak, 3 ounces	210	30%
Egg, 2 hard boiled	200	29%
Chicken breast, 3 ounces	180	26%
Roasted turkey, 3 ounces	180	26%
Pot roast, 3 ounces	170	24%
Lean ham, 3 ounces	165	24%
American cheese, 1 slice	155	22%

Key:
- Grains
- Vegetables
- Fruits
- Dairy
- Protein

ChooseMyPlate.gov

*For adults; see the DRI table in the back of this book for age-specific recommendations.

CONCEPT CHECK

Phosphorus absorption is efficient and is enhanced by the active vitamin D hormone. Urinary excretion mainly controls body content. Phosphorus aids enzyme function and is part of key metabolic compounds and cell membranes. No distinct deficiency symptoms caused by an inadequate phosphorus intake have been reported. Food sources for phosphorus include dairy products, baked goods, and meat. The RDA is met by most North Americans. An excess intake of phosphorus can compromise bone health, if sufficient calcium is not otherwise consumed, and can impair kidney function.

Vitamin D (Calciferol or Calcitriol)

Vitamin D is a unique nutrient in that it can be efficiently produced in the skin when the skin is exposed to ultraviolet light. Cholesterol is the building block or precursor of vitamin D found in the skin. Regardless of whether the body manufactures vitamin D or obtains it from food, chemical modifications of the vitamin D precursor must occur before the vitamin D becomes active. One chemical reaction occurs in the liver, followed by another in the kidney. The definition of a hormone is a compound manufactured by one organ of the body that then enters the bloodstream and has a physiological effect on another organ or tissue. The cells that participate in the synthesis of vitamin D are different from the cells that respond to vitamin D, namely bone and intestinal cells; therefore, vitamin D is considered a hormone. A precursor to vitamin D (7-dehydrocholesterol) is synthesized by cells in the skin. This precursor then travels via the blood to the liver and finally to the kidney where it is chemically converted into the most active form of vitamin D (calcitriol) (Fig. 11-14). This active form of vitamin D then enters the blood and has a physiological effect on cells throughout the body. Overall, sun exposure provides about 80% to 100% of vitamin D requirements.

The amount of sun exposure needed by individuals to produce vitamin D depends on skin color, age, time of day, season, and location. Exposure of hands, face, and arms for about 15 minutes daily will provide the required amount of ultraviolet light (UVB rays) to synthesize an adequate amount of the vitamin D precursor to meet weekly requirements for children and adults. However, seniors and persons with dark skin would need about three to five times this amount of sun exposure to synthesize an equivalent amount of vitamin D. The pigment that imparts color to skin, melanin, is a potent natural sunscreen.

The season of the year, geographic latitude, cloud cover, window glass, obesity, and intestinal and kidney diseases are but a few of the conditions that affect your ability to absorb UVB rays or to absorb dietary vitamin D and convert it to active vitamin D. Something as simple as complete cloud cover reduces UVB rays by 50%. Severe pollution reduces penetration by 60%. Table 11-4 summarizes the various factors that can inhibit vitamin D synthesis, absorption, and activation.

Sunlight is the best source of vitamin D. Unlike with supplements, you can never receive a toxic dose. However, unless you live in a year-round sunny climate and find yourself outside most days some time between 10 A.M. and 3 P.M., you are not maximizing your UVB exposure. We rely on the vitamin D we synthesize from our exposure on sunny days to support us during the days and months of limited exposure (Fig. 11-15).

Vitamin D synthesized in the warm summer months is stored in the liver and adipose cells; however, it is advised that people residing in northern climates should find alternative (dietary) sources in the winter months. Overall, anyone who does not receive enough direct exposure to sunshine to synthesize an adequate amount of vitamin D must have a dietary source of the vitamin. Many tanning machines produce ultraviolet light of the appropriate wavelength to cause vitamin D synthesis in the skin. Relying on tanning machines is not recommended by the Food and Drug Administration and American Academy of Dermatology because of the potential health hazards (burns, damage to eyes, and skin cancer) associated with this practice.

Functions of Vitamin D. The main function of vitamin D (calcitriol) is to maintain the normal range of calcium and phosphorus in the blood. In concert with the hormones parathyroid hormone (PTH) and calcitonin, vitamin D closely maintains blood calcium in a narrow range. This tight regulation of blood calcium level ensures that an appropriate amount of calcium is available to all cells. Vitamin D functions to regulate calcium by three methods: (1) regulates absorption of calcium and phosphorus from the small intestine; (2) in combination with PTH and calcitonin, it regulates calcium excretion via the kidney; and (3) through bone remodeling.

When blood levels of calcium begin to drop from the normal range, PTH stimulates the synthesis of the most active form of vitamin D (calcitriol) by the kidney. The calcitriol increases the production of proteins in the small intestine required for calcium absorption from the gut. The subsequent effect is to increase the amount of calcium absorbed from the intestinal tract. Vitamin D also functions in concert with PTH to (1) cause the kidneys to reduce calcium excretion in the urine and (2) release calcium from bone by stimulating osteoclast activity. When blood calcium levels reach the normal range, PTH release is inhibited and calcitonin is released, which has the opposite effects of PTH. One way to think about PTH and calcitonin is that they have opposing effects similar to insulin and glucagon in the regulation of blood glucose levels in the normal range.

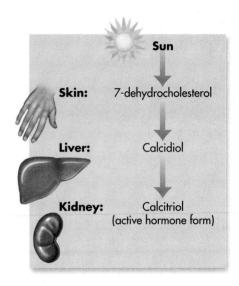

FIGURE 11-14 ▶ A precursor to vitamin D is synthesized when skin is exposed to sunlight. Previtamin D must be further modified by the liver and kidney for maximal activity.

TABLE 11-4 Factors That Impair Vitamin D Status

Factor	Description
Inadequate sun exposure • Northern latitudes • Excess clothing (e.g., robes/veils) • Air pollution (i.e., smog) • SPF >8 • Excessive time spent indoors (e.g., due to health, work, or environmental conditions)	Limited exposure to UVB reduces the skin's ability to synthesize vitamin D.
Age	Vitamin D synthesis by the skin decreases. Vitamin D activation by the kidneys decreases.
Dark skin pigmentation	Melanin reduces the skin's ability to produce vitamin D, particularly for older adults and especially among women.
Inadequate dietary intake	Dietary intake of vitamin D is unable to compensate for inadequate skin synthesis of vitamin D
Exclusive breastfeeding or low consumption of infant formula	Infants typically have limited sun exposure. Breast milk is a poor source of vitamin D. Infant formula contains vitamin D, but young infants may not consume adequate quantities to meet needs.
Fat malabsorption • Liver disease • Cystic fibrosis • Weight-loss medications	Poor absorption of dietary fat limits absorption of vitamin D from the small intestine.
Obesity	Release of vitamin D stored in subcutaneous fat is inefficient.
Liver diseases	Vitamin D activation by the liver decreases.
Kidney diseases	Vitamin D activation by the kidneys decreases.

FIGURE 11-15 ▶ Seasonal variations to sunlight intensity. If you live north of 42° N latitude, the angle of the winter sun is such that the sun's rays must pass through more of the atmosphere than at other times of the year. As a result, skin forms less pro-hormone vitamin D in the winter. The 42nd parallel crosses North America at the northern border of California on the West Coast and Boston on the East Coast. In the far North (e.g. Alaska), this effect can last up to 6 months. Living below the 34th parallel (i.e., south of Los Angeles to Columbia, South Carolina), UVB exposure is adequate year-round.

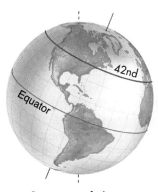

Summer solstice
(Northern Hemisphere tilts toward the sun)

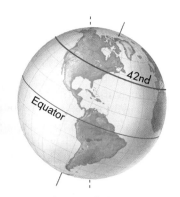

Winter solstice
(Northern Hemisphere tilts away from the sun)

It has been discovered that vitamin D has other critical functions in many cells throughout the body. Vitamin D binds to and subsequently affects cells of the immune system, brain and nervous system, pancreas, skin, muscles, and reproductive organs (see Further Reading 8). Of particular interest, vitamin D is capable of influencing normal development of some cells, such as skin, colon, prostate, and breast cells, in turn reducing cancer risk in these sites. Emerging data suggest that vitamin D has a protective role in colon cancer, but for prostate and breast cancer, the data are not as convincing. Vitamin D also controls the growth of the parathyroid gland, aids in the function of the immune system, and contributes to skin cell development. Studies have shown that vitamin D deficiency can be a problem in individuals with dark skin, the elderly, young infants without supplementation, insufficient exposure to sunlight, and with the use of nonfortified food (e.g., cereal and dairy products).

Without adequate levels of vitamin D in the blood, calcium absorption from the small intestine decreases. Subsequently, calcium and phosphorus deposition during bone synthesis is reduced, resulting in weak bones, especially in the legs where a characteristic bowed leg appearance is observed. Symptoms also include an enlarged head, joints, and rib cage and a deformed pelvis. A child with these symptoms has the disease **rickets** (Fig. 11-16). For the prevention of rickets, infants should be provided supplemental vitamin D (under a physician's guidance). Keep in mind, however, that supplements need to be used carefully to avoid vitamin D toxicity in the infant. Rickets in children is also associated with fat malabsorption, which can occur in children with cystic fibrosis.

Osteomalacia, which means soft bone, is an adult disease comparable to rickets. It results from inadequate calcium intake, inefficient calcium absorption in the intestine, or poor conservation of calcium by the kidneys. This condition leads to a decrease in bone mineral density and subsequently, bones become porous and weak and break easily. One study showed that treatment with 10 to 20 micrograms (400 to 800 IU) per day of vitamin D, in conjunction with adequate dietary calcium, greatly decreased fracture risk in older people in nursing homes. Follow-up studies support this role of vitamin D in reducing hip fracture risk. Meeting the RDA for vitamin D is no less important than calcium adequacy for bone health. An analysis of many human studies concluded that vitamin D decreases the incidence of vertebral fractures and may decrease nonvertebral fractures, as well. Vitamin D supplementation was also found to reduce the risk of fracture from falls among institutionalized elderly by more than 20%. Aging decreases production of vitamin D in the skin by about 70% by age 70.

Osteomalacia in adults occurs most commonly in people with kidney, stomach, gallbladder, or intestinal disease (especially when most of the intestine has been removed) and in people with cirrhosis of the liver. These diseases affect both vitamin D activation and calcium absorption. Adults with limited sun exposure and/or dark skin are more prone to develop this disease. The combination of sun exposure and adequate dietary intake can prevent this problem.

Vitamin D Sources and Needs. Dietary sources of vitamin D are limited. Rich sources are fatty fish (e.g., salmon and sardines), fortified dairy products, and many breakfast cereals (Fig. 11-17). In the United States and Canada, milk is usually fortified with 10 micrograms (400 IU) per quart. Consumption of at least 2 cups of vitamin-D-fortified milk a day is advisable for people at risk for vitamin D deficiency. Although eggs, butter, liver, and a few brands of margarine contain some vitamin D, large servings must be eaten to obtain an appreciable amount of the vitamin; therefore, these foods are not considered significant sources. Without adequate exposure to direct sunlight, consumption of fortified foods, or supplementation, a vegan diet cannot meet vitamin D requirements. It is advisable for vegans to consume vitamin-D-fortified soy milk. Meeting the vitamin D RDA may also be difficult for people with milk allergies or lactose intolerance.

The Food and Nutrition Board established the first RDA for vitamin D in 2010. The RDA for healthy people ages 1 to 70 is 15 micrograms (600 IU) per day, based on a

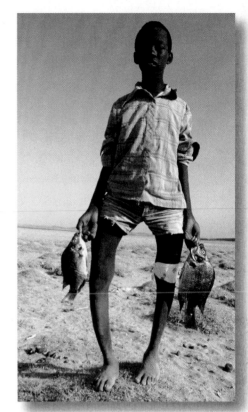

FIGURE 11-16 ▶ Vitamin D deficiency causes rickets, in which the bones and teeth do not develop normally.

rickets The vitamin A deficiency disease observed in infants and children. Mineral content of the bones is markedly reduced.

osteomalacia Adult form of rickets. The bones have low mineral density and subsequently are at risk for fracture.

The 2010 Dietary Guidelines for Americans recommend that all children over age 9 and adults should choose more foods that provide vitamin D, which is a nutrient of concern in American diets (see Further Reading 1).

Food Sources of Vitamin D

Food Item and Amount	Vitamin D (micrograms) Daily Value = 10 micrograms	Vitamin D (IU)	Adult Male and Female RDA = 15 micrograms %RDA
RDA	15	600	100%
Baked herring, 3 ounces	44.4	1775	296%
Smoked eel, 1 ounce	25.5	1020	170%
Baked salmon, 3 ounces	6.0	238	40%
Sardines, 1 ounce	3.4	136	23%
Canned tuna, 3 ounces	3.4	136	23%
1% milk, 1 cup	2.5	99	17%
Nonfat milk, 1 cup	2.5	98	17%
Soft margarine, 1 teaspoon	1.5	60	10%
Italian pork sausage, 3 ounces	1.1	44	7%
Soy milk, 1 cup	1.0	40	7%
Raisin Bran cereal, 3/4 cup	1.0	38	7%
Baked bluefish, 3 ounces	0.9	34	6%
Special K cereal, 3/4 cup	0.8	30	5%
Cooked egg yolk, 1	0.6	25	4%

Key:
- Grains
- Vegetables
- Fruits
- Dairy
- Protein
- Oils

ChooseMyPlate.gov

FIGURE 11-17 ▶ Food sources of vitamin D compared to the Recommended Dietary Allowance up to age 70 for adults.

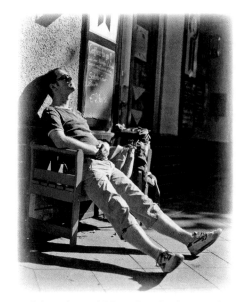

▲ Solar radiation (UVB rays) on the skin provides about 80% to 100% of the vitamin D humans use. This is also the most reliable way to maintain vitamin D status. In the absence of adequate sun exposure, the body must rely on dietary sources of vitamin D to meet needs.

daily intake that is sufficient to maintain bone health and normal calcium metabolism. This recommendation assumes minimal sun exposure. The RDA increases to 20 micrograms per day for those over age 70, because of the reduced ability to absorb vitamin D from the intestine and decreased ability to synthesize it in the skin. The DV used on food and supplement labels is still 10 micrograms (400 IU). As mentioned, young, light-skinned people can synthesize all the vitamin D needed from casual sun exposure. A number of experts suggest older adults, especially those over age 70 who have limited sun exposure or dark skin, receive about 25 micrograms (1000 IU) from a combination of vitamin-D-fortified foods and a multivitamin and mineral supplement, with an individual supplement of vitamin D added if needed (see Further Reading 11).

The American Academy of Pediatrics recommends that all infants, children, and adolescents should consume a minimum of 400 IU of vitamin D daily. Until such intake can be obtained from foods, vitamin D supplementation is endorsed. This recommendation includes all infants (exclusively breastfed, partially breastfed, or formula-fed). As you will learn in Chapter 18, breast milk is a poor source of vitamin D and exclusively breastfed infants with limited sun exposure are at risk for developing rickets. Even though infant formula contains vitamin D (60 IU per 100 kcal), the total intake of formula among young infants may not provide adequate vitamin D to meet needs. Evidence from clinical trials and historical precedence support this dosage of vitamin D for infants and children (see Further Reading 17).

Upper Level for Vitamin D. The UL for vitamin D is 100 micrograms (4000 IU) per day. Too much vitamin D taken regularly can create serious health consequences in infants and children. Due to the role of vitamin D in calcium absorption, excretion, and release of calcium from bone, supplementation with high doses of vitamin D can cause calcium levels in the blood to increase above the normal range. The UL is based on the risk of overabsorption of calcium and eventual calcium deposits in the kidneys and other organs. Toxicity symptoms also include weakness, loss of appetite, diarrhea, vomiting, mental confusion, and increased urine output. Calcium deposits in organs can cause metabolic disturbances and cell death. Vitamin D toxicity does not result from excessive exposure to the sun because the body regulates the amount made in the skin (i.e., as exposure to sunlight increases, vitamin D synthesis decreases).

CONCEPT CHECK

Vitamin D is a true vitamin only for people who fail to produce enough from sunlight, such as some older adults or institutionalized people. Humans synthesize vitamin D from a cholesterol-like substance by the action of sunlight on their skin. The vitamin D is later acted on by the liver and kidneys to form the hormone calcitriol. This hormone increases calcium absorption in the intestines and works with another hormone, PTH, to maintain blood calcium levels within a narrow range. Statistics indicating that 36% of Americans are vitamin D difi-cient led to a recent increase in vitamin D recommendations. Rich food sources of vitamin D are fish oils and fortified milk. Megadose vitamin D intake can be toxic, especially in infancy and early childhood.

Magnesium (Mg)

Magnesium is important for nerve and heart function and aids in many enzyme reactions. Magnesium is similar to calcium and phosphorus in that most of the magnesium in the body is found in bones. Bone contains 60% of the body's magnesium. Magnesium serves a structural role in bones to help provide rigidity, and it also functions as a storage site drawn upon by other tissues when dietary intake is inadequate to meet the body's needs. Magnesium deficiency in animals has been shown to result in decreased bone strength and volume, poor bone development, reduced bone formation, and increased bone resorption. Conversely, magnesium supplementation may improve bone density. Magnesium functions to relax muscles after contraction. It promotes resistance to tooth decay by stabilizing calcium in tooth enamel. Over 300 enzymes use magnesium, and many energy-yielding compounds in cells require magnesium to function properly (e.g., ATP). Magnesium plays a critical role in the synthesis of DNA and protein. Another notable function of magnesium as it relates to bone health is that magnesium is required for the synthesis of vitamin D in the liver.

In humans, a magnesium deficiency causes an irregular heartbeat, sometimes accompanied by weakness, muscle pain, disorientation, and seizures. Other possible benefits of magnesium in relation to cardiovascular disease include decreasing blood pressure by dilating arteries and preventing heart abnormalities. People with cardiovascular disease should closely monitor magnesium intake, especially because they are often on medications such as diuretics that reduce magnesium status. A diet rich in food sources of magnesium and calcium is associated with lower risk of type 2 diabetes in some populations (see Further Reading 16). Keep in mind that a magnesium deficiency develops slowly because our bodies store it readily.

Magnesium Sources and Needs. Magnesium is found in the plant pigment chlorophyll, so rich sources for magnesium are plant products, such as squash, whole grains (like wheat bran), beans, nuts, seeds, and broccoli (Fig. 11-18). Animal products, such as milk and meats, and chocolate supply some magnesium, although less than the foods in the magnesium MyPlate (Fig. 11-19). Two other sources of magnesium are hard tap water, which contains a high mineral content, and coffee (espresso, not brewed).

Food Sources of Magnesium

Food Item and Amount	Magnesium (milligrams)	Adult Male RDA = 400 milligrams		Adult Female RDA = 310 milligrams	
		Daily Value = 400 milligrams			
		%RDA		%RDA	
RDA	310-400		100%		100%
Spinach, 1 cup	157		39%		51%
Squash, 1 cup	105		26%		34%
Wheat germ, ¼ cup	90		23%		29%
Raisin Bran cereal, 1 cup	90		23%		29%
Navy beans, ½ cup	54		14%		17%
Peanut butter, 2 tablespoons	51		13%		16%
Black-eyed peas, ½ cup	46		12%		15%
Plain yogurt, 1 cup	43		11%		14%
Kidney beans, ½ cup	43		11%		14%
Sunflower seeds, ¼ cup	41		10%		13%
Broccoli, 1 cup	37		9%		12%
Banana, 1 medium	34		9%		11%
1% milk, 1 cup	34		9%		11%
Watermelon, 1 slice	32		8%		10%
Oatmeal, ½ cup	28		7%		9%
Whole-wheat bread, 1 slice	25		6%		8%

Key:
- Grains
- Vegetables
- Fruits
- Dairy
- Protein

FIGURE 11-18 ▶ Food sources of magnesium compared to the RDA for adult males and females.

FIGURE 11-19 ▶ Sources of magnesium from MyPlate. The fill of the background color (none, 1/3, 2/3, or completely covered) within each group on the plate indicates the average nutrient density for magnesium in that group. Overall, the vegetables group provides the richest sources. Whole-grain choices in the grains group are also rich sources. With regard to physical activity, magnesium is especially needed for the carbohydrate metabolism that takes place in such endeavors.

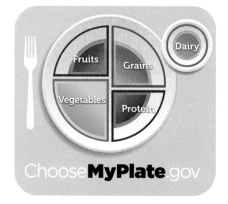

ChooseMyPlate.gov

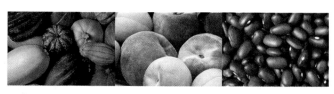

MyPlate: Sources of Magnesium

Grains
- Wheat bran
- Wheat germ
- Whole-grain products

Vegetables
- Avocados
- Spinach
- Greens
- Broccoli
- Lima beans
- Potatoes
- Squash

Fruits
- Figs
- Peaches
- Bananas
- Berries

Dairy
- Milk
- Yogurt

Protein
- Tofu
- Nuts
- Shrimp
- Kidney beans
- Sunflower seeds

The adult RDA for magnesium is about 400 milligrams per day for men and about 310 milligrams per day for women. This value is based on the amount needed to offset daily losses. The DV used on food and supplement labels is 400 milligrams. Adult men consume on average 320 milligrams daily, whereas women consume closer to 220 milligrams daily, suggesting that many of us should improve our intakes of magnesium-rich foods, such as whole-grain breads and cereals. The refined grain products that dominate the diets of many North Americans are poor sources of this mineral as refining reduces the magnesium content by as much as 80%. This low value also reflects poor intake of green and other brightly colored vegetables. If dietary intake of magnesium is inadequate, a balanced multivitamin and mineral supplement containing approximately 100 milligrams of magnesium can help close the gap between intake and needs.

Nutrient-nutrient interactions can reduce magnesium absorption. Diets very high in phosphorus or fiber (phytate) limit intestinal absorption, as do diets too low in protein. Poor magnesium status is especially found among users of certain diuretics. In addition, heavy perspiration for weeks in hot climates and bouts of long-standing diarrhea or vomiting cause significant magnesium loss. Alcoholism increases the risk of a deficiency because dietary intake may be poor and because alcohol increases magnesium excretion in the urine. The disorientation and weakness associated with alcoholism closely resembles the behavior of people with low blood magnesium.

Upper Level for Magnesium. The UL for magnesium intake is 350 milligrams per day, based on the risk of developing diarrhea. This guideline refers only to nonfood sources such as antacids, laxatives, or supplements (see Further Reading 11). Food sources are not known to cause toxicity. Magnesium toxicity especially occurs in people who have kidney failure or who overuse over-the-counter medications that contain magnesium, such as certain antacids and laxatives (e.g., milk of magnesia). Older people are at particular risk, as kidney function may be compromised.

CONCEPT CHECK

Magnesium is required for nerve and heart function; it also aids activity for many enzymes. Food sources of magnesium are whole grains (wheat bran), vegetables, beef, coffee, beans, nuts, and seeds. People taking certain diuretics and people with alcoholism are at greatest risk of developing a deficiency. Magnesium toxicity is most likely in people with kidney failure or people using certain forms of laxatives and antacids.

Fluoride (F)

The fluoride ion (F^-) is the form of this trace mineral essential for human health. Nearly all (about 95%) of the fluoride in the body is found in the teeth and skeleton. Dentists in the early 1900s noticed a lower rate of dental caries (cavities) in the southwestern United States. These areas contained high amounts of fluoride in the water. The amounts of fluoride were sometimes so high that small spots developed on the teeth (mottling). Even though mottled teeth were discolored, they contained few dental caries. Experiments in the early 1940s showed that fluoride in the water decreased the incidence of dental caries by 20% to 80% in children. Fluoridation of public water supplies in many parts of the United States has since been instituted (see Further Reading 14).

Dentists can provide topical fluoride treatments and schools can provide fluoride tablets, but the most economical distribution method is to add fluoride to a community's drinking water. Numerous products are available to topically apply fluoride to teeth. These include gels applied at a dentist's office, toothpaste, and mouth rinses. These products are essential in

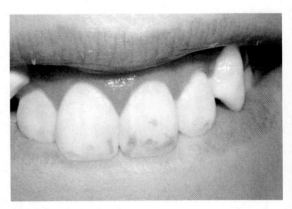

▲ Example of mottling (brown spots) in a tooth caused by overexposure to fluoride.

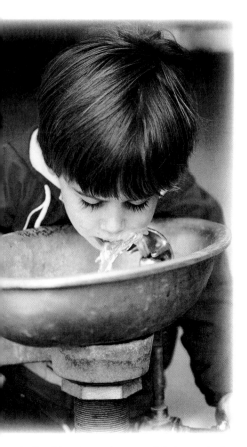

▲ Fluoridated water is responsible for much of the decrease in dental caries throughout North America.

fluorosis Discoloration of tooth enamel sometimes accompanied with pitting due to consuming a large amount of fluoride for an excessive period.

combating dental decay in children who live in homes that use well water rather than the public water supply. When water fluoridation and fluoridated topical products are used in combination, the reductions in dental caries are additive.

Functions of Fluoride. Fluoride functions in the following ways to prevent dental caries: (1) fluoride incorporated into the tooth structure, causing it to be stronger and more resistant to acid degradation from bacteria found in plaque; (2) stimulation of remineralization of enamel and inhibition of tooth demineralization; and (3) antibacterial effect on acid-producing microorganisms found in plaque.

Fluoride has been shown to increase protein synthesis in the osteoblast and subsequently have an effect on the production of new bone. The combination of calcium and fluoride supplementation has been investigated regarding increasing bone mass; however, to date, the studies have been inconclusive.

Fluoride Sources and Needs. Marine fish, clams, lobster, crab, shrimp, tea, seaweed, and some natural water sources are the only good food sources of fluoride. Most fluoride intake comes from fluoride added to drinking water and topical treatments. Fluoride is generally not added to bottled water. Frequent use of bottled water or a household reverse osmosis water purification system significantly restricts fluoride intake. A refrigerator or Brita filter does not remove fluoride.

The AI for fluoride for adults is 3.1 to 3.8 milligrams per day. This range of intake provides the benefits of resistance to dental caries without causing ill effects. Typical fluoridated water contains about 1 milligram per liter, which works out to about 0.25 milligrams per cup.

Upper Level for Fluoride. The UL for fluoride is set at 1.3 to 2.2 milligrams per day for young children and 10 milligrams per day for children over 9 years of age and adults, based on skeletal and tooth damage seen with higher doses. Children may swallow large amounts of fluoride toothpaste as part of daily tooth care and develop **fluorosis.** During tooth development (first decade of life), fluorosis permanently damages teeth. Fluorosis leads to stained and pitted teeth. Not swallowing toothpaste and limiting the amount used to "pea" size are the best ways to prevent this problem. In addition, children under 6 years should have tooth brushing supervised by an adult and should never use fluoride mouthwash. In adults, fluorosis is associated with hip fractures, weak/stiff joints, and chronic stomach inflammation. There have been opponents to the fluoridation of public water supplies. These individuals claim that high fluoride intake can lead to a host of medical problems, including cancer, bone disease, and Alzheimer's disease. These claims have been thoroughly investigated by independent researchers and government health organizations, and none of the claims can be substantiated (see Further Reading 2).

CONCEPT CHECK

Fluoride becomes incorporated into teeth during development and is present in salivary secretions. The presence of this trace mineral makes teeth resistant to acid and bacterial growth, in turn reducing development of dental caries. Fluoride also aids in the remineralization of teeth once decay begins. Most of us receive adequate amounts of fluoride from that added to drinking water and toothpaste. An excessive fluoride intake during tooth development can lead to spotted (i.e., mottled) teeth and possibly bone damage.

11.7 Other Nutrients Involved in Bone Health

In addition to those we have already discussed, there are several other vitamins and minerals that contribute to bone health (Table 11-5). For some, including vitamin K and boron, research clearly links dietary intake or blood nutrient levels to bone

TABLE 11-5 Micronutrients That Function in Bone Health

Nutrient	Primary Function in Bone	Common Food Sources
Calcium	Provides rigidity to bone; 99% of calcium in the human body is found in bones and teeth	Milk, yogurt, fortified orange juice, sardines, canned salmon, fortified cereals
Phosphorus	Critical component of hydroxyapatite crystals in bone	Yogurt, almonds, milk, cheese, salmon, meats, eggs
Vitamin D	Regulates calcium and phosphorus levels for bone integrity and maintenance	Fish, milk, fortified cereals; best source is sunlight
Magnesium	Promotes resistance to tooth decay by holding calcium in tooth enamel; stored in bone like calcium; works like calcium in blood-clot formation; necessary for hundreds of enzymatic reactions within the body	Dark-green leafy vegetables, peanut butter, beans and peas, bananas, almonds
Fluoride	Strengthens bones and teeth; stimulates osteoblasts	Seafood, seaweed, tea; community water supplies have added fluoride; may not be present in bottled drinking water
Vitamin C	Participates in collagen synthesis; may protect bone from oxidative damage	Citrus fruits, strawberries, broccoli, leafy green vegetables
Vitamin K	Imparts calcium-binding ability to the bone protein osteocalcin	Green vegetables, liver, some plant oils, some calcium supplements
Zinc	Cofactor for enzymes in bone remodeling; contributes to collagen synthesis	Seafood, meats, green vegetables, whole grains
Copper	Contributes to collagen synthesis	Liver, cocoa, beans, nuts, whole grains, dried fruits
Iron	Cofactor in vitamin D activation; contributes to collagen synthesis	Meats, seafood, broccoli, peas, bran, enriched bread
Manganese	Cofactor for bone-remodeling enzymes	Nuts, oats, beans, tea
Potassium	Maintains alkaline blood pH which prevents withdrawal of bone minerals for use as buffers	Spinach, squash, bananas, orange juice, milk, meat, legumes, whole grains
Boron	Influences osteoblast and osteoclast activity; participates in calcium transport; involved in synthesis of vitamin D	Fruits, vegetables, nuts, whole grains
Silicon	Contributes to collagen synthesis	Beer, bananas, string beans

health outcomes. Others are still topics of current investigation (see Further Readings 12 and 15).

Micronutrients that participate in the synthesis of collagen are important to support bone health. Vitamin C, iron, zinc, copper, and silicon are important in this regard. Iron is also required by an enzyme that converts vitamin D to its active form in the body. Manganese and zinc are examples of minerals that are required as cofactors for enzymes of bone remodeling. Iron, zinc, copper, and manganese will be explored further in Chapter 12.

Aside from its role in collagen synthesis, vitamin C has been proposed to promote bone health through its antioxidant activity. High levels of oxidative stress contribute to bone resorption. Therefore, nutrients such as vitamin C and the carotenoids may preserve bone mineral density by limiting oxidative stress. Observational and experimental data regarding the antioxidant roles of vitamin C and carotenoids in bone health have mixed results and may depend on other factors, such as gender, smoking, and intake of other bone-building nutrients. Vitamin C and the carotenoids were discussed in relation to their antioxidant roles in Chapter 10.

Vitamin K activates proteins that are present in bone, muscle, and kidneys, thereby imparting calcium-binding potential to these organs. Vitamin K chemically modifies the protein osteocalcin, which is required for calcium to be added to and removed from bone. In one large study, men and women with the highest vitamin K intakes had 65% lower risk of hip fractures compared to those with the lowest vitamin K intakes. Another study showed a relationship between high blood levels of vitamin K and reduced risk of vertebral fracture. Vitamin K will be discussed in more depth regarding its role in blood health in Chapter 12.

Protein metabolism can lower the pH of body fluids, which then requires some minerals to be released from bone to act as buffers. Nutrients that maintain an alkaline environment may therefore preserve bone mineral density by reducing the need for buffers. Potassium and magnesium may contribute to bone health by maintaining an alkaline environment in the blood (see Further Reading 6). Potassium was covered in detail in Chapter 9.

Two ultratrace minerals—boron and silicon—have been implicated in bone health. Recall that ultratrace minerals have no known dietary requirements, but they are present in the body in small amounts and participate in some body functions.

Boron contributes to bone structure and strength due to its influences on osteoblast and osteoclast activity, transport of calcium across membranes, and vitamin D synthesis. Elderly women fed a low-boron diet had low blood levels of calcium and magnesium. Some studies indicate boron also participates in brain and immune functions, and other studies have examined a relationship between boron intake and cancer risk. There is no AI or RDA set, but an estimated daily requirement is 1 milligram per day. The UL for boron is 20 milligrams per day (see Further Reading 10).

Silicon, as already noted, participates in collagen synthesis. No UL for silicon has been established. Toxicity of silicon has been observed in people taking large amounts of silicon-containing antacids over a long time period. The consequences are an increased incidence of kidney stones and decreased levels of some antioxidant enzymes. A serious respiratory condition called silicosis occurs with the inhalation of silicon dust.

As you can see, dietary recommendations for bone health should extend beyond dairy products. Indeed, a diet rich in fruits and vegetables contains ample potassium, magnesium, vitamin C, vitamin K, and several key trace minerals. Overall, following a dietary pattern that matches MyPlate will promote optimal bone health.

Case Study Worried About Grandma

Grace, a 23-year-old woman of Korean descent, is in her final year of nursing school in Boston. She also works 20 hours per week at a local pharmacy. Grace is worried about a phone call she just received from her mom. While out on her walk yesterday, Grandmother Kyon caught her toe on an uneven section of the sidewalk, fell, and broke her hip. The doctor diagnosed Grandmother Kyon with osteoporosis, and the family is worried about the long recovery ahead. As a nursing student, Grace knows how devastating a hip fracture can be. She also knows that osteoporosis can run in families. Grace resolves to do whatever she can to learn about osteoporosis and strengthen her bones now.

She starts by searching the Internet for a website that can help her determine if she is at high risk for osteoporosis. The New York State Department of Health Osteoporosis Education Prevention Program, www.health.state. ny.us/diseases/conditions/osteoporosis/ index.htm, offers a risk assessment for premenopausal women like her, plus one for her dad and another for her mom, who is postmenopausal. For herself, Grace sees a few risk factors that she cannot change, but there are a few that are glaringly obvious. She uses this website to "bone up" on ways to promote her bone health while she is still young.

Grace discovers she is probably pretty low in vitamin D intake. She also does not have much free time for exercise. She cooks traditional Korean dishes for half of her meals, but eats fast food or sandwiches for the rest. Daily, she takes a multivitamin/mineral pill plus one calcium carbonate pill. She generally takes them when she brushes her teeth at night before bed. On weekends, she does get out with friends or her boyfriend and has a glass or two of wine. Grace does not smoke.

Answer the following questions about Grace's situation and check your responses in Appendix A.

1. Go to the URL that Grace visited and click on the link for Osteoporosis Risk Assessment for Premenopausal Women. What risk factors do you see for Grace? Which ones do you feel are critical to know? For which do you not have adequate information?
2. Grace went to the section "Promoting Healthy Bones" to determine key actions she can take to strengthen her bones now. Which ones does she already do? Which lifestyle actions could Grace integrate into her daily life right now?
3. What are the environmental conditions that inhibit Grace from adequately synthesizing vitamin D? How can she overcome some of them?
4. What are some calcium and vitamin D sources in traditional Korean dishes?
5. Give Grace some tips to increase her calcium and vitamin D intake at fast-food restaurants without significantly increasing costs or calories.
6. Would you recommend any changes to her supplement regimen?

Summary (Numbers refer to numbered sections in the chapter.)

11.1 The outermost layer of bone is the periosteum, a specialized type of connective tissue that covers most bone surfaces. Cortical and trabecular bone work together to provide strength, stability, and flexibility. Cortical bone is dense and compact, providing strength and stability in the shafts of long bones. Trabecular bone is spongy and open, allowing for some flexibility and shock absorption. Bone marrow is the spongy tissue inside bones that contains stem cells, which can become blood, fat, cartilage, or bone cells. Teeth are bones covered with a protective layer of enamel.

11.2 Bone remodeling is the continuous process of bone degradation and resynthesis of bone. Osteoclasts break down bone tissue by a process called resorption, which releases bone minerals into the blood. Osteoblasts synthesize new bone tissue from collagen and hydroxyapatite. Bone synthesis exceeds bone resorption until about age 30, after which bone mineral density is gradually lost throughout the rest of life.

11.3 Biological (i.e., nonmodifiable) factors that influence bone health include sex, age, ethnicity, and frame size. Lifestyle (i.e., modifiable) factors associated with bone status include several dietary components, body weight, normal menses, weight-bearing physical activity, smoking, certain medications, and exposure to UVB sunlight.

11.4 Osteoporosis is diagnosed when the T-score (a comparison of individual bone mineral density to age- and gender-specific averages) is −2.5 or lower or by the presence of a stress-induced fracture. Osteopenia is low bone mineral density that does not meet the diagnostic criteria of osteoporosis. Aside from bone fractures, osteoporosis causes kyphosis, pain, loss of mobility and independence, decreased lung capacity, fear of falling, and mortality. Women suffer greater loss of bone mineral density because they typically achieve lower peak bone mass during young adulthood and they lose more trabecular bone due to the hormonal effects of menopause. Type 1 osteoporosis is loss of trabecular bone that follows menopause. Type 2 osteoporosis is loss of cortical and trabecular bone that occurs in both men and women over age 60. Lifestyle factors (e.g., adequate dietary calcium, phosphorous, and vitamin D; exposure to UVB sunlight; and weight-bearing physical activity) are encouraged for prevention of osteoporosis. When lifestyle factors are not enough, medications (e.g., antiresorptive drugs and hormone therapies) may be used to prevent bone loss, but they are not without side effects.

11.5 The gold standard of bone health assessment is central dual energy X-ray absorptiometry (DEXA). Other methods of bone health assessment include peripheral DEXA, peripheral quantitative computed tomography, and quantitative ultrasound.

11.6 Calcium forms a part of bone structure and plays a role in blood clotting, muscle contractions, nerve transmission, and cell metabolism. Calcium absorption is enhanced by stomach acid and the active vitamin D hormone. Dairy products are important calcium sources. Women are particularly at risk for not meeting calcium needs.

Phosphorus aids enzyme function and forms part of key metabolic compounds, cell membranes, and bone. It is efficiently absorbed, and deficiencies are rare, although there is some concern about possible poor intake by some older women. Good sources are dairy products, bakery products, and meats.

Vitamin D is both a hormone and a vitamin. Human skin synthesizes it using sunshine and a cholesterol-like substance. If we do not spend enough time in the sun, such foods as fish and fortified milk can supply the vitamin. The active hormone form of vitamin D helps regulate blood calcium in part by increasing calcium absorption from the intestine. Infants and children who do not get enough vitamin D may develop rickets, and adults with

inadequate amounts in the body develop osteomalacia. Older people and infants often need a supplemental source. Toxicity may lead to calcification of soft tissue, weakness, and gastrointestinal disturbances.

Magnesium contributes to bone mineralization and vitamin D synthesis. It is also important for nerve and heart function and as an activator for many enzymes. Whole-grain breads and cereals (bran portion), vegetables, nuts, seeds, milk, and meats are good food sources.

Fluoride as part of regular intake of food sources and fluoridated water, as well as dental applications, makes teeth resistant to dental caries.

11.7 Trace minerals that participate in maintenance of bone health include boron, which affects calcium transport and vitamin D synthesis, and silicon, which influences connective tissue. In addition, vitamin C and protein are also required for proper synthesis of connective tissue in bone.

Check Your Knowledge (Answers to the following multiple choice questions are on the next page.)

1. Vitamin D is called the sunshine vitamin because
   a. it is available in orange juice.
   b. exposure to sunlight converts a precursor to vitamin D.
   c. it can be destroyed by exposure to sunlight.
   d. All of the above.

2. The most accurate measurement of bone mineral density is
   a. central DEXA.
   b. peripheral DEXA.
   c. peripheral QCT.
   d. QUS.

3. Which of the following is a lifestyle factor that increases bone mineral density?
   a. smoking
   b. physical activity

   c. large frame size
   d. use of SPF 50 sunscreen

4. At the end of long bones, inside the spinal vertebrae, and inside the flat bones of the pelvis, is a spongy type of bone known as _____ bone.
   a. osteoclastic
   b. osteoblastic
   c. trabecular
   d. compact

5. Individuals in which of the following groups are most likely to develop osteoporosis?
   a. premenopausal women athletes
   b. women taking estrogen replacement therapy
   c. slender, inactive women who smoke
   d. women who eat a lot of high-fat dairy products

6. Vitamin D enhances absorption of
   a. calcium.
   b. phosphorus.
   c. both calcium and phosphorus.
   d. neither calcium nor phosphorus.

7. Fatty fish is a source of
   a. calcium.
   b. vitamin D.
   c. vitamin K.
   d. magnesium.

8. All of the following sources of drinking water are poor sources of fluoride, except
   a. commercial bottled water.
   b. city household reverse osmosis water purification system.
   c. city household refrigerator water filter system.
   d. well water from most regions in the United States.

9. Synthesis of the collagen matrix of bone requires all of the following, except
   a. silicon.
   b. boron.
   c. vitamin C.
   d. protein.

10. Which of the following hormones acts to increase calcium loss?
    a. parathyroid hormone
    b. calcitriol
    c. estrogen
    d. calcitonin

Answer Key: 1. b (LO 11.6), 2. a (LO 11.5),
3. b (LO 11.3), 4. c (LO 11.1),
5. c (LO 11.7), 6. c (LO 11.4),
7. b (LO 11.6), 8. c (LO 11.6),
9. b (LO 11.4), 10. d (LO 11.2)

Study Questions (Numbers refer to Learning Outcomes)

1. What are the differences between cortical and trabecular bone? **(LO11.1)**

2. What are osteoclasts and osteoblasts? Describe the process of bone remodeling. **(LO11.2)**

3. Describe the functions of two hormones that affect bone metabolism. **(LO11.3)**

4. What is peak bone mass? At what age is peak bone mass achieved? List three lifestyle factors that affect peak bone mass. **(LO11.3)**

5. Other than its role in bone structure, what are three functions of phosphorus? List three food sources of this mineral. **(LO11.4)**

6. List three roles of magnesium in the body. Identify two chronic diseases that may be affected by magnesium status. **(LO11.4)**

7. Describe the functions of fluoride in the body. List three sources of fluoride. **(LO11.4)**

8. Describe two methods that can be used to assess bone density. What demographic groups should have bone density measured? **(LO11.5)**

9. List three sources of dietary calcium. Identify two factors that negatively influence the absorption of calcium. Identify two factors that positively influence the absorption of calcium. **(LO11.6)**

10. List and describe two vitamin-D-deficiency diseases. Which groups of people likely need to supplement their diets with vitamin D, and on what do you base your answer? **(LO11.7)**

What Would You Choose Recommendations

Vitamin D is important for regulation of calcium balance in the body—it increases absorption of calcium from the small intestine and helps to regulate the deposition of calcium into bones. For this reason, milk is fortified with vitamin D. For young adults, the RDA for vitamin D is now 15 micrograms per day.

Many people associate vitamin D with whole milk—and whole milk *is* a rich source of this nutrient. However, if you compare the Nutrient Facts panels from the various types of milk (Fig. 11-20), you will see that all commercial brands of milk contain about 250 mg of calcium and are fortified with 2.5 micrograms of vitamin D

(25% Daily Value). Note that the Daily Value for vitamin D listed on food labels is still 10 micrograms (400 IU).

Is calcium-fortified orange juice a good source of vitamin D? Because vitamin D is so integral to calcium absorption, many calcium-fortified fruit juices, such as orange juice, also contain vitamin D (Fig. 11-20). The level of fortification of orange juice with calcium and vitamin D varies by brand, but the calcium and vitamin D contents per serving are typically similar to those of milk.

Now that you have completed Chapter 11, you know that vitamin D is fat soluble. Does this mean you need the fat in whole

milk to absorb the vitamin D? Researchers at Boston University compared the bioavailability of vitamin D from whole milk and skim milk and found no differences. Vitamin D bioavailability from calcium and vitamin-D-fortified orange juice was also high. In addition, in the context of a meal, there are bound to be other sources of fat (egg yolk, vegetable oil) to aid fat-soluble vitamin absorption.

To sum up, milks with various fat contents and orange juice fortified with calcium and vitamin D are all rich sources of vitamin D and can help protect against bone loss. For the highest nutrient density, choose skim milk or fortified orange juice.

Skim Milk

Nutrition Facts
Serving Size 1 cup (240ml)

Amount Per Serving

Calories 90	Calories from Fat 0

	% Daily value*
Total Fat 0g	**0%**
Saturated Fat 0g	**0%**
Trans Fat 0g	**0%**
Cholesterol <5mg	**1%**
Sodium 125mg	**5%**
Potassium 410mg	**12%**
Total Carbohydrate 13g	**4%**
Dietary Fiber 0g	
Sugars 13g	
Protein 8g	**17%**

• Vitamin A 10%	• Vitamin C 4%

• Calcium 30% • Iron 0% • Vitamin D 25%

*Percent Daily Values are based on a 2000 calorie diet.

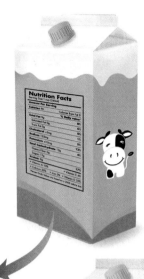

2% Milk

Nutrition Facts
Serving Size 1 cup (240ml)

Amount Per Serving

Calories 120	Calories from Fat 45

	% Daily value*
Total Fat 5g	**8%**
Saturated Fat 3g	**15%**
Trans Fat 0g	**0%**
Cholesterol 20mg	**7%**
Sodium 125mg	**5%**
Potassium 400mg	**11%**
Total Carbohydrate 12g	**4%**
Dietary Fiber 0g	
Sugars 12g	
Protein 8g	**16%**

• Vitamin A 10%	• Vitamin C 4%

• Calcium 30% • Iron 0% • Vitamin D 25%

*Percent Daily Values are based on a 2000 calorie diet.

Whole Milk

Nutrition Facts
Serving Size 1 cup (240ml)

Amount Per Serving

Calories 150	Calories from Fat 70

	% Daily value*
Total Fat 8g	**12%**
Saturated Fat 5g	**25%**
Trans Fat 0g	**0%**
Cholesterol 35mg	**11%**
Sodium 125mg	**5%**
Potassium 400mg	**11%**
Total Carbohydrate 12g	**4%**
Dietary Fiber 0g	
Sugars 12g	
Protein 8g	**16%**

• Vitamin A 6%	• Vitamin C 4%

• Calcium 30% • Iron 0% • Vitamin D 25%

*Percent Daily Values are based on a 2000 calorie diet.

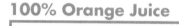

100% Orange Juice

Nutrition Facts
Serving Size 8 fl oz (240ml)
Servings Per Container 8

Amount Per Serving

Calories 110

	% Daily value*
Total Fat 0g	**0%**
Sodium 15mg	**1%**
Potassium 450mg	**13%**
Total Carb 27g	**9%**
Sugars 24g	

Protein 2g Not a significant source of protein

• Vitamin C 120%	• Calcium 35%
• Vitamin D 25%	• Thiamin 10%
• Niacin 2%	• Vitamin B6 4%
• Folate 15%	• Magnesium 6%

Not a significant source of calories from fat, saturated fat, trans fat, cholesterol, dietary fiber, vitamin A and iron.

*Percent Daily values are based on a 2000 calorie diet.

FIGURE 11-20 ▶ Milks of varying fat contents all contain the same amount of vitamin D. Many brands of orange juice are also fortified with calcium and vitamin D to match the nutritian found in milk.

Further Readings

1. Adams JS and Hewison M: Update in vitamin D. *Journal of Clinical Endocrinology and Metabolism* 95:471, 2010.

   The prevalence of vitamin insufficiency has dramatically increased in recent years such that an estimated 75% of white and more than 90% of populations with darker skin pigmentation have low (<30 nanograms/milliliter) serum vitamin D. Aside from decreasing bone mass, low vitamin D has been associated with declines in immune function; increased mortality, especially from cardiovascular diseases; and increased obesity. The inverse relationship between BMI and serum vitamin D is a particularly interesting area of research: vitamin D insufficiency may be both a cause and an effect of increased BMI. Restoring and maintaining serum vitamin D within a healthy range should be a primary goal of therapies to treat patients with bone loss, impaired immunity, and obesity.

2. ADA Reports: Position of the American Dietetic Association: The impact of fluoride on health. *Journal of the American Dietetic Association* 105:1620, 2005.

   The American Dietetic Association reaffirms that fluoride is an important element for all mineralized tissues in the body. Appropriate fluoride intake is beneficial to bone and tooth health.

3. Burge R and others: Incidence and economic burden of osteoporosis-related fractures in the United States, 2005–2025. *Journal of Bone and Mineral Research* 22:465, 2007.

   In 2005, osteoporosis led to more than 2 million fractures and cost at least $17 billion in the United States. Using statistical models, the researchers project a 50% increase in total fractures and costs from 2005 to 2025. Men account for about 30% of fractures and 25% of total costs. An important trend is that nonwhite populations, such as Hispanic-Americans, are anticipated to bear a greater portion of the burden of osteoporosis over the next 20 years.

4. Heaney RP: Absorbability and utility of calcium in mineral waters. *American Journal of Clinical Nutrition* 84(2):371, 2006.

   Published absorbability and utility of high-calcium mineral waters are summarized in this article. The absorbability of all the high-calcium mineral waters was equal to or slightly better than milk calcium. The utility of calcium as measured by increased urinary calcium, decreased serum parathyroid hormone, decreased bone resorption biomarkers, and protection of bone mass indicated that a significant

   quantity of calcium was absorbed. High-calcium mineral waters, therefore, appear to provide useful quantities of bioavailable calcium.

5. Jackson RD and others: Calcium plus vitamin D supplementation and the risk of fractures. *The New England Journal of Medicine* 354(7):669, 2006.

   Postmenopausal women, 50 to 79 years of age, enrolled in a Women's Health Initiative (WHI) clinical trial were assigned to receive daily doses of 1000 mg of elemental calcium as calcium carbonate (with 400 IU of vitamin D) or a placebo. Fracture occurrence and bone density were determined over 7 years. Calcium with vitamin D supplementation resulted in a small but significant increase in hip bone density but did not significantly reduce hip fracture and increased the risk of kidney stones.

6. Lanham-New SA: The balance of bone health: Tipping the scales in favor of potassium-rich, bicarbonate-rich foods. *Journal of Nutrition* 137:1725, 2008.

   About 10 million Americans have osteoporosis. This review article summarizes the current evidence linking potassium-rich, bicarbonate-rich foods (e.g., fruits and vegetables) to osteoporosis prevention.

7. Lewiecki EM: Current and emerging pharmacological therapies for the management of postmenopausal osteoporosis. *Journal of Women's Health* 19(10):1615, 2009.

   The author reviews of the impact of osteoporotic fractures on health outcomes (i.e., effect on physical, emotional, and mental health) of postmenopausal women. Lifestyle strategies to manage osteoporosis as well as optional medications to control the disease are described. Side effects, tolerance, and compliance issues with these medications are discussed.

8. Mark BL and Carson JS: Vitamin D and autoimmune disease—implications for practice from the multiple sclerosis literature. *Journal of the American Dietetic Association* 106:418, 2006.

   Vitamin D is under study for its anti-inflammatory properties in many diseases, including arthritis, cancer, and some autoimmune diseases. Some evidence from studies conducted with multiple sclerosis (MS) patients suggests that vitamin D may be therapeutic, possibly lessening nerve damage and decreasing symptoms of MS. However, vitamin D is not currently a prescribed therapy because the high doses of vitamin D required to produce such effects may induce hypercalcemia. More

   research will be required before vitamin D may be prescribed for the treatment of autoimmune or other inflammatory disorders, but in the meantime, assessing dietary and supplemental vitamin D intake and promoting adequate consumption of this fat-soluble vitamin will support bone health with the possible benefit of reducing inflammation.

9. National Osteoporosis Foundation: *Clinician's guide to prevention and treatment of osteoporosis*. Washington, DC: National Osteoporosis Foundation; January 2010. available at: www.nof.org/professionals/clinical-guidelines.

   This guide provides recommendations for physicians on issues of osteoporosis and low bone mass for postmenopausal women and all women and men over age 50. It reviews the impact of osteoporosis on the individual and community, risk factors, diagnosis, treatment, and rehabilitation. This guideline is updated frequently.

10. Nielsen FH: Is boron nutritionally relevant? *Nutrition Reviews* 66:183, 2008.

    Boron participates in bone health, brain function, and immunity. Although no RDA or AI has been set, studies of boron intake indicate that many Americans consume less than optimal levels of this ultratrace mineral. Several experts encourage consumption of a diet rich in fruits, vegetables, nuts, and grains as rich dietary sources of boron to promote bone and brain health.

11. Office of Dietary Supplements, National Institutes of Health: Dietary supplement fact sheet: vitamin D. Updated 6/24/11. Available at: http://ods.od.nih.gov/factsheets/vitamind; Magnesium fact sheet. Updated 7/13/2009. Available at: http://ods.od.nih.gov/factsheets/magnesium; and Calcium fact sheet. Updated 08/31/2011. Available at: http://ods.od.nih.gov/factsheets/calcium.

    These reader-friendly fact sheets provide the most recent information on supplements. Food sources, deficiencies, at-risk groups, and nutrient-drug interactions are highlighted. Current research and controversial areas are discussed.

12. Palacios C: The role of nutrients in bone health, from A to Z. *Critical Reviews in Food Science and Nutrition* 46:621, 2006.

    Adequate protein is required for formation of collagen in bone and the synthesis of hormones that affect bone health. Calcium, phosphorus, magnesium, and fluoride contribute to bone mineralization. Other minerals, including iron, zinc, copper, manganese, and boron, function as cofactors for enzymes that participate in bone metabolism. Potassium promotes an alkaline environment, which may reduce the use of bone minerals as buffers. Vitamin C is important for the formation of collagen. Vitamin K is required for the binding of calcium to osteocalcin, a bone protein. Vitamin A participates in bone remodeling through its effects on expression of genes that lead to osteoblast and osteoclast formation. Overall, a diet rich in low-fat or fat-free dairy products and fruits and vegetables promotes bone health.

13. Park Y and others: Dairy food, calcium, and risk of cancer in the NIH-AARP diet and health study. *Archives of Internal Medicine* 169:391, 2009.

The 7-year study of 493,000 older men and women provides evidence that diets rich in calcium may lower risk of total cancer and cancers of the digestive system, especially colorectal cancer. Benefits were mostly associated with foods high in calcium, rather than calcium supplements. Getting more than the recommended 1200 milligrams of calcium for older people did not result in greater cancer protection.

14. Pizzo G and others: Community water fluoridation and caries prevention:

A critical review. *Clinical Oral Investigation* 11:189, 2007.

Over the past 50 years, community water fluoridation has been a successful public health measure to reduce dental caries. However, now that oral hygiene has improved, access to regular dental care is widespread, and other sources of fluoride are widely available, fluorosis is the emerging problem. The authors suggest that community water fluoridation may only now be necessary in disadvantaged communities.

15. Tucker KL: Osteoporosis prevention and nutrition. *Current Osteoporosis Reports* 7:111, 2009.

A diet high in fruits and vegetables is just as important as inclusion of low-fat and fat-free dairy products. Fruits and vegetables supply magnesium, potassium, vitamin C, vitamin K, and carotenoids, all of which are implicated in prevention of osteoporosis. Either too high or too low protein intake negatively affects bone health. Intake of soft drinks decreases bone mineral density, whereas moderate alcohol intake is positively associated with bone mineral density.

16. Van Dam RM and others: Dietary calcium and magnesium, major food sources, and risk of type 2 diabetes in U.S. black women. *Diabetes Care* 29:2238, 2006.

Magnesium and calcium intakes have been inversely associated with risk of type 2 diabetes in predominantly white populations. The results of this study of 41,186 participants of the Black Women's Health Study indicated that a diet high in magnesium-rich foods, particularly whole grains, is associated with a significantly lower risk of type 2 diabetes in U.S. black women.

17. Wagner CL and Greer FR: Prevention of rickets and vitamin D deficiency in infants, children, and adolescents. American Academy of Pediatrics Section on Breastfeeding, American Academy of Pediatrics Committee on Nutrition. *Pediatrics* 122:1142, 2008.

In this statement, the American Academy of Pediatrics publishes vitamin D supplement recommendations for exclusively and partially breastfed infants. Also recommended are supplements for older children and adolescents who do not obtain 400 IU/day through vitamin-D-fortified milk and foods. This recommendation by the academy is based on clinical trials and a history of safe use of 400 IU vitamin D by this age group.

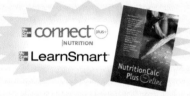

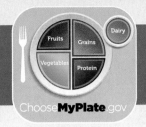

RATE YOUR PLATE

I. Working for Denser Bones

Osteoporosis and related low bone mass affect many adults in North America, especially older women. One-third of all women experience fractures because of this disease, amounting to about 2 million bone fractures per year.

Osteoporosis is a disease you can do something about. Some risk factors cannot be changed, but others, such as poor calcium intake, can. Is this true for you? To find out, complete this tool for estimating your current calcium intake. For all the following foods, write the number of servings you eat in a day. Total the number of servings in each category and then multiply the total number of servings by the amount of calcium for each category. Finally, add the total amount for each category to estimate your calcium intake for that day.

Does your intake meet your RDA set for calcium?

Food	Serving Size	Number of Servings	Calcium (mg)	Total Calcium (mg)
Plain low-fat yogurt	1 cup	_____		
Fat-free dry milk powder	½ cup	_____		
	Total servings	_____	X 400	= _____ mg
Canned sardines (with bones)	3 ounces	_____		
Fruit-flavored yogurt	1 cup	_____		
Milk: fat-free, reduced-fat, whole, chocolate, buttermilk	1 cup	_____		
Calcium-fortified soy milk (e.g., Silk)	1 cup	_____		
Parmesan cheese (grated)	¼ cup	_____		
Swiss cheese	1 ounce	_____		
	Total servings	_____	X 300	= _____ mg
Cheese (all other hard cheese)	1 ounce	_____		
Pancakes	3	_____		
	Total servings	_____	X 200	= _____ mg
Canned pink salmon	3 ounces	_____		
Tofu (processed with calcium)	4 ounces	_____		
	Total servings	_____	X 150	= _____ mg
Collards or turnip greens, cooked	½ cup	_____		
Ice cream or ice milk	1 ounce	_____		
Almonds	Total servings	_____	X 75	= _____ mg
Chard, cooked	½ cup	_____		
Cottage cheese	½ cup	_____		
Corn tortilla	1 medium	_____		
Orange	1 medium	_____		
	Total servings	_____	X 50	= _____ mg
Kidney, lima, or navy beans, cooked	½ cup	_____		
Broccoli	½ cup	_____		
Carrot, raw	1 medium	_____		
Dates or raisins	¼ cup	_____		
Egg	1 large	_____		
Whole-wheat bread	1 slice	_____		
Peanut butter	2 tablespoons	_____		
	Total servings	_____	X 25	= _____ mg
Calcium-fortified orange juice	6 ounces	_____		
Calcium-fortified snack bars	1 each	_____		
Calcium-fortified breakfast bars	½ bar	_____		
	Total servings	_____	X 200	= _____ mg
Calcium-fortified chocolate candies	1 each	_____		
Calcium supplements*	1 each	_____	X 500	
	Total servings	_____	Total calcium intake	= _____ mg
				= _____ mg

Other calcium sources to consider include many breakfast cereals (100–250 mg per cup) and some vitamin/mineral supplements (200–500 mg or more per tablet).
*Amount varies, so check the label for the amount in a specific product and then adjust the calculation as needed.
Reprinted with permission from *Topics in Clinical Nutrition*, "Putting Calcium into Perspective for Your Clients," G. Wardlaw and N. Weese, 11:1, © 1995 Aspen Publishers, Inc.

Chapter 12 Micronutrient Function in Energy Metabolism and Blood Health

Student Learning Outcomes

Chapter 12 is designed to allow you to:

12.1 Describe how vitamins and minerals function as coenzymes that allow chemical reactions in metabolism to occur.

12.2 List and describe the functions of the B vitamins, especially how they relate to energy metabolism.

12.3 Describe food sources, dietary requirements, deficiency, and toxicity of the nutrients involved in energy metabolism.

12.4 Describe the composition of blood.

12.5 List and describe the functions of vitamins and minerals in the maintenance of blood health.

12.6 Describe food sources, dietary requirements, deficiency, and toxicity of the nutrients involved in blood health.

12.7 Describe how nutrients influence the many forms of anemia observed.

What Would You Choose?

Congratulations! The pregnancy test was positive, and your family will soon need to ditch the sports car for a four-door sedan! You have heard that one of the B vitamins, folic acid, is especially important during pregnancy because it helps to prevent birth defects. Besides the prenatal vitamin the doctor recommends, what would you choose as a rich source of folic acid?

a Spinach salad with strawberries

b Quaker Oats® Oatmeal Squares Brown Sugar cereal

c Cooked lentils

d Low-fat yogurt

Think about your choice as you read Chapter 12, then see our recommendations at the end of the chapter. To learn more about nutrient needs during pregnancy, check out the Connect site: www.mcgrawhillconnect.com

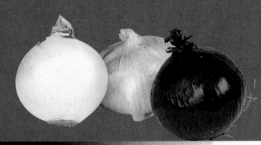

How does the body convert the energy found in food into a form that the cells can use? Cells obtain energy from the chemical bonds found in the macronutrients (carbohydrates, lipids, and protein). You learned previously that during the process of digestion, these macronutrients are broken down chemically into smaller substances (monosaccharides, fatty acids, monoglycerides, glycerol, and amino acids). These smaller substances can be absorbed into the body via the small intestine. The circulatory system then transports these nutrients to the trillions of cells in the body. The cells use chemical reactions to further break down these substances into carbon dioxide and water. In the process, large amounts of energy are converted into a form that the cells can use to perform work (ATP). The chemical processes used by cells to extract energy from these nutrients are termed *metabolism*. A major function of the micronutrients (vitamins and minerals) is to assist enzymes in the chemical reactions in energy metabolism. These micronutrients are called **coenzymes** (vitamins) or **cofactors** (minerals) because they activate the enzymes and thus allow them to become functional.

This chapter is divided into three main sections. The first section will provide an overview of the B vitamins. The second section will discuss the roles that vitamins and minerals have in energy metabolism. The third section provides a detailed look at the vitamins and minerals that function in the maintenance of blood health.

coenzyme An organic compound that combines with an inactive enzyme to form a catalytically active form. In this manner, coenzymes aid in enzyme function.

cofactor An inorganic compound (e.g., mineral) that combines with an inactive enzyme to form a catalytically active form.

bioavailability The degree to which an ingested nutrient is absorbed and utilized by the body.

 Refresh Your Memory

As you begin your study of nutrients that function in energy metabolism and blood health in Chapter 12, you might want to review:

- Implications of the Dietary Supplement Health and Education Act (DSHEA) in Chapter 1
- The gastrointestinal system for the digestion and absorption of nutrients in Chapter 3
- Carbohydrate metabolism in Chapter 4
- Lipid metabolism in Chapter 5
- Amino acid metabolism and protein synthesis in Chapter 6

12.1 The Roles of B Vitamins in Energy Metabolism

The B vitamins and some minerals play key roles in metabolism as coenzymes or cofactors, respectively (recall Fig. 8-5). Many B vitamins are interdependent because they participate in the same metabolic pathways that convert macronutrients into usable energy (Fig. 12-1). Early symptoms of micronutrient deficiency typically occur in the brain and nervous system, skin, and gastrointestinal (GI) tract because cells in these tissues are metabolically active. Cells in the skin and GI tract are also constantly being replaced.

After being ingested, the B vitamins are first broken down from their coenzyme forms into free vitamins in the stomach and small intestine. The vitamins are then absorbed, primarily in the small intestine. Typically, about 50% to 90% of the B vitamins in the diet are absorbed, demonstrating their relatively high **bioavailability.** Once inside cells, the coenzyme forms are resynthesized. Health-food stores sell the coenzyme forms of some vitamins. These more expensive forms of vitamins are unnecessary. The body makes all the coenzymes it needs from vitamin precursors.

B Vitamin Intakes of North Americans

The nutritional health of most North Americans with regard to the B vitamins is good. Typical diets contain plentiful and varied natural sources of these vitamins. In addition, many common foods, such as ready-to-eat breakfast cereals, are fortified

How do the calories in food turn into fuel in my body? Is a dietary deficiency causing me to feel fatigued? Which breakfast cereals provide the nutrients I need? Is it okay to take mineral supplements? Chapter 12 provides some answers.

www.CartoonStock.com

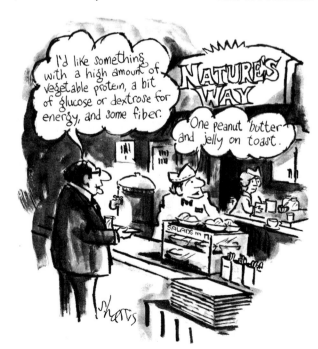

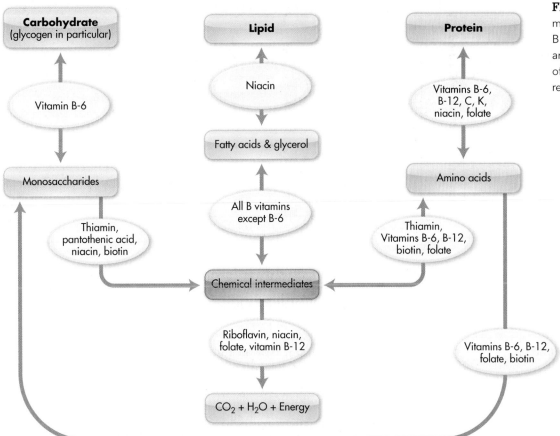

FIGURE 12-1 ▶ Examples of metabolic pathways for which B vitamins and other vitamins are essential. The metabolism of energy-yielding nutrients requires vitamin input.

with one or more of the B vitamins. In some developing countries, however, deficiencies of the B vitamins are more common, and the resulting deficiency diseases pose significant health problems. (A discussion of nutritional deficiencies worldwide is presented in Chapter 15.)

Because B vitamins are water soluble, any excess ends up in the urine or stool and little is stored. Vitamin losses (10% to 25%) occur during food processing and preparation because they dissolve in water. Light cooking methods, such as stir-frying, steaming, and microwaving, best preserve vitamin content (review Table 8-3).

Despite good B vitamin status of North Americans, marginal deficiencies of these vitamins may occur in some cases, especially among older adults who eat little food and in people with poor dietary patterns. In the short run, such a marginal deficiency in most people likely leads only to fatigue or other bothersome and unspecified physical effects. However, the long-term effects of such marginal deficiencies are yet unknown, but increased risk of cardiovascular disease, cancer, and cataracts of the eye is suspected. With rare exceptions, healthy adults do not develop the more serious B-vitamin-deficiency diseases from dietary inadequacy alone. The main exceptions are people with alcoholism. The combination of extremely unbalanced diets and alcohol-induced alterations of vitamin absorption and metabolism creates significant risks for serious nutrient deficiencies among people with alcoholism.

The manufacturing process of refining grains leads to the loss of B vitamins as well as other vitamins and minerals. In milling grains, seeds are crushed and the germ, bran, and husk layers are discarded, leaving just the starch-containing endosperm in the refined grains. This starch is used to make flour, bread, and cereal products. Unfortunately, many nutrients are lost along with the discarded germ, bran, and husk materials. To counteract these losses, in the United States, bread and cereal products

▲ Rapid cooking of vegetables in minimal fluids aids in preserving vitamin content. Steaming is one effective method.

FIGURE 12-2 ▶ Compare the relative nutrient contents of refined versus whole grains. Nutrients are expressed as a percentage of the nutrient contribution of the whole grain product.

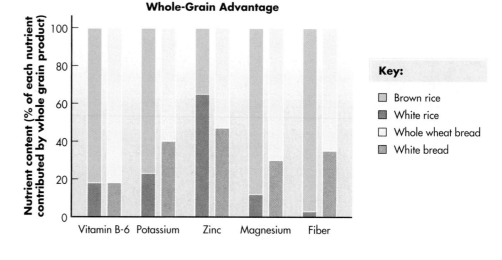

Whole-Grain Advantage

Key:
- ▢ Brown rice
- ◼ White rice
- ▢ Whole wheat bread
- ▨ White bread

anemia A decreased oxygen-carrying capacity of the blood. This can be caused by many factors, such as iron deficiency or blood loss.

goiter An enlargement of the thyroid gland; this is often caused by insufficient iodide in the diet.

made from milled grains are enriched with four B vitamins (thiamin, riboflavin, niacin, and folic acid) and with the mineral iron.

Food enrichment was initiated by a legislative act in the 1930s to help combat nutrient deficiencies like pellagra (niacin deficiency) and iron-deficiency **anemia.** Federal regulations added folate to the list of nutrients required to be added to refined grain products in 1998. Not all nutrients lost in milling are added back through enrichment; these products remain lower in vitamins E and B-6, potassium, magnesium, fiber, and other nutrients than the whole grains. Nutrition experts and the Dietary Guidelines advocate daily consumption of whole-grain products, such as whole-wheat bread and brown rice, rather than refined grain products (Fig. 12-2).

12.2 Vitamins and Minerals Involved in Energy Metabolism

Iodide (I)

During World War I, a link was discovered between a deficiency of iodide and the production of a **goiter,** an enlarged thyroid gland. Men drafted from areas such as the Great Lakes Region of the United States had a much higher rate of goiter than did men from other areas of the country. The soils in these areas have low iodide contents. In the 1920s, a researcher in Ohio found that low doses of iodide given to children over a 4-year period could prevent goiter. That finding led to the addition of iodide to salt beginning in the 1920s, the first time a nutrient was purposely added to food to prevent a disease.

Today, many nations, such as Canada, require iodide fortification of salt. In the United States, salt can be purchased either iodized or plain. Check for this on the label when you purchase salt. Some areas of Europe, such as northern Italy, have very low soil levels of iodide but have yet to adopt an iodide-fortification program. People in these areas, especially women, still suffer from goiter, as do people in areas of Latin America, the Indian subcontinent, Southeast Asia, and Africa. About 2 billion people worldwide are at risk of iodide deficiency, and approximately 800 million of these people have suffered the widespread effects of such a deficiency. Eradication of iodide deficiency is a goal of many health-related organizations worldwide.

Functions of Iodide. The thyroid gland actively accumulates and traps iodide from the bloodstream to support thyroid hormone synthesis. Thyroid hormones are synthesized using iodide and the amino acid, tyrosine. Because these hormones help regulate metabolic rate and promote growth and development throughout the body, iodide adequacy is important for overall energy metabolism.

If a person's iodide intake is insufficient, the thyroid gland enlarges as it attempts to take up more iodide from the bloodstream. This eventually leads to goiter. Simple goiter is a painless condition but, if uncorrected, can lead to pressure on the trachea (windpipe), which may cause difficulty in breathing. Although iodide can prevent goiter formation, it does not significantly shrink a goiter once it has formed. Surgical removal may be required in severe cases.

If a woman has an iodide-deficient diet during the early months of her pregnancy, the fetus suffers iodide deficiency because the mother's body uses up the available iodide. The infant then may be born with short length and develop intellectual delays (Fig. 12-3). Collectively, the stunted growth and developmental delays that result are known as **cretinism.** Cretinism appeared in North America before iodide fortification of table salt began. Today, cretinism still appears in Europe, Africa, Latin America, and Asia.

Iodide Sources and Needs. Iodized salt, dairy products, and grain products contain various forms of iodide (Fig. 12-4). Sea salt and kosher salt found in health-food stores, however, are not good sources because the iodide is lost during processing.

The RDA for iodide for adults is 150 micrograms to support thyroid gland function. This is the same as the DV used on food and supplement labels. A half teaspoon of iodide-fortified salt (about 2 grams) supplies that amount. Most North American adults consume more iodide than the RDA—an estimated 190 to 300 micrograms daily, not including that from use of iodized salt at the table. This extra amount adds up because dairies use it as a sterilizing agent, bakeries use it as a dough conditioner, food producers use it as part of food colorants, and it is added to salt. There is concern, however, that vegans may not consume enough unless iodized salt is used.

Upper Level for Iodide. The UL for iodide is 1.1 milligrams per day. When high amounts of iodide are consumed, thyroid hormone synthesis is inhibited, as in a deficiency. This can appear in people who eat a lot of seaweed, because some seaweeds contain as much as 1% iodide by weight. Total iodide intake then can add up to 60 to 130 times the RDA.

cretinism The stunting of body growth and poor development in the offspring that result from inadequate maternal intake of iodide during pregnancy.

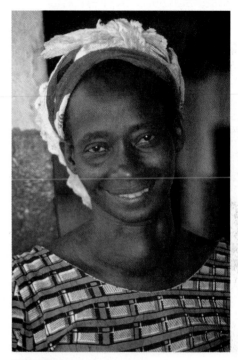

FIGURE 12-3 ▶ This woman has an enlargement of the thyroid gland also known as a goiter caused by insufficient iodide in the diet.

FIGURE 12-4 ▶ Food sources of iodide compared to the RDA.

Food Sources of Iodide

Food Item and Amount	Iodide (micrograms)	Adult Male and Female RDA = 150 micrograms Daily Value = 150 micrograms %RDA	
RDA*	150		100%
Iodized table salt, ½ tsp	195		130%
Cod, haddock fillet, 3½ ounces	116		114%
Plain yogurt, ½ cup	87		56%
1% milk, 1 cup	59		39%
Luna bar, 1	38		25%
Soy protein bar, 1	38		25%
Egg, 1 large	35		23%
1% cottage cheese, ½ cup	28		19%
Mozzarella cheese, 1 ounce	10		7%

Key:
- ■ Grains
- ■ Vegetables
- ■ Fruits
- ■ Dairy
- ■ Protein

*For adults; see the DRI table in the back of this book for gender- and age-specific recommendations.

Thiamin (Vitamin B-1)

Thiamin was the first water-soluble vitamin to be discovered. A primary function is to help release energy from carbohydrate. Its coenzyme form participates in reactions in which carbon dioxide (CO_2) is released from a substrate. This reaction is particularly important in the body's ATP-producing energy pathways, which involve the breakdown of carbohydrates and certain amino acids (see Fig. 12-1). Thiamin also functions in chemical reactions that make RNA, DNA, and neurotransmitters.

Thousands of years ago, the life-threatening condition of thiamin deficiency was described. The thiamin-deficiency disease is called **beriberi,** a word that means "I can't, I can't" in the Sri Lanka language of Sinhalese. The symptoms include weakness, loss of appetite, irritability, nervous tingling throughout the body, poor arm and leg coordination, and deep muscle pain in the calves. A person with beriberi often develops an enlarged heart and sometimes severe edema.

Beriberi is seen in areas where rice is a staple and polished (white) rice is consumed rather than brown (whole-grain) rice. In most parts of the world, brown rice has had its bran and germ layer removed to make white rice, a poor source of thiamin, unless it is enriched.

Beriberi results when glucose, the primary fuel for brain and nerve cells, cannot be metabolized to release energy. Because the thiamin coenzyme participates in glucose metabolism, problems with body functions associated with brain and nerve action are the first signs of a thiamin deficiency. Symptoms can develop in just 10 days on a thiamin-free diet.

Thiamin Sources and Needs. Major sources of thiamin include pork products, whole grains (wheat germ), ready-to-eat breakfast cereals, enriched grains and flour, green beans, milk, orange juice, organ meats, peanuts, dried beans, and seeds (Fig. 12-5).

beriberi The thiamin-deficiency disorder characterized by muscle weakness, loss of appetite, nerve degeneration, and sometimes edema.

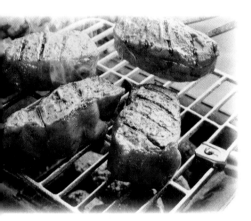

▲ Pork is an excellent source of thiamin.

Food Sources of Thiamin

Food Item and Amount	Thiamin (milligrams)	Adult Male RDA = 1.2 milligrams		Adult Female RDA = 1.1 milligrams	
		Daily Value = 1.5 milligrams			
		%RDA		%RDA	
RDA	1.1-1.2		100%		100%
Canned lean ham, 3 ounces	0.9		75%		82%
Pork chops, 4 ounces	0.6		50%		55%
Wheat germ, ¼ cup	0.5		42%		45%
Canadian bacon, 2 ounces	0.5		42%		45%
Acorn squash, 1 cup	0.4		33%		36%
Soy milk, 1 cup	0.4		33%		36%
Flour tortilla, 1	0.4		33%		36%
Ham lunch meat, 2 pieces	0.3		25%		27%
Watermelon, 1 slice	0.2		17%		18%
Fresh orange juice, 1 cup	0.2		17%		18%
Cooked green peas, ½ cup	0.2		17%		18%
Baked beans, ½ cup	0.2		17%		18%
Navy beans, ½ cup	0.2		17%		18%
Corn, ½ cup	0.2		17%		18%

Key:
- Grains
- Vegetables
- Fruits
- Dairy
- Protein

ChooseMyPlate.gov

FIGURE 12-5 ▶ Food sources of thiamin compared to the RDA for adult males and females.

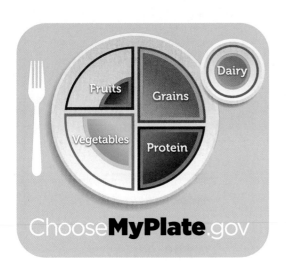

MyPlate: Sources of Thiamin, Riboflavin, and Niacin

FIGURE 12-6 ▶ Sources of thiamin, riboflavin, and niacin from MyPlate. The fill of the background color (none, 1/3, 2/3, or completely covered) within each group on the plate indicates the average nutrient density for these vitamins in that group. Overall, the protein group and the grains group contain many foods that are nutrient-dense sources of thiamin, riboflavin, and niacin. As well, foods from the dairy group are especially rich sources of riboflavin. With regard to physical activity, these vitamins play key roles in the increased energy metabolism that takes place during such endeavors.

The adult RDA for thiamin is 1.1 to 1.2 milligrams per day. The Daily Value (DV) used on food and supplement labels is 1.5 milligrams. Average daily intakes for men exceed the DV by 50% or more, and women generally meet the RDA. Low-income adults and older people may barely meet their needs for thiamin. Potential contributors to thiamin deficiency are diets dominated by highly processed and unenriched foods, sugar, and fat; and heavy alcohol intake combined with a poor diet (Fig. 12-6). Oral thiamin supplements are typically nontoxic because thiamin is rapidly lost in the urine. Thus, no Upper Level (UL) has been set for thiamin.

MAKING DECISIONS

Alcohol Reduces Thiamin Status

People with alcoholism are at greater risk for thiamin deficiency. Absorption and use of thiamin are profoundly diminished and excretion is increased by consumption of alcohol. Furthermore, the low-quality diet that often accompanies severe alcoholism makes matters worse. There is limited storage in the body; therefore, an alcoholic binge lasting 1 to 2 weeks may quickly deplete already diminished amounts of the vitamin and result in deficiency symptoms. The beriberi associated with alcoholism is also called Wernicke-Korsakoff syndrome.

Riboflavin (Vitamin B-2)

Riboflavin derives its name from its yellow color (*flavus* means yellow in Latin). The coenzyme forms of riboflavin participate in many energy-yielding metabolic pathways, such as the breakdown of fatty acids (see Fig. 12-1). Some vitamin and mineral metabolism also requires riboflavin. Indirectly, riboflavin also has an antioxidant role in the body through its support of the enzyme glutathione peroxidase.

Symptoms associated with riboflavin deficiency (ariboflavinosis) include inflammation of the mouth and tongue, dermatitis, cracking of tissue around the corners of the mouth (called cheilosis), various eye disorders, sensitivity to the sun, and confusion (Fig. 12-7). Such symptoms develop after approximately 2 months on a riboflavin-poor diet. Riboflavin deficiencies probably do not exist by themselves. Instead, a riboflavin deficiency would occur jointly with deficiencies of niacin, thiamin, and vitamin B-6 because these nutrients often occur in the same foods.

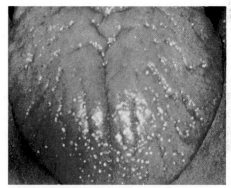

(a)

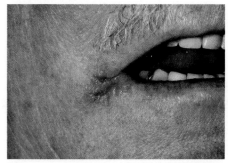

(b)

FIGURE 12-7 ▶ (a) Glossitis is a painful, inflamed tongue that can signal a deficiency of riboflavin, niacin, vitamin B-6, folate, or vitamin B-12. (b) Angular cheilitis, also called cheilosis or angular stomatitis, is another result of a riboflavin deficiency. It causes painful cracks at the corners of the mouth. Both glossitis and angular cheilitis can be caused by other medical conditions; thus, further evaluation is required before diagnosing a nutrient deficiency.

Food Sources of Riboflavin

Food Item and Amount	Riboflavin (milligrams)	Adult Male RDA = 1.3 milligrams		Adult Female RDA = 1.1 milligrams	
		Daily Value = 1.7 milligrams			
		%RDA		%RDA	
RDA	1.1-1.3	▬▬▬▬▬▬▬	100%	▬▬▬▬▬▬▬	100%
Multigrain Cheerios, ¾ cup	1.3	▬▬▬▬▬▬▬	100%	▬▬▬▬▬▬▬	110%
Fried beef liver, 1 ounce	1.2	▬▬▬▬▬▬	92%	▬▬▬▬▬▬▬	109%
Steamed oysters, 10	1.1	▬▬▬▬▬▬	85%	▬▬▬▬▬▬▬	100%
Plain yogurt, 1 cup	0.5	▬▬	38%	▬▬	45%
Raw mushrooms, 5	0.5	▬▬	38%	▬▬	45%
Braunschweiger sausage,1	0.4	▬▬	31%	▬▬	36%
Cooked spinach, 1 cup	0.4	▬▬	31%	▬▬	36%
1% milk, 1 cup	0.4	▬▬	31%	▬▬	36%
Buttermilk, 1 cup	0.4	▬▬	31%	▬▬	36%
Boiled egg, 1	0.3	▬	23%	▬	27%
Sirloin steak, 3 ounces	0.3	▬	23%	▬	27%
Feta cheese, 1 ounce	0.2	▬	15%	▬	18%
Tortilla, 1	0.2	▬	15%	▬	18%
Lean ham, 3 ounces	0.2	▬	15%	▬	18%

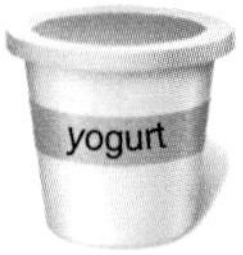

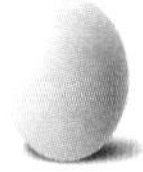

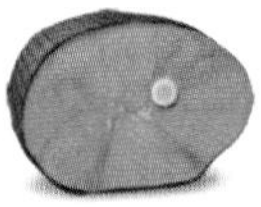

Key:
- ■ Grains
- ■ Vegetables
- ■ Fruits
- ■ Dairy
- ■ Protein

FIGURE 12-8 ▶ Food sources of riboflavin compared to the RDA for adult males and females.

Riboflavin Sources and Needs. Major sources of riboflavin are ready-to-eat break-fast cereals, milk and milk products, enriched grains, meat, and eggs (Fig. 12-8). Vegetables such as asparagus, broccoli, and various greens (e.g., spinach) are also good sources. Riboflavin is a relatively stable water-soluble vitamin; however, it is destroyed by light. Milk is sold in paper or opaque plastic containers rather than clear glass to protect the riboflavin.

The adult RDA of riboflavin is 1.1 to 1.3 milligrams per day. The DV used on food and supplement labels is 1.7 milligrams. On average, daily intakes of riboflavin are slightly above the RDA. As with thiamin, people with alcoholism risk riboflavin deficiency because they eat nutrient-poor diets. No specific symptoms indicate that riboflavin taken in **megadoses** is toxic, so no UL has been set. Riboflavin supplementation can cause the urine to become bright yellow.

Niacin (Vitamin B-3)

Niacin functions in the body as one of two related compounds: nicotinic acid and nicotinamide. The coenzyme forms of niacin function in many cellular metabolic pathways. When energy is being used, a niacin coenzyme is used. Synthetic pathways in the cell—those that make new compounds—also often use a niacin coenzyme. This is especially true for fatty-acid synthesis (see Fig. 12-1).

A coenzyme in over 200 enzymatic reactions, niacin deficiency causes widespread changes in the body. The group of niacin-deficiency symptoms is known as pellagra, which means rough or painful skin. The symptoms of the disease are **dementia,** diarrhea, and dermatitis (especially on areas of skin exposed to the sun) (Fig. 12-9). Left untreated, death often results. Early symptoms include poor appetite, weight loss, and weakness.

megadose Intake of a nutrient beyond estimates of needs to prevent a deficiency or what would be found in a balanced diet; 2 to 10 times human needs is a starting point for such a dose.

dementia A general loss or decrease in mental function.

Pellagra is the only dietary deficiency disease ever to reach epidemic proportions in the United States. It became a major problem in the southeastern United States in the late 1800s and persisted until the 1930s, when standards of living and diets improved. Today, pellagra is rare in Western societies but can be seen in the developing world.

MAKING DECISIONS

Making Niacin Available

Niacin in corn is bound by a protein that hampers its absorption, making it less bioavailable. Soaking corn in an alkaline solution, such as lime water (water with calcium hydroxide), releases bound niacin and renders it more bioavailable. Hispanic people in North America traditionally soak corn in lime water before making tortillas. This treatment is one reason this Hispanic population never experienced much pellagra.

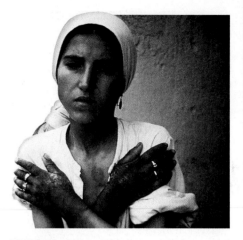

FIGURE 12-9 ▶ The dermatitis of a niacin deficiency is called pellagra. Dermatitis on both sides of the body (bilateral) is a typical symptom. Sun exposure worsens the condition.

Niacin Sources and Needs. Major sources of niacin are tuna, poultry, peanuts, fish, ready-to-eat cereals, beef, and asparagus (Fig. 12-10). Coffee and tea also contribute some niacin to the diet. Niacin is heat stable; little is lost in cooking.

Besides the preformed niacin found in protein foods, we can synthesize niacin from the amino acid tryptophan: 60 milligrams of tryptophan in a diet yield about 1 milligram of niacin. In this manner, we synthesize about 50% of the niacin required each day. This reaction requires two other vitamins (riboflavin and vitamin B-6) to function as coenzymes in this chemical conversion.

Food Sources of Niacin

Food Item and Amount	Niacin (milligrams)	Adult Male RDA = 16 milligrams %RDA	Adult Female RDA = 14 milligrams %RDA
RDA	14-16	100%	100%
Tuna, 3 ounces	11.3	71%	81%
Roasted chicken, 3 ounces	10.1	63%	72%
Peanuts, ½ cup	9.9	62%	71%
Baked salmon, 3 ounces	8.6	54%	61%
Turkey lunch meat, 3 ounces	5.4	34%	39%
Ground beef, 3 ounces	5.0	31%	36%
Raw mushrooms, 5	4.7	29%	34%
Lean steak, 4 ounces	4.5	28%	32%
Chunky peanut butter, 2 tablespoons	4.4	28%	31%
Fried beef liver, 1 ounce	4.1	26%	29%
Raisin Nut Bran cereal, ¾ cup	3.8	24%	27%
Tortilla, 1	2.6	16%	19%
Baked cod, 3 ounces	2.1	13%	15%
Potato, 1	2.1	13%	15%
Broiled halibut, 3 ounces	1.6	10%	11%

Daily Value = 20 milligrams

Key:
- Grains
- Vegetables
- Fruits
- Dairy
- Protein

ChooseMyPlate.gov

FIGURE 12-10 ▶ Food sources of niacin compared to the RDA for adult males and females.

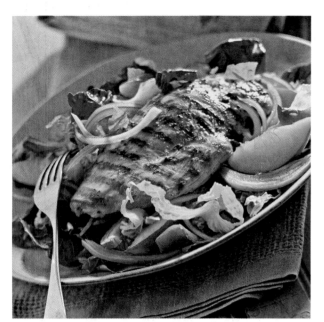

▲ Chicken is a good source of niacin. The tryptophan in chicken can also be metabolized to niacin.

The adult RDA of niacin is 14 to 16 milligrams per day. The RDA is expressed as niacin equivalents (NE) to account for niacin received intact from the diet, as well as that synthesized from tryptophan. The DV used on food and supplement labels is 20 milligrams. Intakes of niacin by adults are about double the RDA, without considering the contribution from tryptophan. (Tables of food composition values also ignore tryptophan contribution.) Although pellagra was once common, today it is typically only seen associated with chronic alcoholism in conjunction with poverty and malnutrition and in those with rare disorders of tryptophan metabolism (for example, Hartnup disease).

Upper Level for Niacin. The UL for niacin is 35 milligrams per day of the nicotinic acid form. Side effects include headache; itching; and increased blood flow to the skin, causing blood vessel dilation or flushing in various parts of the body. These symptoms are especially seen when intakes are above 100 milligrams per day. In the long run, GI tract and liver damage are possible, so any use of megadoses, including large doses recommended for treatment for cardiovascular disease, requires close medical monitoring. Nicotinic acid has been promoted as a natural method to lower blood lipids; however, due to potential adverse side effects, its use is discouraged.

CONCEPT CHECK

The B vitamins thiamin, riboflavin, and niacin are important in the metabolism of carbohydrates, protein, and lipids. Deficiency symptoms typically occur in the brain and nervous system, skin, and GI tract. Cells in these tissues are highly metabolically active, and those in the skin and GI tract are also constantly being replaced. Enriched grains are adequate sources of all three vitamins, as are ready-to-eat breakfast cereals. Otherwise, pork is an excellent source of thiamin; milk is an excellent source of riboflavin; and protein foods in general, such as chicken, are excellent sources of niacin. Deficiencies of all three vitamins can occur with alcoholism; a thiamin deficiency is the most likely of the three.

Pantothenic Acid (Vitamin B-5)

Pantothenic acid functions as a coenzyme in chemical reactions that allow the release of energy from carbohydrates, lipids, and protein. It activates fatty acids so they can yield energy (see Fig. 12-1). It is also used in the initial steps of fatty-acid synthesis. Pantothenic acid is so widespread in foods that a nutritional deficiency among healthy people who eat varied diets is unlikely. *Pantothen* means "from every side" in Greek.

Pantothenic Acid Sources and Needs. Rich sources of pantothenic acid are sunflower seeds, mushrooms, peanuts, and eggs (Fig. 12-11). Other rich sources are meat, milk, and many vegetables.

The Adequate Intake (AI) set for pantothenic acid is 5 milligrams per day for adults. Average consumption is well in excess of this amount. The DV on food and supplement labels is 10 milligrams. A deficiency of pantothenic acid might occur in alcoholism along with a nutrient-deficient diet. However, the symptoms would probably be hidden among deficiencies of thiamin, riboflavin, vitamin B-6, and folate, so the pantothenic acid deficiency might be unrecognizable. No toxicity is known for pantothenic acid, so no UL has been set.

Food Sources of Pantothenic Acid

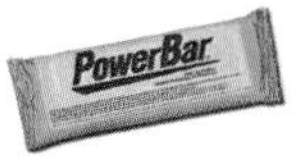

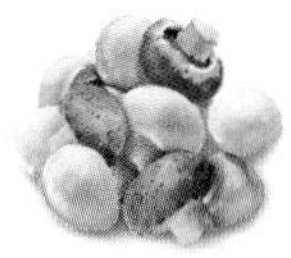

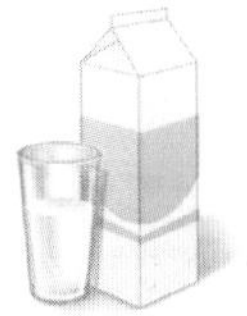

Food Item and Amount	Pantothenic Acid (milligrams)	Adult Male and Female AI = 5 milligrams Daily Value = 10 milligrams %AI
AI	5	100%
Total corn flakes cereal, ¾ cup	11.8	236%
Power bar, 1	10.0	200%
Luna bar, 1	9.9	198%
Sunflower seeds, ¼ cup	2.3	46%
Fried beef liver, 1 ounce	1.7	34%
Raw mushrooms, 5	1.7	34%
Plain yogurt, 1 cup	1.5	30%
Acorn squash, 1 cup	1.2	24%
Peanuts, ½ cup	1.0	20%
1% milk, 1 cup	0.9	18%
Roasted chicken breast, 3 ounces	0.8	16%
Broccoli, 1 cup	0.8	16%
Baked potato, 1	0.7	14%
Legumes, ½ cup	0.7	14%
Cooked egg yolk, 1	0.6	12%

Key:
- Grains
- Vegetables
- Fruits
- Dairy
- Protein

FIGURE 12-11 ▶ Food sources of pantothenic acid compared to the Adequate Intake for adults.

Biotin (Vitamin B-7)

In its coenzyme form, biotin aids in dozens of chemical reactions. Biotin assists in the addition of carbon dioxide to other compounds, a reaction critical in synthesizing glucose and fatty acids, as well as breaking down certain amino acids. Symptoms of biotin deficiency include a scaly inflammation of the skin, changes in the tongue and lips, decreased appetite, nausea, vomiting, a form of anemia, depression, muscle pain and weakness, and poor growth.

Biotin Sources and Needs. Protein sources, such as egg yolks, peanuts, and cheese, are good sources of biotin (Fig. 12-12). Biotin is not often measured and reported in foods. We do not know the content for several foods. Because intestinal bacteria synthesize and supply some biotin, a biotin deficiency is unlikely. Scientists are not sure how much of the bacteria-synthesized biotin in our intestines is absorbed, so we still need to consume some in our diet. If intestinal bacteria synthesis is not sufficient, as in people who are missing a large part of the colon or who take antibiotics for many months, special attention must be paid to meeting biotin needs. Biotin's bioavailability varies significantly among foods based on its biotin-protein complex. In raw egg whites, biotin is bound to avidin, which inhibits absorption of the vitamin. Consuming many raw egg whites can eventually lead to biotin-deficiency disease. Cooking denatures the protein avidin in eggs so it cannot bind biotin. As long as you avoid raw eggs, you are fine.

The AI set for biotin is 30 micrograms per day for adults; our food supply is thought to provide 40 to 60 micrograms per person per day. The DV used on food and supplement labels is 300 micrograms—10 times the estimate of needs. The DV for biotin was set years before the vitamin had an AI level set, and is based on outdated recommendations.

FIGURE 12-12 ▶ Food sources of biotin compared to the Adequate Intake for adults.

Food Sources of Biotin

Food Item and Amount	Biotin (micrograms)	Adult Male and Female AI = 30 micrograms Daily Value = 300 micrograms %AI
AI	30.0	100%
Smooth peanut butter, 2 tablespoons	30.1	100%
Cooked lamb liver, 1 ounce	11.6	39%
Boiled egg, 1	9.3	31%
Cooked egg yolk, 1	8.1	27%
Yogurt, 1 cup	7.4	25%
Wheat germ, ¼ cup	7.2	24%
Roasted peanuts, 5	6.5	22%
Wheat bran, ¼ cup	6.4	21%
Nonfat milk, 1 cup	4.9	16%
Salmon, 3 ounces	4.3	14%
Egg noodles, 1 cup	4.0	13%
Swiss cheese, 2 ounces	2.2	7%
Cheddar cheese, 2 ounces	1.7	6%
Raw cauliflower, 1 cup	1.5	5%
American cheese, 2 ounces	1.4	5%

Key:
- Grains
- Vegetables
- Fruits
- Dairy
- Protein

ChooseMyPlate.gov

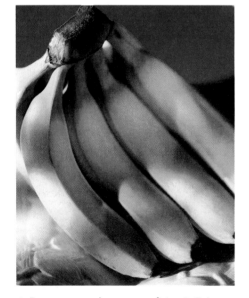

▲ Bananas are a plant source of vitamin B-6.

However, biotin is relatively nontoxic. Large doses (up to 1 milligram/day) have been given over an extended period without harmful side effects to children who exhibit defects in biotin metabolism. Thus, no UL for biotin has been set.

Vitamin B-6 (Pyridoxine)

This vitamin is known by its number, rather than its general name. Vitamin B-6 is a family of three structurally similar compounds. All can be converted into the active vitamin B-6 coenzyme.

Functions of Vitamin B-6. The coenzymes of vitamin B-6 are needed for the activity of numerous enzymes involved in carbohydrate, protein, and lipid metabolism. Vitamin B-6 is required in so many areas of metabolism that a deficiency results in widespread symptoms, including depression, vomiting, skin disorders, irritation of the nerves, anemia, and impaired immune response.

A primary function of vitamin B-6 concerns protein because it functions as a coenzyme in over 100 chemical reactions that involve the metabolism of amino acids and protein (see Fig. 12-1). By helping split the nitrogen group ($-NH_2$) from an amino acid and making it available to another amino acid, the B-6 coenzyme participates in reactions that allow the synthesis of nonessential (dispensable) amino acids.

Among the other important functions of vitamin B-6 are synthesis of neurotransmitters such as serotonin and gamma aminobutyric acid (GABA); conversion of tryptophan to niacin; breakdown of stored glycogen to glucose; and synthesis of hemoglobin and white blood cells. Vitamin B-6 also plays a role in

Food Sources of Vitamin B-6

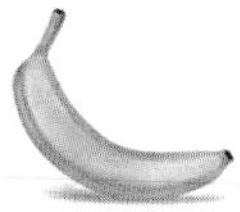

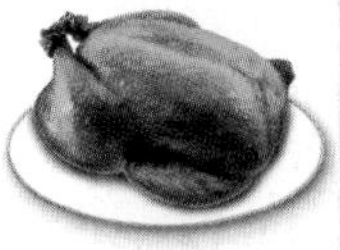

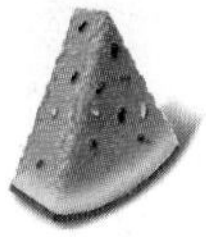

Food Item and Amount	Vitamin B-6 (milligrams)	Adult Male and Female RDA = 1.3 milligrams Daily Value = 2 milligrams %RDA
RDA	1.3	100%
Baked salmon, 3 ounces	0.8	62%
Baked potato, 1 medium	0.7	54%
Banana, 1	0.7	54%
Avocado, 1	0.6	46%
Roasted chicken breast, 3 ounces	0.5	38%
Acorn squash, 1 cup	0.5	38%
Special K cereal, ¾ cup	0.5	38%
Fried beef liver, 1 ounce	0.4	31%
Roasted turkey lunch meat, 3 ounces	0.4	31%
Sirloin steak, 3 ounces	0.4	31%
Lean ham, 3 ounces	0.4	31%
Watermelon, 1 slice	0.3	23%
Sunflower seeds, ¼ cup	0.3	23%
Cooked spinach, ½ cup	0.2	15%

Key:
- Grains
- Vegetables
- Fruits
- Dairy
- Protein

ChooseMyPlate.gov

FIGURE 12-13 ► Food sources of vitamin B-6 compared to the RDA for adults.

homocysteine metabolism (see Further Readings 6, 7, and 11). As you can see, a deficiency in vitamin B-6 would affect multiple body systems, including the cardiovascular, immune, and nervous systems, as well as overall energy metabolism.

Vitamin B-6 is important for the synthesis of the heme portion of **hemoglobin.** A deficiency of vitamin B-6 results in small red blood cells with reduced hemoglobin concentration. This condition (microcytic hypochromic anemia) decreases a cell's ability to produce ATP because aerobic metabolism is limited.

Vitamin B-6 Sources and Needs. Major sources of vitamin B-6 are animal products and fortified ready-to-eat breakfast cereals (Fig. 12-13). Other sources are vegetables and fruits such as potatoes, spinach, bananas, and cantaloupes (Fig. 12-14). Overall, animal sources and fortified grain products are the most reliable because the vitamin B-6 they contain is more absorbable than that in plant foods.

The adult RDA of vitamin B-6 is 1.3 to 1.7 milligrams per day. The DV used on food and supplement labels is 2 milligrams. Average daily consumption of vitamin B-6 for men and women is greater than the RDA.

Athletes may need slightly more vitamin B-6 than sedentary adults. The athlete's body processes large quantities of glycogen and protein, and the metabolism of these compounds requires vitamin B-6. However, unless athletes restrict their food intake, they are likely to consume plenty of protein—enough to supply needed amounts of vitamin B-6.

People with alcoholism are susceptible to a vitamin B-6 deficiency. A metabolite formed in alcohol metabolism can displace the coenzyme form of B-6, increasing its tendency to be destroyed. In addition, alcohol decreases the absorption of vitamin B-6 and decreases the synthesis of its coenzyme form. Cirrhosis and hepatitis (both can accompany alcoholism) also destroy healthy liver tissue. Thus, a cirrhotic liver

homocysteine An amino acid that arises from the metabolism of methionine. Vitamin B-6, folate, vitamin B-12, and choline are required for its metabolism. Elevated levels are associated with an increased risk of cardiovascular disease.

hemoglobin The iron-containing part of the red blood cell that carries oxygen to the cells and carbon dioxide away from the cells. The heme iron portion is also responsible for the red color of blood.

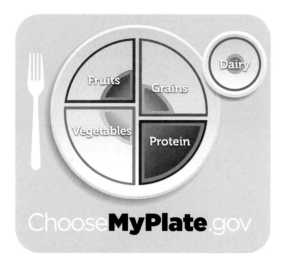

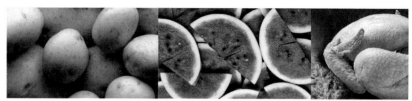

MyPlate:
Sources of Vitamin B-6

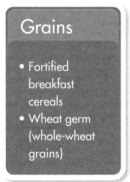

Grains

- Fortified breakfast cereals
- Wheat germ (whole-wheat grains)

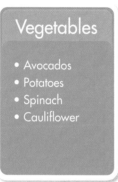

Vegetables

- Avocados
- Potatoes
- Spinach
- Cauliflower

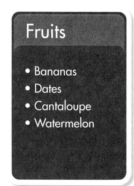

Fruits

- Bananas
- Dates
- Cantaloupe
- Watermelon

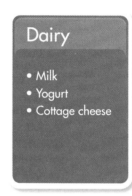

Dairy

- Milk
- Yogurt
- Cottage cheese

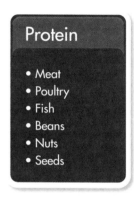

Protein

- Meat
- Poultry
- Fish
- Beans
- Nuts
- Seeds

FIGURE 12-14 ▶ Sources of vitamin B-6 from MyPlate. The fill of the background color (none, 1/3, 2/3, or completely covered) within each group on the plate indicates the average nutrient density for vitamin B-6 in that group. Overall, the protein group especially contains many foods that are nutrient-dense sources of vitamin B-6. With regard to physical activity, vitamin B-6 participates in the related energy metabolism during such endeavors.

cannot adequately metabolize vitamin B-6 or synthesize its coenzyme form. Vitamin B-6 is rather unstable; heating and freezing can easily destroy it.

Upper Level for Vitamin B-6. The UL for vitamin B-6 is 100 milligrams per day, based on the risk of developing nerve damage. Studies have shown that intakes of 2 to 6 grams of vitamin B-6 per day for 2 or more months can lead to irreversible nerve damage. Symptoms of vitamin B-6 toxicity include walking difficulties and hand and foot tingling and numbness. Some nerve damage in individual sensory neurons is probably reversible, but damage to the ganglia (where many nerve fibers converge) appears to be permanent. With 500-milligram tablets of vitamin B-6 available in health-food stores, taking a toxic dose is easy (see Further Reading 8).

CONCEPT CHECK

Pantothenic acid and biotin both participate in the metabolism of carbohydrate and fat. A deficiency of either vitamin is unlikely; pantothenic acid is found widely in foods, and our need for biotin is partially met by intestinal synthesis from bacteria. Vitamin B-6 is important for protein metabolism, neurotransmitter synthesis, homocysteine metabolism, and other key metabolic functions. Headache, a form of anemia, nausea, and vomiting can result from a vitamin B-6 deficiency. Increased risk of cardiovascular disease is also likely. Animal foods, ready-to-eat breakfast cereals, broccoli, spinach, and bananas are some food sources of vitamin B-6. Megadose supplements of vitamin B-6 can lead to nerve damage.

Chromium (Cr)

Chromium is required for glucose uptake into cells by aiding insulin function. Low or marginal chromium intakes may contribute to an increased risk for developing type 2 diabetes, but opinions are mixed on the true degree of this effect.

A chromium deficiency is characterized by impaired blood glucose control and elevated blood cholesterol and triglycerides. The mechanism by which chromium influences cholesterol metabolism is not known but involves enzymes that control cholesterol synthesis. Chromium deficiency appears in people maintained on intravenous total parenteral nutrition solutions not supplemented with chromium and in children with malnutrition. Marginal deficiencies may go undetected, because sensitive measures of chromium status are not available.

Chromium absorption is quite low, at a rate of only 0.4% to 2.5% of the amount consumed. The remainder is excreted in the feces. It is stored in the liver, spleen, soft tissue, and bone. Enhancers to aid absorption are vitamin C and niacin. Certain conditions can enhance urinary excretion of chromium: diets high in simple sugars (more than 35% of total calories), significant infection, acute prolonged exercise, pregnancy and lactation, and major physical trauma. If chromium intakes are already low, these states potentially can lead to deficiency.

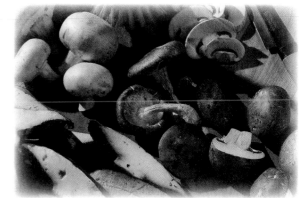

▲ Mushrooms are a good source of chromium.

Chromium Sources and Needs. Specific data regarding the chromium content of various foods are scant, and most food-composition tables do not include values for this trace mineral. Because of two major limits, we really cannot accurately determine the amount of chromium in food: (1) The content is significantly affected by agricultural and manufacturing processes; and (2) when foods are analyzed, they may be "contaminated" by the chromium in the instruments themselves. Meat and whole-grain products, eggs, mushrooms, nuts, beer, and spices are relatively good sources of chromium. Brewer's yeast is also a very good source.

The Adequate Intake (AI) for chromium is 25 to 35 micrograms per day, based on the amount present in a balanced diet. The DV used on food and supplement labels is 120 micrograms. Average adult intakes in North America are estimated at about 30 micrograms per day but could be somewhat higher.

No UL for chromium has been set because toxicity for that present in foods has not been observed. Chromium toxicity, however, has been reported in people exposed to industrial waste and in painters who use art supplies with high chromium content. Liver damage and lung cancer can result. Use of any supplement should normally not exceed the DV unless supervised by a physician, because of the risk of toxicity.

Manganese (Mn)

The mineral manganese is easily confused with magnesium (Mg). Not only are their names similar, but they also often substitute for each other in metabolic processes. Manganese is needed by some enzymes, such as those used in free-radical metabolism (via superoxide dismutase). Manganese is also important in bone formation. As a participant in energy metabolism, manganese is required as a cofactor for synthesis of glucose and metabolism of some amino acids.

Manganese deficiency does not develop in humans unless the mineral is purposely removed from the diet. Animals on manganese-deficient diets suffer alterations in brain function, bone formation, and reproduction. If human diets were low in manganese, these symptoms would probably appear as well. As it happens, our need for manganese is very low, and our diets tend to be adequate in this trace mineral.

Good food sources of manganese are nuts, rice, oats, and other whole grains, beans, and leafy vegetables. The AI for manganese is 1.8 to 2.3 milligrams to

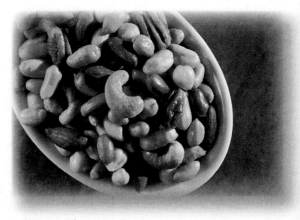

▲ Nuts are rich in manganese.

offset daily losses. Average intakes fall within this range. The DV used on food and supplement labels is 2 milligrams. Manganese is toxic at high doses. Supplements are not recommended, as large doses can decrease absorption of other minerals. People with low iron stores must avoid manganese supplements or risk worsening anemia.

Upper Level for Manganese. The UL is 11 milligrams per day. This value is based on the development of nerve damage. Miners who have inhaled dust fumes high in manganese experience symptoms that mimic Parkinson's disease, including cognitive and muscular dysfunction.

Molybdenum (Mo)

Several human enzymes use molybdenum, including some involved in metabolism of amino acids that contain sulfur. No molybdenum deficiency has been reported in people who consume diets orally. Deficiency symptoms have appeared in people maintained on intravenous total nutrition devoid of this trace mineral. Symptoms include increased heart and respiratory rates, night blindness, mental confusion, edema, and weakness.

Good food sources of molybdenum include milk and dairy products, beans, whole grains, and nuts. The RDA for molybdenum is 45 micrograms to offset daily losses. The DV used on food and supplement labels is 75 micrograms. Our daily intakes average 76 micrograms (for women) and 109 micrograms (for men).

Upper Level for Molybdenum. The Upper Level for molybdenum is 2 milligrams per day. When consumed in high doses, molybdenum causes toxicity in laboratory animals, resulting in weight loss and decreased growth. Toxicity risk in humans is quite low.

Table 12-1 summarizes much of what we know about the energy-related B vitamins.

12.3 Vitamins and Minerals Involved in Blood Health

The human body has a number of elaborate systems to keep its roughly 100 trillion cells alive and properly functioning. One of these marvels is the circulatory system. As you learned in Chapter 3, the circulatory system delivers oxygen and nutrients to the cells. Blood is the conduit through which nutrients are disseminated throughout the body. Blood consists of four distinct elements: white cells, red cells, platelets, and plasma.

All blood cells are formed in bone marrow. As shown in Figure 12-15, these bone marrow stem cells, called **pluripotential stem cells,** are self-renewing. They also have the potential to become any type of blood cell. While in the bone marrow, these stem cells and their subsequent **progenitor cells** separate into the various types of cells found in circulating blood. Once these progenitor cells mature into more defined cells, they are committed to that cell and pass into circulating blood.

What we commonly call white blood cells, or **leukocytes,** are actually five types of cells, each with its own function: **neutrophils, lymphocytes, monocytes, eosinophils,** and **basophils. Erythrocytes** (red blood cells) and **platelets** also result from bone marrow stem cells. Erythrocytes are the most prevalent component of blood. Platelets function in blood clotting; they clump together at the site of an injury, forming a plug to slow the rate of bleeding until a permanent clot can form. If your platelet count is low, your clotting time is prolonged. The fourth component of blood, **plasma,** is the extracellular portion devoid of these cells. It is the largest portion of blood, approximately 55% of the total volume. Often, when you have blood tests done, it is your plasma levels that are measured. Plasma contains proteins, carbohydrates, lipids, hormones, enzymes, and electrolytes.

basophil The WBC that controls inflammation; level increases with poisoning.

eosinophil This WBC is a type of phagocyte that increases in number during allergic attacks.

erythrocyte Red blood cell (RBC); transports oxygen to cells.

leukocyte White blood cell (WBC); cell of the immune system.

lymphocyte The WBC responsible for the immune response; regulates antibody production.

monocyte The WBC that ingests foreign cells; called a phagocyte.

neutrophil A common WBC that fights infections; levels rise during bacterial or fungal infections.

plasma The fluid, extracellular portion of blood.

platelet A protoplasmic disc smaller than an RBC that promotes coagulation.

pluripotential stem cells Self-renewing cells that have the potential to become various kinds of cells.

progenitor cells Like stem cells, can self-renew but are more defined and cannot differentiate into as many types of cells.

TABLE 12-1 Summary of the Vitamins and Minerals Involved in Energy Metabolism

Vitamin	Major Functions	Adult RDA or AI	Dietary Sources*	Deficiency Symptoms	Toxicity Symptoms
Iodide	• Component of thyroid hormones	150 micrograms	• Iodized salt • White bread • Saltwater fish • Dairy products	• Goiter • Mental retardation • Poor growth in infancy when mother is iodide deficient during pregnancy	Upper Level is 1.1 milligrams, based on inhibition of thyroid gland function.
Thiamin	• Coenzyme of carbohydrate metabolism • Nervous function	1.1–1.2 milligrams	• Sunflower seeds • Pork • Whole and enriched grains • Dried beans • Peas	*Beriberi* • Nervous tingling • Poor coordination • Edema • Heart changes • Weakness	None
Riboflavin	• Coenzyme of carbohydrate metabolism	1.1–1.3 milligrams	• Milk • Mushrooms • Spinach • Liver • Enriched grains	• Inflammation of the mouth and tongue • Cracks at the corners of the mouth • Eye disorders	None
Niacin	• Coenzyme of energy metabolism • Coenzyme of fat synthesis • Coenzyme of fat breakdown	14–16 milligrams (niacin equivalents)	• Mushrooms • Bran • Tuna • Salmon • Chicken • Beef • Liver • Peanuts • Enriched grains	*Pellagra* • Diarrhea • Dermatitis • Dementia • Death	Upper Level is 35 milligrams from supplements, based on flushing of skin.
Pantothenic acid	• Coenzyme of energy metabolism • Coenzyme of fat synthesis • Coenzyme of fat breakdown	5 milligrams	• Mushrooms • Liver • Broccoli • Eggs *Most foods have some*	• No natural deficiency disease or symptoms	None
Biotin	• Coenzyme of glucose synthesis • Coenzyme of fatty acid synthesis • Coenzyme of protein breakdown	30 micrograms	• Peanut butter • Lamb liver • Eggs • Milk • Whole grains	• Inflammation of the skin and mouth • Nausea/vomiting • Anemia • Depression • Muscle pain/weakness	None
Vitamin B-6	• Coenzyme of energy metabolism • Coenzyme of protein synthesis • Synthesis of heme	1.3–1.7 milligrams	• Salmon • Potato • Banana • Avocado • Chicken • Fortified cereal	• Irritability • Insomnia • Muscle weakness • Anemia	Upper Level is 100 milligrams, based on risk of developing nerve damage.
Chromium	• Aids insulin function	25–35 micrograms	• Meats • Whole grains • Brewer's yeast	• Impaired glucose tolerance • Elevated blood lipids	None from foods; environmental exposure leads to liver damage and lung cancer.
Manganese	• Cofactor for glucose synthesis • Cofactor for amino acid metabolism • Cofactor for antioxidant systems	1.8–2.3 milligrams	• Nuts • Whole grains • Beans • Leafy vegetables	None observed in humans	Upper Level is 11 milligrams based on development of nervous system disorders.
Molybdenum	• Cofactor for amino acid metabolism	45 micrograms	• Beans • Grains • Nuts	None observed in healthy humans	Upper Level is 2 milligrams based on poor laboratory growth in animals.

*Fortified ready-to-eat breakfast cereals are good and readily available sources of vitamins and minerals for many of us.

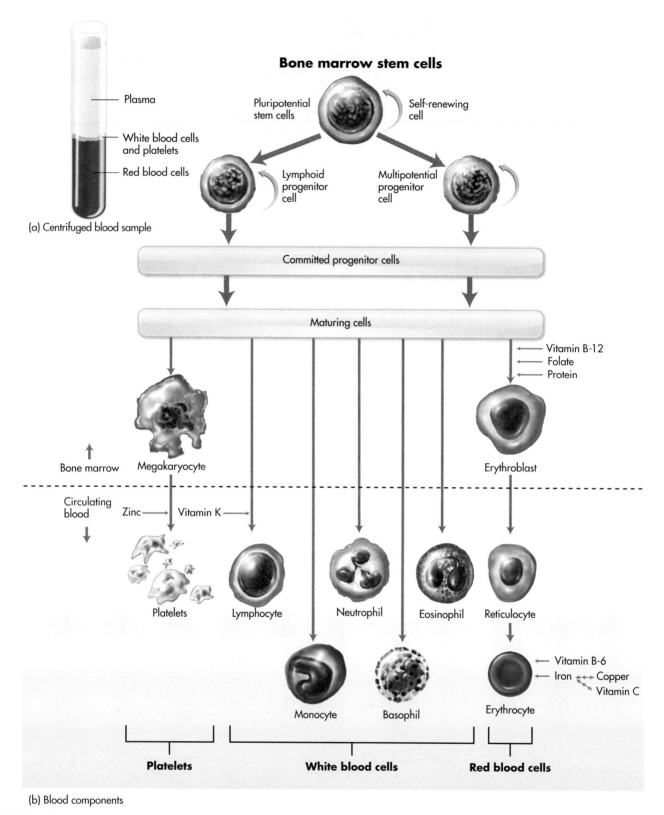

(a) Centrifuged blood sample

(b) Blood components

FIGURE 12-15 ▶ (a) When placed in a centrifuge, whole blood separates into its four components: red blood cells, white blood cells, platelets, and plasma. (b) Blood cells from formation to circulation and nutrients that affect their formation.

The Roles of Vitamins and Minerals in Blood Health

Vitamins and minerals provide critical functions for maintenance of blood health. In this section, we will address the vitamins and minerals most directly concerned with preserving blood health. Vitamin K is essential for clotting. Two B vitamins—folate, and B-12—are essential for RBC formation. Without iron, the RBCs would not be able to deliver oxygen to the cells. Copper is essential for ceruloplasmin, an enzyme that releases iron from storage. Without adequate intake of these nutrients, blood health is compromised.

Vitamin K (Quinone)

A family of compounds known collectively as vitamin K is found in plants, plant oils, fish oils, and animal products. Vitamin K is also synthesized by bacteria in the human colon, which normally fulfills approximately 10% of human requirements. Vitamin K has three forms. The naturally occurring form (phylloquinone) is synthesized by green plants. Gut bacteria synthesize menaquinone, and menadione is the synthetic form found in supplements. Interestingly, this synthetic, menadione form of vitamin K is twice as biologically available as the other two!

Functions of Vitamin K. In concert with a number of proteins and calcium, vitamin K is vital for the life-and-death process of blood clotting (Fig. 12-16). Danish researchers first noted the relationship between vitamin K and blood clotting. The "K" stands for *koagulation* in the Danish language.

Serum is plasma from which clotting factors have been removed.

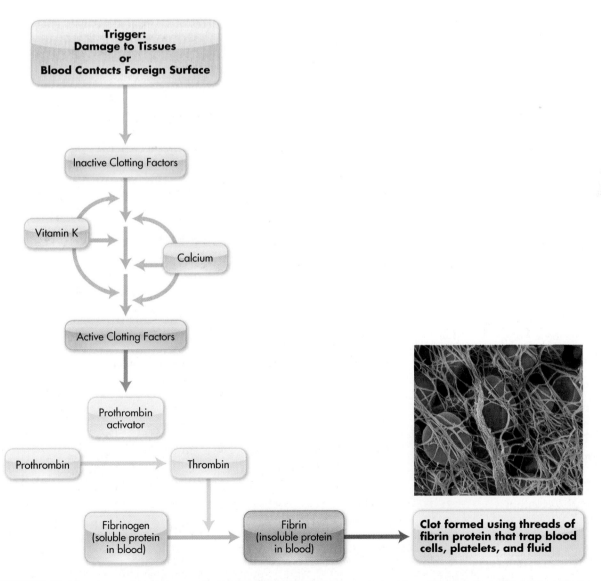

FIGURE 12-16 ▶ Vitamin K works to activate clotting factors, which are then able to bind calcium. This calcium binding to clotting factors is necessary for clot formation.

As you can see in Figure 12-16, vitamin K and calcium keep the clotting factors active. They help activate prothrombin into thrombin, a critical protein to convert soluble fibrinogen into insoluble fibrin (i.e., the clot). Adults who have had a stroke or a heart valve replacement, or have problems with blood circulation, may be placed on Coumadin or what are called "blood thinners." This name is a misnomer. Coumadin (or warfarin) does not thin blood; it is an anticoagulant, inhibiting vitamin-K-dependent coagulation factors. When taking Coumadin or any other anticoagulant, it is important to keep vitamin K intake consistent from day to day (see Further Reading 10).

In addition to its role in formation of blood clots, vitamin K is needed for the addition of CO_2 molecules to various proteins in the body and enables proteins to bind calcium. Binding of calcium to osteocalcin is important for bone health.

At birth, a newborn has what is termed a "sterile gut," that is, an intestinal tract with an insufficient amount of bacteria. In turn, newborns cannot produce enough vitamin K to allow for effective blood clotting if the infant is injured or needs surgery. Therefore, vitamin K is routinely administered by injection shortly after birth. In adults, deficiencies of vitamin K have occurred when a person takes antibiotics for an extended time (this destroys the bacteria that normally produce some of the vitamin K subsequently absorbed) and when fat absorption is limited.

Vitamin K Sources and Needs. Major food sources of vitamin K are liver, green leafy vegetables, broccoli, asparagus, and peas (Fig. 12-17). Vitamin K is widespread in foods; therefore, a deficiency is rare. Vitamin K is resistant to cooking losses. Like other

Food Sources of Vitamin K

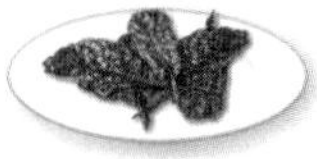

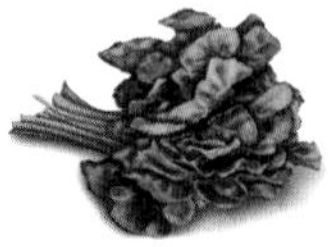

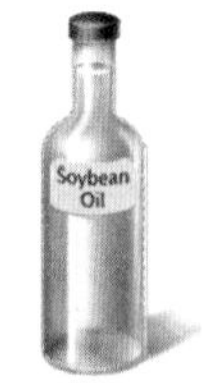

Food Item and Amount	Vitamin K (micrograms)	Adult Male AI = 120 micrograms %AI	Adult Female AI = 90 micrograms %AI
RDA	90-120	100%	100%
Cooked kale, ½ cup	530	442%	589%
Cooked turnip greens, 1 cup	520	433%	578%
Cooked spinach, 1 cup	480	400%	533%
Cooked Brussels sprouts, ½ cup	150	125%	167%
Raw spinach, 1 cup	144	120%	160%
Cooked asparagus, 1 cup	144	120%	160%
Cooked broccoli, ½ cup	110	92%	122%
Looseleaf lettuce, 1 cup	97	81%	108%
Cooked green beans, ½ cup	49	41%	54%
Raw cabbage, 1 cup	42	35%	47%
Sauerkraut, ½ cup	30	25%	33%
Green peas, ½ cup	26	22%	29%
Soybean oil, 1 tablespoon	25	21%	28%
Cooked cauliflower, 1 cup	20	17%	22%
Canola oil, 1 tablespoon	17	14%	19%

Daily Value = 80 micrograms

Key:
- Grains
- Vegetables
- Fruits
- Dairy
- Protein
- Oils

FIGURE 12-17 ▶ Food sources of vitamin K compared to the Adequate Intake for adult males and females.

fat-soluble vitamins, absorption of vitamin K relies on consuming some dietary fat and having adequate liver and pancreatic secretions.

The AI for vitamin K is 90 to 120 micrograms per day for adults. The DV used on food labels is 80 micrograms. Intake of an adequate amount of vitamin K can be a problem in the elderly due to low consumption of vegetables. A UL has not been established for vitamin K because no reports of toxicity have been published.

Anatomy of a Red Blood Cell

Vitamins and minerals are key to erythropoiesis, or the formation of red blood cells (RBCs). The primary function of RBCs is to carry oxygen from your lungs to the tissues. A secondary function is to carry the waste product, carbon dioxide, from the tissues to your lungs. Unlike most cells, RBCs have no nucleus (Fig. 12-18). During maturation, the nucleus is lost to make room for **hemoglobin,** a large protein containing iron. The iron in hemoglobin binds and carries four molecules of oxygen.

RBCs have a flattened concave surface to increase surface area. This allows more oxygen to diffuse through the membrane to bind to the iron. Red cells are also very flexible, allowing them to squeeze through the tiny capillaries of the circulatory system.

Anemia

Anemia develops due to inadequate healthy red blood cells. There are two reasons anemia may occur: (1) a decrease in production of red blood cells or of the hemoglobin in the cells, or (2) a loss or destruction of blood. Symptoms of anemia are associated with inadequate oxygen to the various organs. When anemia develops and RBCs are evaluated, they are described based on size and color. Normal RBCs are called normocytic (normal size) and normochromic (normal color). When there are

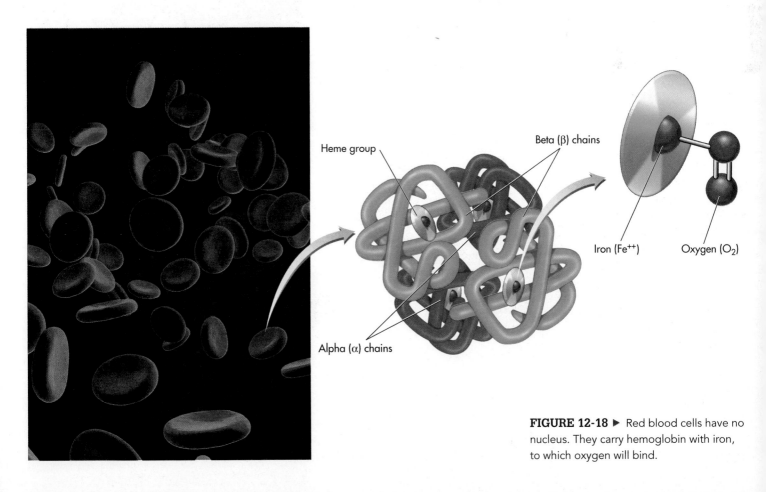

FIGURE 12-18 ▶ Red blood cells have no nucleus. They carry hemoglobin with iron, to which oxygen will bind.

nutrient deficiencies, the size and/or color of the red blood cells may be affected. Examining the size and color of the RBCs helps an observer to determine the cause of the anemia. The following sections present the vitamins and minerals that contribute to blood health. Deficiencies are leading causes for anemia.

Folate (Vitamin B-9)

The term *folate* encompasses a variety of food forms of the vitamin. Folate is the form occurring naturally in food. Folic acid is the synthetic form added to fortified foods and present in supplements.

Functions of Folate. A key role of the folate coenzyme is to supply or accept single carbon compounds. In this role, folate coenzymes help form DNA and metabolize amino acids and their derivatives, such as homocysteine.

One major result of a folate deficiency is that in the early phases of red blood cell synthesis, the immature cells cannot divide because they cannot form new DNA. The cells grow progressively larger because they can still synthesize enough protein and other cell parts to make new cells. When the time comes for the cells to divide, the amount of DNA is insufficient to form two nuclei. The cells then remain in a large immature form, known as a **megaloblast** (Fig. 12-19).

Few mature red blood cells **(erythrocytes)** arrive in the bloodstream because the bone marrow of a folate-deficient person produces mostly immature megaloblast

megaloblast A large, immature red blood cell that results from the inability of the cell to divide normally (*megalo* = large; *blast* = primitive or immature).

erythrocyte Mature red blood cell. Erythrocytes have no nucleus and a life span of about 120 days; they contain hemoglobin, which transports oxygen and carbon dioxide.

FIGURE 12-19 ▶ Megaloblastic anemia occurs when blood cells are unable to divide, leaving large, immature red blood cells. Either a folate or vitamin B-12 deficiency may cause this condition. Measurements of blood concentrations of both vitamins are taken to help determine the cause of the anemia.

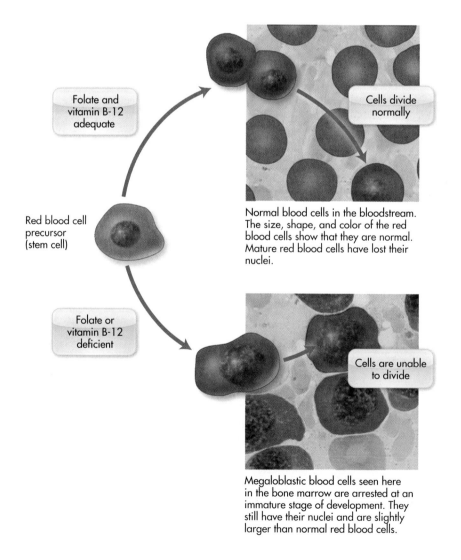

Folate and vitamin B-12 adequate

Cells divide normally

Red blood cell precursor (stem cell)

Normal blood cells in the bloodstream. The size, shape, and color of the red blood cells show that they are normal. Mature red blood cells have lost their nuclei.

Folate or vitamin B-12 deficient

Cells are unable to divide

Megaloblastic blood cells seen here in the bone marrow are arrested at an immature stage of development. They still have their nuclei and are slightly larger than normal red blood cells.

cells. When fewer mature red blood cells are present, the blood's capacity to carry oxygen decreases, causing a form of anemia. In short, a folate deficiency causes **megaloblastic anemia** (also called macrocytic or large-cell anemia).

Changes in red blood cell formation occur after 7 to 16 weeks on a folate-free diet, depending on the person's folate stores. White blood cell formation is also affected but to a lesser degree. In addition, cell division throughout the entire body is disrupted. Clinicians focus primarily on red blood cells because they are easy to collect and examine. Other symptoms of folate deficiency are inflammation of the tongue, diarrhea, poor growth, mental confusion, depression, and problems in nerve function.

megaloblastic (macrocytic) anemia Anemia characterized by the presence of abnormally large red blood cells.

neural tube defect A defect in the formation of the neural tube occurring during early fetal development. This type of defect results in various nervous system disorders, such as spina bifida. Folate deficiency in the pregnant woman increases the risk that the fetus will develop this disorder.

MAKING DECISIONS

Some forms of cancer therapy provide a vivid example of the effects of a folate deficiency on DNA metabolism. A cancer drug, methotrexate, closely resembles a form of folate but cannot act in its place. When methotrexate is taken in high doses, because of this resemblance, it hampers folate metabolism. Methotrexate crowds out folate in the metabolic pathways. As a consequence, DNA synthesis is retarded and cell division decreases. Cancer cells are among the most rapidly dividing cells in the body, so they are among those first affected. However, other rapidly dividing cells, such as intestinal cells and skin cells, are also affected. Not surprisingly, typical side effects of methotrexate therapy are diarrhea, vomiting, and hair loss. These are also typical symptoms of folate deficiency. Today, when patients are given methotrexate, they need to consume a folate-rich diet or take folic-acid supplements in order to reduce the toxic side effects of the drug. High supplemental doses have little or no influence on methotrexate's effectiveness as a cancer therapy.

Maternal deficiency of folate along with a genetic abnormality related to folate metabolism have been linked to development of **neural tube defects** in the fetus (Fig. 12-20). These defects include spina bifida (spinal cord or spinal fluid bulge through the back) and anencephaly (absence of a brain). Annually, about 1500 infants are affected with neural tube defects in the United States (see Further Reading 9). Victims of spina bifida exhibit paralysis, incontinence, learning disabilities, and other health problems. Children born with anencephaly die shortly after birth. Adequate folate status is crucial for all women of childbearing age because the neural tube

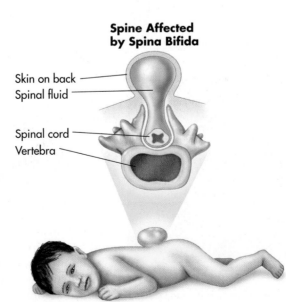

Healthy Spine

Skin on back

Spinal cord
Spinal fluid
Vertebra

Spine Affected by Spina Bifida

Skin on back
Spinal fluid

Spinal cord
Vertebra

FIGURE 12-20 ▶ Neural tube defects result from a developmental failure affecting the spinal cord or brain in the embryo. Very early in fetal development, a ridge of neural-like tissue forms along the back of the embryo. As the fetus develops, this material develops into both the spinal cord and nerves at the lower end and into the brain at the upper end. At the same time, the bones that make up the back gradually surround the spinal cord on all sides. If any part of this sequence goes awry, many defects can appear. The worst case is total lack of a brain (anencephaly). Spina bifida, in which the back bones do not form a complete ring to protect the spinal cord, is much more common. Deficient folate status in the mother during the beginning of pregnancy, especially in combination with a genetic abnormality in folate metabolism, greatly increases the risk of neural tube defects.

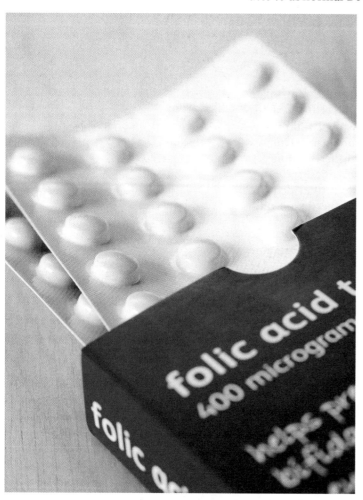

▲ An objective of *Healthy People 2020* is to increase by 10% the proportion of women of childbearing potential who take supplements containing folic acid prior to pregnancy.

closes within the first 28 days of pregnancy, a time when many women are not even aware that they are pregnant. Hence, a recommendation is made that ample folate, specifically 400 micrograms of folic acid per day, be consumed at least 6 weeks before conception. Folic acid is more than twice as biologically available as folate (see Making Decisions on page 440).

Almost all related research has been done with folic acid supplementation. It appears that even women with varied diets may not consume adequate folic acid to prevent neural tube defects unless specific attention to rich sources is given. As many as 70% of these defects could be avoided by adequate folate status before conception. Whereas most pregnant women are advised to consume 600 micrograms of folic acid, women who have had a child with a neural tube defect are advised to consume 4000 micrograms per day of folic acid. They are to begin supplementation at least 1 month before any future pregnancy. This must be done under strict physician supervision.

Along with vitamin B-6 (discussed in the previous section) and vitamin B-12 (see page 441), folate is required for the metabolism of homocysteine (see Further Reading 11). Blood homocysteine levels have been associated with cardiovascular risk; elevated homocysteine is considered an independent risk factor for atherosclerosis. Research is ongoing to examine the impact of folate (and other B vitamins) on cardiovascular disease risk.

Research is also underway on the link between folate and cancer protection. Folate aids in DNA synthesis, so it is hypothesized that even mild folate deficiency contributes to abnormal DNA integrity, which in turn affects certain cancer-producing genes. Meeting the RDA for folate is thought to be one way to reduce cancer risk.

A final function of folate is the formation of neurotransmitters in the brain. Meeting folate needs can improve the depressed state in some cases of mental illness.

Consuming fortified ready-to-eat breakfast cereals that contain 100% of the DV for folate (this is the same as the RDA) is a good practice for meeting the goal for folic acid intake. A multivitamin and mineral supplement can also be used to supply adequate folic acid. Women must be careful to monitor the amount of any accompanying preformed vitamin A content (do not exceed 100% of the DV).

Folate Sources and Needs. Green, leafy vegetables (folate is derived from the Latin word *folium*, which means foliage or leaves); other vegetables; orange juice; dried beans; and organ meats are the richest sources of folate (Fig. 12-21). The vitamin C in orange juice also reduces folate destruction. Fortified ready-to-eat breakfast cereals, bread, and milk are important sources of folic acid for many adults (Fig. 12-22).

Folate is susceptible to destruction by heat. Food processing and preparation destroy 50% to 90% of the folate in food. This underscores the importance of regularly eating fresh fruits and raw or lightly cooked vegetables.

The RDA of folate for adults is 400 micrograms per day, as is the DV used on food and supplement labels. Folate recommendations for all but women of childbearing age are based on dietary folate equivalents (DFE). The DFE takes into account the bioavailability of folate in food and folic acid added to food and present in supplements. See Making Decisions, below, to learn how to calculate folate intake.

Pregnant women need extra folate (a total of 600 micrograms DFE) to accommodate the increased rates of cell division and DNA synthesis in their bodies and in the developing fetus.

Food Sources of Folate

Food Item and Amount	Folate (micrograms)	Adult Male and Female RDA = 400 micrograms Daily Value = 400 micrograms %RDA	
RDA	400		100%
Asparagus, 1 cup	263		66%
Cooked spinach, 1 cup	262		66%
Cooked lentils, ½ cup	179		45%
Black-eyed peas, ½ cup	179		45%
Romaine lettuce, 1½ cups	114		29%
Great Grains cereal, ¾ cup*	114		29%
Tortilla, 1*	89		22%
Cooked turnips, ½ cup	85		21%
Cooked broccoli, 1 cup	78		20%
Sunflower seeds, ¼ cup	76		19%
Fresh orange juice, 1 cup	75		19%
Cooked beets, ½ cup	68		17%
Kidney beans, ½ cup	65		16%
Fried beef liver, 1 ounce	62		16%

Key:
- ■ Grains
- ■ Vegetables
- ■ Fruits
- ■ Dairy
- ■ Protein

* Folic acid.

FIGURE 12-21 ▶ Food sources of folate compared to the RDA for adults.

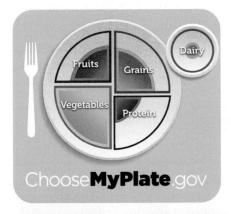

ChooseMyPlate.gov

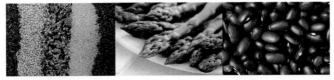

MyPlate: Sources of Folate

Grains*
- Fortified breakfast cereals
- Wheat germ (whole-wheat grains)
- Enriched grains

Vegetables
- Asparagus
- Leafy green vegetables

Fruits
- Oranges
- Strawberries
- Cantaloupes and other melons

Dairy
- Cottage cheese
- Yogurt

Protein
- Liver
- Eggs
- Beans
- Sunflower seeds

* Folic acid in fortified grain products.

FIGURE 12-22 ▶ Sources of folate from MyPlate. The fill of the background color (none, 1/3, 2/3, or completely covered) within each group on the plate indicates the average nutrient density for folate in that group. Overall, the vegetables group provides the richest sources, but the fruits group and the grains group contain some foods that are nutrient-dense sources of folate. With regard to physical activity, folate is especially important for red blood cell synthesis, which is essential for transporting oxygen and carbon dioxide to and from exercising muscles.

A healthy diet can supply this much. Still, prenatal care often includes a specially formulated multivitamin and mineral supplement enriched with folic acid to help compensate for the extra needs associated with pregnancy.

Prior to 1998, average daily folate intakes in the United States were approximately 320 micrograms for men and 220 micrograms for women. In 1998, the Food and Drug Administration (FDA) mandated the fortification of grain products with folate with the aim of reducing birth defects of the spine. With this mandate, average intakes have increased by about 200 micrograms per day. Studies have shown this practice has decreased rates of neural tube defects in infants by an estimated 15% to 30% in the United States (see Further Reading 1). Other factors (genetics, environment) play a role in the development of neural tube defects.

The mandated folic-acid enrichment of grains has also been accompanied by a noticeable decline in cardiovascular risk, especially risk for stroke, due to a drop in blood homocysteine levels among U.S. adults. Supplements of folic acid, B-12, and B-6 have been promoted to help lower homocysteine and decrease cardiac and stroke risk. Recent large and well-controlled studies and analyses of several other studies indicate that low-dose folate treatment (such as the food fortification) just may reduce cardiovascular risk in people with elevated blood homocysteine levels. However, taking supplemental doses at pharmacological levels is not likely to benefit people who have blood homocysteine levels in the normal range.

Older people may be at risk for folate deficiency, possibly due to a combination of inadequate folate intake and decreased absorption. Perhaps these people fail to consume sufficient amounts of fruits and vegetables because of poverty or physical problems, such as poor dental health. In addition, folate deficiencies often occur with alcoholism, due mostly to poor intake and absorption. Symptoms of a folate-related anemia can alert a physician to the possibility of alcoholism.

MAKING DECISIONS

Food Folate Content

Using the dietary folate equivalent (DFE) will enhance your awareness of the difference in bioavailability of folate and folic acid. Here's how:

1 DFE = 1 microgram folate from food
      = 0.6 microgram folic acid from food
      = 0.5 microgram folic acid from a supplement on an empty stomach

So, a breakfast of toast with peanut butter and a glass of orange juice would contain a rich source of folate (OJ) and folic acid (fortified flour in the toast). Peanut butter would not add significantly.

Upper Level for Folate. The UL for folate is 1 milligram (1000 micrograms) but only refers to folic acid; you cannot buy folate supplements, only folic acid. This is because folate, the natural form in food, has limited absorption. Large doses of folate can hide the signs of vitamin B-12 deficiency and therefore complicate its diagnosis. Specifically, regular consumption of large amounts of folate can prevent the appearance of an early warning sign of vitamin B-12 deficiency—enlarged red blood cell size. To prevent such masking of vitamin B-12 deficiency, it is the goal of the FDA, through its enactment of folate fortification of grains, to increase the folate status of women of childbearing age without causing excessive intake (over 1 milligram of folic acid per day) by other groups. Also, because of risk of masking a vitamin B-12 deficiency, FDA limits supplements for nonpregnant adults and food fortification to 400 microgram amounts.

Folate is needed for cell division because it is required for DNA synthesis. A folate deficiency results in megaloblastic (macrocytic) anemia, as well as elevated homocysteine, inflammation of the tongue, diarrhea, and poor growth. Excess folate intake can mask a vitamin B-12 deficiency because these vitamins work together in metabolism. Folate is found in fruits and vegetables, beans, and organ meats. Emphasizing fresh and lightly cooked vegetables in the diet is important because much folate is lost during cooking. Women of childbearing age should meet needs by consuming a source of synthetic folic acid. Folate needs during pregnancy are especially high; a deficiency around the time of conception and in the first month of pregnancy may lead to neural tube defects in the fetus.

Vitamin B-12 (Cobalamin or Cyanocobalamin)

Vitamin B-12 represents a family of compounds that contain the mineral cobalt. Vitamin B-12 compounds are synthesized by bacteria, fungi, and other lower organisms.

The body's complex means of absorbing vitamin B-12 is unique to this vitamin. A combination of the vitamin itself (often called the extrinsic factor because it comes from outside your body) plus a protein produced in the stomach (the **intrinsic factor**) must be present in adequate quantities and in the proper environmental conditions. Following are the steps for B-12 absorption:

1. Vitamin B-12 from food is bound to protein. It must be liberated from this protein in an acid environment. Stomach acid must be high enough to free B-12.
2. Intrinsic factor is secreted by cells lining the stomach.
3. B-12 and intrinsic factor (EF/IF) complex travels to the lower small intestine (ileum) for absorption. Here, 50% of B-12 is absorbed, depending on the body's needs.

> **intrinsic factor** A proteinlike compound produced by the stomach that enhances vitamin B-12 absorption in the ileum.

If any of Steps 1 through 3 fail or are altered, absorption can drop to 1% to 2%.

If a defect in the digestion and absorption of vitamin B-12 develops, the person usually takes monthly injections of vitamin B-12, uses nasal gels of the vitamin to bypass the need for absorption, or takes megadoses of a supplemental form (300 times the RDA). In this latter case, the vitamin B-12 absorption defect is overcome by providing enough of the vitamin via simple diffusion across the intestinal tract.

About 95% of cases of vitamin B-12 deficiencies in healthy people result from defective absorption, rather than from inadequate intakes. This is especially true for older people. As we age, stomach acid production declines and our stomachs have a decreased ability to synthesize the intrinsic factor needed for vitamin B-12 absorption.

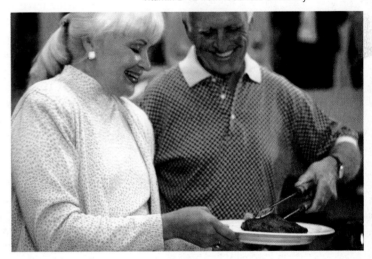

▼ As we age, our digestive system absorbs vitamin B-12 from food less efficiently.

Functions of Vitamin B-12. Vitamin B-12 participates in a variety of cellular processes. The most important function is folate metabolism. B-12 is required to convert folate coenzymes to the active forms needed for metabolic reactions, such as DNA synthesis. Without vitamin B-12, reactions that require certain active forms of folate do not take place in the cell. Thus, a deficiency of vitamin B-12 can result in symptoms of a folate deficiency including elevated homocysteine levels in the blood (see Further Reading 11).

Another vital function of vitamin B-12 is maintaining the myelin sheath that insulates neurons from each other. Initial neurological symptoms of B-12 deficiencies include irregular muscular actions and impaired reflexes. Eventual destruction of the myelin sheath causes paralysis and, perhaps, even death. In the past, vitamin B-12 deficiencies eventually led to death, mainly due to the destruction of nerves. Clinically, the anemia looks much like folate-deficiency anemia, characterized by the appearance of many large red blood cells in the bloodstream. However, the true cause of **pernicious anemia** is poor vitamin B-12 absorption rather than inadequate folate intake. Some symptoms of pernicious anemia include weakness, tongue inflammation, back pain, apathy, and tingling in the extremities.

Because we are able to store some vitamin B-12, symptoms of nerve destruction do not develop until after about 3 years from the onset of the disease. Unfortunately, substantial nerve destruction often occurs before the anemia is detected, and this destruction is irreversible. Pernicious anemia and its accompanying nerve destruction start after middle age, affecting up to 20% of older adults. The explanation for this age-associated pernicious anemia is twofold. First, aging is often associated with reduced production of stomach acid. Thus, vitamin B-12 is not cleaved from substances to which it is bound. Second, aging may be accompanied by reduced output of intrinsic factor. Because of decreased resistance with aging, older adults may develop an autoimmune disease causing the stomach lining to waste away, limiting the production of intrinsic factor.

Infants breastfed by vegetarian mothers are at risk for vitamin B-12 deficiency accompanied by anemia and long-term nervous system problems, such as diminished brain growth, degeneration of the spinal cord, and poor intellectual development. The problems may have their origins during pregnancy, when the mother is deficient in vitamin B-12. Vegan diets supply little vitamin B-12 unless they include vitamin B-12-enriched food (e.g., soymilk) or supplements, so achieving an adequate vitamin B-12 intake is a key diet-planning goal for vegans.

Some medications interact to reduce B-12 absorption or create an environment to lower absorption. Antacids or other medications used to inhibit acid secretions will increase the pH within the stomach, thereby limiting release of B-12 from protein. People who have ulcers, heartburn, or reflux may take these drugs. Metformin, a popular medication for controlling diabetes, may reduce B-12 absorption. With any of these medications, you should check with your physician to see if supplemental B-12 is recommended.

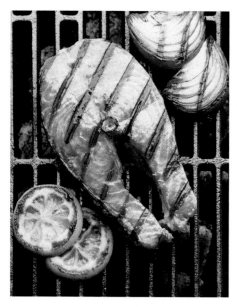

▲ Salmon, rainbow trout, and other types of seafood are excellent sources of B-12.

Vitamin B-12 Sources and Needs. Organ meats (especially liver, kidneys, and heart) are especially rich sources of vitamin B-12. Other major sources of vitamin B-12 include meat, salmon, seafood, ready-to-eat breakfast cereals, milk, and eggs (Fig. 12-23). Adults over age 50 are encouraged to seek a synthetic vitamin B-12 source to increase absolute absorption, which can be limited due to both reduced intrinsic factor and stomach acid output. Synthetic vitamin B-12 is not food-bound, so it does not need stomach acid to release it from foods. It will be more readily absorbed than the form found in food. Ready-to-eat breakfast cereals and multivitamin and mineral supplements are two possible synthetic sources.

The RDA of vitamin B-12 for adults is 2.4 micrograms per day. The DV used on food and supplement labels is 6 micrograms. On average, adults consume two times the RDA or more. This high intake provides the average meat-eating person with 2 to 3 years' storage of vitamin B-12 in the liver.

A person would have to consume a diet essentially free of vitamin B-12 for approximately 20 years before exhibiting nerve destruction caused by a dietary deficiency. Still, vegans, who eat no animal products, should find a reliable source of vitamin B-12, such as fortified soy or rice milk, ready-to-eat breakfast cereals, and a form of yeast grown on media rich in vitamin B-12. Use of a multivitamin and mineral supplement containing vitamin B-12 is another option (see Further Reading 8). Pernicious anemia most frequently develops after a few years of the loss of vitamin B-12 absorption capacity. The quicker appearance is because of the reduced ability to reabsorb vitamin B-12 excreted into the GI tract during digestion, coupled with reduced absorption of dietary sources. Vitamin B-12 supplements are essentially nontoxic, so no UL has been set.

Food Sources of Vitamin B-12

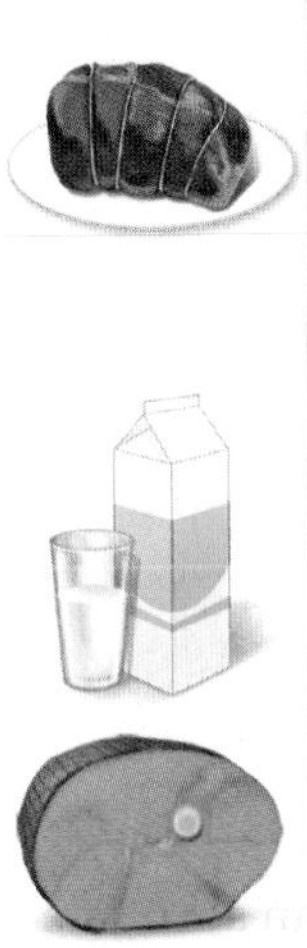

Food Item and Amount	Vitamin B-12 (micrograms)	Adult Male and Female RDA = 2.4 micrograms		
		Daily Value = 6 micrograms %RDA		
RDA	2.4	100%		
Fried beef liver, 1 ounce	31.7	1321%		
Baked clams, 1 ounce	15.7	654%		
Boiled oysters, 2	14.4	600%		
Salmon, 3 ounces	4.9	167%		
Pot roast, 3 ounces	2.5	104%		
Plain yogurt, 1 cup	1.4	58%		
Corn Flakes cereal, ¾ cup	1.1	46%		
Shrimp, 3 ounces	1.0	42%		
1% milk, 1 cup	0.9	38%		
Soy milk, 1 cup	0.8	33%		
Boiled egg, 1	0.6	25%		
Lean ham, 3 ounces	0.6	25%		
Beef hot dog, 1	0.5	21%		
Ham lunch meat, 2 ounces	0.4	17%		

Key: ChooseMyPlate.gov
- Grains
- Vegetables
- Fruits
- Dairy
- Protein

FIGURE 12-23 ▶ Food sources of vitamin B-12 compared to the RDA for adults.

Following the success of folate fortification, some experts advocate widespread fortification of the food supply with vitamin B-12 (see Further Reading 3).

CONCEPT CHECK

Vitamin B-12 is necessary for folate metabolism. Without dietary vitamin B-12, folate-deficiency symptoms, such as macrocytic anemia, develop. In addition, vitamin B-12 is necessary for maintaining the nervous system. Paralysis can develop from a prolonged vitamin B-12 deficiency. The vitamin also participates in homocysteine metabolism. The absorption of vitamin B-12 requires an acidic environment in the stomach and binding to intrinsic factor. If absorption is inhibited, the resulting deficiency can lead to pernicious anemia and nerve destruction. Concentrated amounts of vitamin B-12 are found only in animal foods; meat-eaters generally have a 2- to 3-year supply stored in the liver. Vegans need to find an alternate source. Vitamin B-12 absorption may decline as we age. Monthly injections, nasal gels, or megadoses can make up for this.

Iron (Fe)

Although the importance of dietary iron has been recognized for many years, iron deficiency is the most common nutrient deficiency worldwide. About 30% of the world's population are anemic, and half of these cases are caused by iron deficiency. Iron is the only nutrient for which young women have a greater RDA than do adult men.

Functions of Iron. Iron is part of the hemoglobin in red blood cells and myoglobin in muscle cells (see Fig. 12-24). Hemoglobin molecules in red blood cells transport oxygen (O_2) from the lungs to cells and then transport carbon dioxide (CO_2) from

hematocrit The percentage of blood made up of red blood cells.

heme iron Iron provided from animal tissues in the form of hemoglobin and myoglobin. Approximately 40% of the iron in meat, fish, and poultry is heme iron; it is readily absorbed.

myoglobin Iron-containing protein that binds oxygen in muscle tissue.

nonheme iron Iron provided from plant sources, supplements, and animal tissues other than in the forms of hemoglobin and myoglobin. Nonheme iron is less efficiently absorbed than heme iron; absorption is closely dependent on body needs.

phytic acid A constituent of plants that binds positive ions to its multiple phosphate groups.

oxalic acid An organic acid found in spinach and rhubarb that can depress the absorption of certain minerals present in the food, such as calcium and iron.

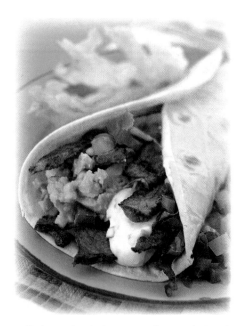

▲ Red meat is a major source of iron in the North American diet. The heme iron present is better absorbed than the nonheme iron found in meats and plants.

cells to the lungs for excretion. In addition, iron is used as part of many enzymes, some proteins, and compounds that cells use in energy production. Iron also is needed for brain and immune function, drug detoxification in the liver, and synthesis of collagen for bone health.

If neither the diet nor body stores can supply the iron needed for hemoglobin synthesis, the concentration of hemoglobin and red blood cells decreases. Medical professionals use both the percentage of blood that consists of red blood cells (**hematocrit**) and the hemoglobin concentration to assess iron status. Other measures indicative of poor iron status include the concentration of iron and iron-containing proteins in blood (serum iron, ferritin, or transferrin). When hematocrit and hemoglobin fall, an iron deficiency is suspected. In severe deficiency, hemoglobin and hematocrit fall so low that the amount of oxygen carried in the bloodstream is decreased. This condition is called iron-deficiency anemia.

Iron deficiency can be categorized into three stages:

- In the first stage, iron stores become depleted but no physiological impairment is observed.
- The second stage involves depletion of circulating iron in transferrin, and some physiological impairment occurs. Heme production is decreased, and activity of enzymes that require iron as a cofactor are limited.
- The last stage is iron-deficiency anemia, in which the red blood cells are small (microcytic) and pale (hypochromic) and their number is reduced.

There are many conditions that lead to an anemic state; iron-deficiency anemia is the most prevalent worldwide. Probably about 10% of North Americans in high-risk categories have iron-deficiency anemia. This appears most often in infancy, the preschool years, and at puberty for both males and females. Growth, with accompanying expansion of blood volume and muscle mass, increases iron needs, making it difficult to consume enough iron. Women are vulnerable to anemia during childbearing years from blood loss during menstruation; anemia is also found in pregnant women. Iron-deficiency anemia in adult men is usually caused by blood loss from ulcers, colon cancer, or hemorrhoids. Athletes can have increased iron requirements due to increased blood loss in feces and urine and chronic lysis of red blood cells in the feet due to the trauma of running.

Absorption and Distribution of Iron. Iron absorption is tightly regulated. Controlling absorption is important because the human body highly conserves iron; approximately 90% is recovered and reused every day. Overall, iron absorption depends on three factors: (1) its form in food, (2) the person's iron status, and (3) other dietary components found in food. Relative to most other nutrients, iron absorption is low. If iron status is normal, absorption can be as low as 2%; however, if iron status is low, or needs are high, as in pregnancy and growth, absorption can be as high as 50%. Healthy people with adequate iron stores absorb between 5% and 15% of dietary iron.

Next to iron stores being the greatest influence in the rate of iron absorption, the other big influence is the form of iron in the food. **Heme** iron, derived from **hemoglobin** and **myoglobin,** comprises 40% of the iron in meat, fish, and poultry (MFP). Absorption of heme iron ranges from about 15% to 35%. Almost nothing affects its absorption. **Nonheme iron,** on the other hand, is subject to many conditions, that can either enhance or inhibit its absorption, which ranges from 2% to 8%. Nonheme iron is found in MFP (the remaining 60%), dairy, eggs, fruit, vegetables, grains, fortified foods, and supplements. Because most of our diet is from nonheme iron, our overall dietary iron absorption is 5% to 15%.

As mentioned, there are dietary enhancers and inhibitors to nonheme absorption. These dietary factors affect the bioavailability of the nonheme iron. Table 12-2 summarizes dietary factors that affect nonheme bioavailability.

TABLE 12-2 Dietary Iron Enhancers and Inhibitors

Nonheme Enhancers	Nonheme Inhibitors

• Vitamin C
  • Add marinara sauce to your spaghetti noodles.
• MFP (meat, fish, poultry) meat protein
  • Add some tuna to your snack of crackers.
	• Tannins (found in tea)
	  • Can lower absorption up to 60%, so drink tea between meals. Does not apply to herbal "tea," which contains no tea leaves.
	• Oxalates (spinach, rhubarb, chard)
	• Phytates (whole grain, bran, soybean)
	• Megadoses of zinc, calcium, or copper

Other inhibitors include taking antacids that are all calcium, as well as medications that control stomach acid secretion 'round the clock. The acidic environment of the stomach solubilizes iron and keeps it in a form more readily absorbed. Also, as people age, gastric acid becomes less efficient; therefore, iron-deficiency anemia tends to become more prevalent with older adults. Megadoses of zinc, copper, or calcium compete for absorption and inhibit absorption of iron. On the other hand, vitamin C is a powerful enhancer. Doses of 75 milligrams can increase nonheme absorption by 4%—a lot for nonheme! One of the best ways to boost iron intake is to drink a glass of orange juice when you take your multivitamin pill.

How do you balance inhibitors and enhancers? The best thing to do is look at your meal. Is it a high-iron meal? If there are a few good sources of nonheme iron, and you have some vitamin C with it (e.g., green beans or red pepper strips), then that would be a meal in which to avoid iced tea, which contains tannins (see Table 12-2) If, on the other hand, it is a meal of peanut butter on whole wheat with an apple, this is not a high-iron meal, and a glass of iced tea would not do much damage.

The most important factor influencing nonheme iron absorption is body need. Iron needs are increased during pregnancy and growth. At high altitudes, the lower oxygen concentration of the air causes an increase in the hemoglobin concentration of blood and thus an increase in iron needs. When iron stores are inadequate, the main protein that carries iron (transferrin) readily binds more iron, shifting it from intestinal cells into the bloodstream. If iron stores are adequate and the iron-binding protein in the blood is fully saturated with iron, absorption from the intestinal cells is minimal. The iron remains in the intestinal cells. This mechanism allows iron to be absorbed as needed. High doses of iron can still be toxic, but absorption is carefully regulated under most dietary conditions. Except for bleeding associated with menstruation, injury, or childbirth, body loss of iron is minimal. The principal mechanism to regulate iron content in the body is tight control of absorption.

Clinical symptoms of iron-deficiency anemia are associated with the lack of oxygen to the tissues. One experiences pale skin, fatigue upon exertion, poor temperature regulation (always cold, especially toes and fingers), loss of appetite, and apathy. Poor iron stores may decrease learning ability, attention span, work performance, and immune status even before a person is anemic. Children with chronic anemia have abnormal cognitive development (see Further Reading 4). More North Americans have an iron deficiency without anemia than have iron-deficiency anemia. Their blood hemoglobin values are still normal, but they have no stores to draw from in times of pregnancy or illness, and basic functioning may be at decreased levels. That could mean anything from too little energy to perform everyday tasks in an efficient manner to difficulties staying mentally alert.

To cure iron-deficiency anemia, a person needs to take iron supplements (see Further Reading 8). A physician should also find the cause so that the anemia does not reoccur. Changes in diet may prevent iron-deficiency anemia, but supplemental iron is the only reliable cure once it has developed. Supplements must be taken for 3 to 6 months or perhaps longer. Hemoglobin levels respond quickly to dietary changes and supplementation, but terminating supplements too soon means that iron stores

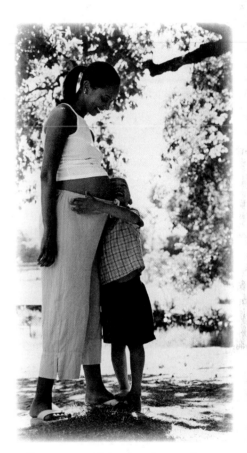

▲ Pregnancy greatly increases iron needs, as does growth in childhood.

The iron added to foods and in most dietary supplements is nonheme iron.

Food Sources of Iron

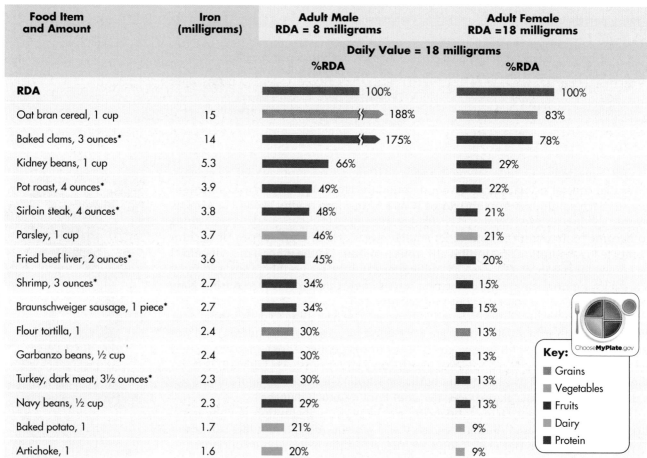

Food Item and Amount	Iron (milligrams)	Adult Male RDA = 8 milligrams %RDA	Adult Female RDA =18 milligrams %RDA
RDA		100%	100%
Oat bran cereal, 1 cup	15	188%	83%
Baked clams, 3 ounces*	14	175%	78%
Kidney beans, 1 cup	5.3	66%	29%
Pot roast, 4 ounces*	3.9	49%	22%
Sirloin steak, 4 ounces*	3.8	48%	21%
Parsley, 1 cup	3.7	46%	21%
Fried beef liver, 2 ounces*	3.6	45%	20%
Shrimp, 3 ounces*	2.7	34%	15%
Braunschweiger sausage, 1 piece*	2.7	34%	15%
Flour tortilla, 1	2.4	30%	13%
Garbanzo beans, ½ cup	2.4	30%	13%
Turkey, dark meat, 3½ ounces*	2.3	30%	13%
Navy beans, ½ cup	2.3	29%	13%
Baked potato, 1	1.7	21%	9%
Artichoke, 1	1.6	20%	9%

Daily Value = 18 milligrams

Key: ChooseMyPlate.gov
- Grains
- Vegetables
- Fruits
- Dairy
- Protein

* Contains heme iron.

FIGURE 12-24 ▶ Food sources of iron compared to the RDA for adult males and females.

(blood, bone marrow, etc.) will not be replenished. It takes time to replenish these stores. So, let's say you feel better after a month on iron therapy, then you quit taking your supplements because of the side effects (e.g., stomach upset, constipation). You slip back to your former eating habits. Within a few weeks, you will start to experience the symptoms of anemia again—"brain fog," cold, fatigue. What happened? Only your superficial (hemoglobin) stores of iron were replenished. You needed the full 3 to 6 months of supplementation to replenish all of your stores. Remember, it did not take just 1 month to become anemic, so it will not take just 1 month to cure it.

Iron Sources and Needs. Animal sources contain approximately 40% heme iron, the most bioavailable form. The major iron sources in the adult diet are ready-to-eat breakfast cereals, beans, and animal products (Fig. 12-24). Iron is added to flour during the enrichment process. Other iron sources are peas and legumes, but the absorption of nonheme iron found in these products is relatively low (Fig. 12-25).

Milk and eggs are poor sources of iron. A common cause of iron-deficiency anemia in children is high consumption of milk coupled with insufficient meat intake. Vegans are particularly susceptible to iron-deficiency anemia because of their lack of dietary heme iron.

The adult RDA is based on a 10% absorption rate to cover average losses of about 0.8 milligrams per day. Thus, the RDA for men is 8 milligrams. Menstrual loss is variable, with a 1-gram loss per day considered average for women ages 19 to 50 years.

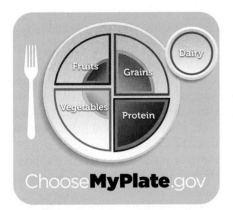
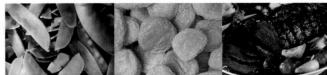

**MyPlate:
Sources of Iron**

Grains	Vegetables	Fruits	Dairy	Protein
• Whole grains • Enriched grains • Wheat germ • Oatmeal	• Spinach • Peas • Potatoes • Green beans • Broccoli	• Peaches • Prune juice • Dried apricots	• None	• Beef • Tofu • Beans • Seafood • Organ meats

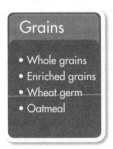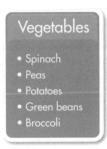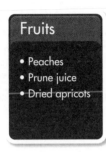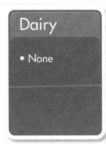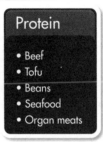

FIGURE 12-25 ▶ Sources of iron from MyPlate. The fill of the background color (none, 1/3, 2/3, or completely covered) within each group on the plate indicates the average nutrient density for iron in the group. Overall, the protein group and the grains group contain many foods that are nutrient-dense sources of iron. Still, the iron content of a food containing mostly nonheme iron is only an approximate measure of the amount delivered to body cells, as body need greatly influences the absorption of nonheme iron. With regard to physical activity, iron is especially needed as part of the hemoglobin that carries oxygen in the red blood cells to muscle (and other) cells.

Thus, the RDA for women in this age range is 18 milligrams. Postmenopausal women's RDA is the same as that of men, 8 milligrams. The DV used on food and supplement labels is 18 milligrams.

Most women do not consume 18 milligrams of iron daily. The average daily amount consumed by women is closer to 13 milligrams, while in men it is about 18 milligrams per day. Women in this age group can close this gap between average daily intakes and needs by seeking out iron-fortified foods, such as ready-to-eat breakfast cereals that contain at least 50% of the DV. Use of a balanced multivitamin and mineral supplement containing up to 100% of the DV for iron is another option. Consuming more than that much iron is not advised unless recommended by a physician.

MAKING DECISIONS

Blood Donation

The adult human body contains about 21 cups (5 liters) of blood. Blood donations are 2 cups (500 milliliters). Thus, a blood donor gives about 10% of the total blood found in the body. Healthy people can generally donate blood two to four times a year without harmful consequences. As a precaution, blood banks first screen potential donors' blood for the presence of anemia. Red blood cells contain about two-thirds of total body iron and have a life span of about 120 days. At the end of the life span of a red blood cell, the iron is efficiently recycled or stored for later use.

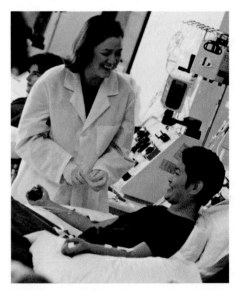

▲ Young adult women should limit frequent blood donations because a significant amount of iron is lost in each donation.

Upper Level for Iron. The UL for iron is 45 milligrams per day. Higher amounts can lead to stomach irritation. Although iron overload is not as common as iron deficiency, it can be a serious result of misuse because it can easily build up in the body

hemochromatosis A disorder of iron metabolism characterized by increased iron absorption and deposition in the liver and heart. This eventually poisons the cells in those organs.

phlebotomy Therapeutic blood removal, as a blood donation, for the purpose of ridding the body of excess iron.

and lead to toxic symptoms. Even a large single dose of 60 milligrams of iron can be life threatening to a 1-year-old. Children are frequently victims of iron poisoning (acute toxicity) because iron pills and supplements containing iron are tempting and available when accessible on kitchen tables and even from cabinets. The FDA requires that all iron supplements carry a warning about toxicity, and those with 30 milligrams of iron or more per tablet must be individually wrapped.

Iron toxicity accompanies the genetic disease, hereditary **hemochromatosis** (see Further Reading 2). The disease is associated with a substantial increase in iron absorption from both food and supplements. Most affected are iron-storing organs such as the liver and heart. Infections are likely. Some iron is deposited in the pancreas and muscles. Blood levels remain high, too. If not treated, iron can be deposited to dangerously high levels to cause severe organ damage.

Development of hereditary hemochromatosis requires that a person carry two defective copies of a particular gene. People with one defective gene and one normal gene, called carriers, may also absorb too much dietary iron but not to the same extent as those with two defective genes. About 5% to 10% of North Americans of Northern European descent are carriers of hemochromatosis. Approximately 1 in 250 North Americans has both hemochromatosis genes. These numbers are high considering that many physicians regard hemochromatosis as a rare disease and therefore do not routinely test for it.

Anyone who has a blood relative (even including uncles, aunts, and cousins) who has hemochromatosis or is a carrier should be screened for iron overload. At your next visit to a physician, ask for a transferrin-saturation test to assess iron stores. A ferritin test may also be added to assess your stores. Hemochromatosis can go undetected until a person is in his 50s or 60s, so some experts recommend screening for anyone over the age of 20. If the disease goes untreated, iron overload progresses and serious health problems may result, including skin pigmentation, arthritis, heart disease, diabetes, liver disease, and cancer (colon). Even with iron overload, the person may have anemia due to damage to the bone marrow or liver. Treatment of hemochromatosis is relatively easy, but it must be monitored consistently. Routine **phlebotomies** to remove excess iron are essential. One must be very careful about the diet. Few heme iron foods should be eaten and supplements with iron or vitamin C should be avoided. Highly fortified breakfast cereals must also be avoided.

CONCEPT CHECK

Iron absorption depends on its form and the body's need for it. Absorption is affected by iron needs but excess iron intake can override the body's ability to effectively control absorption, leading to toxicity. Nonheme iron absorption increases in the presence of vitamin C and meat protein and decreases in the presence of large amounts of some components of grain, such as fiber and phytic acid. Iron is used in synthesizing hemoglobin and myoglobin, supporting immune function, and metabolizing energy. An iron deficiency can cause decreased red blood cell synthesis, which can lead to anemia. It is particularly important for women of childbearing age to consume adequate iron, primarily to replace that lost in menstrual blood. Sources include red meat, pork, liver, enriched grains and cereals, and oysters. Iron toxicity causes overabsorption and accumulation of iron, which can result in severe liver and heart damage. Any use of iron supplements should be supervised by a physician, because of the risk of toxicity.

Copper (Cu)

Copper and iron are similar in terms of food sources, absorption, and functions. Copper is a component of blood. In the body, it is found in highest concentration in the liver, brain, heart, and kidneys. Yet, muscles contain 40% of all the copper in the body. Copper is a component of ceruloplasmin, a protein with several different functions. In the bone marrow, ceruloplasmin functions as an enzyme to help form red blood cells.

A copper-containing enzyme aids in the release of iron from storage. Copper is needed by enzymes that create cross-links in connective tissue proteins, such as the collagen in bone. Copper is also needed by other enzymes, such as those that defend the body against free-radical damage (e.g., superoxide dismutase) and those that act in the brain and nervous system. Finally, copper performs in immune system function, blood clotting, and blood lipoprotein metabolism. Copper absorption is highly variable, with higher intakes associated with lower absorption efficiency. Absorption takes place in the stomach and upper small intestine. Excess copper is not stored to a great extent, so when intake exceeds needs, the liver incorporates it into bile, which is excreted by the feces. Phytates, fiber, and excessive zinc and iron supplements may all interfere with copper absorption. Symptoms of copper deficiency include a form of anemia, low white blood cell count, bone loss, poor growth, and some forms of cardiovascular disease.

Copper Sources and Needs. Rich sources of copper include liver, legumes, seeds, whole-grain breads and cereals, and cocoa (Fig. 12-26). Milk and dairy products, fruit, and vegetables are generally poor sources of copper.

The RDA for copper is 900 micrograms for adults, based on the amount needed for activity of copper-containing proteins and enzymes. The DV used on food and supplement labels is 2 milligrams. The average adult intake is about 1 milligram for women and 1.6 milligrams for men per day. The form of copper typically found in multivitamin and mineral supplements (copper oxide) is not readily absorbed. It is best to rely on food sources to meet copper needs. The copper status of adults appears to be good, although sensitive laboratory tests to determine copper status are lacking.

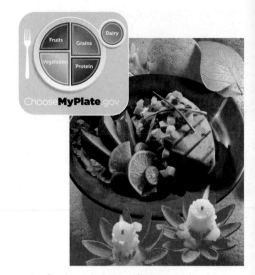

▲ Seafood is one source of copper in the diet. How does this meal of grilled tuna steak with peach salsa compare to MyPlate?

Food Sources of Copper

FIGURE 12-26 ▶ Food sources of copper compared to the RDA.

Food Item and Amount	Copper (milligrams)	Adult Male and Female RDA = 900 milligrams — Daily Value = 2 milligrams %RDA
RDA*	900	100%
Fried beef liver, 3 ounces	3800	422%
Power bar, 1	700	78%
Walnuts, ½ cup	600	67%
Kidney beans, ½ cup	500	56%
Lobster, 3 ounces	400	44%
Molasses, 3 tablespoons	300	33%
Sunflower seeds, 2 tablespoons	300	33%
Shrimp, 3 ounces	300	33%
Raisin Bran cereal, 1 cup	300	33%
Great Grains cereal, 1 cup	300	33%
Black-eyed peas, ½ cup cooked	200	22%
Wheat germ, ¼ cup	200	22%
Milk chocolate, 1 ounce	110	12%
Whole-wheat bread, 1 slice	80	9%

Key: ChooseMyPlate.gov
- Grains
- Vegetables
- Fruits
- Dairy
- Protein
- Discretionary calories

*For adults; see the DRI table in the back of this book for gender- and age-specific recommendations.

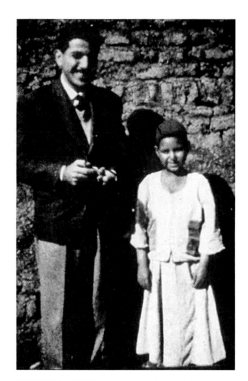

FIGURE 12-27 ▶ Low intakes of zinc limit growth in people worldwide. On the right, an Egyptian farm boy, 16 years old and 49 inches tall, with limited growth and sexual development associated with zinc deficiency.

The groups most likely to develop copper deficiencies are preterm infants recovering from semistarvation on a milk-dominated diet (a poor source of copper) and people recovering from intestinal surgery. A copper deficiency can result from overzealous supplementation of zinc, because zinc and copper compete with each other for absorption.

Upper Level for Copper. The UL for copper is 10 milligrams per day. High doses of copper can cause toxicity with a single dose of greater than 10 milligrams. Consequences of copper toxicity include gastrointestinal distress, vomiting blood, tarry feces, and damage to the liver and kidneys. Toxicity cannot occur with food, just supplements or excessive exposure to copper salts used in agriculture. Wilson's disease is a genetic disease in which the liver cannot synthesize ceruloplasmin. In turn, copper accumulates in such tissues as lungs and liver. A primary treatment for Wilson's disease is a vegan diet, as fruits and vegetables are low in copper.

Zinc (Zn)

Zinc deficiency was first recognized in the early 1960s in Egypt and Iran. Zinc deficiencies were determined to cause growth retardation and poor sexual development in some groups of people (Fig. 12-27). Even though the zinc content of their diets was fairly high, the customary diet contained unleavened bread almost exclusively and little animal protein. Unleavened bread is high in phytic acid and other factors that decrease zinc bioavailability. Parasite infestation and the practice of eating clay and other parts of soil also contributed to the severe zinc deficiency. Adding yeast (leavening) breaks down phytic acid, making zinc in leavened products more bioavailable.

In North America, zinc deficiencies were first observed in the early 1970s in hospitalized patients fed only intravenously via total parenteral nutrition. The protein source in earlier intravenous solutions was based on milk protein or a blood protein, both naturally rich in zinc. When the solutions were changed to include mostly individual amino acids as the protein source, deficiency symptoms quickly developed because of their low zinc content.

Zinc absorption is influenced by the foods a person ingests. About 40% of dietary zinc is absorbed, especially when animal protein sources are used and when the body needs more zinc. Most people worldwide rely on cereal grains (low in zinc) for their source of protein, calories, and zinc. This habit makes consuming adequate zinc a problem. High-dose calcium supplementation with meals decreases zinc availability at the meal. Finally, zinc competes with copper and iron for absorption, and vice versa, when supplemental sources are consumed. Supplements with more than 100% of the Daily Value for individual minerals are not advised without medical supervision.

Functions of Zinc. Approximately 200 enzymes require zinc as a cofactor for activity. Adequate zinc intake is necessary to support many physiological functions, such as:

- DNA synthesis and function
- Protein metabolism, wound healing, and growth
- White blood cell formation and function (intakes in excess of the RDA do not provide any extra benefit to immune function)
- Development of sexual organs and bones
- Storage, release, and function of insulin
- Cell membrane structure and function
- Component of superoxide dismutase (SOD), an enzyme that aids in the prevention of oxidative damage to cells (Zinc, therefore, has an indirect antioxidant function.)

Other possible functions of zinc are slowing the progression of macular degeneration of the eye and reducing the risk for developing certain forms of cancer.

Food Sources of Zinc

Food Item and Amount	Zinc (milligrams)	Adult Male RDA = 11 milligrams %RDA	Adult Female RDA = 8 milligrams %RDA
		Daily Value = 15 milligrams	
RDA		100%	100%
Steamed oysters, 3	24.9	226%	311%
Sirloin steak, 4 ounces	7.4	67%	93%
Pot roast, 3 ounces	4.6	42%	58%
Special K cereal, 1 cup	3.8	35%	48%
Wheat germ, ¼ cup	3.5	32%	44%
Lamb chops, 3 ounces	2.7	25%	34%
Peanuts, ½ cup	2.4	22%	30%
Black-eyed peas, 1 cup	2.2	20%	28%
Plain yogurt, 1 cup	2.2	20%	28%
Lean ham, 3 ounces	1.9	17%	24%
Swiss cheese, 1.5 ounces	1.7	15%	21%
Ricotta cheese, ½ cup	1.7	15%	21%
Sunflower seeds, 1 ounce	1.5	14%	19%
Cheddar cheese, 1.5 ounces	1.3	12%	16%
Enriched white rice, ½ cup	1.1	10%	14%

Key:
- Grains
- Vegetables
- Fruits
- Dairy
- Protein

FIGURE 12-28 ▶ Food sources of zinc compared to the RDA for adult males and females.

Symptoms of adult zinc deficiency include an acnelike rash, diarrhea, lack of appetite, delayed wound healing, reduced sense of taste (metallic-like) and smell, and hair loss. In children and adolescents with zinc deficiency, growth, sexual development, and learning ability may also be hampered.

Zinc Sources and Needs. Protein-rich diets are high in zinc. Animal foods supply almost half of zinc intake. Major sources of zinc are beef, fortified breakfast cereals, wheat germ, and some cheese (Fig. 12-28). The food source influences bioavailability of zinc. Zinc found in animal foods is better absorbed than that found in plants. Phytic acid binding in whole grains limits zinc, but other plant sources of zinc do contribute to zinc intake (Fig. 12-29). The form generally used in multivitamin and mineral supplements (zinc oxide) is not as well-absorbed as zinc found naturally in foods but still contributes to meeting zinc needs. In North America, almost 80% of zinc is provided by meat, fish, poultry, fortified cereal, and dairy products.

The adult RDA for zinc is 11 milligrams for men and 8 milligrams for women, based on the amount to cover daily losses of zinc. The DV used on food and supplement labels is 15 milligrams. The average North American consumes 10 to 14 milligrams of zinc a day, with men consuming the higher values. There are no indications of moderate or severe zinc deficiencies in an otherwise healthy adult population. It is likely, however, that some North Americans—especially some poor children, vegans, and older people with alcoholism—have a marginal zinc status (see Further Reading 5). These and other people who show deterioration in taste sensation, recurring infections, poor growth, or depressed wound healing should have their zinc status checked.

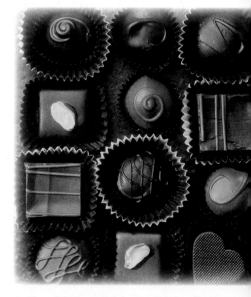

▲ Chocolate is a good source of zinc and magnesium. Eaten in moderation, chocolate, like other foods, can be part of a healthy diet.

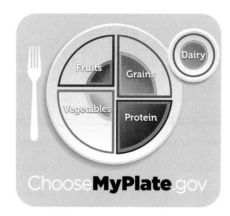

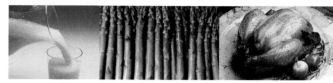

MyPlate:
Sources of Zinc

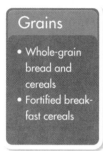

Grains

- Whole-grain bread and cereals
- Fortified breakfast cereals

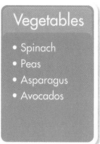

Vegetables

- Spinach
- Peas
- Asparagus
- Avocados

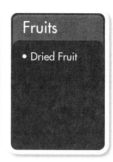

Fruits

- Dried Fruit

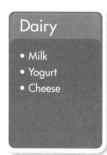

Dairy

- Milk
- Yogurt
- Cheese

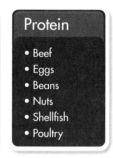

Protein

- Beef
- Eggs
- Beans
- Nuts
- Shellfish
- Poultry

FIGURE 12-29 ▶ Sources of zinc from MyPlate. The fill of the background color (none, 1/3, 2/3, or completely covered) within each group on the plate indicates the average nutrient density for zinc in that group. Overall, the protein group and the grains group contain many foods that are nutrient-dense sources of zinc. With regard to physical activity, zinc is especially needed to support muscle growth and muscle healing.

Upper Level for Zinc. The UL for zinc is 40 milligrams per day. Excessive zinc intake over time can lead to problems by interfering with copper metabolism. The interference with copper metabolism is the basis for setting the UL. Zinc toxicity can occur from zinc supplements and overconsumption of zinc-fortified foods. A person using megadose supplementation should be under close medical supervision and also take a supplement containing copper (2 milligrams per day). Zinc intakes over 100 milligrams result in diarrhea, cramps, nausea, vomiting, loss of appetite, and depressed immune system function, especially if intake exceeds 2000 milligrams per day. Intakes consistently over 2000 milligrams per day can lead to a depressed immune system and decreased high-density lipoproteins (HDLs).

Case Study Anemia

Anita is a 60-year-old woman who prides herself on taking charge of her health. She exercises daily, whether it is walking her dog, playing golf, or a tai chi class at the senior center. She follows the 2010 Dietary Guidelines for Americans, choosing a variety of whole grains; eating at least five servings per day of fruits and vegetables; and keeping her saturated fat, *trans* fat, cholesterol, and sodium intakes to a minimum. She eats lean sources of protein, choosing poultry, fish, or vegetable sources of protein instead of red meat. She maintains a healthy body weight, has never had high blood pressure or high blood sugar, and does not take any medications or supplements.

Last week, she went to a blood drive at her church with the intent of donating blood, but she was turned away because her hematocrit (a measure of the percentage of red blood cells in the blood) was slightly below the requirements for donation. Anita was surprised because she had never had a problem donating blood before. The nurse told Anita that her low hematocrit level was indicative of anemia, which has many possible causes. As Anita

thought about it, she realized that she had been feeling more tired than usual.

Answer the following questions and check your responses in Appendix A.

1. Iron deficiency is the most common form of anemia. What role does iron play in the health of red blood cells? From the description, is it possible that Anita has low iron stores? What dietary changes could Anita make to improve her iron status?

2. A deficiency of vitamin B-6 is another possible cause of anemia. What role does vitamin B-6 play in the health of red blood cells? From the description, is it likely that Anita is deficient in vitamin B-6?

3. Folate deficiency may lead to anemia. What role does folate play in the health of red blood cells? From the description, is it likely that Anita is deficient in folate?

4. Low vitamin B-12 may result in anemia. What role does vitamin B-12 play in the health of red blood cells? Suggest an explanation for why Anita may have low

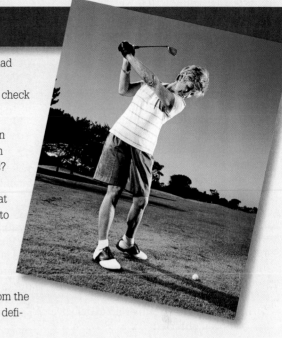

vitamin B-12 status even with adequate dietary intake of vitamin B-12. What dietary changes could Anita make to improve her vitamin B-12 status?

5. What should Anita do now that she knows she is anemic? Will changes to her food choices suffice to resolve the problem?

Summary (Numbers refer to numbered sections in the chapter.)

12.1 The B vitamins yield no energy directly, but they contribute to energy-yielding chemical reactions in the body by virtue of their coenzyme functions. B vitamins are highly bioavailable. North American diets are typically adequate in B vitamins except in cases of poverty, metabolic disorders, or alcoholism. Whole grains are more nutrient-dense sources of B vitamins (as well as other nutrients) than refined grains.

12.2 Several B vitamins function as coenzymes in energy metabolism. In addition, iodide, chromium, manganese, and molybdenum participate in various aspects of metabolism of carbohydrates, lipids, and protein.

Iodide is necessary for the synthesis of thyroid hormones, which regulate metabolism, growth, and development.

Iodized salt, some seafood, dairy products, and grain products are dietary sources of iodide. A dietary deficiency of iodide can lead to enlargement of the thyroid gland (goiter) or, for the offspring of deficient mothers, impaired physical and mental development (cretinism). Toxicity of iodide, like deficiency, also inhibits thyroid hormone synthesis.

Thiamin's coenzyme form is involved in metabolism of carbohydrates and proteins as well as synthesis of RNA, DNA, and neurotransmitters. Rich food sources of thiamin include pork, enriched or fortified grain products, and milk. Beriberi, the thiamin-deficiency disease, leads to muscle weakness and nerve damage. Thiamin toxicity is unknown, and no UL has been set.

The coenzyme form of riboflavin participates in catabolism of fatty acids, metabolism of other vitamins and minerals, and

the antioxidant activity of glutathione peroxidase. Dairy products, enriched and fortified grain products, meat, and eggs are rich food sources of riboflavin. Symptoms of ariboflavinosis include glossitis and angular cheilitis. There is no evidence of toxicity with high doses of riboflavin; no UL has been set.

Niacin's coenzyme form functions in many synthetic reactions, especially fatty-acid synthesis. Rich food sources include seafood, poultry, meats, peanuts, and enriched or fortified grains. Pellagra, the disease of niacin deficiency, results in dermatitis; diarrhea; dementia; and, eventually, death. Megadoses of niacin have been used to lower blood lipids; but they cause side effects, such as flushing of the skin.

Pantothenic acid functions as a coenzyme in reactions that yield energy from carbohydrates, lipids, and protein, as well as fatty acid synthesis. It is widely distributed among foods, with sunflower seeds, mushrooms, peanuts, and eggs among the richest sources. A deficiency of pantothenic acid is unlikely, but symptoms would be similar to those seen with deficiencies of other B vitamins. There is no known toxicity and no UL for pantothenic acid.

Biotin's coenzyme form aids in reactions that synthesize glucose and fatty acids and in the metabolism of amino acids. Egg yolks, peanuts, and cheese provide dietary biotin, but this vitamin is also synthesized by bacteria in the intestines. Consuming raw egg whites may lead to a biotin deficiency because avidin in egg whites binds biotin and reduces its bioavailability. Biotin deficiency can lead to inflammation of the skin and mouth, gastrointestinal symptoms, muscle pain and weakness, poor growth, and anemia. No UL has been set for biotin as no toxicity has ever been observed.

Vitamin B-6 coenzymes activate many enzymes of carbohydrate; lipid; and, especially, protein metabolism. They also help synthesize neurotransmitters and participate in homocysteine metabolism. Rich food sources include animal products and enriched or fortified grain products, as well as some fruits and vegetables. A deficiency of vitamin B-6 leads to headaches, depression, gastrointestinal symptoms, skin disorders, nerve problems, anemia, and impaired immunity. Vitamin B-6 toxicity can result in nerve damage.

Chromium participates in carbohydrate metabolism by aiding insulin function. Meat, whole-grain products, and Brewer's yeast are good sources of chromium, but data on chromium content of foods are limited. A chromium deficiency leads to impaired glucose tolerance and elevated blood lipids. There is no UL for chromium as toxicity has only been reported from exposure to environmental contamination.

Manganese is a cofactor for glucose synthesis and amino acid metabolism. It also contributes to bone formation and antioxidant functions. Food sources include nuts, whole grains, beans, and leafy vegetables. Manganese deficiency is unknown in humans but would likely impair brain function, bone formation, and reproduction. Nerve damage may occur with manganese toxicity.

Molybdenum is a cofactor for enzymes that function in amino acid metabolism. Food sources include dairy products, beans, whole grains, and nuts. A deficiency, which has only been observed in people on total parenteral nutrition devoid of molybdenum, leads to problems with heart rate and respiration, mental confusion, and weakness. Risk for molybdenum toxicity in humans is low.

12.3 Blood contains white cells, red cells, platelets, and plasma. Vitamin K, folate, vitamin B-12, iron, copper, and zinc contribute to the blood cells. Deficiencies may lead to various types of anemia or immune dysfunction.

Vitamin K is essential for blood clotting and also imparts calcium-binding ability to various proteins, including those in bone. Rich food sources include liver, leafy green vegetables, and plant oils. A deficiency of vitamin K could lead to hemorrhage. Infants routinely receive vitamin K injections after birth. Although vitamin K is fat soluble, no toxicity is known and no UL exists.

Folate plays an important role in DNA synthesis and homocysteine metabolism. Food sources are leafy vegetables, organ meats, and orange juice. Symptoms of a deficiency include poor cell division, megaloblastic anemia, tongue inflammation, diarrhea, and poor growth. Folate requirements during pregnancy are high; deficiency during the first month of pregnancy can result in neural tube defects in offspring. A deficiency can also occur in people with alcoholism. Women of childbearing age need to meet the RDA with synthetic folic acid. Excess folate in the diet can mask a vitamin B-12 deficiency.

Vitamin B-12 is needed to metabolize folate and homocysteine and to maintain the insulation surrounding nerves. A deficiency results in anemia and nerve degeneration. Older people often suffer from inefficient absorption of vitamin B-12 and may require injections or megadoses of the vitamin. A dietary deficiency is unlikely because vitamin B-12 is highly concentrated in animal products, which constitute a major part of the North American diet. Vitamin B-12 does not occur naturally in plant foods. Vegans need a supplemental source, as found in fortified breakfast cereals. No UL has been set.

Iron is part of hemoglobin, which functions to transport oxygen and carbon dioxide in the blood. Also, iron participates as a cofactor for many enzymes. It is important for brain and immune function, detoxification of drugs, and bone health. Heme iron comprises 40% of the iron found in meat, fish, and poultry and is more readily absorbed than nonheme iron, which makes up the other 60% of iron in animal products and all of the iron in plant sources, enriched and fortified foods, and most dietary supplements. Food sources include meat, poultry, seafood, whole grains, fortified grain products, and legumes. Iron deficiency leads to anemia, poor growth, impaired immunity, and delayed cognitive development. Iron toxicity leads to stomach irritation and liver damage. Hereditary hemochromatosis is a genetic condition that increases iron absorption, leading to buildup of toxic levels of iron in the blood and tissues. Routine phlebotomy and avoidance of rich sources of iron are advised for people with hemochromatosis.

Copper participates as a cofactor for enzymes with a broad range of functions: formation of red blood cells, release of iron from storage, antioxidant function, and synthesis of collagen in bone. It also participates in immune function, blood clotting, and blood lipid metabolism. Food sources of copper include beef liver, legumes, seeds, whole grains, and cocoa. Copper deficiency leads to anemia, low white blood cell count, bone loss, poor growth, and cardiovascular disease. Toxicity results in gastrointestinal distress and organ damage. Wilson's disease leads to accumulation of copper in tissues.

Zinc is a cofactor for more than 200 enzymes. It participates in DNA synthesis, protein metabolism, immune function, normal growth and development, insulin function, cell membrane structure and function, and antioxidant systems. Food sources of zinc include beef, fortified grain products, and many other protein-rich foods. Severe zinc deficiency leads to growth retardation and delayed sexual development, dermatitis, poor appetite, reduced senses of taste and smell, hair loss, and impaired immunity. Toxicity can lead to gastrointestinal distress, depressed immune function, and decreased HDL and can interfere with copper absorption.

Check Your Knowledge (Answers to the following questions are below.)

1. An inorganic compound that is required for activation or function of an enzyme is called
   a. a collagen.
   b. an organophosphate.
   c. a coenzyme.
   d. a cofactor.

2. Thiamin, riboflavin, and niacin are called the "energy" vitamins because they
   a. can be broken down to provide energy.
   b. are coenzymes needed for release of energy from carbohydrates, fats, and proteins.
   c. are ingredients in energy drinks such as Powerade.
   d. are needed in large amounts by competitive athletes.

3. A deficient intake of _____ has been shown to increase the risk of having a baby with a neural tube defect such as spina bifida.
   a. thiamin
   b. biotin
   c. iron
   d. folic acid

4. Dietary heme iron is derived from
   a. elemental iron in food.
   b. animal flesh.
   c. breakfast cereal.
   d. vegetables.

5. An erythrocyte
   a. is a red blood cell.
   b. requires iron.
   c. transports carbon dioxide.
   d. All of the above.

6. Strict vegetarians (vegans) are at risk for deficiency of which of the following micronutrients?
   a. vitamin B-6
   b. vitamin B-12
   c. folate
   d. thiamin

7. Avidin, a component of raw egg whites, may decrease the absorption of
   a. biotin.
   b. iron.
   c. thiamin.
   d. riboflavin.

8. Which of the following micronutrients participates in DNA synthesis?
   a. folate
   b. riboflavin

   c. biotin
   d. All of the above.

9. Anemia may result from deficiency of all of the following micronutrients except
   a. copper.
   b. chromium.
   c. vitamin B-6.
   d. vitamin B-12.

10. Noodles, spaghetti, and bread are all made from wheat flour. This flour is enriched with all of the following nutrients except
    a. vitamin B-6.
    b. thiamin.
    c. niacin.
    d. iron.
    e. folic acid.

Answer Key: 1. d (LO 12.1), 2. b (LO 12.2), 3. d (LO 12.3), 4. b (LO 12.6), 5. d (LO 12.4), 6. b (LO 12.6), 7. a (LO 12.3), 8. a (LO 12.5), 9. b (LO 12.7), 10. a (LO 12.3)

Study Questions (Numbers refer to Learning Outcomes)

1. Describe how the RDA, DV, and UL for vitamin B-6 should be used in everyday life. How do the RDA and DV for vitamin B-6 differ? **(LO 12.3)**

2. Describe the four main components of blood. Where do blood cells come from? Which micronutrients affect blood cell formation? **(LO 12.4)**

3. Take one of the B vitamins that might be low in the North American diet and explain why a deficiency might occur. **(LO 12.3)**

4. Milling (refining) grains removes which vitamins and minerals? Which of these are replaced during processing? **(LO 12.3)**

5. Why does the FDA limit the amount of folate that may be included in supplements and fortified foods? **(LO 12.2)**

6. What are the best food sources for copper? **(LO 12.6)**

7. Describe the symptoms of iron-deficiency anemia and explain possible reasons they occur. **(LO 12.7)**

8. List two different types of anemia. Identify a nutrient deficiency that could be responsible for each of these types of anemia. **(LO 12.5)**

9. Name two vitamins that function as coenzymes. How do the deficiency diseases (if any) associated with inadequate supply of these micronutrients relate to their coenzyme functions? **(LO 12.1)**

10. Explain the difference between heme and nonheme iron. Name one food source of each. How does the body's need for iron influence the absorption of heme and nonheme iron? **(LO 12.6)**

What Would You Choose Recommendations

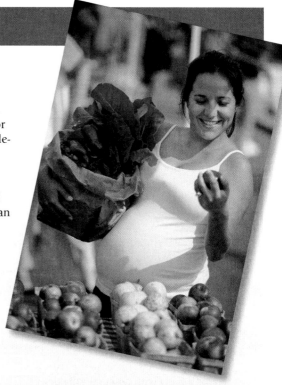

Folate is especially important during pregnancy because it is required for DNA synthesis. During pregnancy, folate needs increase from 400 to 600 micrograms per day. Obstetricians typically prescribe prenatal vitamins that contain 800 micrograms of folic acid, but good food sources of folate have benefits besides the nutrient itself, such as phytochemicals and fiber.

Meats and other animal products are not particularly good sources of folate. Dairy foods do contribute some—your low-fat yogurt supplies about 27 micrograms of folate per 1-cup container. Other dairy products, such as skim milk, provide about 12 micrograms of folate. To find more folate, seek out plant sources.

Lentils and other dried beans are among the richest sources of folate. A 1/2-cup serving of cooked lentils provides about 179 micrograms of folate. Beans are also great sources of other nutrients that are typically low in American diets, such as fiber, potassium, and magnesium. Plus, they are low in fat and are cholesterol-free.

Spinach and other leafy green vegetables are excellent sources of folate. Two cups of fresh, chopped spinach provides 116 micrograms of folate. Half a cup of sliced strawberries adds an additional 20 micrograms, so this delicious spinach salad supplies almost 25% of the RDA for folate during pregnancy. Even with 1 tablespoon of low-fat vinaigrette, this salad is a very nutrient-dense source of folate (recall Chapter 2)—136 micrograms of folate compared to only 50 kcal. Cooked spinach, as presented in Figure 12-21, is an even more concentrated source of folate because greens cook down to a smaller volume, so you are actually consuming more vegetables per cup.

Recall that grain products, such as the whole-wheat bread in your turkey sandwich, are fortified with folic acid. Fortified breakfast cereals are a fabulous source of synthetic folic acid. One cup of Oatmeal Squares cereal contains 400 micrograms (100% of the DV) of folic acid in one serving! Also, the synthetic folic acid incorporated into fortified foods is more bioavailable than natural sources of folate. During pregnancy—or any life stage—a fortified, whole-grain, ready-to-eat breakfast cereal is an excellent way to start the day.

Your next choice—should you decorate the nursery pink or blue?

Further Readings

1. Bentley TGK and others: Population-level changes in folate intake by age, gender, and race/ethnicity after folic acid fortification. *American Journal of Public Health* 96:2040, 2006.

   The impact of the 1998 U.S. FDA folic-acid-fortification policy was quantified by estimating folate intake at the population level. After fortification, mean food and total folate intake increased by about 100 µg/day. The number of women of childbearing age who consume more than 400 µg/day of folate increased after fortification but has not yet reached the FDA's target of 50%. Although folic acid intake has increased among the U.S. population since fortification, there are substantial variations by age, gender, and race/ethnicity.

2. Franchini M and Veneri D: Hereditary hemochromatosis. *Hematology* 10(2):145, 2005.

   Hereditary hemochromatosis is a disorder of iron metabolism characterized by progressive tissue iron overload, which leads to irreversible organ damage if not treated in time. Transferrin saturation and serum ferritin are the most reliable tests for the detection of subjects with hereditary hemochromatosis. Therapeutic phlebotomy is the mainstay of treatment. If phlebotomy is started before the onset of irreversible organ damage, the life expectancy of these patients is similar to that of the normal population.

3. Green R: Is it time for vitamin B-12 fortification? What are the questions? *American Journal of Clinical Nutrition* 89:712S, 2009.

   The success of folate fortification of grains over the past decade leads to consideration of other common nutrient deficiencies that may be corrected by widespread fortification of the food supply. Vitamin B-12 deficiency is of greatest concern among infants and older adults. Inadequate vitamin B-12 may be at the root of some birth defects. For older adults, decreased absorption of vitamin B-12 can lead to anemia and nerve damage. Research remains to answer questions about optimal dose, potential toxic effects, impact on microbial growth, and whether or not fortification would be adequate to overcome the malabsorption experienced by older adults.

4. Hubbs-Tait L and others: Zinc, iron, and lead: Relations to Head Start children's cognitive scores and teachers' ratings of behavior. *Journal of the American Dietetic Association* 107:128, 2007.

   Research points to interactions between essential micronutrients (e.g., iron and zinc) and toxic elements (e.g., lead) and their effects on cognition and behavior. In this small study, higher levels of lead were associated with lower levels of iron and zinc. Low zinc levels were associated with higher anxiety in boys. High lead levels were associated with lower social skills in girls. This study emphasizes the importance of micronutrient status for learning and behavior among young children and also highlights the detrimental effect of lead exposure.

5. King JC: Zinc: An essential but elusive nutrient. *American Journal of Clinical Nutrition* 94:679S, 2011.

   Zinc is essential for many biochemical functions. When zinc is insufficient in the diet, body stores give up zinc immediately to conserve the nutrient. There is probably a small zinc reserve in all cells in addition to the zinc in the blood.

Zinc concentrations in blood decline quickly with severe deficiencies and more slowly with marginal depletion. Blood zinc concentrations also decrease with conditions such as infection, trauma, stress, and steroid use due to redistribution of zinc from blood to tissues. This redistribution confuses the interpretation of low blood zinc concentrations.

6. Larsson SC and others: Vitamin B-6 and risk of colorectal cancer: A meta-analysis of prospective studies. *Journal of the American Medical Association* 303:1077, 2010.

Elevated levels of homocysteine have been linked to risk for several chronic diseases, including cancer. Vitamin B-6 is involved in more than 100 enzymatic reactions, including those that metabolize homocysteine. Vitamin B-6 intake may be inadequate for older adults. This meta-analysis of research that measured serum vitamin B-6 (pyridoxal 5' phosphate) in comparison to cancers of the colon and rectum found that colorectal cancer risk is decreased in subjects with high blood levels of vitamin B-6.

7. McCormick DB: The dubious use of vitamin-mineral supplements in relation to cardiovascular disease. *American Journal of Clinical Nutrition* 84(4):680, 2006.

This editorial supports the findings of studies, including a meta-analysis by Bleys and others, that antioxidants and B vitamins should not be used to prevent cardiovascular disease. The author hopes that these recent findings, "which carefully separate fact from faith," will decrease the extensive use of vitamin-mineral supplements.

8. Office of Dietary Supplements, National Institutes of Health: Dietary supplement fact sheet: Iron. Updated 8/24/2007. Available at: http://ods.od.nih.gov/factsheets/iron.; vitamin B-6 fact sheet. Updated 8/24/2007. http://ods.od.nih.gov/factsheets/vitaminb6.; vitamin B-12 fact sheet. Updated 06/24/2011. http://ods.od.nih.gov/factsheets/vitaminb12.

These reader-friendly fact sheets provide the most recent information on supplements. Food sources, deficiencies, at-risk groups, and nutrient-drug interactions are highlighted. Current research as well as controversial areas are discussed.

9. Pitkin RM: Folate and neural tube defects. *American Journal of Clinical Nutrition* 85:285S, 2007.

The ability of adequate folic acid during the periconceptional period to prevent neural tube defects is well-established. This article reviews important research that has led to advancements in the prevention of neural tube defects, discusses recommendations for intake (0.4 mg/d for all women of childbearing age or 4 mg/d for high-risk women), and examines the success of the folic-acid-fortification program instituted in 1998 in the United States.

10. Warren Grant Magnusen Clinical Center. National Institutes of Health: Important information to know when you are taking: Coumadin and vitamin K. December 2003. Available in pdf form through the Office of Dietary Supplements, National Institutes of Health. Available at: http://ods.od.nih.gov/pubs/factsheets/coumadin1.pdf.

This very helpful pamphlet discusses the nutrient-drug interaction between a commonly prescribed anticlotting medication and vitamin K, a key vitamin to promote clotting. Foods identified as low, moderate, and high in vitamin K are provided in order to keep vitamin K intake consistent and allow Coumadin to function as prescribed.

11. Zhang SM and others: Effect of combined folic acid, vitamin B-6, and vitamin B-12 on cancer risk in women: A randomized trial. *Journal of the American Medical Association* 300:2012, 2008.

Use of a combined supplement of folic acid, vitamin B-6, and vitamin B-12 had no significant effect on overall risk of total invasive cancer or breast cancer in a 7-year study of 5442 women. This was the longest-running trial of its kind and occurred at the time that background fortification of the food supply with folic acid had begun.

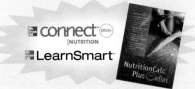

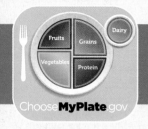

RATE YOUR PLATE

Boosting Your Micronutrient Intake

For each of the following meal options, choose the one that would supply the most of the given micronutrient.

1. Which meal supplies the most iron?

A	B
• Roast beef sandwich on whole-grain bread with lettuce, tomato, and mustard • Grapes • Skim milk	• Roast beef sandwich on whole-grain bread with lettuce, tomato, and mustard • Grapes • Orange juice

2. Which meal supplies the most vitamin K?

A	B
• Pasta with shrimp, tomatoes, and spinach • Italian bread with olive oil • White wine	• Pasta with shrimp, tomatoes, and feta cheese • Italian bread with butter • White wine

3. Which meal supplies the most copper?

A	B
• Cheerios • Banana • Orange juice	• Blueberry bagel with cream cheese • Banana • Orange juice

4. Which meal supplies the most vitamin B-12?

A	B
• Cheeseburger • Baked potato with sour cream • Diet cola	• Veggie burger • Baked potato with sour cream • Iced tea

Answers

1. B: The vitamin C in orange juice enhances absorption of the iron in the roast beef and enriched bread.
2. A: Spinach is a source of vitamin K, whereas cheese is not.
3. A: Fortified breakfast cereals are a good source of many trace minerals; although breads are enriched with some vitamins and minerals lost during the refining process, copper is not one of those.
4. A: Animal products are sources of vitamin B-12.

Chapter 16 Safety of Our Food Supply

Student Learning Outcomes

Chapter 16 is designed to allow you to:

16.1 List some of the types and common sources of viruses, bacteria, fungi, and parasites that can make their way into food.

16.2 Compare and contrast food-preservation methods.

16.3 Understand the foodborne illnesses caused by bacteria, viruses, and parasites.

16.4 Describe the main reasons for using chemical additives in foods, the general classes of additives, and the functions of each class.

16.5 Identify sources of toxic environmental contaminants in food and the consequences of their ingestion.

16.6 Understand the reasons behind pesticide use, the possible long-term health complications, and the safety limits set for their use.

16.7 Understand the effects of conventional and sustainable agriculture on our food choices.

16.8 Describe the procedures that can be used to limit the risk of foodborne illness.

What Would You Choose?

By now, you have learned the importance of including more fruits and vegetables in your diet. You are choosing fresh or frozen produce more often than canned to cut back on sodium and other preservatives. You are steaming or stir-frying your vegetables to retain nutrients and avoid adding too much fat during preparation. In the grocery store, you have seen the growing selection of organic products including produce. Do they have health benefits that make them worth the extra cost? If cost was not a concern, what type of fruits and vegetables would you choose from the following list to satisfy your desire for increased nutritional value, decreased exposure to preservatives, lower risk for foodborne illness, and decreased exposure to pesticides?

a Canned low-sodium

b Organically grown

c Frozen

d Fresh

 | NUTRITION Think about your choice as you read Chapter 16, then see our recommendations at the end of the chapter. To learn more about organic foods, check out the Connect site: www.mcgrawhillconnect.com

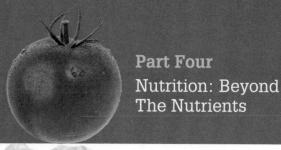

Over 100 years ago, in 1906, increasing public pressure forced the passage of the first Food and Drug Act in the United States and generally improved food preparation standards. Today, warnings about the safety of food and water appear everywhere. Attention has turned to more contemporary concerns, such as microbial and chemical contamination. Whereas we are told to eat more fruits, vegetables, fish, and poultry and to drink more water, we are also warned that these may contain dangerous substances. We still must ask, "How safe is our food and water?"

Scientists and health authorities agree that North Americans enjoy a relatively safe food supply, especially if foods are stored and prepared properly. Over the past 100 or so years, tremendous progress has been made to allow for this. Nonetheless, microorganisms and certain chemicals in foods still can pose a health risk. Thus, the nutritional and health benefits of food must be balanced against any food-related hazards. Chapter 16 focuses on these hazards—how real they are and how you can minimize their effect on your life. As the comic in the chapter suggests, you bear some responsibility for this—government agencies and industry can only do so much. Recall from Chapter 2 that the 2010 Dietary Guidelines for Americans encourage us to prepare and store foods safely.

pasteurizing The process of heating food products to kill pathogenic microorganisms and reduce the total number of bacteria.

virus The smallest known type of infectious agent, many of which cause disease in humans. A virus is essentially a piece of genetic material surrounded by a coat of protein. They do not metabolize, grow, or move by themselves. They reproduce only with the aid of a living cellular host.

bacteria Single-cell microorganisms; some produce poisonous substances, which cause illness in humans. Bacteria can be carried by water, animals, and people. They survive on skin, clothes, and hair and thrive in foods at room temperature. Some can live without oxygen and survive by means of **spore** formation.

spores Dormant reproductive cells capable of turning into adult organisms without the help of another cell. Various bacteria and fungi form spores.

fungi Simple parasitic life forms, including molds, mildews, yeasts, and mushrooms. They live on dead or decaying organic matter. Fungi can grow as single cells, like yeast, or as a multicellular colony, as seen with molds.

parasite An organism that lives in or on another organism and derives nourishment from it.

foodborne illness Sickness caused by the ingestion of food containing harmful substances.

 Refresh Your Memory

As you begin your study of food safety in Chapter 16, you may want to review:

- Alternative sweeteners in Chapter 4
- The disease phenylketonuria (PKU) in Chapter 4
- Fat substitutes in Chapter 5
- Food biotechnology in Chapter 15

16.1 Food Safety: Setting the Stage

During the early stages of urbanization in North America, contaminated water and food—notably, milk—were responsible for many large outbreaks of typhoid fever, septic sore throat, scarlet fever, diphtheria, and other devastating human diseases. These experiences led to the development of processes for purifying water, treating sewage, and **pasteurizing** milk. Since that time, safe water and milk have become universally available, with only occasional problems from either.

The greatest health risk from food today is contamination by **viruses** and **bacteria** and, to a lesser extent, by various forms of **fungi** and **parasites**. These microorganisms can all cause **foodborne illness.** In a recent outbreak in the United States, 199 persons in 26 states were infected with *Escherichia coli* (*E. coli*) bacteria O157:H7 from fresh spinach. Of these ill persons, 102 were hospitalized, 31 developed kidney failure, and 22 were children under 5 years. Three deaths were associated with the outbreak. A deadlier outbreak of Escherichia coli O104:H4 occurred in Germany during the summer of 2011, resulting in over 3000 infections, hundreds of cases of kidney failure, and a death toll of at least 36. Read more about this outbreak that was linked to sprouts in Table 16.1.

Although microbial contamination is the cause of most incidents of foodborne illness, North Americans seem more concerned about health risks from chemicals in foods. In the long run, this concern has some merit. On a day-to-day basis, however, food additives cause only about 4% of all cases of foodborne illness in North America. Microbial contamination of food is by far the more important issue for our day-to-day health, so it will be discussed first. Chapter 16 will then cover chemical food safety hazards, including the use and safety of food additives, and discuss the risks of pesticides in foods.

Garfield ® by Jim Davis

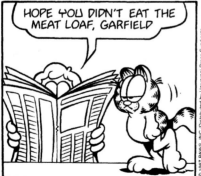
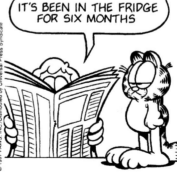
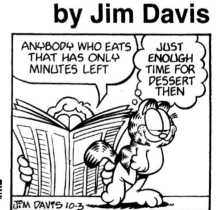

Which foods pose the greatest risk for foodborne illness? Is any food safe after being stored in the refrigerator for 6 months? Are food additives and pesticides an even greater day-to-day concern? Chapter 16 provides some answers.

Effects of Foodborne Illness

According to the U.S. Centers for Disease Control and Prevention, foodborne illness causes 48 million illnesses, 128,000 hospitalizations, and 3000 deaths in the United States each year. Some people are particularly susceptible to foodborne illness, including the following:

- Infants and children
- Older adults
- Those with liver disease, diabetes, HIV infection (and AIDS), or cancer
- Postsurgical patients
- Pregnant women
- People taking immunosuppressant agents (e.g., transplant patients)

Some bouts of foodborne illness, especially when coupled with ongoing health problems, are lengthy and lead to food allergies, seizures, blood poisoning (from **toxins** or microorganisms in the bloodstream), or other illnesses. Foodborne illnesses often result from the unsafe handling of food at home, so we each bear some responsibility for preventing them (see Further Readings 2 and 10). You can't usually tell so by taste, smell, or sight that a particular food contains harmful microorganisms; therefore, you might not even be aware that food has caused your distress. In fact, your last case of diarrhea may have been caused by foodborne illness (Table 16-1). In response to the significant public health burden of foodborne illness that is largely preventable, the FDA Food Safety Modernization Act was signed into law by President Obama on January 4, 2011. This new law strengthens the food safety system, enabling FDA to better protect public health. It allows FDA to focus on prevention of food safety problems before they occur. The law also provides new tools for inspection and compliance and for holding imported foods to the same standards as domestic foods. The law also directs FDA to build a national food safety system that is integrated and in partnership with state and local authorities. Although government agencies are at work on problems regarding food safety, this does not substitute for individual safety efforts (Table 16-2).

toxins Poisonous compounds produced by an organism that can cause disease.

Read more about the Food Safety Modernization Act at www.fda.gov./Food/FoodSafety/FSMA/default.htm.

Why Is Foodborne Illness So Common?

Foodborne illness is carried or transmitted to people by food. Most foodborne illnesses are transmitted through food in which microorganisms are able to grow rapidly. These foods are generally moist, rich in protein, and have a neutral or slightly acidic pH. Unfortunately, this describes many of the foods we eat every day, such as meats, eggs, and dairy products.

Our food industry tries whenever possible to increase the shelf life of food products; however, a longer shelf life allows more time for bacteria in foods to multiply. Some bacteria even grow at refrigeration temperatures. Partially cooked—and some fully cooked—products pose a particular risk because refrigerated storage may only slow, not prevent, bacterial growth. The risk of contracting foodborne illness also is high because of consumer trends. First, there is greater consumer interest in eating raw or undercooked animal products. In addition, more people receive medication that suppresses their ability to combat foodborne infectious agents. Another factor is the continuing increase in the number of older adults in the population.

The risk of illness from foodborne microorganisms increases as more of our foods are prepared in kitchens outside the home. Supermarkets have become an alternative to cooking at home by offering a variety of prepared foods from specialty meat shops, salad bars, and bakeries. With the increasing number of two-income families, more people are looking for convenient, easy-to-prepare, nutritious foods. Supermarkets offer entrées that can be served immediately or reheated. The foods are usually prepared in central kitchens or processing plants and shipped to individual stores.

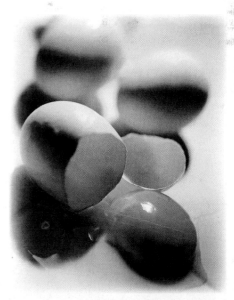

▲ Some restaurants that serve requested undercooked food are now warning patrons (on the menu) of the health risks of ordering such foods, particularly with undercooked eggs and meats.

TABLE 16-1 Some Examples of Cases of Foodborne Illness. We generally have a safe food supply, but there are occasional instances of foodborne illnesses, such as those listed.

Viruses

- *Norovirus:* Over 380 passengers and crew members of the largest cruise ship, Royal Caribbean's Freedom of the Seas, were sickened by *Norovirus*. The ship was sanitized, but one week later a second outbreak of the gastrointestinal illness afflicted 97 passengers and 11 crew members.

- *Hepatitus A:* Over 500 adults in the United States contracted hepatitis A after eating raw green onions in a Mexican restaurant. These were contaminated during growth in Mexico and not properly washed by food service workers.

Bacteria

- *Salmonella:* In 2008–2009, two outbreaks of salmonella cost their industries millions of dollars. The first outbreak was traced to imported jalapeno and serrano peppers from one Mexican farm. Illnesses led to 282 hospitalizations and 2 deaths. The second outbreak, traced to peanut butter from a processing plant in Georgia may have caused at least eight deaths.

- *Shigella:* More than 600 people on a cruise ship developed shigellosis and one person died.

- *Listeria:* Forty-eight deaths were associated with foodborne illness caused by *Listeria* organisms in soft, Mexican-style cheeses. A listeriosis outbreak associated with undercooked hot dogs and cold cuts resulted in more than 82 illnesses and 17 deaths in 19 states.

- *E. coli:* The world's deadliest outbreak of *Escherichia coli* occurred during the summer of 2011 with 3332 persons infected, more than 600 in intensive care, and a death toll of 36. The outbreak occurred mainly in Germany and involved the rare *E.coli* O104:H4 strain. Several hundred also contracted its potentially fatal kidney complication. The *E.coli* infection was caused by tainted vegetable sprouts from a small, rather traditional organic sprout farm. The sprout seeds were mostly imported from overseas and the *E.coli* bacteria were antibiotic

resistant. In the United States, the largest *E. coli* O157:H7 outbreak on record infected more than 1000 people in upstate New York at a county fair. The bacterium was found in infected well water. It killed a 79-year-old man and a 4-year-old girl, and it caused 10 other children to undergo kidney dialysis. Six adults and a 2-year-old child were killed after an *E. coli* outbreak from contaminated drinking water in Canada. The bacteria entered the water supply from animal manure after flooding from a heavy storm. In an outbreak of 199 persons infected with *E. coli* from fresh spinach, *E. coli* O157:H7 was isolated from 13 packages of fresh spinach in 10 states.

- *C. botulinum:* A man in Arkansas developed botulism after eating stew that was cooked and then kept at room temperature for 3 days. He spent—42 days on mechanical ventilation.

- *Vibrio:* Since 1992, 17 people in Florida have died of *Vibrio vulnificus* infections after eating raw oysters.

- *B. cereus:* A teenage boy and his father experienced abdominal pain, vomiting, and diarrhea within 30 minutes of eating 4-day-old homemade pesto that had been reheated and left out a number of times and was apparently contaminated with *Bacillus cereus*. The boy died of liver failure.

Parasites

- *Cryptosporidium:* A group attending a banquet developed diarrhea 3 to 9 days after eating green onions. Stool specimens were positive for *Cryptosporidium*. Restaurant workers reported they did not consistently wash green onions before using them.

Risks from Seafood

- *Ciguatera:* An outbreak of ciguatera fish poisoning involved 17 crew members of a cargo ship that caught, cooked, and ate a barra-cuda in the Bahamas. All became ill with nausea, vomiting, abdominal cramps, and diarrhea within hours of eating the fish. Within 2 days, all suffered from muscle pain and weakness; dizziness; and numb or itchy feet, hands, and mouth.

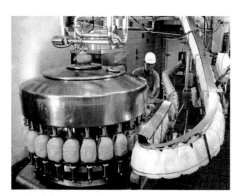

▲ Food contaminated in a central plant can go on to produce illness in people across the nation. In the case of juices, pasteurization is an effective method of reducing the risk of foodborne illness.

This centralization of food production by the food-processing and restaurant industry enhances the risk of foodborne illness. If a food product is contaminated in a central processing plant, consumers over a wide area can suffer foodborne illness. For example, a malfunction in an ice cream plant in Minnesota resulted in 224,000 suspected cases of *Salmonella* bacterial infections, which were linked to use of contaminated ice cream mix. At least 4 people died and 700 became ill in Washington and surrounding western states after eating at a chain of fast-food restaurants. The source of the problem was undercooked hamburger contaminated with the bacterium *E. coli* O157:H7. Restaurants are inspected by health departments only about every 6 months so we must rely on each restaurant to practice good food safety.

Greater consumption of ready-to-eat foods imported from foreign countries is still another cause of increased foodborne illness in North America. In the past, food imports were mostly raw products processed here under strict sanitation standards. Now, however, we import more ready-to-eat processed foods—such as berries from Guatemala and shellfish from Asia—some of which are contaminated. U.S. authorities are re-examining inspection procedures for these imports.

TABLE 16-2 Agencies Responsible for Monitoring the Food Supply in the United States

Agency Name	Responsibilities	Methods	How to Contact
United States Department of Agriculture (USDA)	• Enforces wholesomeness and quality standards for grains and produce (while in the field), meat, poultry, milk, eggs, and egg products	• Inspection • Grading • "Safe Handling Label"	www.fsis.usda.gov
Bureau of Alcohol, Tobacco, Firearms and Explosives (ATF)	• Enforces laws on alcoholic beverages	• Inspection	www.atf.gov
Environmental Protection Agency (EPA)	• Regulates pesticides • Establishes water quality standards	• Approval required for all U.S. pesticides • Sets pesticide residue limits in food	www.epa.gov
Food and Drug Administration (FDA)	• Ensures safety and wholesomeness of all foods in interstate commerce (except meat, poultry, and processed egg products) • Regulates seafood • Controls product labels	• Inspection • Food sample studies • Sets standards for specific foods	www.fda.gov or call 1-800-FDA-4010
Centers for Disease Control and Prevention (CDC)	• Promotes food safety	• Responds to emergencies concerning foodborne illness • Surveys and studies environmental health problems • Directs/enforces quarantines • National programs for prevention and control of foodborne and other diseases	www.cdc.gov
National Marine Fisheries Service or NOAA Fisheries	• Domestic and international conservation and management of living marine resources	• Voluntary seafood inspection program • Can use mark to show federal inspection	www.nmfs.noaa.gov
State and local governments	• Milk safety • Monitors food industry within their borders	• Inspection of food-related establishments	Government pages of telephone book

Government agencies responsible for monitoring food safety in Canada and the specific laws followed are listed in Appendix C.

The use of antibiotics in animal feeds is also increasing the severity of cases of foodborne illness. This antibiotic use encourages bacteria such as *E.coli* O157:H7 and O104:H4 to develop antibiotic-resistant strains, those that can grow even if exposed to typical antibiotic medicines. This issue is receiving considerable attention by scientists in the field.

Finally, more cases of foodborne disease are reported now because scientists are more aware of the roles of various players in the process. Every decade the list of microorganisms suspected of causing foodborne illness lengthens. In addition, physicians are more likely to suspect foodborne contaminants as a cause of illness. Furthermore, we now know that food, besides serving as a good growth medium for some microorganisms, transmits many others as well. Seafood is receiving greater scrutiny and surveillance by FDA as a cause of foodborne illness. For more information about food safety, contact FDA's Center for Food Safety and Applied Nutrition information line at 1-888-SAFEFOOD or log on to www.FoodSafety.gov (see Further Reading 5).

One tool in the battle against foodborne illness is HACCP, or Hazard Analysis Critical Control Point. By applying the principles of HACCP, food handlers critically analyze how they approach food preparation and what conditions may exist that might allow pathogenic microorganisms to enter and thrive in the food system. Once specific hazards and critical control points (potential problems) are identified, preventive measures can be used to reduce specific sources of contamination.

16.2 Food Preservation—Past, Present, and Future

For centuries, salt, sugar, smoke, fermentation, and drying have been used to preserve food. Ancient Romans used sulfites to disinfect wine containers and preserve wine. In the age of exploration, European adventurers traveling to the New World preserved their meat by salting it. Most preserving methods work on the principle of decreasing water content. Bacteria need abundant stores of water to grow; yeasts and molds can grow with less water, but some is still necessary. Adding sugar or salt binds water and so decreases the water available to these microbes. The process of drying evaporates off free water.

Decreasing the water content of some high-moisture foods, however, would cause them to lose essential characteristics. To preserve such foods—cucumber pickles, sauerkraut, milk (yogurt), and wine—fermentation has been a traditional alternative. Selected bacteria or yeast are used to ferment or pickle foods. The fermenting bacteria or yeast make acids and alcohol, which minimize the growth of other bacteria and yeast.

Today we can add pasteurization, sterilization, refrigeration, freezing, food **irradiation,** canning, and chemical preservation to the list of food preservation techniques. An additional method of food preservation—**aseptic processing**—simultaneously sterilizes the food and package separately before the food enters the package. Liquid foods, such as fruit juices, are especially easy to process in this manner. With aseptic packaging, boxes of sterile milk and juices can remain on supermarket shelves, free of microbial growth, for many years.

Food irradiation uses minimal doses of radiation to control pathogens such as *E. coli* O157:H7 and *Salmonella*. The radiation energy used does not make the food radioactive. The energy essentially passes through the food, as in microwave cooking, and no radioactive residues are left behind. However, the energy is strong enough to break chemical bonds, destroy cell walls and cell membranes, break down DNA, and link proteins together. Irradiation thereby controls growth of insects, bacteria, fungi, and parasites in foods.

FDA approved the use of irradiation for raw red meat to reduce risk of *E. coli* and other infectious microorganisms. Other additions to the approved list are shell eggs and seeds. Prior to this, the only animal products so treated were pork and chicken. Irradiation also extends the shelf life of spices, dry vegetable seasonings, meats, and fresh fruits and vegetables.

Irradiated food, except for dried seasonings, must be labeled with the international food irradiation symbol, the Radura, and a statement that the product has been treated by irradiation. Foods treated in this way are safe in the opinion of FDA and many other health authorities, including the American Academy of Pediatrics. Although the demand for irradiated foods is still low in the United States, other countries, including Canada, Japan, Italy, and Mexico, all use food irradiation technology widely. Certain consumer groups continually try to block its use in the United States, claiming that irradiation diminishes the nutritional value of food and that it can lead to the formation of harmful compounds, such as carcinogens. Future research should be able to sort out this controversy, but in any case the risk is very low. Keep in mind that, even when foods, especially meats, have been irradiated, it is still important to follow basic food-safety procedures, as later contamination during food preparation is possible.

16.3 Foodborne Illness Caused by Microorganisms

Most cases of foodborne illness are caused by specific viruses, bacteria, and other fungi. Prions—proteins involved in maintaining nerve cell function—can also turn infectious and lead to diseases such as mad cow disease. Bacteria specifically cause health problems either directly by invading the intestinal wall and producing an *infection* via a toxin contained in the organism, or indirectly by producing a toxin

irradiation A process in which **radiation** energy is applied to foods, creating compounds (free radicals) within the food that destroy cell membranes, break down DNA, link proteins together, limit enzyme activity, and alter a variety of other proteins and cell functions of microorganisms that can lead to food spoilage. This process does not make the food radioactive.

radiation Literally, energy that is emitted from a center in all directions. Various forms of radiation energy include X-rays and ultraviolet rays from the sun.

aseptic processing A method by which food and container are separately and simultaneously sterilized; it allows manufacturers to produce boxes of milk that can be stored at room temperature.

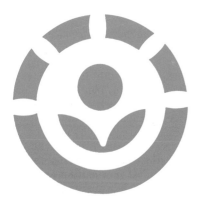

▲ This is the Radura, the international label denoting prior irradiation of the food product.

secreted into the food, which later harms us (called an *intoxication*). The main way to distinguish an infectious route from an intoxication is time: If symptoms appear in 4 hours or less, it is an intoxication.

Bacteria

Bacteria are single-cell organisms found in the food we eat, the water we drink, and the air we breathe. Many types of bacteria cause foodborne illness, including *Bacillus, Campylobacter, Clostridium, Escherichia, Listeria, Vibrio, Salmonella,* and *Staphylococcus* (Table 16-3). Bacteria are everywhere: each teaspoon of soil contains about 2 billion bacteria. Luckily, only a small number of all bacteria pose a threat. Some foodborne bacteria cause infections, whereas others cause intoxications. *Salmonella,* for example, causes an infection because the bacteria cause the illness. *Clostridium botulinum, Staphylococcus aureus,* and *Bacillus cereus* produce toxins and therefore cause illness from intoxication. In addition, while most strains of *E. coli* are harmless, *E. coli* O157:H7 and O104:H4 produce a toxin that can cause severe illness, including severe bloody diarrhea and hemolytic uremic syndrome (HUS). Bacterial foodborne illnesses typically cause gastrointestinal symptoms such as vomiting, diarrhea, and abdominal cramps. *Salmonella, Listeria, E. coli* O157:H7 and O104:H4, and *Campylobacter* are the bacterial foodborne illnesses of particular interest because they are the ones most often associated with death. *E. coli* O157:H7 and O104:H4 has caused deaths when HUS has developed. Of the 1600 cases of Listeriosis in the United States each year, 255 cases are fatal. Listeriosis is of particular concern for pregnant women because they are about 20 times more likely to get this infection than other healthy adults, and Listeriosis can cause spontaneous abortion or stillbirth because the *Listeria* bacteria can cross the placenta and infect the fetus.

To proliferate, bacteria require nutrients, water, and warmth. Most grow best in **danger zone** temperatures of 40° to 140°F (4° to 60°C) (Fig. 16-1). Pathogenic bacteria

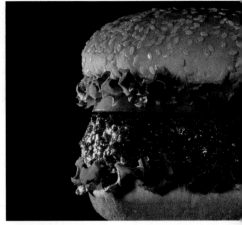

▲ Ground meats are a typical source of foodborne infection because bacteria on the surface of whole meats are distributed throughout the meat during grinding.

FIGURE 16-1 ▶ Effects of temperature on microbes that cause foodborne illness.

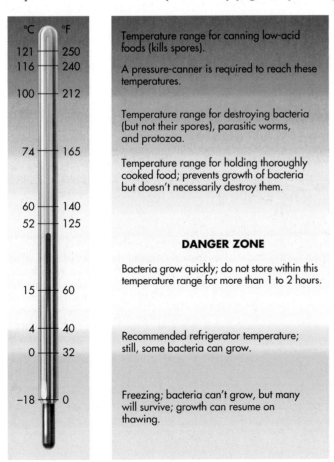

°C / °F	
121 — 250	Temperature range for canning low-acid foods (kills spores).
116 — 240	A pressure-canner is required to reach these temperatures.
100 — 212	
74 — 165	Temperature range for destroying bacteria (but not their spores), parasitic worms, and protozoa.
	Temperature range for holding thoroughly cooked food; prevents growth of bacteria but doesn't necessarily destroy them.
60 — 140	
52 — 125	**DANGER ZONE**
	Bacteria grow quickly; do not store within this temperature range for more than 1 to 2 hours.
15 — 60	
4 — 40	Recommended refrigerator temperature; still, some bacteria can grow.
0 — 32	
−18 — 0	Freezing; bacteria can't grow, but many will survive; growth can resume on thawing.

TABLE 16-3 Bacterial Causes of Foodborne Illness

Bacteria	Typical Food Sources	Symptoms	Additional Information
Salmonella species	Raw and undercooked meats, poultry, eggs, and fish; produce, especially raw sprouts; peanut butter; unpasteurized milk (see Further Reading 4.)	Onset: 12–72 hours; nausea, fever, headache, abdominal cramps, diarrhea, and vomiting; can be fatal in infants, the elderly, and those with impaired immune systems; lasts 4–7 days	Estimated 1 million infections/year; bacteria live in the intestines of animals and humans; food is contaminated by infected water and feces; about 2000 strains of *Salmonella* bacteria can cause disease, but 3 strains account for almost 50% of cases; *Salmonella enteritidis* infects the ovaries of healthy hens and contaminates eggs; almost 20% of cases are from eating undercooked eggs or egg-containing dishes; reptiles, such as turtles, also spread the disease
Campylobacter jejuni	Raw and undercooked meat and poultry (more than half of raw poultry in the United States is contaminated), unpasteurized milk, contaminated water	Onset: 2–5 days; muscle pain, abdominal cramping, diarrhea (sometimes bloody), fever; lasts 2–7 days	Estimated 845,000 infections/year; produces a toxin that destroys intestinal mucosal surfaces; can cause Guillain-Barré syndrome, a rare neurological disorder that causes paralysis
Escherichia coli (O157:H7 O104:H4 and other strains)	Undercooked ground beef; produce—lettuce, spinach, sprouts; unpasteurized juice and milk	Onset: 1–8 days; bloody diarrhea, abdominal cramps; in children under age 5 and the elderly, hemolytic uremic syndrome (HUS) is a serious complication; red blood cells are destroyed and kidneys fail; can be fatal; lasts 5–10 days	Leading cause of bloody diarrhea in the United States; estimated 73,000 cases/year; lives in the intestine of healthy cattle; cattle and cattle manure are chief sources; illness caused by a powerful toxin made by the bacteria; petting zoos, lakes, and swimming pools can contain pathogenic *E. coli*
Shigella species	Fecal/oral transmission; water supplies, produce, and other foods contaminated by infected food handlers with poor hygiene	Onset: 1–3 days; abdominal cramps, fever, diarrhea (often bloody); lasts 5–7 days	Estimated 448,000 cases/year; humans and primates are the only sources; common in day-care centers and custodial institutions from poor hygiene; traveler's diarrhea often caused by *Shigella dysenteriae*
Staphylococcus aureus	Ham, poultry, egg salads, cream-filled pastries, custards, whipped cream	Onset: 1–6 hours; diarrhea, vomiting, nausea, abdominal cramps; lasts 1–3 days	Bacteria on skin and nasal passages of up to 25% of people; can be passed to foods; multiplies rapidly when contaminated foods are held for extended time at room temperature; illness caused by a heat-resistant toxin that cannot be destroyed by cooking

TABLE 16-3 *(continued)*

Bacteria	Typical Food Sources	Symptoms	Additional Information
Clostridium perfringens	Beef, poultry, gravy, Mexican food	Onset: 8–24 hours; abdominal pain and diarrhea, usually mild; can be more serious in elderly or ill persons; lasts 1 day or less	Estimated 966,000 cases/year; anaerobic bacteria widespread in soil and water; multiplies rapidly in prepared foods, such as meats, casseroles, and gravies, held for extended time at room temperature
Listeria monocytogenes	Unpasteurized milk and soft cheeses, raw meats, uncooked vegetables, ready-to-eat deli meats and hotdogs, refrigerated smoked fish (see Further Reading 6.)	Onset: 9–48 hours for early symptoms, 14–42 days for severe symptoms; fever, muscle aches, headache, vomiting; can spread to nervous system, resulting in stiff neck, confusion, loss of balance, or convulsion; can cause premature birth and stillbirth	Estimated 1600 cases with 260 fatalities/year; widespread in soil and water and can be carried in healthy animals; grows at refrigeration temperatures; about one-third of cases occur during pregnancy; high-risk persons should avoid uncooked deli meats, soft cheeses (e.g., feta, Brie, and Camembert), blue-veined cheeses, Mexican-style cheeses (e.g., queso blanco made from unpasteurized milk), refrigerated meat spreads or pates, uncooked refrigerated smoked fish
Clostridium botulinum	Incorrectly home-canned vegetables, meats, and fish; incorrectly canned commercial foods; herb-infused oils; bottled garlic; potatoes baked in foil and held at room temperature; honey	Onset: 18–36 hours but can be 6 hours to 10 days; neurological symptoms—double and blurred vision, drooping eyelids, slurred speech, difficulty swallowing, muscle weakness, and paralysis of face, arms, respiratory muscles, trunk, and legs; can be fatal; lasts days to weeks	Estimated 100 cases/year; caused by a neurotoxin; *C. botulinum* grows only in the absence of air in non-acidic foods; incorrect home canning causes most botulism, but in 2007 commercially canned chili sauce caused an outbreak; honey can contain botulism spores and should not be given to infants younger than 1 year of age
Vibrio	*V. parahemolyticus:* raw and undercooked shellfish, especially oysters	Onset: 24 hours; watery diarrhea, nausea, vomiting, fever, chills; lasts 3 days	Found in coastal waters; more infections in summer; number of infections hard to determine because it is difficult to isolate in the lab
	V. vulnificus: raw and undercooked shellfish, especially oysters	Onset: 1–2 days; vomiting, diarrhea, abdominal pain; in more severe cases, bloodstream infection with fever, chills, decreased blood pressure, blistering skin lesions; lasts 3 or more days	Estimated 95 cases/year; found in coastal waters; more infections in summer; those with impaired immune systems and liver disease at higher risk of infection; fatality rate of 50% with bloodstream infection
	V. cholerae: contaminated water and food, human carriers	Onset: 2–3 days; severe, dehydrating diarrhea, vomiting; dehydration, cardiovascular collapse, and death can occur	Occurs mainly in countries without adequate water purification and sewage treatment
Yersinia enterocolitica	Raw or undercooked pork, particularly pork intestines (chitterlings); tofu; water; unpasteurized milk	Onset: 4–7 days; fever, abdominal pain, diarrhea (often bloody); lasts 1–3 weeks or longer	Yersinosis most common in children under age 5 years; relatively rare; bacteria live mainly in pigs but can be found in other animals

typically do not multiply when food is held at temperatures above 140°F (60°C) or stored at safe refrigeration temperatures, 32° to 40°F (0° to 4.4°C). One important exception is *Listeria* bacteria, which can multiply at refrigeration temperatures. Also note that high temperatures can kill toxin-producing bacteria, but any toxin produced in the food will not be inactivated by high temperatures. Most pathogenic bacteria also require oxygen for growth, but *Clostridium botulinum* and *Clostridium perfringens* grow only in anaerobic (oxygen-free) environments, such as those found in tightly sealed cans and jars. Food acidity can affect bacterial growth, too. Although most bacteria do not grow well in acidic environments, some, such as disease-causing *E. coli*, can grow in acidic foods, such as fruit juice.

Viruses

Viruses, like bacteria, are widely dispersed in nature. Unlike bacteria, however, viruses can reproduce only after invading body cells, such as those that line the intestines. Experts speculate that about 70% of foodborne illness cases go un-diagnosed because they result from viral causes, and there is no easy way to test for these pathogens. Table 16-4 describes the two most common viral causes of foodborne illness and describes typical food sources and symptoms of the illnesses they cause. Norovirus is the number one pathogen contributing to domestically acquired foodborne illnesses. It causes an illness commonly misdiagnosed as the "stomach flu." Norovirus infection has a sudden onset and usually a short duration of only one to two days. Noroviruses have become a problem on cruise ships. They are hardy and survive freezing, relatively high temperatures, and chlorination up to 10 ppm. A website coordinating the U.S. efforts on food safety is the www.FoodSafety.gov site mentioned earlier. Another useful website is www.homefoodsafety.org.

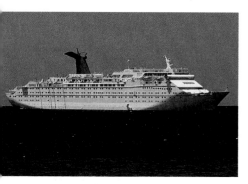

▲ Norovirus epidemics commonly occur on cruise ships. Noroviruses were originally called "Norwalk viruses" from Norwalk, Ohio, where they were first known to cause an epidemic of gastroenteritis.

TABLE 16-4 Viral Causes of Foodborne Illness

Viruses	Typical Food Sources	Symptoms	Additional Information
Norovirus (Norwalk and Norwalk-like viruses), human rotavirus	Foods prepared by infected food handlers; shellfish from contaminated waters; vegetables and fruits contaminated during growing, harvesting, and processing (see Further Reading 13.)	Onset: 1–2 days; "stomach flu"—severe diarrhea, nausea, vomiting, stomach cramping, low-grade fever, chills, muscle aches; lasts 1–2 days or longer	Estimated over 5 million cases per year and 150 deaths. Viruses found in stool and vomit of infected persons; food handlers can contaminate foods or work surfaces; noroviruses are very infectious—as few as 10–100 particles can lead to infection; workers with norovirus symptoms should not work until 2 or 3 days after they feel better.
Hepatitis A virus	Foods prepared by infected food handlers, especially uncooked foods or those handled after cooking, such as sandwiches, pastries, and salads; shellfish from contaminated waters; vegetables and fruits contaminated during growing, harvesting, and processing	Onset: 15–50 days; anorexia, diarrhea, fever, jaundice, dark urine, fatigue; may cause liver damage and death; lasts several weeks up to 6 months	Infected food handlers contaminate food and transmit the disease to dozens of persons; children and young adults are more susceptible; a vaccine is available, decreasing the number of infections dramatically; immunoglobulin given within 1 week to those exposed to hepatitis A virus can also decrease infection.

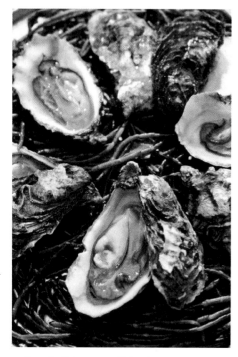

▲ Raw shellfish, especially bivalves (e.g., oysters and clams), present a particular risk related to foodborne viral disease. These animals filter feed, a process that concentrates viruses, bacteria, and toxins present in the water as it is filtered for food. Adequate cooking of shellfish will kill viruses and bacteria, but toxins may not be affected. It's important to buy shellfish from reliable sources who have harvested these foods from safe areas.

Parasites

Parasites live in or on another organism, known as the host, from which they absorb nutrients. Humans may serve as a host to parasites. These tiny ravagers rob millions of people around the globe of their health and, in some cases, their lives. Those hardest hit live in tropical countries where poor sanitation fosters the growth of parasites.

The more than 80 foodborne parasites known to affect humans include mainly **protozoa** (one-celled animals), such as *Cryptosporidium* and *Cyclospora*, and **helminths,** such as tapeworms and the roundworm *Trichinella spiralis.* Table 16-5 describes common parasites and typical food sources and symptoms of the illnesses they cause. Parasitic infections spread via person-to-person contact and contaminated food, water, and soil.

16.4 Food Additives

By the time you see a food on the market shelf, it usually contains substances added to make it more palatable or increase its nutrient content or shelf life. Manufacturers also add some substances to foods to make them easier to process. Other substances may have accidentally found their way into the foods you buy. All of these extraneous substances are known as **additives,** and, although some may be beneficial, others, such as sulfites, may be harmful for some people. All purposefully added substances must be evaluated by FDA.

protozoa One-celled animals that are more complex than bacteria. Disease-causing protozoa can be spread through food and water.

helminth Parasitic worm that can contaminate food, water, feces, animals, and other substances.

additives Substances added to foods, such as preservatives.

preservatives Compounds that extend the shelf life of foods by inhibiting microbial growth or minimizing the destructive effect of oxygen and metals.

sequestrants Compounds that bind free metal ions. By so doing, they reduce the ability of ions to cause rancidity in foods containing fat.

Why Are Food Additives Used?

Most additives are used to limit food spoilage. Common food additives serve the general function of **preservatives,** including acidic or alkaline agents, antioxidants, antimicrobial agents, curing and pickling agents, and **sequestrants.** Table 16-6 helps you to understand exactly why these are used and to learn more about the specific substances used. Food additives, such as potassium sorbate, are used to maintain the safety and acceptability of foods by retarding the growth of microbes implicated in foodborne illness.

Additives are also used to combat some enzymes that lead to undesirable changes in color and flavor in foods but don't cause anything as serious as foodborne illness. This second type of food spoilage occurs when enzymes in a food react to oxygen—for example, when apple and peach slices darken or turn rust color as they are exposed to air. Antioxidants are a type of preservative that slow the action of oxygen-requiring enzymes on food surfaces. These preservatives are not necessarily novel chemicals. They include vitamins E and C and a variety of sulfites.

Without the use of some food additives, it would be impossible to produce massive quantities of foods and safely distribute them nationwide or worldwide, as is now done. Despite consumer concerns about the safety of food additives, many have been extensively studied and proven safe when FDA guidelines for their use are followed.

TABLE 16-5 Parasitic Causes of Foodborne Illness

Parasite	Typical Food Sources	Symptoms	Additional Information
Trichinella spiralis	Pork, wild game	Onset: weeks to months; GI symptoms followed by muscle weakness, fluid retention in the face, fever, flulike symptoms	The number of trichinosis infections has decreased greatly because pigs are now less likely to harbor this parasite; cooking pork to 160°F (72°C) will kill *trichinella*, as will freezing it for 3 days at −4°F (−20°C).
Anisakis	Raw or undercooked fish	Onset: 12 hours or less; violent stomach pain, nausea, vomiting	Caused by eating the larvae of roundworms; the infection is more common where raw fish is routinely consumed.
Tapeworms	Raw beef, pork, and fish	Abdominal discomfort, diarrhea	
Toxoplasma gondii	Raw or undercooked meat, unwashed fruits and vegetables	Onset: 5–20 days; most people are asymptomatic; those with symptoms have fever, headache, sore muscles, diarrhea; can be fatal to the fetus of pregnant women	Parasite is spread to humans from animals, including cats, the main reservoir of the disease; humans acquire the disease from ingesting contaminated meat or from fecal contamination from handling cat litter.
Cyclospora cayetanensis	Water, contaminated food	Onset: 1 week; watery diarrhea, vomiting, muscle aches, fatigue, anorexia, weight loss; lasts 10–12 weeks	Most common in tropical and subtropical areas, but since 1990 about a dozen outbreaks, affecting 3600 people, have occurred in the United States and Canada.
Cryptosporidium	Water, contaminated food	Onset: 2–10 days; watery diarrhea, abdominal pain, fever, nausea, vomiting, weight loss; those with impaired immune systems become more ill; lasts 1–2 weeks in otherwise healthy persons	Outbreaks occur worldwide; the largest U.S. outbreak was in 1993 in Milwaukee, with more than 443,000 persons affected; also can be spread in water parks and community swimming pools.

TABLE 16-6 Types of Food Additives—Sources and Related Health Concerns

Food Additive Class	Attributes	Health Risks
Acidic or alkaline agents, such as citric acid, calcium lactate, and sodium hydroxide	Acids impart a tart taste to soft drinks, sherbets, and cheese spreads; inhibit mold growth; lessen discoloration and rancidity. They also reduce the risk of botulism in naturally low-acid vegetables, such as canned green beans. Alkaline agents neutralize acids produced during fermentation, and so improve flavor.	No known health risks when used properly.
Alternative low-calorie sweeteners, such as saccharin, sucralose, ascesulfame potassium, aspartame, neotame, and tagatose	Sweeten foods without adding more than a few calories	Moderate use of these alternative sweeteners is considered safe (except for use of aspartame by people with the disease PKU).
Anticaking agents, such as calcium silicate, magnesium stearate, and silicon dioxide	Absorb moisture to keep table salt, baking powder, or powdered sugar and powdered food products free-flowing and prevent caking and lumping	No known health risks when used properly.
Antimicrobial agents, such as salt, sodium benzoate, sorbic acid, and calcium propionate	Inhibit mold and fungal growth	Salt increases the risk of developing hypertension, especially in some individuals. No known health risks from other agents when used properly.
Antioxidants, such as BHA (butylated hydroxyanisole), BHT (butylated hydroxytoluene), alpha-tocopherol (vitamin E), ascorbic acid (vitamin C), and sulfites	Delay food discolorations from oxygen exposure; Reduce rancidity from the breakdown of fats; Maintain the color of luncheon meats; Prevent the formation of cancer-causing nitrosamines	Sulfites can cause an allergic reaction in about 1 in every 100 people. Symptoms include difficulty breathing, wheezing, hives, diarrhea, abdominal pain, cramps, and dizziness. Salad bars, dried fruit, and wine are typical sources of sulfites.
Color additives, such as tartrazine	Make foods more appealing	Tartrazine (FD&C yellow number 5) can cause allergic symptoms such as hives and nasal discharge in some people, especially those allergic to aspirin. FDA requires manufacturers to list all forms of synthetic colors on the labels of foods that contain them.
Curing and pickling agents, such as salt, nitrates, and nitrites	Nitrates and nitrites act as preservatives, especially to prevent the growth of *Clostridium botulinium;* often used in conjunction with salt	Salt increases the risk of developing hypertension, especially in some individuals. Nitrate and nitrite consumption from both cured foods and that found naturally in some vegetables has been associated with synthesis of nitrosamines. (An adequate

Sugar, salt, corn syrup, and citric acid constitute 98% of all additives (by weight) used in food processing.

▲ Soft drinks are typical sources of alternative sweeteners for many of us. Moderate use of these products generally poses no health risk in most people.

You might wonder why, if nitrates and nitrites form chemical substances that can cause cancer, they aren't banned by the Delaney Clause. In the United States, USDA regulates the use of chemicals in meats. The laws that govern USDA regulation of foods are separate from those that govern FDA regulation. Because of this, the Delaney Clause does not apply to USDA actions. USDA sees no clear threat to public safety from the regulated use of nitrates and nitrites in meats, so no action has been taken.

TABLE 16-6 *(continued)*

Food Additive Class	Attributes	Health Risks
		vitamin C intake may reduce this synthesis.) Some nitrosamines are cancer-causing agents, particularly for the stomach, esophagus, and colon, but the risk is low. The National Cancer Institute advises consuming these foods in moderation.
Emulsifiers, such as monoglycerides and lecithins	Suspend fat in water to improve uniformity, smoothness, and body of foods, such as baked goods, ice cream, and mayonnaise	No known health risks when used properly.
Fat replacements, such as Paselli SA2, Dur-Low, Oatrim, Sta-Slim 143, Stellar, and Olean	Limit calorie content of foods by reducing some of the fat content	Generally no known health risks when used properly.
Flavor and flavoring agents (such as natural and artificial flavors), sugar, and corn syrup	Impart more or improve flavor of foods	Sugar and corn syrup can increase risk for dental caries. Generally no known health risks for flavoring agents when used properly.
Flavor enhancers, such as monosodium glutamate (MSG) and salt	Help bring out the natural flavor of foods, such as meats	Some people (especially infants) are sensitive to the glutamate portion of MSG and after exposure experience flushing, chest pain, facial pressure, dizziness, sweating, rapid heart rate, nausea, vomiting, increase in blood pressure, and headache. Those so affected should look for the word glutamate on food labels, as well as isolated protein, yeast extract, bullion, and soup stock. Salt increases the risk of developing hypertension, especially in some people.
Humectants, such as glycerol, propylene glycol, and sorbitol	Retain more moisture, texture, and fresh flavor in foods such as candies, shredded coconut, and marshmallows	No known health risk when used properly.
Leavening agents, such as yeast, baking powder, and baking soda	Introduce carbon dioxide into food products	No known health risk when used properly.
Maturing and bleaching agents, such as bromates, peroxides, and ammonium chloride	Shorten the time needed for maturation of flour to become usable for baking products	No known health risk when used properly.
Nutrient supplements, such as vitamin A, vitamin D, and potassium iodide	Enhance the nutrient content of foods such as margarine, milk, and ready-to-eat breakfast cereals	No known health risk if intake from such supplemental sources combined with other natural food sources of a nutrient does not exceed the Upper Level set for a particular nutrient (iron may be one exception; review Chapter 12).

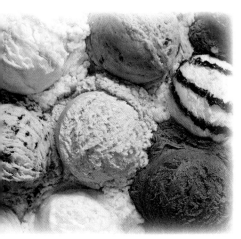

▲ Emulsifiers improve the texture of foods such as ice cream, baked goods, and cookies.

CRITICAL THINKING

Recognizing that Joseph is taking a nutrition class, his roommate asks him, "What is more risky: the bacteria that can be present in food or the additives listed on the label of my favorite snack cake?" How should Joseph respond? On what information should he base his conclusions?

TABLE 16-6 *(continued)*

Food Additive Class	Attributes	Health Risks
Stabilizers and thickeners, such as pectins, gums, gelatins, and agars	Impart a smooth texture and uniform color and flavor to candies, ice cream and other frozen desserts, chocolate milk, and beverages containing alternative sweeteners. Prevent evaporation and deterioration of flavorings used in cakes, puddings, and gelatin mixes	No known health risk when used properly.
Sequestrants, such as EDTA and citric acid	Bind free ions, helping preserve food quality by reducing ability of ions to cause rancidity in products containing fat	No known health risk when used properly.

Intentional Versus Incidental Food Additives

Food additives are classified into two types: **intentional food additives** (directly added to foods) and **incidental food additives** (indirectly added as contaminants). Both types of agents are regulated by FDA in the United States. Currently, more than 2800 different substances are intentionally added to foods. As many as 10,000 other substances enter foods as contaminants. This includes substances that may reasonably be expected to enter food through surface contact with processing equipment or packaging materials.

The GRAS List

In 1958, all food additives used in the United States and considered safe at that time were put on a **generally recognized as safe (GRAS)** list. The U.S. Congress established the GRAS list because it believed manufacturers did not need to prove the safety of substances that had been used for a long time and were already generally recognized as safe. Since that time, FDA has been responsible for proving that a substance does not belong on the GRAS list. Substances may be added to the GRAS list if data and information about the use of the substance are known and accepted widely by qualified experts, and establish that the substance is safe under the conditions of its intended use.

Since 1958, some substances on the list have been reviewed. A few, such as cyclamates, failed the review process and were removed from the list. The additive red dye #3 was removed because it is linked to cancer. Many chemicals on the GRAS list have not yet been rigorously tested, primarily because of expense. These chemicals have received a low priority for testing, mostly because they have long histories of use without evidence of toxicity or because their chemical characteristics do not suggest they are potential health hazards.

Are Synthetic Chemicals Always Harmful?

Nothing about a natural product makes it inherently safer than a synthetic product. Many synthetic products are laboratory copies of chemicals that also occur in nature (see the discussion in Chapter 15 on biotechnology for some examples). Moreover, although human endeavors contribute some toxins to foods, such as synthetic pesticides and industrial chemicals, nature's poisons are often even more potent and

intentional food additives Additives knowingly (directly) incorporated into food products by manufacturers.

incidental food additives Additives that appear in food products indirectly, from environmental contamination of food ingredients or during the manufacturing process.

generally recognized as safe (GRAS) A list of food additives that in 1958 were considered safe for consumption. Manufacturers were allowed to continue to use these additives, without special clearance, when needed for food products. FDA bears responsibility for proving they are not safe, but can remove unsafe products from the list.

Some important definitions:

toxicology	Scientific study of harmful substances
safety	Relative certainty that a substance won't cause injury
hazard	Chance that injury will result from use of a substance
toxicity	Capacity of a substance to produce injury or illness at some dosage

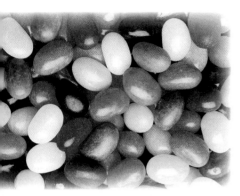

▲ Color additives make some foods more desirable.

The 100-fold margin of safety is 25 times less than that for vitamin A, when you compare the RDA for healthy women (700 micrograms) to a potentially harmful dose of vitamin A for pregnant women (3000 micrograms).

Delaney Clause A clause to the 1958 Food Additives Amendment of the Pure Food and Drug Act in the United States that prevents the intentional (direct) addition to foods of a compound shown to cause cancer in laboratory animals or humans.

widespread. Some cancer researchers suggest that we ingest at least 10,000 times more (by weight) natural toxins produced by plants than we do synthetic pesticide residues. (Plants produce these toxins to protect themselves from predators and disease-causing organisms.) This comparison does not make synthetic chemicals any less toxic, but it does put them in a more accurate perspective.

Consider vitamin E, often added to food to prevent rancidity of fats. This chemical is safe when used within certain limits. However, high doses have been associated with health problems, such as interfering with vitamin K activity in the body (review Chapter 10). Thus, even well-known chemicals we are comfortable using can be toxic in some circumstances and at some concentrations.

Tests of Food Additives for Safety

Food additives are tested by FDA for safety on at least two animal species, usually rats and mice. Scientists determine the highest dose of the additive that produces *no observable effects* in the animals. These doses are proportionately much higher than humans are ever exposed to. The maximum dosage that produced no observable effects is then divided by at least 100 to establish a margin of safety for human use. This 100-fold margin is used because it is assumed that we are at least 10 times more sensitive to food additives than are laboratory animals and that any one person might be 10 times more sensitive than another. This broad margin essentially ensures that the food additive in question will cause no harmful health effects in humans. In fact, many synthetic chemicals are probably less dangerous at these low doses than some of the natural compounds in common foods such as apples or celery.

One important exception applies to the schema for testing intentional food additives: If an additive is shown to cause cancer, even though only in high doses, no margin of safety is allowed. The food additive cannot be used, because it would violate the **Delaney Clause** in the 1958 Food Additives Amendment. This clause prohibits intentionally adding to foods a compound introduced after 1958 and that causes cancer at any level of exposure. Evidence for cancer could come from either laboratory animal or human studies. Few exceptions to this clause are allowed; exceptions are discussed regarding curing and pickling agents in Table 16-6.

Incidental food additives are another matter. FDA cannot ban various industrial chemicals, pesticide residues, and mold toxins from foods, even though some of these contaminants can cause cancer. These products are not purposely added to foods. FDA sets an acceptable level for these substances. An incidental substance found in a food cannot contribute to more than one cancer case during the lifetimes of 1 million people. If a higher risk exists, the amount of the compound in a food must be reduced until the guideline is met.

In general, if you consume a variety of foods in moderation, the chances of food additives jeopardizing your health are minimal. Pay attention to your body. If you suspect an intolerance or a sensitivity, consult your physician for further evaluation. Remember that in the short run, you are more likely to suffer either from foodborne illness due to poor food-handling practices that allow viral and bacterial contamination in food, or from the consumption of raw animal foods, than from consuming additives. Excess calories, saturated fat, cholesterol, *trans* fat, salt, and other potential "problem" nutrients in our diets pose the greatest long-term health risk.

Approval for a New Food Additive

Before a new food additive can be added to foods, FDA must approve its use. Besides rigorously testing an additive to establish its safety margins, manufacturers must give FDA information that (1) identifies the new additive, (2) gives its chemical composition, (3) states how it is manufactured, and (4) specifies laboratory methods used to measure its presence in the food supply at the amount of intended use.

Manufacturers must also offer proof that the additive will accomplish its intended purpose in a food, that it is safe, and that it is to be used in no higher amount than needed. Additives cannot be used to hide defective food ingredients, such as rancid oils; to deceive customers; or replace good manufacturing practices. A manufacturer must establish that the ingredient is necessary for producing a specific food product.

MAKING DECISIONS

Processed or Whole Foods?

If you are bewildered or concerned about all the additives in your diet, you can easily avoid most of them by consuming unprocessed whole foods. However, no evidence shows that this will necessarily make you healthier, nor can you avoid all additives, because some are used even on whole foods, such as with pesticides. It amounts to a personal decision. Do you have confidence that FDA and food manufacturers are adequately protecting your health and welfare, or do you want to take more personal control by minimizing your intake of compounds not naturally found in foods?

CONCEPT CHECK

Food additives are used to reduce spoilage from microbial growth, oxygen, metals, and other compounds. Additives are also used to adjust acidity, improve flavor and color, leaven, provide nutritional fortification, thicken, and emulsify food components. Additives are classified as intentional (direct; purposely added to foods), and incidental (indirect; present in foods from environmental contamination or various manufacturing practices). The amount of an additive allowed in a food is limited to one-one-hundredth of the highest amount that has no observable effect when fed to animals. The Delaney Clause allows FDA to limit intentional addition of cancer-causing compounds to food in the United States under its jurisdiction. Also set by law in the United States are the permissible amounts of carcinogens that incidentally enter foods.

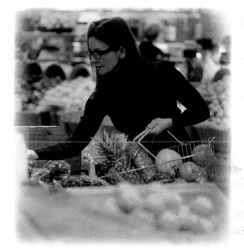

▲ Depending on whether you choose fresh versus processed foods, a diet can be either essentially free of or contain food additives. For most of us, this specific concern regarding food choice is not worth worrying about.

16.5 Substances That Occur Naturally in Foods and Can Cause Illness

Foods contain a variety of naturally occurring substances that can cause illness. Here are some of the more important examples:

- *Safrole*—found in sassafras, mace, and nutmeg; causes cancer when consumed in high doses
- *Solanine*—found in potato shoots and green spots on potato skins; inhibits the action of neurotransmitters
- *Mushroom toxins*—found in some species of mushrooms such as aminita; can cause stomach upset, dizziness, hallucinations, and other neurological symptoms. The more lethal varieties can cause liver and kidney failure, coma, and even death. FDA regulates commercially grown and harvested mushrooms. These are cultivated in concrete buildings or caves. However, there are no systematic controls on individual gatherers harvesting wild species, except in Illinois and Michigan.
- *Avidin*—found in raw egg whites (cooking destroys avidin); binds the vitamin biotin in a way that prevents its absorption, so a biotin deficiency may ultimately develop over the long term
- *Thiaminase*—found in raw fish, clams, and mussels; destroys the vitamin thiamin
- *Tetrodotoxin*—found in puffer fish; causes respiratory paralysis
- *Oxalic acid*—found in spinach, strawberries, sesame seeds, and other foods; binds calcium and iron in the foods, and so limits absorption of these nutrients
- *Herbal teas* containing senna or comfrey—can cause diarrhea and liver damage

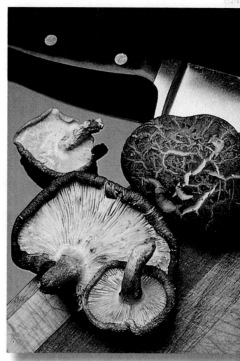

▲ When hunting wild mushrooms, know what you are looking for. Many varieties contain deadly toxins.

People have coexisted for centuries with these naturally occurring substances and have learned to avoid some of them and limit intake of others. They pose little health risk. Farmers know potatoes must be stored in the dark, so that solanine won't be synthesized. Furthermore, we've developed cooking and food-preparation methods to limit the potency of other substances, such as thiaminase. Spices are used in such small amounts that health risks don't result. Nevertheless, it's important to understand that some potentially harmful chemicals in foods occur naturally.

Is Caffeine a Cause for Concern?

Why all the controversy over a cup of coffee? Researchers have spent a great deal of time on the study of caffeine, the substance of greatest concern in the favorite beverage of many of us. So why do caffeine recommendations change from year to year?

Caffeine is a stimulant found as a natural or added ingredient in many beverages and chocolate. On average, we consume 75% of our caffeine intake as coffee, 15% as tea, 10% as soft drinks, and 2% as chocolate (Table 16-7). (For teenagers and young adults this ratio is often relatively higher for soft drinks and lower for coffee.)

Caffeine is not often consumed by itself. With the popularity of trendy coffee shops that serve everything from mocha java to flavored lattes, it is difficult to separate caffeine intake from cream, sugar, alternative sweeteners, and flavorings. So what is the conscientious coffee drinker to think? Let's explore the myths and facts of caffeine intake.

Caffeine does not accumulate in the body and is normally excreted within several hours following consumption. Caffeine can cause anxiety, increased heart rate, insomnia, increased urination (possibly resulting in dehydration), diarrhea, and gastrointestinal upset in high doses. In addition, those already suffering from ulcers may experience irritation due to increased acid production; those who have anxiety

TABLE 16-7 Caffeine Content of Common Sources

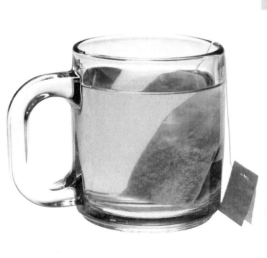

Item	Milligrams of Caffeine	
	Typical	Range*
Coffee (8 fl oz)		
Brewed, drip method	85	65–120
Brewed, percolator	75	60–85
Decaffeinated, brewed	3	2–4
Espresso (1 fl oz serving)	40	30–50
Teas (8 fl oz)		
Brewed, Black tea	40	20–90
Brewed, Green tea	20	8–30
Iced	25	9–50
Instant	28	24–31
Some soft drinks (8 fl oz)	24	20–40
"Energy drinks" such as Red Bull (8.3 fl oz)	80	0–80
Cocoa beverage (8 fl oz)	6	3–32
Chocolate milk beverage (8 fl oz)	5	2–7
Milk chocolate (1 oz)	6	1–15
Dark chocolate, semi-sweet (1 oz)	20	5–35
Baker's chocolate (1 oz)	26	26
Chocolate-flavored syrup (1 fl oz)	4	4

*For the coffee and tea products, the range varies due to brewing method, plant variety, brand of product, and so on.

Source: International Food Information Council. *Caffeine and women's health*, August 2002.

or panic attacks may find that caffeine worsens their symptoms; and those prone to heartburn may find that caffeine worsens this symptom because it relaxes sphincter muscles in the esophagus. Some people need little caffeine to feel such effects, and the dosage for children is likely even lower than that for adults.

Withdrawal symptoms are also real. Former coffee drinkers may experience headache, nausea, and depression for a short time after discontinuing use. These symptoms can be expected to peak at 20 to 48 hours following the last intake of caffeine. Symptoms hold true even for those trying to quit as little as one cup of coffee per day. Slow tapering of use over a few days is recommended to avoid these problems.

Are there more serious consequences of consuming caffeine regularly? It has been hypothesized that caffeine consumption can lead to certain types of cancer, such as pancreatic and bladder cancers. The association of caffeine with cancer has not been supported in recent literature. In fact, regular coffee consumption has been linked to a decreased risk of colon cancer.

Negative press has dwindled with regard to a link between cardiovascular disease and moderate coffee consumption. Heavy use does increase blood pressure for a short period of time. Coffee consumption also has been linked to increased LDL-cholesterol and triglycerides in the blood. This association was found to be caused by cafestol and kahweol, two oils in ground coffee. However, filtered and instant coffees do not contain the harmful oils. It is prudent, though, to limit the amount of coffee in general, especially from French coffee presses and from espresso as these beverages are not filtered.

Women are thought to be at higher risk for a variety of deleterious effects with caffeine consumption, including miscarriages, osteoporosis, and birth defects in their offspring. It is true that heavy caffeine use mildly increases the amount of calcium excreted in urine. For this reason, it is important that heavy coffee drinkers check their diets for adequate calcium sources. Some studies do show a higher likelihood for miscarriages in women consuming more than 500 milligrams of caffeine per day (about five 8-ounce cups of coffee). FDA warns women to consume caffeine in moderation (no more than the equivalent of one to two 8-ounce cups of coffee per day).

In contrast to these possibly harmful effects of caffeine consumption, many people are convinced of the benefits of a "cup of joe." Though some women testify to the idea that caffeine improves premenstrual symptoms, no study proves this theory. Some weight-loss drugs previously contained caffeine, under the assumption that it made the drugs more effective. FDA has since banned this use as it was found to be ineffective. Some newer research findings suggest caffeine may reduce the risk of developing headaches, cirrhosis of the liver, some forms of kidney stones, gallbladder stones, some nerve-related diseases, and furthermore, that it aids in blood glucose regulation. You may have heard that caffeine can improve physical performance. This has been shown in highly trained athletes; recall that use of large amounts of caffeine is banned by the NCAA (review Chapter 13). For those below professional status, though, no benefit has been shown. Also keep in mind that coffee will not "sober up" a person who is drunk.

Though the debate over caffeine will likely continue as long as North Americans drink coffee, research does not support many of the concepts previously thought of as fact. These studies are reinforcing the idea of moderation—the equivalent of about two to three 8-ounce cups of coffee per day. A prudent dose of caffeine is 200 to 300 milligrams per day. Review Table 16-7 concerning the caffeine content of typical sources.

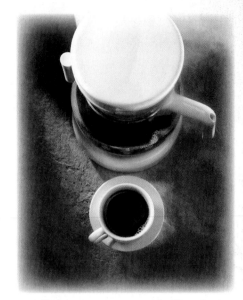

▲ Coffee is a common source of caffeine for many adults.

16.6 Environmental Contaminants in Food

A variety of environmental contaminants can be found in foods. Aside from pesticide residues, other potential contaminants that deserve attention are listed in Table 16-8. To reduce exposure to environmental toxins present in our foods that cause disease, find out which foods pose a risk. In addition, emphasize variety and moderation in food selection. Tips provided in Tables 16-8 and 16-9 also apply to reducing exposure to environmental contaminants.

Genetic alteration of foods such as corn and soybeans has created concern, especially in Europe. FDA considers genetically altered products safe if approval for human use has been granted (see Chapter 15 for details).

TABLE 16-8 Potential Environmental and Other Contaminants in Our Food Supply

Chemical Substance	Sources	Toxic Effects	Preventive Measures
Acrylamide	Fried foods rich in carbohydrate cooked at high temperatures for extended periods, such as French fries and potato chips	Potential neurotoxin and carcinogen. Known carcinogen for laboratory animals; however, studies have not clearly proven the relationship between acrylamide ingestion and the development of cancer in humans.	Limit intake of deep-fat fried foods rich in carbohydrate.
Cadmium	Plants in general if much cadmium is in the soil Clams, shellfish, tobacco smoke Occupational exposure in some cases	Kidney disease Liver disease Prostate cancer (debatable) Bone deformities Lung disease (when inhaled)	Consume a wide variety of foods, including seafood sources.
Dioxin	Trash-burning incinerators Bottom-feeding fish from the Great Lakes Animal fats from animals exposed to such contamination via water or soil	Abnormal reproduction and fetal/infant development Immune suppression Cancer (to date only clearly shown in laboratory animals)	Pay attention to warnings of dioxin risks from local fish; if risk exists, limit intake as suggested on the fishing license. Consume a variety of fish from local waters rather than mostly one specific species.
Lead	Lead-based paint chips and related dust in older homes Occupational exposure (e.g., radiator repair) Lead caps on wine bottles Fruit juices and pickled vegetables stored in galvanized or tin containers or leaded glass Some types of solder used in joining copper pipes (mostly in older homes) Mexican pottery dishes Koo Soo herbal remedies Leaded glass containers (see Further Reading 8.)	Anemia Kidney disease Nervous system damage (tiredness and changes in behavior are symptoms) Reduced learning capacity in childhood (even from mild lead exposure)	Avoid paint chips and related dust in older homes; regular cleaning of these homes is also important (see **www.hud.gov/offices/lead**). Meet iron and calcium needs to reduce lead absorption. Wipe the inside and outside neck of wine bottles before use if the bottle has a lead cap. Store fruit juices and pickled vegetables in glass or plastic or waxed paper containers. Let water run 1 minute or so if off for more than 2 hours, and use only cold water for cooking; do not soften drinking water. Do not store alcoholic beverages in leaded glass containers.
Mercury	Swordfish, shark, king mackerel, and tilefish. Fresh and canned albacore tuna also is a possible source. (In contrast, the more typical light chunk tuna is very low in mercury.)	Reduced fetal/child development and birth defects; toxic to nervous system	Consume these sources no more than once per week, no more than two times per week for albacore tuna. Pregnant women should avoid these species of fish, but some albacore tuna consumption is fine. Two to three fish meals per week is appropriate for pregnant (and nursing) women if different types of fish are eaten.
Polychlorinated biphenyls (PCBs)	Fish from the Great Lakes and Hudson River Valley (e.g., coho salmon) Farmed salmon are a possible source, but less so	Cancer (to date only clearly shown in laboratory animals), as well as a potential for liver, immune, and reproductive disorders	Pay attention to warnings of PCB contamination from local fish; if risk exists, limit intake as suggested on the fishing license or on state advisories. Vary the type of fish eaten during a specific week.
Urethane	Alcoholic beverages such as sherry, bourbon, sake, and fruit brandies	Cancer (to date only clearly shown in laboratory animals)	Avoid generous amounts of typical sources.

A general program to minimize exposure to environmental contaminants includes knowing which foods pose greater risks and consuming a wide variety of foods in moderation.

Pesticides in Food

Pesticides used in food production produce both beneficial and unwanted effects (see Further Reading 3). Most health authorities believe that the benefits outweigh the risks. Pesticides help ensure a safe and adequate food supply and help make foods available at reasonable cost. However, there is sentiment nationwide that pesticides pose avoidable health risks. Consumers have come to assume that synthetic is dangerous and organic is safe. Some researchers believe this sentiment is grounded in fear and fueled by unbalanced reports. Other researchers say concern about pesticides is valid and overdue.

Most concern about pesticide residues in food appropriately focuses on chronic rather than acute toxicity because the amounts of residue present, if any, are extremely small. These low concentrations found in foods are not known to produce adverse effects in the short term, although harm has been caused by the high amounts that occasionally result from accidents or misuse. For humans, pesticides pose a danger mainly in their cumulative effects, so their threats to health are difficult to determine. However, growing evidence, including the problems of the contamination of underground water supplies and destruction of wildlife habitats, indicates that North Americans would probably be better off if we could reduce our use of pesticides. Both the U.S. federal government and many farmers are working toward that end. Chapter 15 discussed the lastest use of biotechnology to reduce pesticide use.

One of the problems with pesticides is that they create new pests because they destroy the predators (spiders, wasps, and beetles) that naturally keep most plantfeeding insect populations in check. The brown plant hopper, which has plagued Indonesian rice fields, was not a serious problem before heavy pesticide use began to kill its predators in the early 1970s. In the United States, such major pests as spider mites and the cotton bollworm were merely nuisances until pesticides decimated their predators.

What Is a Pesticide?

Federal law defines a pesticide as any substance or mixture of substances intended to prevent, destroy, repel, or mitigate any pest. The built-in toxic properties of pesticides lead to the possibility that other, nontarget organisms, including humans, might also be harmed. The term *pesticide* tends to be used as a generic reference to many types of products, including insecticides, herbicides, fungicides, and rodenticides. A pesticide product may be chemical or bacterial, natural or synthetic. For agriculture, EPA allows about 10,000 pesticides to be used, containing some 300 active ingredients. About 1.2 billion pounds of pesticides are used each year in the United States, much of which is applied to agricultural crops.

Once a pesticide is applied, it can turn up in a number of unintended and unwanted places. It may be carried in the air and dust by wind currents, remain in soil attached to soil particles, be taken up by organisms in the soil, decompose to other compounds, be taken up by plant roots, enter groundwater, or invade aquatic habitats. Each is a route to the food chain; some are more direct than others.

Why Use Pesticides?

In the United States, pests destroy nearly $20 billion of food crops yearly, despite extensive pesticide use. The primary reason for using pesticides is economic—the use of agricultural chemicals increases production and lowers the cost of food, at least in the short run. Many farmers believe that it would be impossible to stay in business without pesticides, which help protect farmers from ruinous losses.

Consumer demands also have changed over the years. At one time, we wouldn't have thought twice about buying an apple with a worm hole; we took it home, cut out

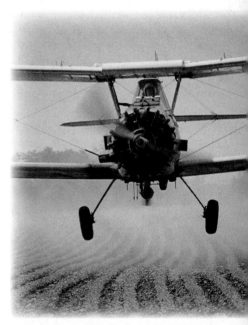

▲ Pesticide use poses a risk-versus-benefit question. Each side has points that deserve to be considered. Rural communities, where exposure is more direct, experience the greatest short-term risk.

the wormy part, and ate the apple. Today, consumers find worm holes less acceptable, so farmers rely more on pesticides to produce cosmetically attractive fruits and vegetables. On the practical side, pesticides can protect against the rotting and decay of fresh fruits and vegetables. This is helpful because our food distribution system doesn't usually permit consumer purchase within hours of harvest. Also, food grown without pesticides can contain naturally occurring organisms that produce carcinogens at concentrations far above current standards for pesticide residues. For example, fungicides help prevent the carcinogen aflatoxin (caused by growth of a fungus) from forming on some crops. Thus, although some pesticides may do little more than improve the appearance of food products, others help keep foods fresher and safer to eat.

Regulation of Pesticides

The responsibility for ensuring that residues of pesticides in foods are below amounts that pose a danger to health is shared by FDA, EPA, and the Food Safety and Inspection Service of USDA in the United States. Table 16-2 listed the roles of various food protection agencies. FDA is responsible for enforcing pesticide tolerances in all foods except meat, poultry, and certain egg products, which are monitored by USDA. A newly proposed pesticide is exhaustively tested, perhaps over 10 years or more, before it is approved for use. EPA must decide that the pesticide causes no unreasonable adverse effects on people and the environment and that benefits of use outweigh the risks of using it. However, there is concern about older chemicals registered before 1970, when less stringent testing conditions were permitted. EPA is now asking chemical companies to retest the old compounds using more rigorous tests. Unfortunately, inadequate funding at EPA has hampered the review of older pesticides. The slow pace of this retesting has angered the critics of pesticide use. When weighing whether to approve or cancel a pesticide, EPA considers how much more it would cost the farmer to use an alternative pesticide or process and whether cancellation would decrease productivity. After determining the dollar cost to the farmer, EPA then looks at costs to processors and consumers. Once a pesticide is approved for use, it must follow the margin of safety provisions required of food additives (see previous section, "Tests of Food Additives for Safety").

How Safe Are Pesticides?

Dangers from exposure to pesticides through food depend on how potent the chemical toxin is, how concentrated it is in the food, how much and how frequently it's eaten, and the consumer's resistance or susceptibility to the substance. Accumulating information links pesticide use to increased cancer rates in farm communities. For rural counties in the United States, the incidence of lymph, genital, brain, and digestive tract cancers increases with higher-than-average pesticide use. Respiratory cancer cases increase with greater insecticide use. In tests using laboratory animals, scientists have found that some of the chemicals present in pesticide residues cause birth defects, sterility, tumors, organ damage, and injury to the central nervous system. Some pesticides persist in the environment for years.

Still, some researchers argue that the cancer risk from pesticide residues is hundreds of times less than the risk from eating such common foods as peanut butter, brown mustard, and basil. Plants manufacture toxic substances to defend themselves against insects, birds, and grazing animals (including humans). When plants are stressed or damaged, they produce even more of these toxins. Because of this, many foods contain naturally occurring chemicals considered toxic, and some are even carcinogenic. Other scientists argue that if natural carcinogens are already in the food supply, then we should reduce the number of added carcinogens whenever possible. In other words, we should do what we can to decrease our overall exposure.

Tests of the Amounts of Pesticides in Foods

FDA tests thousands of raw products each year for pesticide residues. (A pesticide is considered illegal in this case if it is not approved for use on the crop in question or

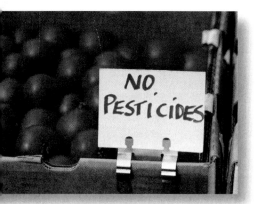

▲ Fruits and vegetables grown without use of pesticides are available and may bear an "organic" label (see Table 2-10 for rules regarding the use of the term "organic" on food labels). These products generally are more expensive than those grown using pesticides. Consumers need to decide if the potential benefits of the products are worth the extra cost.

if the amount used exceeds the allowed tolerance.) The latest FDA studies show no residues in about 60% of samples. Less than 1% of domestic and about 3% of import samples have residues continually over tolerance. These findings continue to support previous FDA studies over the past 10 years that pesticide residues in food are generally well below EPA tolerances, and they confirm the safety of the food supply relative to pesticide residues.

Personal Action

We often take risks in our lives, but we prefer to have a choice in the matter after weighing the pros and cons. With regard to pesticides in food, however, someone else is deciding what is acceptable and what is not. Our only choice is whether to buy or avoid pesticide-containing foods. In reality, it's almost impossible to avoid pesticides entirely, because even organic produce often contains traces of pesticides, probably as the result of cross-contamination from nearby farms.

Short-term studies of the effects of pesticides on laboratory animals cannot precisely pinpoint long-term cancer risks in humans. It should be clearly understood, however, that the presence of minute traces of an environmental chemical in a food does not mean that any adverse effect will result from eating that food.

FDA and other scientific organizations believe that the hazards are comparatively low and in the short run are less dangerous than the hazards of foodborne illness created in our kitchens. We cannot avoid pesticide risks entirely, but we can limit exposure by following some simple advice (Table 16-9).

We can also encourage farmers to use fewer pesticides to reduce exposure to our foods and water supplies, but we'll have to settle for produce that isn't perfect in appearance or that has been grown with the aid of biotechnology (again, see Chapter 15 for details). Are you concerned enough about pesticides on food to change your shopping habits or take more political action?

16.7 Food Production Choices

Agriculture, the production of food and livestock, has supplied humans with food for millennia. At one time, nearly everyone was involved in food production. Only about 1 in 3 people around the globe and far fewer in the United States (less than 1%), is now involved in farming. Today, numerous advances in agricultural sciences are affecting our food supply; of particular note are organic food production and sustainable agriculture.

TABLE 16-9 What You Can Do to Reduce Exposure to Pesticides

FDA's sampling and testing show that pesticide residues in foods do not pose a health hazard. Nevertheless, if you want to reduce dietary exposure to pesticides, follow this advice from the Environmental Protection Agency:

- Consume a wide variety of foods, especially regarding fruits, vegetables, and fish.
- Thoroughly rinse and scrub (with a brush if possible) fruits and vegetables. Peel them, if appropriate—although some nutrients will be peeled away.
- Remove the outer leaves of leafy vegetables, such as lettuce and cabbage.
- Residues of some pesticides in animal feed concentrate in the animals' fat, so trim fat from meat, poultry, and fish; remove skin (which contains most of the fat) from poultry and fish; and discard fats and oils in broths and pan drippings.
- When fishing, throw back the big fish—the little ones have had less time to take up and concentrate pesticides and other harmful residues. In addition, pay attention to any warnings by local authorities (and on the fishing license) about the high risk for contamination in specific waters or species of fish.
- Avoid lawns, gardens, and flower beds that have recently been treated with pesticides and herbicides.

Adapted from Food and Drug Administration: Safety first: Protecting America's food supply, *FDA Consumer*, p. 26, November 1988.

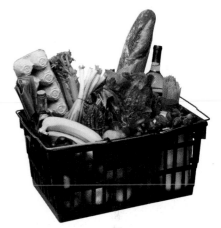

▲ FDA's yearly evaluation of a "market basket" of typical foods shows that pesticide content is minimal in most foods.

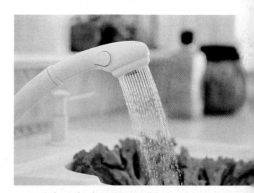

▲ Wash fresh fruits and vegetables under running water to remove bacteria and soil. Special antibacterial washing products are not necessary.

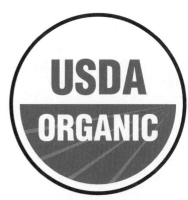

▲ The USDA organic seal identifies organic foods grown on USDA-certified organic farms.

▲ Organic fruits and vegetables experienced the highest growth in food sales at 11.8% over 2009 sales and representing over 11% of all fruit and vegetable sales.

biological pest management Control of agricultural pests by using natural predators, parasites, or pathogens. For example, ladybugs can be used to control an aphid infestation.

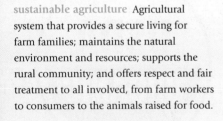

sustainable agriculture Agricultural system that provides a secure living for farm families; maintains the natural environment and resources; supports the rural community; and offers respect and fair treatment to all involved, from farm workers to consumers to the animals raised for food.

Organic Foods

Organic foods are increasingly available in supermarkets, specialty stores, farmers' markets, and restaurants (see Further Readings 11 and 14). Consumers can select organic fruits, vegetables, grains, dairy products, meats, eggs, and many processed foods, including sauces and condiments, breakfast cereals, cookies, and snack chips. Interest in personal and environmental health has contributed to the increasing availability and sales of organic foods. According to the Organic Trade Association, U.S. sales of organic foods reached $26.7 billion by the end of 2010. This was a 7.7% increase over 2009 sales, despite tough economic times. Despite this rapid growth, only 4% of foods sold are organic. Organic foods, because they often cost more to grow and produce, are typically more expensive than comparable conventional foods.

The term **organic** refers to the way agricultural products are produced. Organic production relies on farming practices such as **biological pest management,** composting, manure applications, and crop rotation to maintain healthy soil, water, crops, and animals. Synthetic pesticides, fertilizers, and hormones; antibiotics; sewage sludge (used as fertilizer); genetic engineering; and irradiation are not permitted in the production of organic foods. Additionally, organic meat, poultry, eggs, and dairy products must come from animals allowed to graze outdoors and are fed only organic feed.

The Organic Foods Production Act of 1990 established standards for the production of foods that bear the USDA organic seal. Foods labeled and marketed as organic must be grown on farms that are certified by the USDA as following all of the rules established in the 1990 act. Foods made from multiple ingredients (e.g., breakfast cereal) labeled as organic must have at least 95% of their ingredients (by weight) meet organic standards. The term "made with organic" can be used if at least 70% of the ingredients are organic. Small organic producers and farmers with sales less than $5000 per year are exempt from the certification regulation. Some farmers use organic production methods but choose not to be USDA certified. Their foods cannot be labeled as organic, but many of these farmers market and sell to those seeking organic foods.

The organic food market received a boost in 2009 when USDA offered $50 million in new funding to encourage greater production of organic food in the United States. The Organic Trade Association (www.ota.com/index.html) believes that this funding will further encourage farmers to use organic practices and help increase the U.S. production of organic food to meet growing consumer demand. With tough economic times, consumers have used various strategies in continuing to buy organic products. Because most stores now offer organic products, consumers have the opportunity to shop around. Increased availability and use of coupons, the proliferation of private label and store brands, and better value products offered by major organic brands all have contributed to increased sales.

Organic Foods and Health Consumers may choose to eat organic foods to reduce their pesticide intake, to protect the environment, and to improve the nutritional quality of their diets. Those who consume organic produce do ingest lesser amounts of pesticides (only 1 in 4 organically grown fruits and vegetables contains pesticides and in lower amounts than conventional produce), but it's still not known whether or how this affects the health of most consumers. However, organic foods may be a wise choice for young children because pesticide residues may pose a greater risk to them. Consumers also may opt for organic foods to encourage environmentally friendly **sustainable agriculture** practices.

Most studies do not show that organic foods have higher amounts of vitamins and minerals (see Further Reading 5). However, researchers have found that, in some cases, organic fruits and vegetables contain more vitamin C and antioxidants that help protect cells against damage. At this point, it's not possible to recommend organic foods over conventional foods based on nutrient content—both can meet nutritional needs. A healthy dose of common sense also is important—an "organic" label does not change a less healthy food into a more healthy food. Organic potato chips have the same calorie and fat content as conventional potato chips.

One concern raised about organic foods is that food safety may be jeopardized because animal manures used for fertilizers might cause more pathogen contamination of food. The recent outbreaks of foodborne illness linked to organically grown sprouts in Europe confirm that an organic label does not guarantee good health. However, research does not show that certified organic food has higher contamination with bacterial pathogens. Consumers should wash or scrub all produce—organic as well as conventional—under running water.

The term "natural" is not regulated. Products labeled as "natural" are generally those derived from natural ingredients, such as a plant source, which retain their natural properties in the finished product. Meat or poultry labeled "natural" must be minimally processed, and contain no artificial flavoring, coloring, chemical preservative, or other artificial or synthetic ingredient. No one is really checking these products, and there is some debate over what constitutes "minimally processed." Although all organic products fit this definition of natural, not all natural products are necessarily organic.

Sustainable Agriculture

Conventional agriculture focuses on maximizing production through the use of large acreages, powerful machines, chemicals to control pests, and petroleum-based fertilizers to boost growth. In contrast, sustainable agriculture is an integrated system of plant and animal production that will, over the long-term, satisfy human food needs, enhance environmental quality, efficiently use nonrenewable resources, sustain the economic viability of farm operations, and enhance the quality of life for farmers and society as a whole. A culture of sustainability has emerged, including a clear trend for sustainable food choices manufactured in an environmentally responsible way. The food industry has responded with a move toward "green" initiatives that should be sustainable for the long-term. A new demographic term, LOHAS (Lifestyle of Health and Sustainability), describes a growing demographic group focused on sustainable living. An increasing number of today's college students are joining this market segment and developing behaviors associated with social responsibility. These consumers are driving changes in many areas, including the food industry. Slow Food Nation is an example of a non-profit group dedicated to creating a framework for a deeper environmental connection to our food and aiming to inspire and empower Americans to build a food system that is sustainable, healthy, and delicious.

Locally Grown Foods

With people everywhere more interested in the origins of their food, more grocery store shelves are devoted to "locally grown" products. Consumers are demanding increased transparency with the food supply, and local food helps answer questions about where food comes from and how it was grown. Retailers are using the "locally grown" label to respond to consumer desires for fresh, safe products that also support small, local farmers and help the environment. Local products provide fresher options, do not have the added costs of long transportation, and thus, use less fossil fuel. Foodservice establishments are giving greater emphasis to local producers, focusing on where food was grown and how it was handled.

Farmers' markets are the most obvious way that consumers have access to locally grown, farm-fresh produce. Farmers' markets are also an integral part of the urban/farm linkage and continue to gain popularity. In 2010 there were 6132 farmers' markets operating throughout the United States, which was a 16% increase from 2009.

The interest in "local" foods has become such a phenomenon that the term "locavore" was the 2007 Word of the Year in the New Oxford American Dictionary. **Locavore** is defined as someone who eats food grown or produced locally or within a certain radius such as 50, 100, or 150 miles. The locavore movement has gained prominence due to food-safety concerns by consumers and the search for local, sustainable foods. It encourages consumers to buy from farmers' markets or even to produce their own food, with the argument that fresh, local products are more nutritious and taste better.

CRITICAL THINKING

Stephanie, a college sophomore, is adamant about eating only organic foods. She frequently states that conventionally grown and processed foods are unhealthy, full of harmful chemicals, and almost nutrient-free. Knowing that you are studying nutrition, Stephanie discusses her beliefs with you and asks for your opinion. What are some ways you might respond to her?

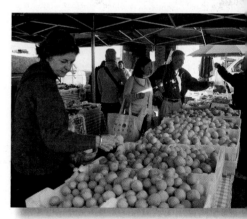

▲ The locavore movement is based on the assumption that local products are more nutritious and taste better and encourages consumers to buy from farmers' markets or even to produce their own food.

locavore Someone who eats food grown or produced locally or within a certain radius such as 50, 100, or 500 miles.

NEWSWORTHY NUTRITION

German organic sprouts cause deadly *E. coli* outbreak

The world's deadliest outbreak of *Escherichia coli* occurred during the summer of 2011. The outbreak occurred mainly in Germany and involved a rare enterohemorrhagic strain of *E. coli* known as O104:H4. In June 2011, 3332 persons had been infected, more than 600 were in intensive care, and the death toll from the outbreak had reached 36. Several hundred also contracted its potentially fatal kidney complication, known as hemolytic uremic syndrome. The European Centre for Disease Prevention and Control concluded that the *E. coli* infection was caused by tainted vegetable sprouts from a small, rather traditional organic sprout farm. The sprout seeds were mostly imported from overseas and the *E. coli* bacteria were antibiotic resistant. Experts say these types of outbreaks are becoming more common due to large-scale industrial farming and the widespread use of antibiotics.

Source: Dempsey J, Neuman W: Deadly *E. coli* outbreak linked to German sprouts. *New York Times*, June 5, 2011.

 connect NUTRITION **Check out the Connect site www.mcgrawhillconnect.com to further explore *E. coli*.**

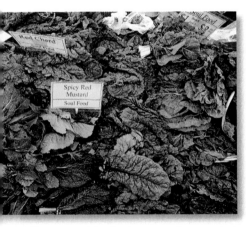

▲ Farmers participating in community supported agriculture (CSA) offer a share of foods from each growing season, to individuals, families or companies who support the CSA financially and/or by working for the CSA.

There is no evidence, however, that locally grown products are safer. Although many small producers have good food-safety practices, they often lack the expensive food-safety audits more common among big producers. Food-safety auditors determine such things as whether or not there is evidence of insects on produce and whether or not producers have enough bathrooms for workers. In addition, undetected foodborne illness outbreaks are more likely with "local" products delivered in small quantities and sold in a small area. Local products are not necessarily pesticide-free and may not be cheaper, given that smaller growers lack the economic advantages of bigger growers. Read about the outbreak of foodborne illness linked to a local organic farm in Newsworthy Nutrition.

Unlike organic products, there are no regulations specifying the meaning of "locally grown." Whole Foods Market, Inc. is the biggest retailer of natural and organic food and probably the best-known for buying and selling locally grown produce. Whole Foods considers local to be anything produced within seven hours of one of its stores, with most local producers within 200 miles of a store. Wal-Mart, the world's largest retailer, has also become a large buyer of locally grown fruits and vegetables and considers anything local if it is grown in the same state as it is sold. Searchable databases and mapping resources such as MarketMaker (http://national.marketmaker.uiuc.edu/) are now available to connect growers with buyers, restaurants with distributors, and consumers with local farmers' markets. These tools make it easier for people to find and sell locally grown foods.

Community Supported Agriculture

Consumers are not only taking comfort in knowing where their food comes from, but are also starting to have interest in community connections with local/regional farmers. Stemming from the interest in locally grown food, there is growing national support for local food collaboratives and community supported agriculture. Community Supported Agriculture programs (CSA) involve a partnership between local food producers and local consumers. During each growing season, CSA farmers offer a share of foods to individuals, families, or companies who have pledged support to the CSA either financially and/or by working for the CSA.

Another example of a farm-community partnership is the National Farm to School Program (www.farmtoschool.org/), a nonprofit effort to connect farmers with nearby school cafeterias. Between 1997 and 2011, this program grew from only six local programs to 2352 programs in 48 states resulting in 9756 schools incorporating the local bounty into their menus. Administrators of the program have found that if kids can meet the farmer who actually grew the food, they are much more likely to eat it.

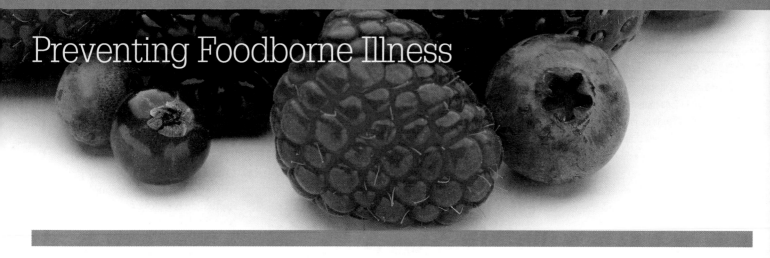

Preventing Foodborne Illness

General Rules for Preventing Foodborne Illness

You can greatly reduce the risk of foodborne illness by following some important rules (see Further Reading 7). It's a long list, because many risky habits need to be addressed.

Purchasing Food

- When shopping, select frozen foods and perishable foods, such as meat, poultry, or fish, last. Always have these products put in separate plastic bags, so that drippings don't contaminate other foods in the shopping cart. Don't let groceries sit in a warm car; this allows bacteria to grow. Get the perishable foods such as meat and egg and dairy products home and promptly refrigerate or freeze them.
- Don't buy or use food from damaged containers that leak, bulge, or are severely dented or from jars that are cracked or have loose or bulging lids. Don't taste or use food that has a foul odor or spurts liquid when the can is opened; the deadly *Clostridium botulinum* toxin may be present.
- Purchase only pasteurized milk and cheese (check the label). This is especially important for pregnant women because highly toxic bacteria and viruses that can harm the fetus thrive in unpasteurized milk.
- Purchase only the amount of produce needed for a week's time. The longer you keep fruits and vegetables, the more time is available for bacteria to grow.
- When purchasing precut produce or salads, avoid those that look slimy,

brownish, or dry; these are signs of improper holding temperatures.
- Observe sell-by and expiration dates on food labels.

Preparing Food

- Thoroughly wash your hands for 20 seconds with hot, soapy water before and after handling food. This practice is especially important when handling raw meat, fish, poultry, and eggs, after using the bathroom, after playing with pets, or after changing diapers (see Further Reading 2).
- Make sure counters, cutting boards, dishes, and other equipment are thoroughly sanitized and rinsed before use. Be especially careful to use hot, soapy water to wash surfaces and equipment that have come in contact with raw meat, fish, poultry, and eggs as soon as possible to remove *Salmonella* bacteria that may be present. Otherwise, bacteria on the surfaces will infect the next foods that come in contact with the surface, a process called cross-contamination. In addition, replace sponges and wash kitchen towels frequently. (Microwaving sponges for 30 to 60 seconds also helps rid them of live bacteria.)
- If possible, cut foods to be eaten raw on a clean cutting board reserved for that purpose. Then clean this cutting board using hot, soapy water. If the same board must be used for both meat and other foods, cut any potentially contaminated items, such as meat, last. After cutting the meat, wash the cutting board thoroughly.

FDA recommends cutting boards with unmarred surfaces made of easy-

to-clean, non-porous materials, such as plastic, marble, or glass. If you prefer a wooden board, make sure it is made of a nonabsorbent hardwood, such as oak or maple, and has no obvious seams or cracks. Then reserve it for a specific purpose; for example, set it aside for cutting raw meat and poultry. Keep a separate wooden cutting board for chopping produce and slicing bread to prevent these products from picking up bacteria from raw meat. Many foods are served raw, so any bacteria clinging to them are not destroyed.

Furthermore, FDA recommends that all cutting boards be replaced when they become streaked with hard-to-clean grooves or cuts, which may harbor bacteria. In addition, cutting boards should be sanitized once a week in a dilute bleach solution. Flood the board with the solution, let it sit a few minutes, then rinse thoroughly.

- When thawing foods, do so in the refrigerator, under cold potable running water, or in a microwave oven. Also, cook foods immediately after thawing under cold water or in the microwave. Never let frozen foods thaw unrefrigerated all day or night. Also, marinate food in the refrigerator.
- Avoid coughing or sneezing over foods, even when you're healthy. Cover cuts on hands with a sterile bandage. This helps stop *Staphylococcus* from entering food.
- Carefully wash fresh fruit and vegetables under running water to remove dirt and bacteria clinging to the surface, using a vegetable brush if the skin is to

▶ The World Health Organization's Golden Rules for Safe Food Preparation

1. Choose foods processed for safety.
2. Cook food thoroughly.
3. Eat cooked foods immediately.
4. Store cooked foods carefully.
5. Reheat cooked foods thoroughly.
6. Avoid contact between raw and cooked foods.
7. Wash hands repeatedly.
8. Keep all kitchen surfaces meticulously clean.
9. Protect foods from insects, rodents, and other animals.
10. Use pure water.

The USDA simplified these rules into four actions as a part of their Fight BAC! Program (check out www.fightbac.org):

1. Clean. Wash hands and surfaces often.
2. Separate. Don't cross-contaminate.
3. Cook. Cook to proper temperatures.
4. Chill. Refrigerate promptly.

The 2010 Dietary Guidelines for Americans also stress the importance of these four actions.

be eaten. People have become ill from *Salmonella* introduced from melons used in making a fruit salad and from oranges used for fresh-squeezed orange juice. The bacteria were on the outside of the melons and oranges (see Further Reading 10).

- Completely remove moldy portions of food or don't eat the food. *When in doubt, throw the food out.* Mold growth is prevented by properly storing food at cold temperatures and using the food promptly.

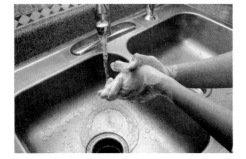

▲ Washing hands thoroughly (for at least 20 to 30 seconds) with hot water and soap should be the first step in food preparation. The 4 "F's" of food contamination are fingers, foods, feces, and flies. Handwashing especially combats the finger and fecal routes.

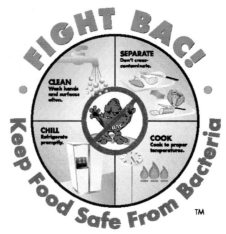

▲ Food safety logo of USDA.

- Use refrigerated ground meat and patties in 1 to 2 days and frozen meat and patties within 3 to 4 months. The 6-month interval mentioned in the comic at the beginning of this chapter is too long a time to be safe.

Cooking Food

- Cook food thoroughly using a bimetallic thermometer to check for doneness, especially for fresh beef and fish (145°F [63°C]), pork (160°F [71°C]), and poultry (165°F [74°C]) (Fig. 16-2). Eggs should be cooked until the yolk and white are hard. Alfalfa sprouts and other types of sprouts should be cooked until they are steaming. Cooking is by far the most reliable way to destroy foodborne viruses and bacteria, such as Norovirus and toxic strains of *E. coli*. Freezing only halts viral and bacterial growth. FDA does not recommend that eggs be prepared sunny-side-up.

As noted, many restaurants now include an advisory on menus stating that an increased risk of foodborne illness is associated with eating undercooked eggs. As long as restaurants provide this warning on their menus, however, they are allowed to cook eggs to any temperature requested by the consumer. FDA warns us not to consume homemade ice cream, eggnog, and mayonnaise if made with unpasteurized, raw eggs because of the risk of *Salmonella* foodborne illness. It is safer to use eggs or egg products that have been pasteurized, which kills *Salmonella* bacteria. Overall, a good general precaution is to eat no raw animal products.

USDA answers questions about the safe use of animal products (800-535-4555, 10 A.M. to 4 P.M. weekdays, Eastern time).

Seafood also poses a risk of foodborne illness, especially oysters. Properly cooked seafood should flake easily and/or be opaque or dull and firm. If it's translucent or shiny, it's not done.

- Cook stuffing separately from poultry (or wash poultry thoroughly, stuff immediately before cooking, and then transfer the stuffing to a clean bowl immediately after cooking). Make sure the stuffing reaches 165°F (74°C). *Salmonella* is the major concern with poultry.
- Once a food is cooked, consume it right away, or cool it to 40°F (4°C) within 2 hours. If it is not to be eaten immediately, in hot weather (80°F and above) make sure this cooling is done within 1 hour. Do this by separating the food into as many shallow pans as needed to provide a large surface area for cooling. Be careful not to recontaminate cooked food by contact with raw meat or juices from hands, cutting boards, dirty utensils, or in other ways.
- Serve meat, poultry, and fish on a clean plate—never the same plate used to hold the raw product. For example, when grilling hamburgers, don't put cooked items on the same plate used to carry the raw product out to the grill.
- For outdoor cooking, cook food completely at the picnic site, with no partial cooking in advance.

Storing and Reheating Cooked Food

- Keep foods out of the "danger zone" (Fig.16-1) by keeping hot foods hot and cold foods cold. Hold food below 40°F (4°C) or above 140°F (60°C). Foodborne microorganisms thrive in more moderate temperatures (60°F to 110°F [16°C to 43°C]). Some microorganisms can even grow in the refrigerator. Again, don't leave cooked or refrigerated foods, such as meats and salads, at room temperature for more than 2 hours (or 1 hour in hot weather) because that gives microorganisms an opportunity to grow. Store dry food at 60°F to 70°F (16°C to 21°C).
- Reheat leftovers to 165°F (74°C); reheat gravy to a rolling boil to kill *Clostridium*

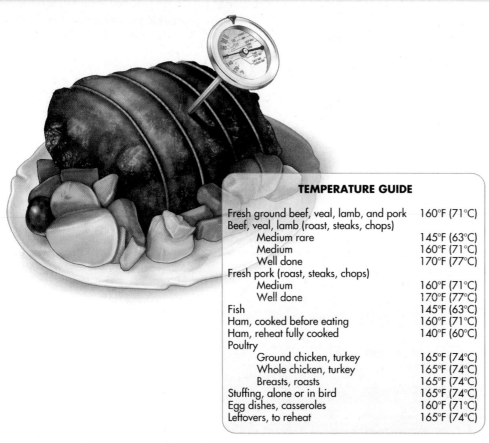

TEMPERATURE GUIDE

Fresh ground beef, veal, lamb, and pork	160°F (71°C)
Beef, veal, lamb (roast, steaks, chops)	
Medium rare	145°F (63°C)
Medium	160°F (71°C)
Well done	170°F (77°C)
Fresh pork (roast, steaks, chops)	
Medium	160°F (71°C)
Well done	170°F (77°C)
Fish	145°F (63°C)
Ham, cooked before eating	160°F (71°C)
Ham, reheat fully cooked	140°F (60°C)
Poultry	
Ground chicken, turkey	165°F (74°C)
Whole chicken, turkey	165°F (74°C)
Breasts, roasts	165°F (74°C)
Stuffing, alone or in bird	165°F (74°C)
Egg dishes, casseroles	160°F (71°C)
Leftovers, to reheat	165°F (74°C)

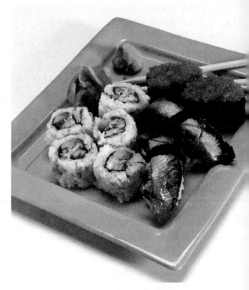

▲ Sushi, like all raw fish or meat dishes, is a high-risk food. For maximum protection from food-borne illness, animal foods should be cooked thoroughly before eating.

FIGURE 16-2 ▶ Minimum internal temperatures when cooking or reheating foods.

Source: USDA "Kitchen's Companion," February 2008.

perfringens bacteria, which may be present. Merely reheating to a good eating temperature isn't sufficient to kill harmful bacteria.

- Store peeled or cut-up produce, such as melon balls, in the refrigerator.
- Make sure the refrigerator stays below 40°F (4°C). Either use a refrigerator thermometer or keep it as cold as possible without freezing milk and lettuce.
- Keep leftovers in the refrigerator only for the recommended length of time (Fig. 16-3).

Cross-contamination is not only a threat during food preparation; it can also become a problem during food storage. Make sure all foods, including leftovers, are contained and covered in the refrigerator to prevent drippings from uncooked and potentially hazardous foods from tainting other foods. It is a good idea to store foods likely to pose risk of foodborne illness on lower shelves of the refrigerator, beneath other foods to be eaten raw.

MAKING DECISIONS

Raw Fish

Raw fish dishes, such as sushi, can be safe for most people to eat if they are made with very fresh fish that has been commercially frozen and then thawed. The freezing is important to eliminate potential health risks from parasites. FDA recommends that the fish be frozen to an internal temperature of −10°F for 7 days. If you choose to eat uncooked fish, purchase the fish from reputable establishments that have high standards for quality and sanitation. If you are at high risk for foodborne illness, it is wise to avoid raw fish products.

▶ **Current Safe Handling Instructions Issued by USDA for Labeling Meat and Poultry Products**

This product was prepared from inspected and passed meat and/or poultry. Some food products may contain bacteria that could cause illness if the product is mishandled or cooked improperly. For your protection, follow these handling instructions.

Keep refrigerated or frozen.

Thaw in refrigerator or microwave.

Keep raw meat and poultry separate from other foods.

Wash working surfaces (including cutting boards), utensils, and hands after touching raw meat or poultry.

Cook thoroughly.

Keep hot foods hot. Refrigerate leftovers immediately or discard.

▶ **Safe Handling Instructions for Eggs**

To prevent illness from bacteria: keep eggs refrigerated, cook eggs until yolks are firm, and cook foods containing eggs thoroughly.

▶ To reduce the risk of bacteria surviving during microwave cooking,

- Cover food with glass or ceramic when possible to decrease evaporation and heat the surface.
- Stir and rotate food at least once or twice for even cooking. Then, allow microwaved food to stand, covered, after heating is completed to help cook the exterior and equalize the temperature throughout.
- Use the oven temperature probe or a meat thermometer to check that food is done. Insert it at several spots.
- If thawing meat in the microwave, use the oven's defrost setting. Ice crystals in frozen foods are not heated well by the microwave oven and can create cold spots, which later cook more slowly.

▶ Regularly cleaning surfaces and equipment with a dilute bleach solution (1:10) is helpful in reducing the risk of cross-contamination of foods.

When in doubt, throw it out!

Food	Refrigerator Storage Time (days)
Meats	
Cooked ground beef/turkey	3–4
Deli meat	2–3
Cooked pork	3–4
Cooked poultry	3–4
Cooked beef, bison, lamb	3–4
Seafood	
Raw (e.g. sushi/sashimi)	Must consume on day of purchase
Cooked	2
Other Entrees	
Pizza	1–2
Pasta/rice	1–2
Casserole	3–4
Soups and Chili	
Chili with meat	2–3
Chili without meat	3–4
Soup/stew	3–4
Side Dishes	
Fresh salad	1–2
Fresh vegetables	1–2
Pasta or potato salad	2–3
Deviled egg	2–3
Hard boiled egg	7
Potato (any style)	3–4
Cooked vegetables	3–4
Dessert	
Cream pie	2–3
Fruit pie	2–3
Pastries	7
Cake	7
Cheesecake	7

FIGURE 16-3 ▶ Length of time to keep leftovers in the refrigerator.

CONCEPT CHECK

Thoroughly cook all meat and poultry to reduce the risk of foodborne illness from *E. coli,* and *Salmonella.* In addition, always separate raw meats and poultry products from cooked foods. To prevent foodborne intoxication from *Staphylococcus* organisms, cover cuts on hands and avoid sneezing on foods. To avoid intoxication from *Clostridium perfringens,* rapidly cool leftover foods and thoroughly reheat them. To avoid intoxication from *Clostridium botulinum,* carefully examine canned foods. Overall, don't allow cooked food to stand for more than 1 to 2 hours at room temperature. For other causes of foodborne illness, precautions already mentioned generally apply as well. In addition, thoroughly cook fish and other seafood; consume only pasteurized dairy products; wash all fruits and vegetables; and thoroughly wash your hands with soap and water before and after preparing food and after using the bathroom.

Case Study Preventing Foodborne Illness at Gatherings

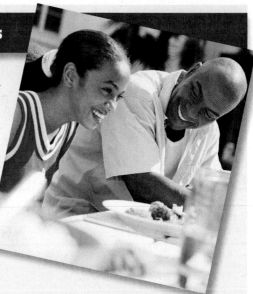

Nicole attended a gathering of her co-workers on a warm Saturday in July. The theme of the party was international dining. Nicole and her husband were asked to bring an Argentinian dish, potato and beef empanadas. They followed the recipe and cooking time carefully, removing the dish from the oven at 1 P.M. and keeping it warm by wrapping the pan in a towel. They traveled in their car to the party and set the dish out on the buffet table at 3 P.M. Dinner was to be served at 4 P.M. However, the guests were enjoying themselves so much lounging around the host's pool and drinking ginger beer (also on the menu) that no one began to eat until 6 P.M. Nicole made sure she sampled the empanadas that she and her husband made, while her husband did not. She also had some salad, garlic bread, and a sweet dessert made with coconut.

The couple returned home at 11 P.M. and went to bed. At about 2 A.M., Nicole knew something was wrong. She had severe abdominal pain and had to make a dash to the bathroom. She spent most of the next 3 hours in the bathroom with severe diarrhea. By dawn, the diarrhea subsided and she started to feel better. After a few cups of tea and a light breakfast, she was feeling like herself by noon.

Answer the following questions, and check your responses in Appendix A.

1. Based on her symptoms, what type of foodborne illness did Nicole contract?
2. Why is the beef the most likely vehicle for this type of foodborne illness?
3. Why is consuming food at large gatherings risky?
4. What precautions for avoiding foodborne illness were ignored by Nicole and the rest of the people at the party?
5. How could this scenario be rewritten to substantially reduce the risk of foodborne illness?

Summary (Numbers refer to numbered sections in the chapter.)

16.1, 16.3 Viruses, bacteria, and other microorganisms in food pose the greatest risk for foodborne illness. Major causes of foodborne illness are Norovirus and the bacteria *Campylobacter jejuni, Salmonella, Staphylococcus aureus,* and *Clostridium perfringens.* In addition, such bacteria as *Clostridium botulinum, Listeria monocytogenes,* and *Escherichia coli* have been found to cause illness.

16.2 In the past, salt, sugar, smoke, fermentation, and drying were used to protect against foodborne illness. Today, careful cooking, pasteurization, keeping hot foods hot and cold foods cold, and thorough handwashing provide additional insurance.

16.4 Food additives are used primarily to extend shelf life by preventing microbial growth and the destruction of food components by oxygen, metals, and other substances. Food additives are classified as those intentionally added to foods and those that incidentally appear in foods. An intentional additive is limited to no more

than one-one-hundredth of the greatest amount that causes no observed symptoms in animals. Under its jurisdiction in the United States, the Delaney Clause allows FDA to ban the use of any intentional food additive that causes cancer.

Antioxidants, such as BHA, BHT, vitamins E and C, and sulfites, prevent oxygen and enzyme destruction of food products. Emulsifiers suspend fat in water, improving the uniformity, smoothness, and body of foods such as ice cream. Common preservatives include salt, sodium benzoate, and sorbic acid, which prevent bacterial growth. Sequestrants bind metals and thus prevent spoilage of food from metal contamination. Various natural products such as natural flavors, sugar, and corn syrup, as well as artificial flavors and sweeteners, such as aspartame, improve the flavor of food.

16.5 Toxic substances occur naturally in a variety of foods, such as green potatoes, raw fish, mushrooms, and raw egg whites. Cooking foods limits their toxic effects in

some cases; others are best to avoid altogether, such as toxic mushroom species and the green parts of potatoes.

16.6 A variety of environmental contaminants and pesticide residues can be found in foods. It is helpful to know which foods pose the greatest risks and act accordingly to reduce exposure, such as washing fruits and vegetables before use.

16.7 Conventional agriculture focuses on maximizing production through the use of large farms, machines, and chemicals. A more recent culture of sustainability demands food choices produced in an environmentally responsible way. U.S. sales of organic foods have grown dramatically in recent years, despite tough economic times. Consumers are more interested in the origins of their food, resulting in grocery stores providing more "locally grown" products. Although there is no evidence that locally grown products are safer, local products provide fresher options and do not have the added transportation costs. Consumers also have an interest in connecting with local/regional farmers, resulting in growing national support for community-supported agriculture.

N&YH To protect against viruses and bacteria, cook susceptible foods thoroughly. In addition, cover cuts on the hands, do not sneeze or cough on foods, avoid contact between raw meat or poultry products

and other food products, rapidly cool and thoroughly reheat leftovers, and use pasteurized dairy products. Overall, be careful when foods are in the "danger zone" (40°F to 140°F).

Cross-contamination commonly causes foodborne illness. It occurs particularly when bacteria on raw animal products

contact foods that can support bacterial growth. Because of the risk of cross-contamination, no perishable food should be kept in the "danger zone" for more than 1 to 2 hours (depending on the environmental temperature), especially if it may have come in contact with raw animal products.

Check Your Knowledge (Answers to the following questions are below.)

1. Nitrite prevents the growth of
   a. *Clostridium botulinum.*
   b. *Escherichia coli.*
   c. *Staphylococcus aureus.*
   d. yeasts.

2. Substances used to preserve foods by lowering the pH are
   a. smoke and irradiation.
   b. baking powder and soda.
   c. salt and sugar.
   d. vinegar and citric acid.

3. Food additives widely used for many years without apparent ill effects are on the _____ list.
   a. FDA
   b. GRAS
   c. USDA
   d. Delaney

4. The foodborne illness organism often associated with small cuts and boils is
   a. *Listeria.*
   b. *Staphylococcus.*
   c. *C. botulinum.*
   d. *Salmonella.*

5. Salmonella bacteria are usually spread via
   a. raw meats, poultry, and eggs.
   b. pickled vegetables.
   c. home-canned vegetables.
   d. raw vegetables.

6. It is unwise to thaw meats or poultry
   a. in a microwave oven.
   b. in the refrigerator.
   c. under cool running water.
   d. at room temperature.

7. Milk that can remain on supermarket shelves, free of microbial growth, for many years has been processed by which of the following methods?
   a. use of humectants
   b. using antibiotics in animal feed
   c. use of sequestrants
   d. aseptic processing

8. Those at greatest risk for food-borne illness include
   a. pregnant women.
   b. infants and children.
   c. immunosuppressed individuals.
   d. All of the above.

9. Pasteurization involves the
   a. exposure of food to high temperatures for short periods to destroy harmful microorganisms.
   b. exposure of food to heat to inactivate enzymes that cause undesirable effects in foods during storage.
   c. fortification of foods with vitamins A and D.
   d. use of irradiation to destroy certain pathogens in foods.

10. Food can be kept for long periods by adding salt or sugar because these substances
    a. make the food too acidic for spoilage to occur.
    b. bind to water, thereby making it unavailable to the microorganisms.
    c. effectively kill microorganisms.
    d. dissolve the cell walls in plant foods.

Answers: 1. a (LO 16.4), 2. d (LO 16.2), 3. b (LO 16.4), 4. b (LO 16.1), 5. a (LO 16.1), 6. d (LO 16.8), 7. d (LO 16.2), 8. d (LO 16.3), 9. a (LO 16.2), 10. b (LO 16.4)

Study Questions (Numbers refer to Learning Outcomes)

1. What three trends in food purchasing and production have led to a greater number of cases of foodborne illness? (**LO 16.1**)

2. Which types of foods are most likely to be involved in foodborne illness? Why are they targets for contamination? (**LO 16.2**)

3. Identify three major classes of microorganisms responsible for foodborne illness. (**LO 16.3**)

4. Define the term *food additive,* and give examples of four intentional food

additives. What are their specific functions in foods? What is their relationship to the GRAS list? (**LO 16.4**)

5. Describe the federal process that governs the use of food additives, including the Delaney Clause. (**LO 16.4**)

6. Put into perspective the benefits and risks of using additives in food. Point out an easy way to reduce the consumption of food additives. Do you think this is worth the effort in terms of maintaining health? Why or why not? (**LO 16.4**)

7. Name some substances that occur naturally in foods but may cause illness (**LO 16.5**).

8. Describe four recommendations for reducing the risk of toxicity from environmental contaminants. (**LO 16.6**)

9. Why is thoroughly cooking food an important practice for reducing the risk of foodborne illness? (**LO 16.8**)

10. List four techniques other than thorough cooking that are important in preventing foodborne illness. (**LO 16.8**)

What Would You Choose Recommendations

Some organic fruits and vegetables do have higher levels of vitamin C, iron, phosphorus, magnesium, and phytochemicals. Exposure to environmental stressors may cause plants to produce more phytochemicals that have a positive impact on human health. However, current research is insufficient to recommend organic over conventional produce on the basis of nutrient content. Canned and frozen fruits and vegetables have greater nutrient content compared to fresh or organic products that are purchased several days or weeks after harvest.

Products labeled organic must comply with standards regarding use of fertilizers, pesticides, hormones, antibiotics, genetic engineering, and irradiation. Organic food producers may use natural preservatives. Most preservatives are used to prevent food spoilage and are not linked to negative health effects. Buying fresh or frozen produce and preparing meals at home are the best ways to avoid excessive preservative intake.

Organic produce is no less likely to be contaminated with microorganisms than conventionally grown foods. Although manure is used as organic fertilizer, statistics show similar levels of foodborne pathogens from either type of food. It is still important to follow food-safety advice, such as washing all fresh produce before eating it.

Exposure to pesticides makes organically grown produce stand apart. Because of

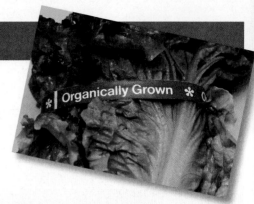

▲ Exposure to pesticides is lower from organic foods.

strict production standards we can expect a dramatically lower intake of pesticides from organic produce compared to conventionally grown produce. The health benefits of lower pesticide intake is greatest for children.

Further Readings

1. ADA Reports: Position of the American Dietetic Association: Food and water safety. *Journal of the American Dietetic Association* 109:1449, 2009.

    The public has a right to a safe food and water supply. The ADA supports collaboration among food and nutrition professionals, academics, representatives of the agriculture and food industries, and appropriate government agencies to ensure the safety of the food and water supply.

2. Anderson JB and others: A camera's view of consumer food-handling behaviors. *Journal of the American Dietetic Association* 104:186, 2004.

    Improper food handling was common in households studied. Implementing Fight BAC! recommendations would improve food handling practices.

3. Calvert GM: Health effects of pesticides. *American Family Physician* 69:1613, 2004.

    Clear cases of disease from high pesticide exposure are seen. Effects of low dose, chronic exposure have been hard to quantify, but most adults have detectable pesticide levels in their blood.

4. Consumers Union: Dirty birds: Even "premium" chickens harbor dangerous bacteria. *Consumer Reports* p. 20, January 2007.

    An analysis of fresh, whole chickens bought in the United States revealed that 83% contained two leading causes of foodborne disease.

5. Dangour AD and others: Nutritional quality of organic foods: A systematic review. *American Journal of Clinical Nutrition* 90:680, 2009.

    This systematic review found there is inadequate evidence of a nutritional benefit to consuming organic foods over conventionally produced foods. Organic and conventional food production methods had minimal impact on the nutrient content and therefore minimal health benefit.

6. Food Safety and Inspection Service: A century of progress in food safety. *Be Food Safe* Fall:12, 2006.

    This article summarizes the 100-year history of federal inspection of meat and poultry.

7. Gerner-Smidt P and others: Invasive listeriosis in Denmark 1994–2003: A review of 299 cases with special emphasis on risk factors for mortality. *Clinical Microbiological Infections* 11:618, 2005.

    Listeria infections lead to death primarily in older people and those with underlying cases of cancer.

8. McCabe-Sellers BJ, Beattie SF: Food safety: emerging trends in foodborne illness surveillance and prevention. *Journal of the American Dietetic Association* 104:1708, 2004.

    Recommendations are given to reduce risk of foodborne illness, with proper personal hygiene being a major focus.

9. Schardt D: Get the lead out—What you don't know can hurt you. *Nutrition Action Healthletter* p. 1, March 2005.

    Hypertension, renal disease, impaired brain function, and cataracts have been linked to lead exposure.

10. Sivapalasingam S and others: Fresh produce: A growing cause of outbreaks of foodborne illness in the United States. *Journal of Food Protection* 67:2342, 2004.

    Caution should be used with fresh produce, just as one would with raw meat and dairy products.

11. Spano M: Organics in overdrive—the explosion of natural food products. *Today's Dietitian* 9:66, October 2007.

    Increased availability of organic products and fear of hormones and antibiotics, has led to a dramatic growth in organic food sales.

12. U.S. Food and Drug Administration: *Food Code.* U.S. Department of Health and Human Services, Public Health Service, Food and Drug Administration: College Park, MD, 2009.

    The FDA Food Code is the model for local, state, tribal, and federal regulators to develop or update their food safety rules consistent with national policy.

13. Widdowson MA and others: Norovirus and foodborne disease, United States, 1991–2000. *Emerging Infectious Diseases* 11:95, 2005.

    The Norovirus leads to more causes of foodborne illness than any other agent.

14. Yeager D: Got organic? *Today's Dietitian* 10:60, October 2008.

    The USDA regulates the organic industry and the National Organic Program certifies that food is produced using organic practices.

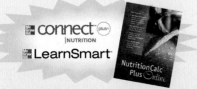

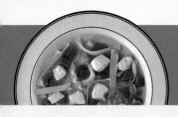
I. Can You Spot the Improper Food-Safety Practices?

In this chapter you learned that (1) foodborne illness strikes up to 76 million U.S. citizens each year and (2) about 5000 deaths each year in the United States are caused by foodborne organisms.

Carefully preparing foods to prevent foodborne illness can minimize its occurrence for most of us. Read the following excerpt and find the food-safety violations that could lead to illness.

A Local Health Department Inspector Gives the Following Account of His Visit to a Local Diner

As I walked through the kitchen of the Morningside Diner, I noticed that all food handlers washed their hands thoroughly with hot, soapy water before handling the food, especially after handling raw meat, fish, poultry, or eggs. Before preparing raw foods, they also thoroughly washed the cutting boards, dishes, and other equipment. As they used their cutting boards after cutting foods, they wiped them with a damp rag and used them again to cut more food.

When preparing fresh fruits and vegetables, they washed them but were careful to leave a little dirt on for fear of washing important nutrients from the outside. The cooks generally cooked meats to an internal temperature of 180°F (82°C). However, to preserve the flavor, pork was cooked to an internal temperature of 140°F (60°C). Some cooked foods to be served later were cooled to below 41°F (5°C) within 2 hours, and foods like beef stew were cooled in shallow pans.

The diner served canned foods, even when the cans were dented. When leftovers were reheated, they were raised to an internal temperature of 130°F (55°C) and served immediately. Food handlers took great care to remove moldy portions of food. The cooks prepared stuffing separately from the poultry. The temperature of refrigerators was approximately 45°F (7°C).

1. List the violations of food-safety practices that could contribute to foodborne illness.

_____

_____

_____

_____

2. If you were writing a report describing ways to correct these practices, what would you say?

_____

_____

_____

_____

_____

3. List the food-safety practices that follow the general rules for preventing foodborne illness.

_____

_____

_____

_____

II. Take a Closer Look at Food Additives

Evaluate a food label of a convenience food item (e.g., frozen entree, ready-to-eat baked good) either in the supermarket or one you have available.

1. Write out the list of ingredients.

   _____

   _____

   _____

   _____

2. Identify the ingredients that you think may be food additives.

   _____

   _____

   _____

   _____

   _____

3. Based on the information available in this chapter, what are the functions of these food additives?

   _____

   _____

   _____

   _____

4. How might this food product differ without these ingredients?

   _____

   _____

   _____

   _____

III. Take a Closer Look at Organic Foods

Visit one or more supermarkets to see what organic foods are available. Note your findings below.

	Available	Not Available
Meat		
Poultry		
Milk		
Eggs		
Cheese		
Lettuce		
Apples		
Bananas		
Broccoli		
Other produce		
Breakfast cereal		
Snack chips		
Crackers		
Bread		
Pasta		
Beer		

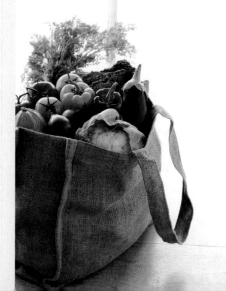

Do you currently purchase organic foods? Why or why not?

Chapter 17 Pregnancy and Breastfeeding

Chapter Outline

Student Learning Outcomes

Chapter 17 is designed to allow you to:

17.1 List major physiological changes that occur in the body during pregnancy and how nutrient needs are altered.

17.2 List factors that predict a successful pregnancy outcome and some that do not.

17.3 Specify the optimal weight gain during pregnancy for a healthy adult woman.

17.4 Design an adequate, balanced meal plan for a pregnant or breastfeeding woman based on the Dietary Guidelines and MyPlate.

17.5 Identify the nutrients that may need to be supplemented during pregnancy and explain the reason for each.

17.6 Explain the typical discomforts of pregnancy that can be minimized by dietary changes.

17.7 Describe the physiological processes involved in breastfeeding, as well as some advantages of breastfeeding for both the infant and mother.

What Would You Choose?

As a pregnant vegetarian, which of the following meals would you choose as the best source of iron?

a Spinach salad with hard boiled eggs and a whole-wheat roll

b Lean hamburger with cheese, lettuce, and tomato and roasted red potatoes

c Bean and cheese soft taco and stewed tomatoes

d Kellogg's Smart Start cereal, fat-free milk, and orange juice

 Think about your choice as you read Chapter 17, then see our recommendations at the end of the chapter. To learn more about pregnancy and vegetarian diets, check out the Connect site: www.mcgrawhillconnect.com

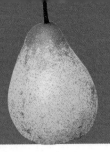

Pregnancy can be a special time. Exhilaration and amazement accompany parents' tremendous responsibility of helping a child develop and grow. Parents-to-be often feel an overriding desire to produce a healthy baby, which can arouse new interest in nutrition and health information. They usually want to do everything possible to maximize their chances of having a robust, lively newborn.

Despite these intentions, the infant mortality rate in North America is higher than that seen in many other industrialized nations. In Canada, about 6.1 of every 1000 infants per year die before their first birthday, while in the United States, it is 6.9. These are alarming statistics for two countries that have such a high per capita expenditure for health care compared to many other countries in the world. Comparatively, the rate of infant mortality in Sweden is roughly 3 of every 1000 infants. In addition, in the United States, about 20% of pregnant women receive inadequate prenatal care in the early months of pregnancy. Expectant teenagers are at the highest risk for this.

Producing a healthy baby is not just a matter of luck. True, some aspects of fetal and newborn health are beyond our control. Still, as the comic in this chapter suggests, conscious decisions about social, health, environmental, and nutritional factors during pregnancy significantly affect the baby's future. Choosing to breastfeed the infant adds further benefits. Let's examine how eating well during pregnancy and breastfeeding can help a baby to have a healthy start in life.

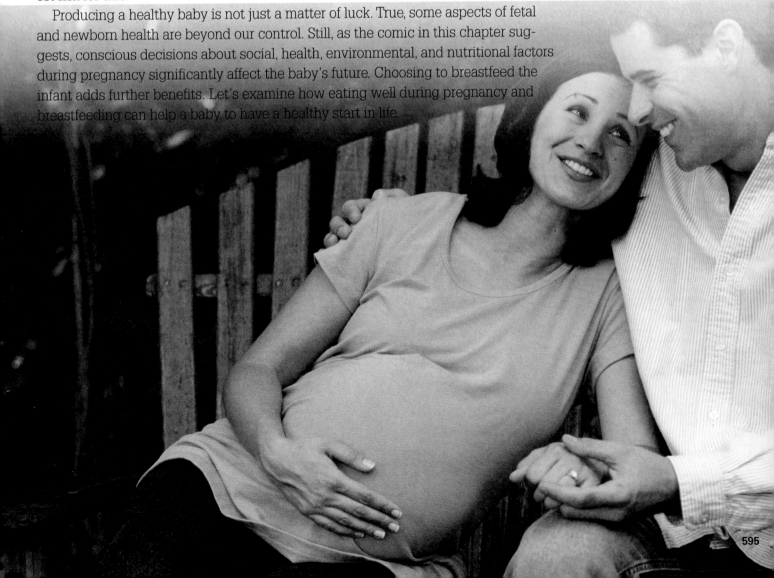

Refresh Your Memory

As you begin your study of nutrition in pregnancy and breastfeeding in Chapter 17, you may want to review:

- Typical fortification in meal replacement bars in Chapter 1 and ready-to-eat breakfast cereals in Chapter 2
- Causes and effects of ketosis in Chapter 4
- Components of the macronutrient classes—carbohydrates, proteins, and lipids—in Chapters 4 to 6, especially omega-3 fatty acids
- Calculation of body mass index in Chapter 7
- Food sources of folate, calcium, iron, and zinc in Chapters 11 and 12.

17.1 Planning for Pregnancy

In an effort to reduce the occurrence of neural tube defects, *Healthy People 2020* includes a goal of increasing by 10% the proportion of women of child-bearing potential who consume at least 400 micrograms of folic acid per day. Currently, about 24% of women of child-bearing potential consume adequate folic acid from fortified foods or dietary supplements.

Controlling or correcting existing health conditions and modifying potentially harmful habits before conception can improve the chances for a successful pregnancy. About 50% of all pregnancies are unplanned. Even when planned, women often do not suspect they are pregnant during the first few weeks after conception. They may not seek medical attention until after the first 2 to 3 months of pregnancy. Still, even without fanfare, the child-to-be grows and develops daily. For that reason, the health and nutrition habits of a woman who is trying to become pregnant—or who has the ability to become pregnant—are particularly important. Although some aspects of fetal and newborn health are beyond the parents' control, a woman's conscious decisions about social, health, environmental, and nutritional factors affect her infant's health and future.

The time to address ongoing health concerns is before conception. Poor control of existing diabetes, hypertension, phenylketonuria, and HIV-positive status or AIDS may lead to serious complications in pregnancy, including birth defects and fetal death. In addition, women should aim to achieve a healthy weight prior to becoming pregnant. Prepregnancy weight and nutrient stores affect the woman's ability to become pregnant. Many underweight women experience amenorrhea, which may reduce their ability to ovulate. The chances of ovulating and becoming pregnant improve when body fat increases to a healthy level.

Infants born to women who began pregnancy substantially above or below a healthy weight are more likely to experience problems than women who began

DOCTOR, THE WAITRESS IS WAITING — AM I EATING FOR TWO, OR WHAT?!

Which diet and lifestyle habits contribute to a successful pregnancy? Which are likely to be harmful?

Why should a woman begin to prepare for pregnancy months before conception of her new baby?

When pregnant, does the mother need to "eat for two?" Chapter 17 provides some answers.

© Rina Piccolo. Reprinted with special permission of King Features Syndicate.

pregnancy at a normal weight. For instance, babies born to obese women are at increased risk of having birth defects, death in the first few weeks after birth, and obesity in childhood. Many obese pregnant women experience high blood pressure, gestational diabetes, and difficult deliveries. At the other extreme, women who begin pregnancy underweight (BMI < 18.5) are more likely to have infants who are low birth weight and premature than women at a normal weight. These differences may be because underweight women tend to have lighter placentas and lower nutrient stores, especially iron, than heavier women, which can affect fetal growth negatively. An underweight woman can improve her nutrient stores and pregnancy outcome by gaining weight before pregnancy or gaining extra weight during pregnancy.

Figure 17-1 depicts how and when toxic agents can harm the developing fetus. To prepare for a healthy pregnancy, the mother should undoubtedly eliminate tobacco, alcohol, and illicit drugs (e.g., marijuana and cocaine). Certain medicines, such as aspirin and related NSAIDs (e.g., ibuprofen [Advil]), as well as typical medicines to treat the common cold and many herbal therapies, have the potential to damage the fetus. Lower doses and/or safer alternatives should be used when planning for pregnancy. Health hazards in the mother's environment, including job-related hazards and exposure to x-rays, should be minimized. Caffeine intake also should be limited.

Much research suggests that an adequate vitamin and mineral intake at least 8 weeks before conception and then during pregnancy can improve outcomes of pregnancy. In particular, meeting folate needs (400 micrograms of synthetic folic acid per day) helps to prevent birth defects such as neural tube defects (review Fig. 12-20 in Chapter 12) and decrease the risk of preterm delivery. Recall from Chapter 12 that adequate folate status before and during pregnancy reduces the risk of neural tube defects by about 70%. Low intakes of calcium and iron or excessive intakes of vitamin A also are cause for concern during pregnancy. Careful dietary choices, often with the help of a balanced multivitamin and mineral supplement, will contribute to a healthy pregnancy for both mother and infant.

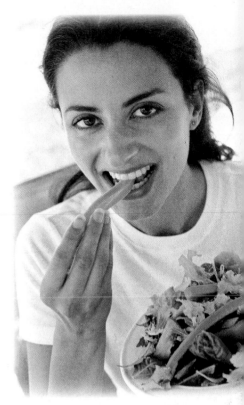

▲ The time to begin thinking about prenatal nutrition is before becoming pregnant. This includes making sure folic acid intake is adequate (400 micrograms of synthetic folic acid per day) and that any supplemental intake of preformed vitamin A does not exceed 100% of the Daily Value (1000 micrograms RAE or 5000 IU).

MAKING DECISIONS

Folate Supplements

Women who have previously given birth to an infant with a neural tube defect such as spina bifida should consult their physician about the need for folate supplementation; an intake of 4 milligrams of synthetic folic acid per day at least one month prior to conception is recommended for these women, but must be taken under a physician's supervision.

17.2 Prenatal Growth and Development

For 8 weeks after conception, a human **embryo** develops from a fertilized **ovum** into a **fetus.** For about another 32 weeks, the fetus continues to develop. When its body finally matures, the infant is born. Until birth, the mother nourishes it via a **placenta,** an organ that forms in her uterus to accommodate the growth and development of the fetus (Fig. 17-2). The role of the placenta is to exchange nutrients, oxygen and other gases, and waste products between the mother and the fetus. This occurs through a network of capillaries that bring the fetal blood close to the maternal blood supply, but the two blood supplies do not mix.

Early Growth—The First Trimester Is a Very Critical Time

In the formation of the human organism, egg and sperm unite to produce the **zygote** (Fig. 17-1). From this point, the reproductive process occurs very rapidly:

- Within 30 hours—zygote divides in half to form 2 cells.
- Within 4 days—cell number climbs to 128 cells.

embryo In humans, the developing offspring in utero from about the beginning of the third week to the end of the eighth week after conception.

ovum The egg cell from which a fetus eventually develops if the egg is fertilized by a sperm cell.

fetus The developing life form from about the beginning of the ninth week after conception until birth.

placenta An organ that forms in the uterus in pregnant women. Through this organ, oxygen and nutrients from the mother's blood are transferred to the fetus, and fetal wastes are removed. The placenta also releases hormones that maintain the state of pregnancy.

zygote The fertilized ovum; the cell resulting from the union of an egg cell (ovum) and sperm until it divides.

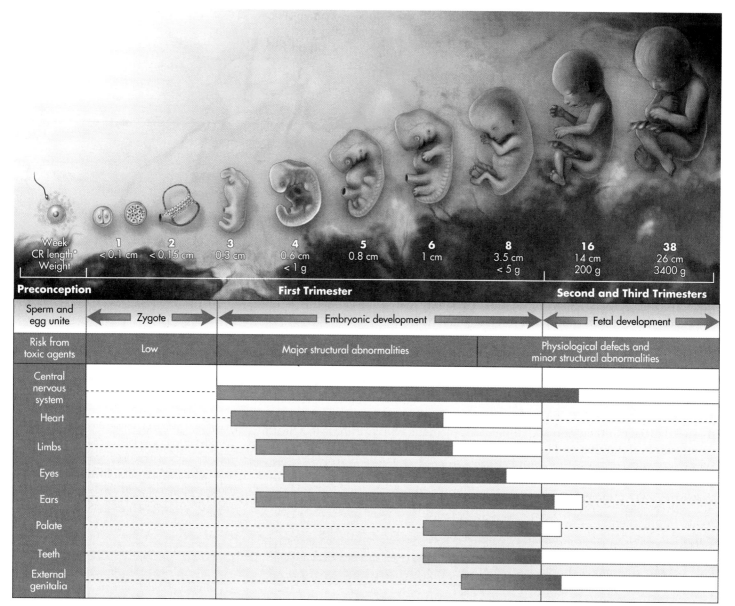

FIGURE 17-1 ▶ Harmful effects of toxic agents during pregnancy. Vulnerable periods of fetal development are indicated with purple bars. The purple shading indicates the time of greatest risk to the organ. The most serious damage to the fetus from exposure to toxins is likely to occur during the first 8 weeks after conception, two-thirds of the way through the first trimester. As the white bars in the chart show, however, damage to vital parts of the body—including the eyes, brain, and genitals—can also occur during the later months of pregnancy.

trimesters Three 13- to 14-week periods into which the normal pregnancy (the length of a normal pregnancy is about 40 weeks, measured from the first day of the woman's last menstrual period) is divided somewhat arbitrarily for purposes of discussion and analysis. Development of the offspring, however, is continuous throughout pregnancy, with no specific physiological markers demarcating the transition from one trimester to the next.

- At 14 days—the group of cells is called an embryo.
- Within 35 days—heart is beating, embryo is 1/30 of an inch (8 millimeters) long, eyes and limb buds are clearly visible.
- At 8 weeks—the embryo is known as a fetus.
- At 13 weeks (end of first trimester)—most organs are formed, and the fetus can move.

For purposes of discussion, the duration of pregnancy—normally, 38 to 42 weeks—is commonly divided into three periods, called **trimesters**. Growth begins in the first trimester with a rapid increase in cell number. This type of growth dominates embryonic and early fetal development. The newly formed cells then begin to grow larger. Further growth is a mix of increases in cell number and cell size. By the end of 13 weeks—the first trimester—most organs are formed and the fetus can move (see Fig. 17-1).

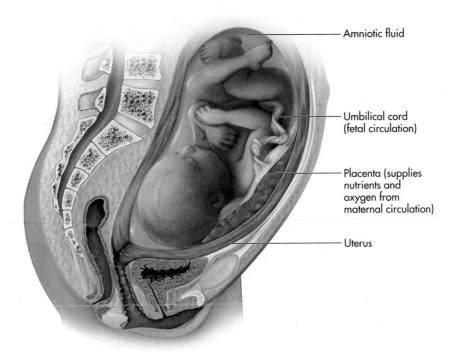

FIGURE 17-2 ▶ The fetus in relationship to the placenta. The placenta is the organ through which nourishment flows to the fetus.

Labels: Amniotic fluid; Umbilical cord (fetal circulation); Placenta (supplies nutrients and oxygen from maternal circulation); Uterus

As the embryo or fetus develops, nutritional deficiencies and other insults have the potential to impose damage or risk to organ systems. For example, adverse reactions to medications, high intakes of vitamin A, exposure to radiation, or trauma can alter or arrest the current phase of fetal development, and the effects may last a lifetime (review Fig. 17-1). The most critical time for these potential problems is during the first trimester. Most **spontaneous abortions**—premature terminations of pregnancy that occur naturally—happen at this time. About one-half or more pregnancies end in this way, often so early that a woman does not even realize she was pregnant. (An additional 15% to 20% are lost before normal delivery.) Early spontaneous abortions usually result from a genetic defect or fatal error in fetal development. Smoking, alcohol abuse, use of aspirin and NSAIDs, and illicit drug use raise the risk for spontaneous abortion.

A woman should avoid substances that may harm the developing fetus, especially during the first trimester. This holds true, as well, for the time when a woman is trying to become pregnant. As previously mentioned, she is unlikely to be aware of her pregnancy for at least a few weeks. In addition, the fetus develops so rapidly during the first trimester that, if an essential nutrient is not available, the fetus may be affected even before evidence of the nutrient deficiency appears in the mother.

For this reason, the *quality*—rather than the *quantity*—of the woman's nutritional intake is most important during the first trimester. In other words, women should consume the same amount of calories, but the foods chosen should be more nutrient dense. Although some women lose their appetite and feel nauseated during the first trimester, they should be careful to meet nutrient needs as much as possible.

Although a mother's decisions, practices, and precautions during pregnancy contribute to the health of her fetus, she cannot guarantee her fetus good health because some genetic and environmental factors are beyond her control. She and others involved in the pregnancy should not hold an unrealistic illusion of total control.

Second Trimester

By the beginning of the second trimester, a fetus weighs about 1 ounce. Arms, hands, fingers, legs, feet, and toes are fully formed. The fetus has ears and begins to form tooth sockets in its jawbone. Organs continue to grow and mature, and, with a stethoscope or Doppler instrument, physicians can detect the fetal heartbeat. Most bones

spontaneous abortion Cessation of pregnancy and expulsion of the embryo or nonviable fetus prior to 20 weeks gestation. This is the result of natural causes, such as a genetic defect or developmental problem; also called *miscarriage*.

► A healthy 1-week-old baby. At birth, a baby usually weighs about 7.5 pounds and is 20 inches long.

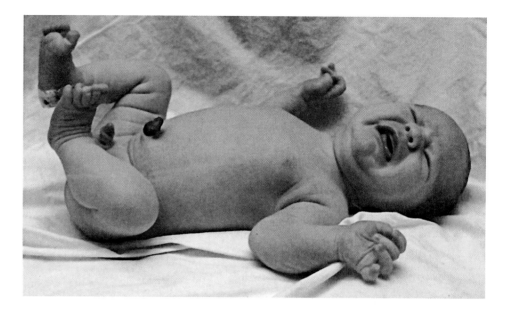

lactation The period of milk secretion following pregnancy; typically called *breastfeeding.*

gestation The period of intrauterine development of offspring, from conception to birth; in humans, gestation lasts for about 40 weeks after the woman's previous menstrual period.

A goal of *Healthy People 2020* is to reduce low birth weight by 5% and preterm births by 10%. Currently about 8% of live births are of low birth weight and about 13% are preterm.

are distinctly evident through the body. Eventually, the fetus begins to look more like an infant. It may suck its thumb and kick strongly enough to be felt by the mother. As was shown in Figure 17-1, the fetus can still be affected by exposure to toxins, but not to the degree seen in the first trimester.

During the second trimester, the mother's breast weight increases by approximately 30% due to the development of milk-producing cells and the deposition of 2 to 4 pounds of fat for **lactation.** This stored fat serves as a reservoir for the extra calories needed to produce breast milk.

Third Trimester

By the beginning of the third trimester, a fetus weighs about 2 to 3 pounds. The third trimester is a crucial time for fetal growth. The fetus will double in length and will increase its weight by three to four times. The fetus takes higher priority than the mother with regard to iron and will deplete the stores of the mother. If the mother is not meeting her iron needs, she can be severely depleted after delivery. An infant born after about 26 weeks of **gestation** has a good chance of survival if cared for in a nursery for high-risk newborns. However, the infant will not contain the stores of minerals (mainly iron and calcium) and fat normally accumulated during the last month of gestation. This and other medical problems, such as a poor ability to suck and swallow, complicate nutritional care for preterm infants.

By full term, the fetus usually weighs about 7 to 9 pounds (3 to 4 kilograms) and is about 20 inches (50 centimeters) long. A soft spot on the top of the head indicates where the skull bones (fontanels) are growing together. The bones finally close by the time the baby is about 12 to 18 months of age.

17.3 Success in Pregnancy

The goal of pregnancy is to achieve optimal health for both the baby and the mother. For the mother, a successful pregnancy is one in which her physical and emotional health is protected so that she can return to her prepregnancy health status. For the infant, two widely accepted criteria are (1) a gestation period longer than 37 weeks and (2) a birth weight greater than 5.5 pounds (2.5 kilograms). Sufficient lung development, likely to have occurred by 37 weeks of gestation, is critical to the survival of a newborn. The longer the gestation, the greater the ultimate birth weight and maturation state, leading to fewer medical problems and better quality of life for the infant. Overall, a successful pregnancy is the outcome of a complex interplay between genes, various lifestyle practices, and the environment.

Infant Birthweight

Low-birth-weight (LBW) infants are those weighing less than 5.5 pounds (2.5 kilograms) at birth. Most commonly, LBW is associated with **preterm** birth. Medical costs during the first year of life for LBW infants are higher than those for normal-weight infants. In fact, hospital-related costs of caring for LBW newborns total more than $4 billion per year in the United States. Full-term and preterm infants who weigh less than the expected weight for their duration of gestation, the result of insufficient growth, are described as **small for gestational age (SGA).** Thus, a full-term infant weighing less than 5.5 pounds at birth is SGA but not preterm, whereas a preterm infant born at 30 weeks' gestation is probably LBW without being SGA. Infants who are SGA are more likely than normal-weight infants to have medical complications, including problems with blood glucose control, temperature regulation, growth, and development in the early weeks after birth.

Prenatal Care and Counseling

Adequate prenatal care is a primary determinant of success in pregnancy. Ideally, women should receive examinations and counseling before becoming pregnant and continue regular prenatal care throughout pregnancy. If prenatal care is inadequate, delayed, or absent, untreated maternal nutritional deficiencies can deprive a developing fetus of needed nutrients. In addition, untreated health conditions, such as anemia, AIDS, hypertension, or diabetes, must be carefully addressed to minimize complications of pregnancy. Treating ongoing infections will also decrease risks of fetal damage. Without prenatal care, a woman is three times more likely to deliver an LBW baby—one who will be 40 times more likely to die during the first 4 weeks of life than a normal-birth-weight infant. According to the Physicians Committee for Responsible Medicine, early and consistent prenatal care could reduce the number of LBW births by 12,600 per year in the United States. Although the ideal time to start prenatal care is before conception, about 20% of women in the United States receive *no* prenatal care throughout the first trimester—a critical time to positively influence the outcome of pregnancy.

Food habits cannot be predicted from income, education, or lifestyle. Although some women already have good dietary habits, most can benefit from nutritional advice. All should be reminded of habits that may harm the growing fetus, such as severe dieting or fasting. By focusing on appropriate prenatal care, nutrient intake, and health habits, parents give their fetus—and later, their infant—the best chance of thriving. Overall, the chances of producing a healthy baby are maximized with education, an adequate diet, and early and consistent prenatal medical care.

Effects of Maternal Age

The age of the mother is another factor that determines pregnancy outcome. The ideal age for pregnancy is between 20 and 35 years of age. Outside that age range—at either extreme—complications are more likely to arise. The rates of teen pregnancy have declined since 1990; still, approximately 400,000 babies are born to teen mothers each year—the highest of any industrialized country. Teen pregnancy increases risk for negative outcomes for both mother and child (Table 17-1) and costs taxpayers an estimated $9.1 billion each year. A portion of these burdens stems from a disadvantaged background, but teenage pregnancy cuts across socioeconomic classes and the effects are evident even after controlling for background factors. Pregnant teens frequently exhibit a variety of risk factors that can complicate pregnancy and pose risk to the fetus. For instance, teenagers are more likely than adult women to be underweight at the start of pregnancy and to gain too little weight during pregnancy. In addition, their bodies lack the physical maturity needed to carry a fetus safely. Even with prenatal care—and 7% of teenage mothers receive none at all—10% of children born to teenage mothers are of low birth weight and 15% are preterm.

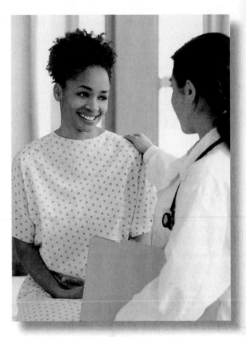

▲ To ensure optimal health and rapid treatment of medical conditions that develop during pregnancy, a pregnant woman should consult with her health-care provider on a regular basis. Ideally, this consultation should begin before she becomes pregnant.

low birth weight (LBW) Referring to any infant weighing less than 2.5 kilograms (5.5 pounds) at birth; most commonly results from preterm birth.

preterm An infant born before 37 weeks of gestation; also referred to as *premature*.

small for gestational age (SGA) Referring to infants who weigh less than the expected weight for their length of gestation. This corresponds to less than 2.5 kilograms (5.5 pounds) in a full-term newborn. A preterm infant who is also SGA will most likely develop some medical complications.

TABLE 17-1 The Burdens of Teenage Pregnancy

For Mother	For Child
↑ Depression and other mental health problems	↓ Birth weight
↑ Use of illicit drugs and alcohol	↑ Premature birth
↑ Poverty and reliance on public assistance	↑ Infant mortality
↓ Graduation rates from high school and college	↑ Hospital admissions during childhood
↑ Single parenthood	↓ Academic performance
	↓ Nutritional status
	↑ Rates of imprisonment during adulthood

At the other end of the spectrum, advanced maternal age poses special risks for pregnancy. The risks of LBW and preterm delivery increase modestly, but progressively, with maternal age beyond 35 years. Given close monitoring, however, a woman older than 35 years has an excellent chance of producing a healthy infant.

Closely Spaced and Multiple Births

Siblings born in succession to a mother with less than a year between birth and subsequent conception are more likely to be born with low birth weights than are those farther apart in age. The risks of low birth weight, preterm birth, or small size for gestational age are 30% to 40% higher for infants conceived less than 6 months following a birth compared to those conceived 18 to 23 months following a birth. These poor outcomes are probably linked to a lack of enough time to rebuild nutrient stores depleted by the pregnancy. Similarly, multiple births (i.e., twins) increase the risk for preterm birth.

Smoking, Medication Use, and Drug Abuse

Smoking, use of some medications, and illicit drug use during pregnancy all lead to harmful effects. Smoking is linked to preterm birth and appears to increase the risk of birth defects, sudden infant death, and childhood cancer. Problem drugs include aspirin (especially when used heavily), hormone ointments, nose drops and related "cold" medications, rectal suppositories, weight-control pills, antidepressants, and medications prescribed for previous illnesses. Illicit drug use is particularly harmful during pregnancy. Many chemicals in recreational drugs cross the placenta and affect the fetus, whose detoxification systems are immature. During organ development, such insults can cause malformations. Marijuana, the most common illegal drug used during the reproductive years, can result in reduced blood flow to the uterus and placenta, leading to poor fetal growth. Low birth weight and higher risk of premature delivery often are seen in infants whose mothers used marijuana during pregnancy. Use of psychoactive drugs, such as cocaine and methamphetamines, restricts fetal growth and brain development, the effects of which may plague the child for a lifetime.

Food Safety

Any foodborne illness during any stage of life is a concern. One type of foodborne illness that poses particular danger for pregnant women is caused by the bacterium *Listeria monocytogenes* (review Chapter 16). Infection with this microorganism typically causes mild flulike symptoms, such as fever, headache, and vomiting, about 7 to 30 days after exposure. However, pregnant women, newborn infants, and people with depressed immune function may suffer more severe symptoms, including spontaneous abortion and serious blood infections. In these high-risk people, 25% of infections may be fatal. Unpasteurized milk, soft cheeses made from raw milk (e.g., brie, Camembert, feta, and blue cheeses), and raw cabbage can be sources of *Listeria* organisms, so it is especially important that pregnant women (and other people at high risk for infection) avoid these products. Experts advise consuming only pasteurized milk products and cooking meat, poultry, and seafood thoroughly to kill this and other foodborne organisms. It is unsafe in pregnancy to eat any raw meats or other raw animal products, uncooked hot dogs, or

Women with acquired immune deficiency syndrome (AIDS) may pass the virus that causes this disease to the fetus during pregnancy or delivery. About one in three infected newborns will develop AIDS symptoms and die within just a few years. Studies show that these odds of mother-infant transmission can be cut significantly if the woman begins taking highly active antiretroviral therapy (HAART) and receiving routine obstetrical care. Before HAART was available, up to 45% of babies born to mothers with the AIDS virus were infected. Now, transmission is less than 2%. Thus, screening pregnant women for AIDS and providing HAART to those with AIDS are advocated by many experts.

The USDA warns pregnant women to thoroughly cook (e.g., microwave) all ready-to-eat meats, including hot dogs and cold cuts, until they are steaming to reduce risk of *Listeria* infections.

undercooked poultry. These food safety recommendations are included in the Dietary Guidelines for Americans discussed later in the chapter (Table 17-3 on page 608).

Nutritional Status

Is attention to good nutrition worth the effort? Yes; evidence shows that the effort is justified (see Further Readings 3, 5, and 19). Extra nutrients and calories are used for fetal growth, as well as for the changes the mother's body undergoes to accommodate the fetus. Her uterus and breasts grow, the placenta develops, her total blood volume increases, the heart and kidneys work harder, and stores of body fat increase.

Although it is difficult to predict to what degree poor nutrition will affect each pregnancy, a daily diet containing only 1000 kcal has been shown to greatly restrict fetal growth and development. Increased maternal and infant death rates seen in famine-stricken areas of Africa provide further evidence.

Genetic background can explain little of the observed differences in birth weight between developed and developing countries. Both environmental factors and nutritional factors are important. The worse the nutritional condition of the mother at the beginning of pregnancy, the more valuable a healthy prenatal diet and/or use of prenatal supplements are in improving the course and outcome of her pregnancy.

Nutrition Assistance for Low-Income Families

A low socioeconomic status is also associated with problems in pregnancy. Typical characteristics of low socioeconomic status include poverty, inadequate health care, poor health practices, lack of education, and unmarried status. In the United States, about 4 of every 10 births are to unwed mothers, and about 25% of unwed mothers and children live in poverty.

Several U.S. government programs provide high-quality health care and foods to reduce infant mortality. These are designed to alleviate the negative impact of poverty, insufficient education, and inadequate nutrient intake on pregnancy outcome. An example of such a program is the Special Supplemental Nutrition Program for Women, Infants, and Children (WIC). This program offers health assessments and vouchers for foods that supply high-quality protein, calcium, iron, and vitamins A and C to pregnant women, infants, and children (up to age 5 years) from low-income populations. The WIC program is available in all areas of the United States and has a staff trained to help women have healthy babies. More than 9 million women, infants, and young children are benefiting from this program, but many eligible pregnant women are not participating.

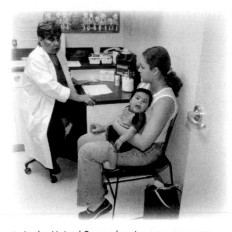

▲ In the United States, low-income pregnant women and their infants (and children) benefit from the nutritional and medical attention provided by the WIC program.

CONCEPT CHECK

To help ensure the optimal health of both the mother and her offspring, adequate nutrition is vital both before and during pregnancy. In particular, meeting folate needs from a synthetic source starting at least 3 months before pregnancy begins, is effective at preventing a variety of fetal malformations. The first trimester is a critical period when inadequate nutrient intake or alcohol and drug use can result in birth defects.

Infants born after 37 weeks of gestation who weigh more than 5.5 pounds (2.5 kilograms) have the fewest medical problems at birth. To reduce infant and maternal medical problems or death, the expectant mother, family, and medical care providers should take the steps necessary to allow the mother to carry the baby in her uterus for the entire 40 weeks. Good nutrition and health practices aid in this goal.

17.4 Increased Nutrient Needs to Support Pregnancy

Pregnancy is a time of increased nutrient needs. It is important to recognize the need for individual assessment and counseling of mothers-to-be, as the nutritional and health status of each woman is different. Still, there are some general principles true for most women with regard to increased nutrient needs.

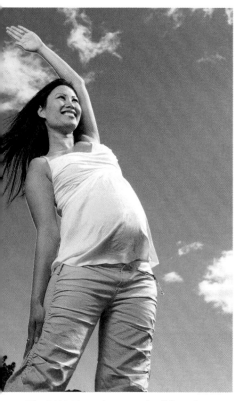

▲ The 2008 Physical Activity Guidelines for Americans recommend that healthy women should get at least 150 minutes of moderate-intensity aerobic activity each week during pregnancy.

Increased Calorie Needs

To support the growth and development of the fetus, pregnant women need to increase their calorie intake. Calorie needs during the first trimester are essentially the same as for nonpregnant women. However, during the second and third trimesters, it is necessary for a pregnant woman to consume approximately 350 to 450 kcal more per day than her prepregnancy needs (the upper end of the range is needed in the third trimester).

Rather than seeing this as an opportunity to fill up on sugary desserts or fat-filled snacks, these extra calories should be in the form of nutrient-dense foods. For example, throughout the day, about six whole-wheat crackers, 1 ounce of cheese, and ½ cup of fat-free milk would supply the extra calories (and also some calcium). Although she "eats for two," the pregnant woman must not double her normal calorie intake. The "eating for two" concept refers more appropriately to increased needs for several vitamins and minerals. Micronutrient needs are increased by up to 50% during pregnancy, whereas calorie needs during the second and third trimesters represent only about a 20% increase.

If a woman is active during her pregnancy, she may need to increase her calorie intake by even more than the estimated 350 to 450 kcal per day. Her greater body weight requires more calories for activity. Many women find that they are inactive during the later months, partly because of their increased size, so an extra 350 to 450 kcal in their daily diets is usually enough.

MAKING DECISIONS

Staying Active During Pregnancy

While pregnancy is not the time to begin an intense fitness regimen, women can generally take part in most low- or moderate-intensity activities during pregnancy. Walking, cycling, swimming, or light aerobics for at least 150 minutes per week is generally advised. Such exercise may prevent pregnancy complications and promote an easier delivery. Some research indicates that regular physical activity during pregnancy lowers a woman's risk of developing gestational diabetes by 50% and preeclampsia by 40%. Women who were highly active prior to pregnancy can maintain their activities as long as they remain healthy and discuss with their health care providers. A few types of activities can potentially harm the fetus and should be avoided, especially those with inherent risk of falls and abdominal trauma. Examples of exercises to avoid, especially during the second and third trimesters, include downhill skiing, weightlifting, soccer, basketball, horseback riding, certain calisthenics (e.g., deep knee bends), any contact sports (e.g., hockey), and SCUBA diving.

Women with high-risk pregnancies, such as those experiencing premature labor contractions, may need to restrict their physical activity. To ensure optimal health for both herself and her infant, a pregnant woman should first consult her physician about physical activity and possible limitations (see Further Reading 13).

Adequate Weight Gain

Key recommendations for weight management during pregnancy and lactation are included in the Dietary Guidelines for Americans (see Table 17-3 on page 608). Healthy prepregnancy weight and appropriate weight gain during pregnancy are excellent predictors of pregnancy outcome (see Further Readings 8, 10, and 11). Her diet should allow for approximately 2 to 4 pounds (0.9 to 1.8 kilograms) of weight gain during the first trimester and then a subsequent weight gain of 0.8 to 1 pound (0.4 to 0.5 kilogram) weekly during the second and third trimesters (Fig. 17-3). A healthy goal for total weight gain for a woman of normal weight (based on BMI; Table 17-2) averages about 25 to 35 pounds (11.5 to 16 kilograms). Pregnant adolescents and women of various racial and ethnic groups are advised to meet these weight gain goals until further research determines any special recommendations. Women of normal prepregnancy BMI carrying twins should aim to gain within the range of 37 to

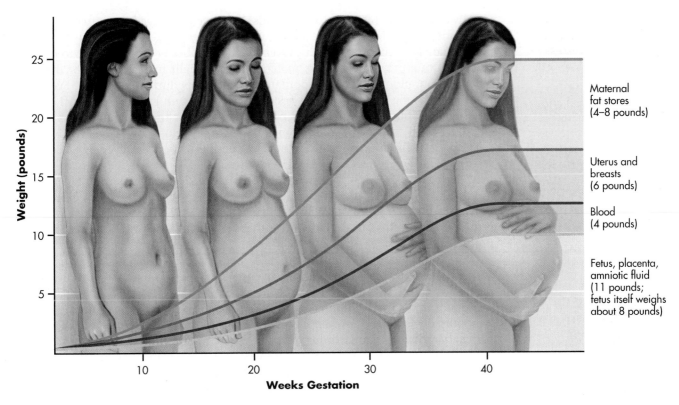

FIGURE 17-3 ▶ The components of weight gain in pregnancy. A weight gain of 25 to 35 pounds is recommended for most women. The various components total about 25 pounds.

54 pounds, whereas overweight or obese women should gain less (31 to 50 pounds or 25 to 42 pounds, respectively).

For women who begin pregnancy with a low BMI, the goal increases to 28 to 40 pounds (12.5 to 18 kilograms). The goal decreases to 15 to 25 pounds (7 to 11.5 kilograms) for overweight women. Target weight gain for obese women is 11 to 20 pounds (5 to 9 kilograms). Figure 17-3 shows why the typical recommendation begins at 25 pounds.

A weight gain of between 25 and 35 pounds for a woman starting pregnancy at normal weight has repeatedly been shown to yield optimal health for both mother and fetus if gestation lasts at least 38 weeks. The weight gain should yield a birth weight of 7.5 pounds (3.5 kilograms). Although some extra weight gain during pregnancy is

TABLE 17-2 Recommended Weight Gain in Pregnancy Based on Prepregnancy Body Mass Index (BMI)

Prepregnancy BMI Category	Total Weight Gain*	
	(pounds)	(kilograms)
Low (BMI less than 18.5)	28 to 40	12.5 to 18
Normal (BMI 18.5 to 24.9)	25 to 35	11.5 to 16
High (BMI 25.0 to 29.9)	15 to 25	7 to 11.5
Obese (BMI greater than 30.0)	11 to 20	5 to 9

*The listed values are for pregnancies with one fetus. For women of normal BMI carrying twins, the range is 37 to 54 pounds (17 to 24.5 kilograms), or less for heavier women.

Reprinted in part with permission from *Weight Gain During Pregnancy: Reexamining the Guidelines,* Copyright 2009 by the Institute of Medicine and National Research Council of the National Academies. Courtesy of the National Academies Press, Washington, DC.

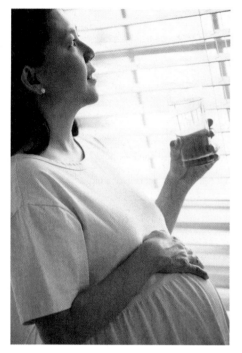

During pregnancy, women in North America are more likely to gain excess weight and make poor food choices than to eat too little.

▲ During pregnancy, the Adequate Intake for total water increases 0.3 liters (1¼ cups) above prepregnancy needs to 3.0 liters (about 12½ cups) per day. For breastfeeding, consume 3.8 liters (16 cups) daily.

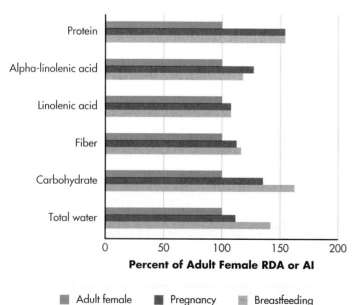

Percent of Adult Female RDA or AI

▪ Adult female ▪ Pregnancy ▪ Breastfeeding

FIGURE 17-4 ▶ Relative macronutrient and water requirements for pregnancy and breastfeeding. Note that there is no RDA or AI for total fat.

usually not harmful (about 5 to 10 pounds), it can set the stage for a pattern of weight gain during the child-bearing years if the mother does not return to her approximate prepregnancy weight after delivery. Overweight and obesity do contribute to complications during pregnancy. Excess maternal body weight increases risk for diabetes, hypertension, blood clots, and spontaneous abortions during pregnancy. Even after childbirth, lasting effects of excess gestational weight gain include high BMI, central body fat distribution, and elevated blood pressure. For the baby, there is a greater chance of birth defects and macrosomia, in which the fetus grows larger than average in utero. Larger infants contribute to a greater need for surgical delivery (i.e., Cesarean sections) among overweight and obese mothers.

Weight gain during pregnancy should generally follow the pattern in Figure 17-3. Monitoring weekly records of a pregnant woman's weight gain helps assess how much to adjust her food intake. Weight gain is a key issue in prenatal care and a concern of many mothers-to-be. Remember that inadequate weight gain can cause many problems.

If a woman deviates from the desirable pattern, she should make the appropriate adjustment. For example, if a woman begins to gain too much weight during her pregnancy, she should not lose weight to get back on track. Even if a woman gains 35 pounds in the first 7 months of pregnancy, she must still gain more during the last 2 months. She should, however, slow the increase in weight to parallel the rise on the prenatal weight gain chart. In other words, the sources of the unnecessary calories should be found and minimized. Alternately, if a woman has not gained the desired weight by a given point in pregnancy, she shouldn't gain the needed weight rapidly. Instead, she should slowly gain a little more weight than the typical pattern to meet the goal by the end of the pregnancy. A registered dietitian can help make any needed adjustments.

Increased Protein and Carbohydrate Needs

The RDA for protein increases by an additional 25 grams per day during pregnancy. A cup of milk alone contains 8 grams. Many nonpregnant women already consume protein in excess of their needs and therefore do not need to increase protein intake any further. However, all women should check to make sure they are eating enough protein as well as enough calories, so this protein is not used to meet energy needs.

The RDA for carbohydrate increases to 175 grams daily, primarily to prevent ketosis. Ketone bodies, a by-product of metabolism of fat for energy, are thought to be poorly used by the fetal brain, implying possible slowing of fetal brain development. Carbohydrate intakes of most women, pregnant or not, already exceed the RDA (Fig. 17-4).

A Word About Lipids

Fat intake should increase proportionally with calorie intake during pregnancy to maintain around 20% to 30% of total calories from fat. Pregnancy is not a time for a low-fat diet, as lipids are a source of extra calories and essential fatty acids needed during pregnancy. Recommendations for the types of lipids during pregnancy are generally the same as for nonpregnant adults. To reduce risk for cardiovascular disease, the American Heart Association recommends no more than 7% of total calories from saturated fat and no more than 1% from *trans* fat. Consumption of dietary cholesterol is not required, but keeping cholesterol intake at a maximum of 300 milligrams per day is also a good goal for maintenance of maternal cardiovascular health.

During pregnancy, it is particularly important to make sure to consume adequate essential fatty acids—linoleic acid (omega-6) and alpha-linolenic acid (omega-3). As you learned in Chapter 5, essential fatty acids cannot be synthesized in the body and must be consumed in the diet. For the developing fetus, essential fatty acids are required for growth, brain development, and eye development. Recommendations are slightly increased by pregnancy: 13 grams per day of omega-6 fatty acids and 1.4 grams per day of omega-3 fatty acids. These needs can be met by consuming 2 to 4 tablespoons per day of plant oils. Consumption of fish at least two times per week is also helpful in meeting needs for essential fatty acids in the diet (see Further Reading 15). (See the "Nutrition and Your Health" section at the end of this chapter for a discussion of mercury in fish.)

Increased Vitamin Needs

Vitamin needs generally increase from prepregnancy RDAs/Adequate Intakes by up to 30% for most of the B vitamins and even greater for vitamin B-6 (45%) and folate (50%) (Fig 17-5). Vitamin A needs only increase by 10%, so a specific focus on this vitamin is not needed. And remember, excess amounts of vitamin A are harmful to the developing fetus.

The extra amount of vitamin B-6 and other B vitamins (except folate) needed in the diet is easily met via wise food choices, such as a serving of a typical ready-to-eat breakfast cereal and some animal protein sources. Folate needs, however, often merit specific diet planning and possible vitamin supplementation. The synthesis of DNA, and therefore cell division, requires folate, so this nutrient is especially crucial during pregnancy. Ultimately, both fetal and maternal growth depend on an ample supply of folate. Red blood cell formation, which requires folate, increases during pregnancy. Serious folate-related anemia therefore can result if folate intake is inadequate. The RDA for folate increases during pregnancy to 600 micrograms DFE per day (review Chapter 12 for calculation of DFE). This is a critical goal in the nutritional care of a pregnant woman. Increasing folate intakes to meet 600 micrograms DFE per day for a pregnant woman can be achieved through dietary sources, a supplemental source of folic acid, or a combination of both. Choosing a diet rich in synthetic folic acid, such as from ready-to-eat breakfast cereals or meal replacement bars (look for approximately 50% to 100% of the Daily Value), is especially helpful in meeting folate needs. Recall from Chapter 12 that synthetic folic acid is much more easily absorbed than the various forms of folate found naturally in foods (see Further Readings 14 and 17).

Increased Mineral Needs

Mineral needs generally increase during pregnancy, especially the requirements for iodide and iron (Fig. 17-6). Zinc needs also increase. (Calcium needs do not increase but still may deserve special attention because many women have deficient intakes.)

Pregnant women need the extra iodide (total of 220 micrograms per day) for prevention of goiter. Typical iodide intakes are enough if the woman uses iodized salt. Animal proteins or a fortified ready-to-eat breakfast cereal in the diet can easily provide enough extra zinc. The extra iron (total of 27 milligrams per day) is needed to synthesize the greater amount of hemoglobin needed during pregnancy and to provide iron stores for the fetus. Women often need a supplemental source of iron, especially if they do not consume iron-fortified foods, such as highly fortified breakfast cereals containing close to 100% of the Daily Value for iron (18 milligrams). Iron supplements decrease appetite and can cause nausea and constipation, so if used, these should be taken between meals or just before going to bed. Milk, coffee, or tea should not be consumed with an iron supplement because these beverages have substances that interfere with iron absorption. Eating foods rich in vitamin C along with nonheme iron-containing foods and iron supplements helps increase iron absorption from those sources. Pregnant women who are not anemic may wait until the second trimester, when pregnancy-related nausea generally lessens, to start iron supplementation if needed.

The consequences of iron-deficiency anemia—especially during the first trimester—can be severe. Negative outcomes include preterm delivery, LBW infants, and increased risk for fetal death in the first weeks after birth.

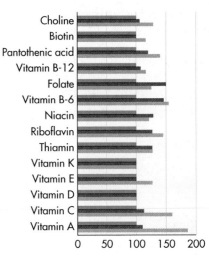

Percent of Adult Female RDA or AI

- Adult female
- Pregnancy
- Breastfeeding

FIGURE 17-5 ▶ Relative vitamin requirements for pregnancy and breastfeeding.

The Dietary Guidelines for Americans recommend that women who may become pregnant eat foods high in iron and consume adequate amounts of the synthetic form of folate (see Table 17-3).

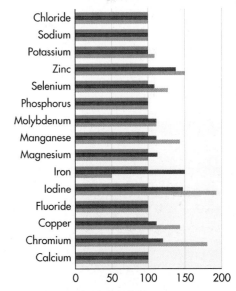

Percent of Adult Female RDA or AI

- Adult female
- Pregnancy
- Breastfeeding

FIGURE 17-6 ▶ Relative mineral requirements for pregnancy and breastfeeding.

NEWSWORTHY
NUTRITION

Experts advocate higher vitamin D for pregnant women

Emerging evidence indicates that low maternal levels of vitamin D during pregnancy affect multiple health parameters in their children. Aside from its well-known role in bone health and prevention of rickets, poor vitamin D status is implicated in serious complications of pregnancy, including higher rates of gestational diabetes, pregnancy-induced hypertension, and a fourfold increased rate of Cesarean section. Vitamin D's role in immune regulation is underscored by higher rates of respiratory infections and mother-to-child transmission of HIV. Because of the ability of vitamin D to modulate gene expression, vitamin D status is critically important during early fetal development through infancy. Diseases that develop later in childhood or adulthood, such as type 1 diabetes, multiple sclerosis, asthma, schizophrenia, and certain types of cancer, are associated with low vitamin D status during gestation. The RDA for pregnant women is 15 micrograms (600 IU) of vitamin D daily, but many experts advocate increasing this recommendation to 25 micrograms (1000 IU) or more.

Source: Dror DK, Allen LH. Vitamin D inadequacy in pregnancy: Biology, outcomes, and interventions. *Nutrition Reviews* 68: 464, 2010.

Connect
NUTRITION
Check out the Connect site www.mcgrawhillconnect.com to further explore vitamin D and pregnancy.

TABLE 17-3 Targeted Recommendations for Women from the Latest Dietary Guidelines for Americans

Balancing Calories to Manage Weight

Women capable of becoming pregnant
- Achieve and maintain a healthy weight before becoming pregnant.

Women who are pregnant
- Gain weight within the 2009 Institute of Medicine gestational weight-gain guidelines (review Table 17-2).

Foods and Food Components to Reduce

Women capable of becoming pregnant and women who are pregnant
- During pregnancy or when conception is possible, avoid alcohol. No safe level of alcohol consumption during pregnancy has been established.

Women who are pregnant
- Only eat foods with seafood, meat, poultry, or eggs that have been cooked to recommended safe minimum internal temperatures.
- Do not consume unpasteurized (raw) juice or milk or foods made from unpasteurized milk, like some soft cheeses (e.g., feta, queso blanco, queso fresco, Brie, Camembert, blue-veined cheeses, and Panela).
- Reheat deli and luncheon meats and hot dogs to steaming hot to kill *Listeria* and do not eat raw sprouts).

Women who are breastfeeding
- Wait at least 4 hours after drinking alcohol before breastfeeding.
- Alcohol should not be consumed at all until consistent latch on and breastfeeding patterns are established.

Foods and Nutrients to Increase

Women capable of becoming pregnant
- Choose foods that supply heme iron, which is more readily absorbed by the body, additional iron sources, and enhancers of iron absorption such as vitamin C–rich foods.
- Consume 400 micrograms per day of synthetic folic acid (from fortified foods and/or supplements) in addition to food forms of folate from a varied diet.

Women who are pregnant
- Take an iron supplement, as recommended by an obstetrician or other health care provider.
- Consume 600 micrograms of dietary folate equivalents daily from all food sources.

Women who are pregnant or breastfeeding
- Consume 8 to 12 ounces of seafood per week from a variety of seafood types.
- Due to their methyl mercury content, limit white (albacore) tuna to 6 ounces per week and do not eat the following four types of fish: tilefish, shark, swordfish, and king mackerel.

Use of Prenatal Vitamin and Mineral Supplements

Special supplements formulated for pregnancy are prescribed routinely for pregnant women by most physicians. Some are sold over the counter, while others are dispensed by prescription because of the high synthetic folic acid content (1000 micrograms), which could pose problems for others, such as older people (see Chapter 19). These supplements are high in iron (27 milligrams per pill). There is no evidence that use of such supplements causes significant health problems in pregnancy, aside perhaps from the combined amounts of supplementary and dietary vitamin A (see Nutrition and Your Health at the end of this chapter).

Instances when prenatal supplements may especially contribute to a successful pregnancy are with poor women, teenagers, those with a generally deficient diet, women carrying multiple fetuses, those that smoke or use alcohol or illegal drugs, and vegans. In other cases, healthy diets can provide the needed nutrients. When choosing a multivitamin, rely on brands that display the USP symbol on their label, signifying that the supplement meets the content, quality, purity, and safety standards of the

U.S. Pharmacopoeia. Also, avoid megadoses of any nutrient. In particular, toxicity of vitamin A is linked with birth defects. Skip supplements containing herbs, enzymes, and amino acids. Many of these ingredients have not been evaluated for safety during pregnancy or breastfeeding and may be toxic to the fetus. Furthermore, discard supplements that are past the expiration date, as some ingredients lose potency over time.

17.5 Food Plan for Pregnant Women

One dietary approach to support a successful pregnancy is based on MyPlate. For an active 24-year-old woman, about 2200 kcal is recommended during the first trimester (the same as recommended for such a woman when not pregnant). The plan should include:

- 3 cups of calcium-rich foods from the dairy group or use of calcium-fortified foods to make up for any gap between calcium intake and need
- 6 ounce-equivalents from the protein group
- 3 cups from the vegetables group
- 2 cups from the fruits group
- 7 ounce-equivalents from the grains group
- 6 teaspoons of vegetable oil

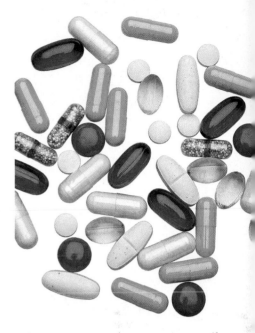

▲ Pregnancy, in particular, is not a time to self-prescribe vitamin and mineral supplements. For example, although vitamin A is a routine component of prenatal vitamins, intakes over three times the RDA for vitamin A have been shown to have toxic effects on the fetus.

MAKING DECISIONS

Cravings During Pregnancy

It is a common myth that women instinctively know what to eat during pregnancy. Cravings of the last two trimesters are often related to hormonal changes in the mother, or family traditions. Such "instinct" cannot be trusted, however, based on observations that some women crave nonfood items (called **pica**) such as laundry starch, chalk, cigarette ashes, and soil (clay). This practice can be extremely harmful to the mother and the fetus. Overall, though women may have a natural instinct to consume the right foods in pregnancy, humans are so far removed from living by instinct that relying on our cravings to meet nutrient needs is risky. Nutrition advice by experts is more reliable.

pica The practice of eating nonfood items, such as dirt, laundry starch, or clay.

At **www.ChooseMyPlate.gov**, moms-to-be can find individualized dietary information by clicking on the link for Daily Food Plans for Moms. Based on age, height, physical activity, and prepregnancy weight, calorie and food group recommendations are generated for each trimester.

Specifically, choices from the dairy group should include low-fat or fat-free versions of milk, yogurt, and cheese. These foods supply extra protein, calcium, and carbohydrate, as well as other nutrients. Choices from the protein group should include both animal and vegetable sources. Besides protein, these foods help provide the extra iron and zinc needed. The vegetables and fruits group choices provide a variety of vitamins and minerals. One cup from this combination should be a good vitamin C source, and 1 cup should be a green vegetable or other rich source of folate. Choices from the grains group should focus on whole-grain and enriched foods. One ounce of a whole-grain, ready-to-eat breakfast cereal significantly contributes to meeting many vitamin and mineral needs. Finally, inclusion of plant oils in the diet contributes essential fatty acids. Calories from solid fats and added sugars should be limited to 270 kcal per day.

In the second and third trimesters, about 2600 kcal is recommended for this woman. The plan should now include:

- 3 cups of calcium-rich foods from the dairy group or use of calcium-fortified foods
- 6 ½ ounce-equivalents from the protein group
- 3 ½ cups from the vegetables group
- 2 cups from the fruits group
- 9-ounce equivalents from the grains group
- 8 teaspoons of vegetable oil

Solid fats and added sugars should contribute no more than 360 kcal per day. Table 17-4 illustrates one daily menu based on the 2600 kcal plan for pregnancy for women in the second or third trimesters. This menu meets the extra nutrient needs associated with pregnancy. Women who need to consume more than this—and some do for various reasons—should incorporate additional fruits, vegetables, and whole-grain breads and cereals, not poor nutrient sources such as desserts and sugared soft drinks.

Pregnant Vegetarians

Women who are either lactoovovegetarians or lactovegetarians generally do not face special difficulties in meeting their nutritional needs during pregnancy. Like

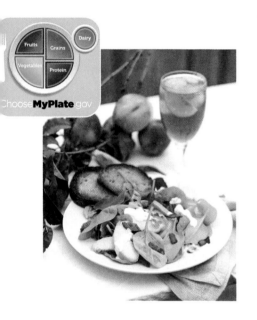

CRITICAL THINKING

How does this lunch of spinach and fruit salad and whole-wheat toast compare to MyPlate? Is iced tea a good beverage choice? Why or why not?

TABLE 17-4 Sample 2600 kcal Daily Menu That Meets the Nutritional Needs of Most Pregnant and Breastfeeding Women

	Vitamin B-6	Folate	Iron	Zinc	Calcium
Breakfast					
1 cup Kellogg's Smart Start cereal	✓	✓	✓	✓	✓
1 cup orange juice		✓			
1 cup fat-free milk	✓				✓
Snack					
2 tbsp peanut butter	✓	✓	✓	✓	
2 stalks of celery		✓			
1 slice whole-wheat toast		✓	✓	✓	
1 cup plain low-fat yogurt	✓				✓
½ cup strawberries		✓			
Lunch					
2 cups spinach and fruit salad with 2 tbsp oil and vinegar dressing		✓			✓
2 slices whole-wheat toast		✓	✓	✓	
1 ½ ounces provolone cheese	✓				✓
Snack					
5 whole-wheat crackers		✓	✓	✓	
1 cup grape juice					
Dinner					
3 ounces lean hamburger, broiled (with condiments)	✓		✓	✓	
½ cup baked beans	✓	✓	✓	✓	
1 hamburger bun		✓	✓		
½ sliced tomato					
1 cup cooked broccoli		✓			✓
1 tsp soft margarine					
Iced tea					
Snack					
Granola bar (2 ounces)		✓	✓	✓	
½ banana	✓				
Foods or beverages containing solid fats or added sugars can be included (up to 360 kcal per day) to support adequate weight gain.					

*Amount of solid fats and added sugars will vary based on the actual food choices made within each MyPlate group.

This diet meets nutrient needs for pregnancy and breastfeeding. Lack of a check (✓) indicates a poor source of the nutrient. The vitamin- and mineral-fortified breakfast cereal used in this example makes an important contribution to meeting nutrient needs. Fluids can be added as desired. Total intake of fluids, such as water, should be 10 cups per day for pregnant women or about 13 cups per day for breastfeeding women.

nonvegetarian women, they should be concerned primarily with meeting vitamin B-6, iron, folate, and zinc needs.

On the other hand, for a vegan, careful diet planning during preconception and pregnancy is crucial to ensure sufficient protein, vitamin D (particularly in the absence of sufficient sun exposure), vitamin B-6, iron, calcium, zinc, and especially a supplemental source of vitamin B-12. The basic vegan diet listed in Chapter 6 should be modified to include more grains, beans, nuts, and seeds to supply the necessary extra amounts of some of these nutrients. As mentioned, use of a prenatal multivitamin and mineral supplement also is generally advocated to help fill micronutrient gaps. However, although these are high in iron, this is not true for calcium (200 milligrams per pill). If iron and calcium supplements are used, they should not be taken together, to avoid possible competition for absorption.

CONCEPT CHECK

Calorie needs increase by an average of about 350 to 450 kcal per day during the second and third trimesters of pregnancy, respectively. Weight gain should be slow and steady up to a total of 25 to 35 pounds for a woman of normal weight (i.e., prepregnancy BMI of 18.5 to 24.9). Protein and certain vitamin and mineral needs increase during pregnancy. Most important to consider are vitamin B-6, folate, iron, iodide, and zinc. A pregnant woman's diet should be varied and generally comply with MyPlate standards. A prenatal multivitamin and mineral supplement is commonly prescribed but may not be necessary, depending on one's diet and health status. Taking too many supplements—especially vitamin A—can be hazardous to the fetus.

17.6 Physiological Changes of Concern During Pregnancy

During pregnancy, the fetus's needs for oxygen and nutrients, as well as excretion of waste products increase the burden on the mother's lungs, heart, and kidneys. Although a mother's digestive and metabolic systems work efficiently, some discomfort accompanies the changes her body undergoes to accommodate the fetus.

Heartburn, Constipation, and Hemorrhoids

Hormones (such as progesterone) produced by the placenta relax muscles in the uterus and the gastrointestinal tract. This often causes heartburn as stomach acid refluxes into the esophagus (review Chapter 3). When this occurs, the woman should avoid lying down after eating, eat less fat so that foods pass more quickly from the stomach into the small intestine, and avoid spicy foods she cannot tolerate. She should also consume most liquids between meals to decrease the volume of food in the stomach after meals, and thus relieve some of the pressure that encourages reflux. Women with more severe cases may need antacids or related medications.

Constipation often results as the intestinal muscles relax during pregnancy. It is especially likely to develop late in pregnancy, as the fetus competes with the GI tract for space in the abdominal cavity. To offset these discomforts, a woman should perform regular exercise and consume more fluid, fiber, and dried fruits, such as prunes (dried plums). The Adequate Intake for fiber in pregnancy is 28 grams, slightly more than for the nonpregnant woman. Fluid needs are 10 cups per day. These practices can help prevent constipation and a problem that frequently accompanies it, hemorrhoids. Straining during elimination can lead to hemorrhoids, which are more likely to occur during pregnancy because of other body changes. A re-evaluation of the need for and dose of iron supplementation also should be considered, as high iron intakes are linked to constipation.

Edema

Placental hormones cause various body tissues to retain fluid during pregnancy. Blood volume also greatly expands during pregnancy. The extra fluid normally causes some swelling (edema). There is no reason to restrict salt severely or use diuretics to limit mild edema. However, the edema may limit physical activity late in pregnancy and occasionally requires a woman to elevate her feet or wear compression stockings to control the symptoms. Overall, edema generally spells trouble only if hypertension and the appearance of extra protein in the urine accompany it (see a following section, "Pregnancy-Induced Hypertension").

Morning Sickness

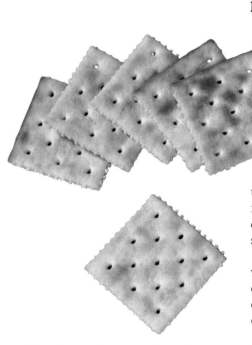

About 70% to 85% of pregnant women experience nausea during the early stages of pregnancy. This nausea may be related to the increased sense of smell induced by pregnancy-related hormones circulating in the bloodstream. Although commonly called "morning sickness," pregnancy-related nausea may occur at any time and persist all day. It is often the first signal to a woman that she is pregnant. To help control mild nausea, pregnant women can try the following: avoiding nauseating foods, such as fried or greasy foods; cooking with good ventilation to dissipate nauseating smells; eating saltine crackers or dry cereal before getting out of bed; avoiding large fluid intakes early in the morning; and eating smaller, more frequent meals. The iron in prenatal supplements triggers nausea in some women, so changing the type of supplement used or postponing use until the second trimester may provide relief in some cases. If a woman thinks her prenatal supplement is related to morning sickness, she should discuss switching to another supplement with her physician.

Overall, if a food sounds good to a pregnant woman with morning sickness, whether it is broccoli, soda crackers, or lemonade, she should eat it and eat when she can, while also striving to follow her prenatal diet. The American College of Obstetricians and Gynecologists recommends the following for the prevention and treatment of nausea and vomiting of pregnancy:

- History of use of a balanced multivitamin and mineral supplement at the time of conception
- Use of megadoses of vitamin B-6 (10–25 milligrams taken three to four times a day), especially coupled with the antihistamine doxylamine (10 milligrams) with each dose
- Ginger may also be helpful (350 milligrams taken three times per day)

Usually, nausea stops after the first trimester; however, in about 10% to 20% of cases, it can continue throughout the entire pregnancy. In cases of serious nausea, the preceding practices offer little relief. Excessive vomiting can cause dangerous dehydration and must be avoided. When vomiting persists (about 0.5% to 2% of pregnancies), medical attention is needed.

▲ A few saltine crackers upon waking or between meals can help lessen pregnancy-related nausea.

Anemia

To supply fetal needs, the mother's blood volume expands to approximately 150% of normal. The number of red blood cells, however, increases by only 20% to 30%, and this occurs more gradually. As a result, a pregnant woman has a lower ratio of red blood cells to total blood volume in her system. This hemodilution is known as **physiological anemia.** It is a normal response to pregnancy, rather than the result of inadequate nutrient intake. If during pregnancy, however, iron stores and/or dietary iron intake are not sufficient to meet needs, any resulting iron-deficiency anemia requires medical attention. The Dietary Guidelines for Americans recommend that women who may become pregnant eat foods high in iron (Table 17-3).

physiological anemia The normal increase in blood volume in pregnancy that dilutes the concentration of red blood cells, resulting in anemia; also called *hemodilution.*

Gestational Diabetes

Hormones synthesized by the placenta decrease the efficiency of insulin. This leads to a mild increase in blood glucose, which helps supply calories to the fetus. If the rise in blood glucose becomes excessive, this leads to **gestational diabetes,** often beginning in weeks 20 to 28, particularly in women who have a family history of diabetes or who are obese. Other risk factors include maternal age over 35 and gestational diabetes in a prior pregnancy. In North America, gestational diabetes develops in about 4% of pregnancies; however, it increases to 7% in the Caucasian population. Today, pregnant women with risk factors for type 2 diabetes (e.g., obesity, family history) should be screened for undiagnosed type 2 diabetes at the first prenatal visit. Pregnant women without type 2 diabetes should be screened for diabetes at 24 to 28 weeks by checking for elevated blood glucose concentration 1 to 2 hours after consuming 75 grams of glucose (see Further Reading 16). If gestational diabetes is detected, a special diet that distributes low glycemic load carbohydrates throughout the day needs to be implemented. Sometimes insulin injections or oral medications are also needed. Regular physical activity also helps control blood glucose.

The primary risk of uncontrolled diabetes during pregnancy is that the fetus can grow quite large. This is a result of the oversupply of glucose from maternal circulation coupled with an increased production of insulin by the fetus, which allows fetal tissues to take up an increased amount of building materials for growth. The mother may require a Cesarean section if the size of the fetus is not compatible with a vaginal delivery. Another threat is that the infant may have low blood glucose at birth, because of the tendency to produce extra insulin that began during gestation. Other concerns are the potential for early delivery and increased risk of birth trauma and malformations. Although gestational diabetes often disappears after the infant's birth, it increases the mother's risk of developing diabetes later in life, especially if she fails to maintain a healthy body weight. Studies show that infants of mothers with gestational diabetes may also have higher risks of developing obesity and type 2 diabetes as they grow to adulthood. For all these reasons, proper control of gestational diabetes (and any diabetes present in the mother before pregnancy) is extremely important.

gestational diabetes A high blood glucose concentration that develops during pregnancy and returns to normal after birth; one cause is the placental production of hormones that antagonize the regulation of blood glucose by insulin.

pregnancy-induced hypertension A serious disorder that can include high blood pressure, kidney failure, convulsions, and even death of the mother and fetus. Although its exact cause is not known, an adequate diet (especially adequate calcium intake) and prenatal care may prevent this disorder or limit its severity. Mild cases are known as *preeclampsia;* more severe cases are called *eclampsia* (formerly called *toxemia*).

CRITICAL THINKING

Sandy, 4 months pregnant, has been having heartburn after meals, constipation, and difficult bowel movements. As a student of nutrition, you understand the digestive system and the role of nutrition in health. What remedies might you suggest to Sandy to relieve her problems?

Pregnancy-Induced Hypertension

Pregnancy-induced hypertension is a high-risk disorder that occurs in about 3% to 5% of pregnancies. In its mild forms, it is also known as *preeclampsia* and, in severe forms, as *eclampsia*. Early symptoms include a rise in blood pressure, excess protein in the urine, edema, changes in blood clotting, and nervous system disorders. Very severe effects, including convulsions, can occur in the second and third trimesters. If not controlled, eclampsia eventually damages the liver and kidneys, and mother and fetus may die. The populations most at risk for this disorder are women under age 17 or over age 35, overweight or obese women, and those who have had multiple-birth pregnancies. A family history of pregnancy-induced hypertension in the mother's or father's side of the family, diabetes, African-American race, and a woman's first pregnancy also raise risk.

Pregnancy-induced hypertension resolves once the pregnancy ends, making delivery the most reliable treatment for the mother. However, because the problem often begins before the fetus is ready to be born, physicians in many cases must use treatments to prevent the worsening of the disorder. Bed rest and magnesium sulfate are the most effective treatment methods, although their effectiveness varies. Magnesium likely acts to relax blood vessels, and so leads to a fall in blood pressure. There is good evidence of the role of adequate calcium intake in reducing incidence of pregnancy-induced hypertension. However, results of a recent trial showed that vitamin C and E supplementation during pregnancy is not effective in preventing the disorder. Several other treatments, such as various antiseizure and antihypertensive medications, fish oils, selenium, and vitamin D are under study (see Further Reading 6).

17.7 Breastfeeding

Many of the benefits of breastfeeding can be found in Table 17-5 and at www .womenshealth.gov/Breastfeeding/ index.cfm, sponsored by the U.S. Surgeon General.

Breastfeeding the new infant further fosters his or her health, and so complements the attention given to diet during pregnancy. The American Dietetic Association and the American Academy of Pediatrics (AAP) recommend breastfeeding exclusively for the first 6 months, with the continued combination of breastfeeding and infant foods until 1 year (see Further Readings 2 and 4). The World Health Organization goes beyond that to recommend breastfeeding (with appropriate solid food introduction; see Chapter 18) for at least 2 years. Still, surveys show that only about 70% of North American mothers now begin to breastfeed their infants in the hospital, and at 4 and 6 months only 33% and 20%, respectively, are still breastfeeding their infants. The number falls to 18% at 1 year of age. These statistics refer to Caucasian women; minority women are even less likely to be breastfeeding at these time intervals.

Women who choose to breastfeed usually find it an enjoyable, special time in their lives that strengthens the bond with their new infant. Although bottle feeding with an infant formula is also safe for infants, as discussed in Chapter 18, it does not equal the benefits derived from human milk in all aspects. If a woman doesn't breastfeed her child, breast weight returns to normal soon after birth.

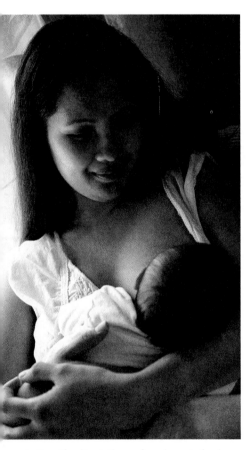

▲ Breastfeeding is the preferred way to feed a young infant.

*H*ealthy People 2020 has set a goal of 82% of women breastfeeding their infants at time of hospital discharge, 60% breastfeeding for 6 months, and 34% still breastfeeding at 1 year.

Planning to Breastfeed

Almost all women are physically capable of breastfeeding their children (see later section "Medical Conditions Precluding Breastfeeding" for exceptions). In most cases, problems encountered in breastfeeding are due to a lack of appropriate information. Anatomical problems in breasts, such as inverted nipples, can be corrected during pregnancy. Breast size generally increases during pregnancy and is no indication of success in breastfeeding. Most women notice a dramatic increase in the size and weight of their breasts by the third or fourth day of breastfeeding. If these changes do not occur, a woman needs to speak with her physician or a lactation consultant.

Breastfed infants must be followed closely over the first days of life to ensure that feeding and weight gain are proceeding normally. Monitoring is especially important with a mother's first child, because the mother will be inexperienced with the technique of breastfeeding. Mothers and healthy infants are commonly discharged from the hospital 1 to 2 days after delivery, whereas 20 years ago they stayed in the hospital for 3 or 4 days or longer. One result of such rapid discharge is a decreased period of infant monitoring by health care professionals. Incidents have been reported of infants developing dehydration and, in turn, blood clots soon after hospital discharge when breastfeeding did not proceed smoothly. Careful monitoring in this first week by a physician or lactation consultant is advised.

First-time mothers who plan to breastfeed should learn as much as they can about the process early in their pregnancy. Interested women should learn the proper technique, what obstacles to anticipate, and how to respond to them. Overall, breastfeeding is a learned skill, and mothers need knowledge to breastfeed, especially with the first child.

Production of Human Milk

During pregnancy, cells in the breast form milk-producing cells called **lobules** (Fig. 17-7). Hormones from the placenta stimulate these changes in the breast. After birth, the mother produces more **prolactin** hormone to maintain the changes in the breast and therefore the ability to produce milk. During pregnancy, breast weight increases by about 1 to 2 pounds.

The hormone prolactin also stimulates the synthesis of milk. Infant suckling stimulates prolactin release from the pituitary gland. Milk synthesis then occurs as an infant nurses. The more the infant suckles, the more milk is produced. Because of this, even twins (and triplets) can be breastfed adequately.

Most protein found in human milk is synthesized by breast tissue. Some proteins also enter the milk directly from the mother's bloodstream. These proteins include immune factors (e.g., antibodies) and enzymes. Fats in human milk come from both the mother's diet and those synthesized by breast tissue. The sugar galactose is synthesized in the breast, whereas glucose enters from the mother's bloodstream. Together, these sugars form lactose, the main carbohydrate in human milk.

Let-Down Reflex

An important brain-breast connection—commonly called the **let-down reflex**—is necessary for breastfeeding. The brain releases the hormone **oxytocin** to allow the breast tissues to let down (release) the milk from storage sites (Fig. 17-8). It then travels to the nipple area. A tingling sensation signals the let-down reflex shortly before milk flow begins. If the let-down reflex doesn't operate, little milk is available to the infant. The infant then gets frustrated, and this can frustrate the mother.

The let-down reflex is easily inhibited by nervous tension, a lack of confidence, and fatigue. Mothers should be especially aware of the link between tension and a weak let-down reflex. They need to find a relaxed environment where they can breastfeed.

lobules Saclike structures in the breast that store milk.

prolactin A hormone secreted by the pituitary gland that stimulates the synthesis of milk in the breast.

let-down reflex A reflex stimulated by infant suckling that causes the release (ejection) of milk from milk ducts in the mother's breasts; also called *milk ejection reflex*.

oxytocin A hormone secreted by the pituitary gland. It causes contraction of the muscle-like cells surrounding the ducts of the breasts and the smooth muscle of the uterus.

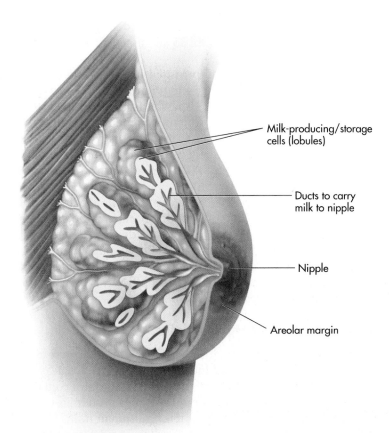

FIGURE 17-7 ▶ The anatomy of the breast. Many types of cells form a coordinated network to produce and secrete human milk.

Milk-producing/storage cells (lobules)

Ducts to carry milk to nipple

Nipple

Areolar margin

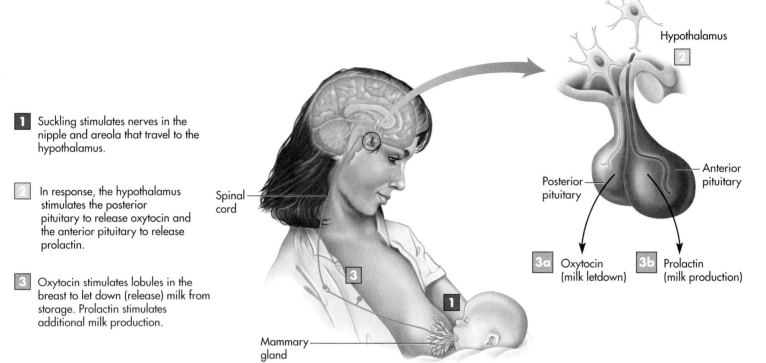

1 Suckling stimulates nerves in the nipple and areola that travel to the hypothalamus.

2 In response, the hypothalamus stimulates the posterior pituitary to release oxytocin and the anterior pituitary to release prolactin.

3 Oxytocin stimulates lobules in the breast to let down (release) milk from storage. Prolactin stimulates additional milk production.

Spinal cord

Mammary gland

Hypothalamus
2

Posterior pituitary

Anterior pituitary

3a Oxytocin (milk letdown)   **3b** Prolactin (milk production)

FIGURE 17-8 ▶ Let-down reflex. Suckling sets into motion the sequence of events that lead to milk let-down, the flow of milk into ducts of the breast.

Disposable diapers can absorb so much urine that it is difficult to judge when they are wet. A strip of paper towel laid inside a disposable diaper makes a good wetness indicator. Alternatively, cloth diapers may be used for a day or two to assess whether nursing is supplying sufficient milk.

After a few weeks, the let-down reflex becomes automatic. The mother's response can be triggered just by thinking about her infant or seeing or hearing another one cry. At first, however, the process can be a bit bewildering. A mother cannot measure the amount of milk the infant takes in, so she may fear that she is not adequately nourishing the infant.

As a general rule, a well-nourished breastfed infant should (1) have three to five wet diapers per day by 3 to 5 days of age and four to six wet diapers per day thereafter, (2) show a normal weight gain, and (3) pass at least one or two stools per day that look like lumpy mustard. In addition, softening of the breast during the feeding helps indicate that enough milk is being consumed. Parents who sense their infant is not consuming enough milk should consult a physician immediately because dehydration can develop rapidly. Losing more than 7% of birth weight is an indicator of a feeding problem that requires intervention.

It generally takes 2 to 3 weeks to fully establish the feeding routine: Infant and mother both feel comfortable, the milk supply meets infant demand, and initial nipple soreness disappears. Establishing the breastfeeding routine requires patience, but the rewards are great. The adjustments are easier if supplemental formula feedings are not introduced until breastfeeding is well established, after at least 3 to 4 weeks. Then it is fine if a supplemental bottle or two of infant formula per day is needed, but supplemental feedings will decrease milk production.

Nutritional Qualities of Human Milk

Human milk is different in composition from cow's milk. Unless altered, cow's milk should never be used in infant feeding until the infant is at least 12 months old. Cow's milk is too high in minerals and protein and does not contain enough carbohydrate to meet infant needs. In addition, the major protein in cow's milk is harder for an infant to digest than the major proteins in human milk. The proteins in cow's milk also may spur allergies in the infant. Finally, certain compounds in human milk presently under study show other possible benefits for the infant.

Colostrum. At the end of pregnancy, the first fluid made by the human breast is **colostrum.** This thick, yellowish fluid may leak from the breast during late pregnancy and is produced in earnest for a few days to a week after birth. Colostrum contains antibodies and immune system cells, some of which pass unaltered through the infant's immature GI tract into the bloodstream. The first few months of life are the only time when we can readily absorb whole proteins across the GI tract. These immune factors and cells protect the infant from some GI tract diseases and other infectious disorders, compensating for the infant's immature immune system during the first few months of life.

One component of colostrum, the *Lactobacillus bifidus* **factor,** encourages the growth of *Lactobacillus bifidus* bacteria. These bacteria limit the growth of potentially toxic bacteria in the intestine. Overall, breastfeeding promotes the intestinal health of the breastfed infant in this way.

colostrum The first fluid secreted by the breast during late pregnancy and the first few days after birth. This thick fluid is rich in immune factors and protein.

Lactobacillus bifidus **factor** A protective factor secreted in the colostrum that encourages growth of beneficial bacteria in the newborn's intestines.

Mature Milk. Human milk composition gradually changes until it achieves the normal composition of mature milk several days after delivery. Human milk looks very different from cow's milk. (Table 18-1 in Chapter 18 provides a direct comparison.) Human milk is thin and almost watery in appearance and often has a slightly bluish tinge. Its nutritional qualities, however, are impressive.

Human milk's proteins form a soft, light curd in the infant's stomach and are easy to digest. Some human milk proteins bind iron, reducing the growth of iron-requiring bacteria, some of which can cause diarrhea. Still other proteins offer the important immune protection already noted.

The lipids in human breast milk are high in linoleic acid and cholesterol, needed for brain development. Breast milk also contains long-chain omega-3 fatty acids, such as docosahexaenoic acid (DHA). This polyunsaturated fatty acid is used for the synthesis of tissues in the brain and the rest of the central nervous system and in the retina of the eye.

The fat composition of human milk changes during each feeding. The consistency of milk released initially (fore milk) resembles that of skim milk. It later has a greater fat proportion, similar to whole milk. Finally, the milk released after 10 to 20 minutes (hind milk) is essentially like cream. Babies need to nurse long enough (e.g., a total of 20 or more minutes) to get the calories in the rich hind milk to be satisfied between feedings and to grow well. The overall calorie content of human milk is about the same as that of infant formulas (67 kcal per 100 milliliters).

Human milk composition also allows for adequate fluid status of the infant, provided the baby is exclusively breastfed. A question commonly asked is whether the infant needs additional water if stressed by hot weather, diarrhea, vomiting, or fever. The AAP recommends against supplemental water or juice during the first 6 months of life. The practice may unnecessarily introduce pathogens or allergens. Excessive water can lead to brain disorders, low blood sodium, and other problems. Thus, supplemental water and juice should be given only with a physician's guidance before 6 months of age.

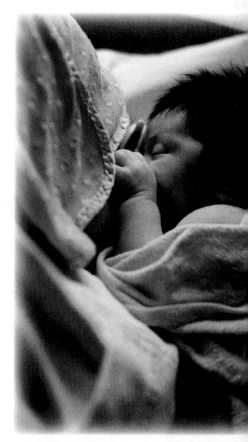

▲ Breastfeeding promotes the intestinal health of the breastfed infant.

Food Plan for Women Who Breastfeed

Nutrient needs for a breastfeeding mother change to some extent from those of the pregnant woman in the second and third trimester (see the inside cover of this book). There is a decrease in folate and iron needs and an increase in the needs for calories, vitamins A, E, and C, riboflavin, copper, chromium, iodide, manganese, selenium, and zinc. Still, these increased needs of the breastfeeding mother will be met by the general diet plan proposed for a woman in the latter stages of pregnancy. Recall that each day of this diet plan includes at least:

- 3 cups of calcium-rich foods such as from the dairy group or use of calcium-fortified foods to make up for any gap between calcium intake and need
- 6 ½ ounce-equivalents from the protein group
- 3 ½ cups from the vegetables group

Most substances that the mother ingests are secreted into her milk. For this reason, she should limit intake of or avoid all alcohol and caffeine and check all medications with a pediatrician. Some mothers believe that certain foods, such as garlic and chocolate, flavor the breast milk and upset the infant. If a woman notices a connection between a food she eats and the infant's later fussiness, she could consider avoiding that food. However, she might experiment again with it later, as infants become fussy for other reasons. Some researchers, on the other hand, feel that the passage of flavors from the mother's diet into her milk affords an opportunity for the infant to learn about the flavor of the foods of its family long before solids are introduced. These researchers suspect that bottle-fed infants are missing significant sensory experiences that, until recent times in human history, were common to all infants.

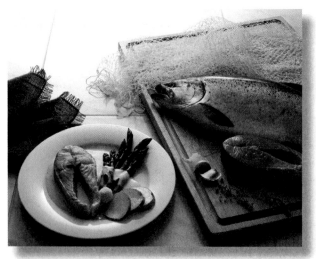

▲ Eating fish at least twice a week will help breastfeeding women ensure that their infants receive important omega-3 fatty acids. It is important, however, to avoid those fish likely to be contaminated with mercury (swordfish, shark, king mackerel, and tile fish).

atopic disease Condition resulting from an inappropriate immune response, such as asthma, allergic rhinitis, food allergies, or eczema.

- 2 cups from the fruits group
- 9 ounce-equivalents from the grains group
- 8 teaspoons of vegetable oil

Foods containing solid fats and added sugars (up to about 360 kcal) can then be added to allow for weight maintenance or gradual weight loss, whichever is needed.

Table 17-4 provided a menu for such a plan. Substituting a soyburger (veggie burger) for the hamburger in that menu would make this a practical guide for a lacto-vegetarian woman as well.

As in pregnancy, a serving of a highly fortified ready-to-eat breakfast cereal (or use of a balanced multivitamin and mineral supplement) is advised to help meet extra nutrient needs. And, as mentioned for pregnant women, breastfeeding mothers should consume fish at least twice a week (or 1 gram per day of omega-3 fatty acids from a fish oil supplement) because the omega-3 fatty acids present in fish are secreted into breast milk and are likely to be important for development of the infant's nervous system.

Milk production requires approximately 800 kcal every day. The Estimated Energy Requirement during lactation is an extra 400 to 500 kcal daily above prepregnancy recommendations. The difference between that needed for milk production and the recommended intake—about 300 kcal—should allow a gradual loss of the extra body fat accumulated during pregnancy, especially if breastfeeding is continued for 6 months or more and the woman performs some physical activity. This shows just one of the natural benefits of following pregnancy with at least several months of breastfeeding.

After giving birth, women are often eager to shed the excess "baby fat." Breastfeeding, however, is no time for crash diets. A gradual weight loss of 1 to 4 pounds per month by the nursing mother is appropriate. At significantly greater rates of weight loss—when calories are restricted to less than about 1500 kcal per day—milk output decreases. A reasonable approach for a breastfeeding mother is to eat a balanced diet that supplies at least 1800 kcal per day; has moderate fat content; and includes a variety of dairy products, fruits, vegetables, and whole grains.

To promote the best possible feeding experience for the infant, there are several other dietary factors to consider. Hydration is especially important during breastfeeding; the woman should drink fluids every time her infant nurses. Drinking about 13 cups of fluids per day encourages ample milk production. Poor health habits, such as smoking cigarettes or drinking more than two alcoholic drinks a day, can decrease milk output. (Even less alcohol can have a deleterious effect on milk output in some women.) To avoid exposure to harmful levels of mercury, precautions concerning fish likely to contain mercury should extend past pregnancy for the breastfeeding mother. There is no evidence that maternal diet restrictions (e.g., peanuts, eggs, fish) during pregnancy or breastfeeding prevent food allergies in their infants. The AAP recommends exclusive breastfeeding and delaying introduction of solid foods until 4 to 6 months of age as the best approaches for preventing **atopic diseases** (see Further Reading 9).

CONCEPT CHECK

Recognition of the importance of breastfeeding has contributed to its greater popularity. Almost all women have the ability to breastfeed. The hormone prolactin stimulates breast tissue to synthesize milk. Infant suckling triggers a let-down reflex, which releases the milk. The more an infant nurses, the more milk is synthesized. Some components of human milk come directly from the mother's bloodstream. The nutrient composition of human milk is different from that of cow's milk and changes as the infant matures. The first fluid produced, colostrum, is rich in immune factors. The mother's diet during breastfeeding is generally similar to that for pregnancy, except for necessary additional fluids.

Breastfeeding Today

As noted, the vast majority of women are capable of breastfeeding and their infants benefit from it (see Table 17-5 and Further Reading 18). Nonetheless, some circumstances may make breastfeeding impractical or undesirable for a woman. Mothers who don't want to breastfeed their infants should not feel pressured to do so. Breastfeeding provides advantages, but none so great that a woman who decides to bottle feed should feel she is compromising her infant's well being.

Advantages of Breastfeeding. Human milk is tailored to meet infant nutrient needs for the first 4 to 6 months of life. However, there are some cases when infant dietary supplements, used under a pediatrician's guidance, are recommended:

- The AAP recommends all infants, including exclusively breastfed infants, be given 400 IU of vitamin D per day, beginning shortly after birth and continuing until the infant consumes that much from food (e.g., at least 2 cups (0.5 liters) of infant formula per day). Some sun exposure also helps in meeting vitamin D needs.
- Iron supplements are generally necessary for infants who were preterm, LBW, have blood disorders, or who were born with low iron stores.
- The AAP does not advise fluoride supplements before 6 months of age. After 6 months, the pediatrician or dentist may recommend supplemental fluoride if the infant's intake of fluoridated water, food sources, and use of toothpaste is insufficient.
- Vitamin B-12 supplements are recommended for the breastfed infant whose mother is a complete vegetarian (vegan).

Fewer Infections. Due in part to the antibodies in human milk, breastfeeding reduces the infant's overall risk of developing infections (see Further Reading 7). Breastfed

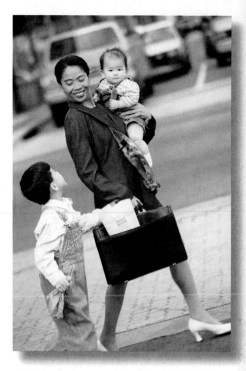

▲ Mothers who return to work outside the home can continue to breastfeed with the aid of a breastpump. In 2010, President Obama signed an amendment to the Fair Labor Standards Act that requires most U.S. employers to allow break time and a private setting for breastfeeding mothers to express milk.

TABLE 17-5 Advantages of Breastfeeding

For Infant
• Bacteriologically safe
• Always fresh and ready to go
• Provides antibodies and substances that contribute to maturation of the immune system
• Contributes to maturation of gastrointestinal tract via *Lactobacillus bifidus* factor; decreases incidence of diarrhea and respiratory disease
• Reduces risk of food allergies and intolerances, as well as some other allergies
• Establishes habit of eating in moderation, linked to 20% lower risk of obesity later in life
• Contributes to proper development of jaws and teeth for better speech development
• Decreases ear infections
• May enhance nervous system development (by providing DHA) and eventual learning ability
• May reduce the risk of chronic diseases (e.g., hypertension and diabetes)

For Mother
• Contributes to earlier recovery from pregnancy due to the action of hormones that promote a quicker return of the uterus to its prepregnancy state
• Decreases the risk of ovarian and premenopausal breast cancer
• Potential for quicker return to prepregnancy weight
• Potential for delayed ovulation, thus reducing chances of pregnancy in the short term

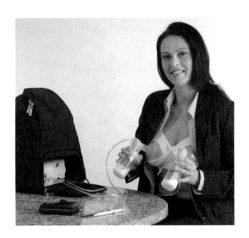

▲ Breast milk can be expressed by the mother using a manual, battery-operated, or electric (shown) breast pump. The expressed milk can be stored for times when the mother is not available to breastfeed the infant.

Useful breastfeeding resources on the Web:

www.lalecheleague.org

www.breastfeeding.com

www.breastfeeding.org

nal.usda.gov/wicworks

www.cdc.gov/breastfeeding

www.usbreastfeeding.org

www.breastfeedinginc.ca

Nipple piercings should have no impact on a woman's ability to breastfeed, but the jewelry should be removed before each feeding. Repeated removal and reinsertion of the jewelry may be inconvenient and irritating, so it may be best to leave the jewelry out for the entire period of breastfeeding. Breast tattoos will not impair breastfeeding, either. However, getting a new nipple piercing or breast tattoo while breastfeeding is not advised due to the pain of healing and possibility of infection. Past breast augmentation or reduction surgeries may impair a woman's ability to breastfeed if milk-producing tissue was damaged during the surgery.

infants also have fewer ear infections (otitis media) because they do not sleep with a bottle in their mouths. Experts strongly discourage allowing any infants to sleep with a bottle in their mouths; milk can pool in the mouth, throat, and inner ear, creating a growth medium for bacteria. By reducing these common infections parents can decrease discomfort for the infant, avoid related trips to the doctor, and prevent possible hearing loss. Tooth decay from nighttime bottles is another likely consequence of sleeping with a bottle in the mouth (see Chapter 18).

Fewer Allergies and Intolerances. Breastfeeding also reduces the chances of some allergies, especially in allergy-prone infants (see Chapter 18). The key time to attain this benefit from breastfeeding is during the first 4 to 6 months of an infant's life. A longer commitment is best, but breastfeeding for even a few weeks is beneficial. Infants are also better able to tolerate human milk than formulas. Formulas sometimes must be switched several times until caregivers find the best one for the infant.

Convenience and Cost. Breastfeeding frees the mother from the time and expense involved in buying and preparing formula and washing bottles. Human milk is ready to go and sterile. This allows the mother to spend more time with her baby.

Possible Barriers to Breastfeeding. Widespread misinformation, the mother's need to return to a job, and social reticence serve as barriers to breastfeeding.

Misinformation. The major barriers to breastfeeding are misinformation, such as the idea that one's breasts are too small, and the lack of role models. One positive note has been the widespread increase in the availability of lactation consultants over the past several years. First-time mothers who are interested in breastfeeding can find invaluable support from lactation consultants or by talking to women who have experienced it successfully. In almost every community, a group called La Leche League offers classes in breastfeeding and advises women who have problems with it (800-LALECHE or www.lalecheleague.org). Online resources are listed in the margin.

Return to an Outside Job. Working outside the home can complicate plans to breastfeed. One possibility after a month or two of breastfeeding is for the mother to express and save her own milk. She can use a breast pump or manually express milk into a sterile plastic bottle or nursing bag (used in a disposable bottle system). Saving human milk requires careful sanitation and rapid chilling. It can be stored in the refrigerator for 3 to 5 days or be frozen for 3 to 6 months. Thawed milk should be used within 24 hours. There is a knack to learning how to express milk, but the freedom can be worth it, because it allows others to feed the infant the mother's milk. A schedule of expressing milk and using supplemental formula feedings is most successful if begun after 1 to 2 months of exclusive breastfeeding. After 1 month or so, the baby is well adapted to breastfeeding and probably feels enough emotional security and other benefits from nursing to drink both ways.

Some women can juggle both a job and breastfeeding, but others find it too cumbersome and decide to formula-feed. A compromise—balancing some breastfeedings, perhaps early morning and night, with infant formula feedings during the day—is possible. However, too many supplemental infant formula feedings decrease milk production.

Social Concerns. Another barrier for some women is embarrassment about nursing a child in public. Historically, our society has stressed modesty and has discouraged public displays of breasts—even for as good a cause as nourishing babies. In the United States, no state or territory has a law prohibiting breastfeeding. However, indecent exposure (including the exposure of women's breasts) has long been a common law or statutory offense. Now, 45 states, the District of Columbia, and the Virgin Islands have specific laws that protect a woman's right to breastfeed in any location. Women who feel reluctant should be reassured that they do have social support and that breastfeeding can be done discreetly with little breast exposure.

Medical Conditions Precluding Breastfeeding. Breastfeeding may be ruled out by certain medical conditions in either the infant or mother. For example, breastfeeding is contraindicated for infants with galactosemia, an inherited disorder in which the body cannot break down galactose. Recall from Chapter 4 that lactose, the main carbohydrate in human breast milk, is made of glucose and galactose. When galactose is not properly broken down, its by-products can damage body organs.

Certain medications, which pass into the milk and adversely affect the nursing infant, are best avoided while breastfeeding. In addition, a woman in North America or other developed region of the world who has a serious chronic disease (such as tuberculosis, AIDS, or HIV-positive status) or who is being treated with chemotherapy medications should not breastfeed.

Environmental Contaminants in Human Milk. There is some legitimate concern over the levels of various environmental contaminants in human milk. However, the benefits of human milk are well established and the risks from environmental contaminants are still largely theoretical. Thus, it is probably best to continue with what has been shown to work until sufficiently strong research data contradict it. A few measures a woman could take to counteract some known contaminants are to (1) consume a variety of foods within each food group; (2) avoid freshwater fish from polluted waters; (3) carefully wash and peel fruits and vegetables; and (4) remove the fatty edges of meat, as pesticides concentrate in fat. In addition, a woman should not try to lose weight rapidly while nursing (more than ¾ to 1 pound per week) because contaminants stored in her fat tissue might then enter her bloodstream and affect her milk. If a woman questions whether her milk is safe, especially if she has lived in an area known to have a high concentration of toxic wastes or environmental pollutants, she should consult her local health department.

Phenylketonuria (PKU), a disorder of phenylalanine metabolism described in Chapter 6, was once thought to be a contraindication for breastfeeding. However, with complementary use of specialized phenylalanine-free formulas, infants with PKU can now enjoy the health and emotional benefits of breastfeeding.

MAKING DECISIONS

Breast Milk for Preterm Infants

There is no universal answer to whether a woman can breastfeed a preterm infant. In some cases, human milk is the most desirable form of nourishment, depending on infant weight and length of gestation. If so, it must usually be expressed from the breast and fed through a tube until the infant's sucking and swallowing reflex develops. This type of feeding demands great maternal dedication. Fortification of the milk with such nutrients as calcium, phosphorus, sodium, and protein is often necessary to meet the needs of a rapidly growing preterm infant. In other cases, special feeding problems may prevent the use of human milk or necessitate supplementing it with specialized formula. Sometimes total parenteral nutrition (intravenous feeding) is the only option. Working as a team, the pediatrician, neonatal nurses, and registered dietitian must guide the parents in this decision.

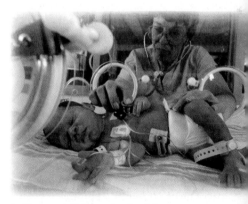

▲ If human milk is used to feed the preterm infant, fortification of the milk with certain nutrients is often needed.

CONCEPT CHECK

Human milk supplies most of an infant's nutritional needs for the first 6 months, although supplementation with vitamin D, iron, and fluoride may be needed. Breastfeeding is often more convenient than formula feeding. Compared with formula-fed infants, breastfed infants have fewer intestinal, respiratory, and ear infections and are less susceptible to some allergies and food intolerances. Despite the advantages of breastfeeding, misinformation, job responsibilities, and social reticence may dissuade a mother from breastfeeding. A combination of breastfeeding and formula feeding is possible when a mother is regularly away from the infant and is not able to express and store her milk for later use. Breastfeeding is not desirable if a mother has certain diseases or must take medication potentially harmful to the infant. The preterm infant, depending on its condition, may benefit from consuming human milk.

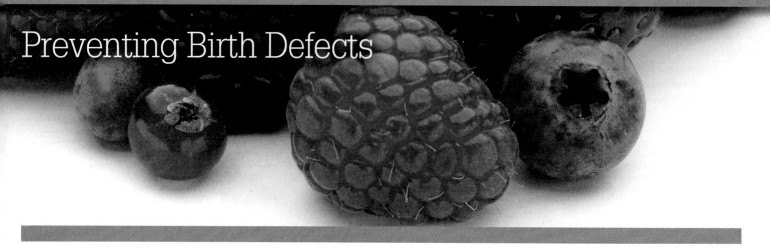

Preventing Birth Defects

Eating well for a healthy pregnancy not only supplies materials for fetal growth and development, but also helps to direct the amazing process of building a new life. Considering the complexity of the human body and its more than 20,000 genes, it's not surprising that abnormalities of structure, function, or metabolism are sometimes present at birth. Birth defects impact one of every 33 babies born in the United States. In some cases, they are so severe that a baby cannot survive or thrive. Birth defects are the presumed cause of many spontaneous abortions and are at the root of about 20% of infant deaths before one year of age. However, with medical intervention, many babies with birth defects can go on to live healthy and productive lives.

A wide range of physical or mental disabilities result from birth defects. Heart defects are present in approximately 1 of every 100 to 200 newborn babies, accounting for a large proportion of infant deaths. Cleft lip and/or cleft palate are malformations of the lip or roof of the mouth and occur in approximately 1 in 700 to 1000 births. Neural tube defects are malformations of the brain or spinal cord that occur in early stages of pregnancy, during embryonic development. Examples include spina bifida, in which all or part of the spinal cord is exposed, and anencephaly, in which some or all of the brain is missing. Babies born with spina bifida can survive to adulthood, but in many cases, have extreme disabilities. Babies born with anencephaly die soon after birth. Neural tube defects occur in 1 in 1000 births. Down syndrome, a condition in which an extra chromosome

leads to mental retardation and other physical alterations, occurs in about 1 in 800 births. Other common birth defects include musculoskeletal defects, gastrointestinal defects, and metabolic disorders.

What causes a birth defect? About 15%–25% of birth defects are known to be genetic (i.e., inherited or spontaneous mutations of the genetic code). Another 10% are due to environmental influences (e.g., exposure to **teratogens**). The specific cause of the remaining 65%–75% of birth defects is unknown. Although the etiology of birth defects is multifactorial and many elements are beyond human control, good nutrition practices are an important way a mother-to-be can have a positive influence on the outcome of her pregnancy.

Folic Acid

During the 1980s, researchers in the United Kingdom noticed a relationship between poor dietary habits and a high rate of neural tube defects among children of impoverished women. Subsequent intervention studies demonstrated that administration of a multivitamin supplement during the periconceptional period— the months before conception and during early pregnancy—reduced the recurrence of these birth defects. The specific link between dietary folic acid and neural tube defects was tested and confirmed in several follow-up studies. As you learned in Chapter 12, folate plays a leading role in the synthesis of DNA and the metabolism of amino acids. The rapid cell growth of pregnancy increases needs for folate during pregnancy to 600 micrograms DFE per day. Some women, for genetic reasons,

may have an even higher requirement. Adequate folic acid in the periconceptional period decreases the risk of neural tube defects by about 70% and has also been associated with decreased risk of cleft lip/palate, heart defects, and Down syndrome.

In 1998, the FDA mandated fortification of grain products to provide 140 micrograms of folic acid per 100 grams of grain consumed. In Canada, the level of fortification is 150 micrograms of folate per 100 grams of grain consumed. In general, this increases the average consumption of dietary folic acid by 100 micrograms per day.

A well-planned diet can meet the RDA for folic acid, but the U.S. Public Health Service and the March of Dimes recommend that all women of childbearing age take a daily multivitamin and mineral supplement that contains 400 micrograms of folic acid. A physician may recommend prenatal vitamins or a higher dose of folic acid for some women, particularly those who have had a prior pregnancy complicated by a neural tube defect. The Dietary Guidelines for Americans recommend that women who may become pregnant and those in the first few months of pregnancy consume an adequate amount of the synthetic form of folate, folic acid (Table 17-3).

teratogen A substance that may cause or increase the risk of a birth defect. Exposure to a teratogen does not always lead to a birth defect; its effects on the fetus depend on the dose, timing, and duration of exposure.

Iodide

The relationship between folic acid and neural tube defects is a dramatic example of how a nutrient deficiency can negatively impact pregnancy outcome, but it is not the only nutrient of concern. Low iodide status during the first trimester of pregnancy—a critical period of brain development—may lead to cretinism (see Further Reading 20). This is a congenital form of hypothyroidism that leads to diminished physical and mental development if left untreated. When the defect is identified early (by newborn screening tests), cretinism can be prevented by treatment with thyroid hormones. With use of iodized salt, however, iodide deficiencies are rare.

Antioxidants

A case can be made for antioxidants in the prevention of birth defects as well. Free radicals are constantly generated within the body as a result of normal metabolic processes. An abundance of free radicals results in damage of cells and their DNA, which can lead to gene mutations or tissue malformations. Some research points to free radicals as a source of damage during embryo development and organogenesis. Antioxidant systems within the body act to minimize the damage caused by free radicals, and researchers hypothesize that dietary sources of antioxidants may aid in the prevention of birth defects. At this time, there is insufficient evidence to support supplementation of individual nutrients that participate in antioxidant systems—vitamin E, vitamin C, selenium, zinc, and copper—for the prevention of birth defects. However, use of a balanced multivitamin and mineral supplement while consuming a diet rich in whole grains, legumes, and a variety of fruits and vegetables will provide enough of these nutrients to meet current recommendations.

Vitamin A

Whereas the needs for most vitamins and minerals increase by about 30% during pregnancy, the requirement for vitamin A increases by only 10%. Studies have shown the teratogenic potential of vitamin A in doses as low as approximately 3000 micrograms RAE per day. This is just over three times the RDA of 770 micrograms RAE/per day for pregnant adult women.

Fetal abnormalities resulting from vitamin A toxicity primarily include facial and cardiac defects, but a wide range of defects have been reported. It is rare that food sources of vitamin A would lead to toxicity. Recall from Chapter 10 that preformed vitamin A is found in liver, fish, fish oils, fortified milk and yogurt, and eggs. Carotenoids, found in fruits and vegetables, are precursors of vitamin A that are converted to vitamin A in the small intestine. However, the efficiency of absorption of carotenoids decreases as intake increases. Vitamin A excesses typically arise from high-dose dietary supplements rather than food sources. Typical North American diets supply adequate vitamin A from foods, so supplemental use is not generally necessary. During pregnancy, supplemental preformed vitamin A should not exceed 3000 micrograms RAE per day (15,000 IU per day). Most multivitamins and prenatal vitamins supply less than 1500 micrograms RAE per day. A balanced diet and prudent use of dietary supplements are actions that can sidestep potential problems with vitamin A toxicity.

Caffeine

Caffeine has been scrutinized for its safety during pregnancy, especially for any link with rate of birth defects. Caffeine decreases the mother's absorption of iron and may reduce blood flow through the placenta. In addition, the fetus is unable to detoxify caffeine. Research shows that as caffeine intake increases, so does the risk of miscarriage or delivering an LBW infant. Heavy caffeine use during pregnancy may also lead to caffeine withdrawal symptoms in the newborn. These risks are reported with caffeine intakes in excess of 500 milligrams, or the equivalent of about 5 cups of coffee per day. Moderate use of caffeine (up to the equivalent of 3 cups of coffee per day), however, is not associated with risk for birth defects. Based on current evidence, drinking no more than three cups of coffee and no more than four cups of caffeinated soft

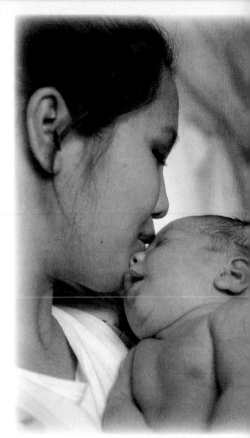

▲ Delivering a healthy baby is more than just luck. Many nutrition- and health-related practices need to be considered.

drinks per day during pregnancy (or when pregnancy is possible) is advocated. Paying attention to caffeine intake from tea, over-the-counter medicines containing caffeine, and chocolate is also important.

Aspartame

Phenylalanine, a component of the artificial sweetener aspartame (NutraSweet® and Equal®), causes concern for some pregnant women. High amounts of phenylalanine in maternal blood disrupt fetal brain development if the mother has a disease known as *phenylketonuria* (see next section). If the mother does not have this condition, however, it is unlikely that the baby will be affected by moderate aspartame use.

For most adults, diet soft drinks are the primary source of artificial sweeteners. Of greater concern than the safety of sweeteners during pregnancy is the quality of foods and beverages consumed. A high intake of diet soft drinks may crowd out healthier beverages, such as water and low-fat milk.

Obesity and Chronic Health Conditions

Even before becoming pregnant, women of childbearing age should have regular medical checkups to keep an eye on any health conditions that already exist or to identify any developing health problems. In some cases, the condition itself increases risk for birth defects. Obesity, high blood pressure, and uncontrolled diabetes are common health problems known to increase the risk for birth defects, including neural tube defects. In other cases, medications used to control illnesses may pose a risk to the developing fetus. Other health issues, such as seizure disorders and metabolic disorders, could also affect fetal development. A preconception visit with a health professional can help to sort out and make plans to minimize such risks. Once a woman has become pregnant, early and regular prenatal care can aid in the success of a pregnancy.

Women with diabetes are two to three times more likely to give birth to a baby with birth defects compared to women with normal glucose metabolism. Examples of birth defects common in this group include malformations of the spine, legs, and blood vessels of the heart. Some experts speculate that the mechanism by which diabetes increases birth defects is via excessive free radicals, which lead to oxidative damage of DNA during early gestation. Careful control of blood glucose drastically lowers risk for women with diabetes. Optimal blood glucose control can be achieved through a combination of dietary modifications and medications. Given that diabetes is on the rise among women of childbearing age, this elevated rate of birth defects has become an area of heightened awareness.

Another health condition for which maternal nutritional control is of utmost importance is PKU. Recall from Chapter 6 that PKU is an error of metabolism in which the liver lacks the ability to process phenylalanine, leading to an accumulation of this amino acid and its metabolites in body tissues. Babies born to women who have phenylketonuria that is not controlled by diet are at heightened risk for brain defects, such as microcephaly and mental retardation (see Further Reading 1).

Alcohol

Conclusive evidence shows that repeated consumption of four or more alcoholic drinks at one sitting harms the fetus (see Further Reading 12). Such binge drinking is especially perilous during the first 12 weeks of pregnancy, as this is when critical early developmental events take place in utero. Although scientists don't know whether pregnant women must totally eliminate alcohol use to avoid risk of damage to the fetus, women are advised not to drink any alcohol during pregnancy or when there is a chance pregnancy might occur—until a safe level can be established. The embryo (and, at later stages, the fetus), has no means of detoxifying alcohol.

Women with chronic alcoholism produce children with a variety of physical and intellectual problems collectively called **fetal alcohol spectrum disorders (FASDs)**. The most severe of these disorders is **fetal alcohol syndrome (FAS)**. A diagnosis of FAS is based mainly on poor fetal and infant growth, physical deformities (especially of facial features), and mental retardation (Fig. 17-9). Irritability, hyperactivity, short attention span, and limited hand-eye coordination are other symptoms of FAS. Defects in vision, hearing, and mental processing may also develop over time. Other FASDs consist of some but not all of the defects of FAS. **Alcohol-related neurodevelopmental disorders (ARNDs)** include behavior and learning problems resulting from exposure to alcohol in utero. **Alcohol-related birth defects (ARBDs)** typically include malformations of the heart, kidneys, bones, and/or ears.

Exactly how alcohol causes these defects is not known. One line of research suggests that alcohol, or products produced by the metabolism of alcohol (e.g., acetaldehyde), cause faulty movement of cells in the brain during early stages of nerve cell development or block the action of certain brain neurotransmitters. In addition, inadequate nutrient intake, reduced nutrient and oxygen transfer across the placenta, cigarette smoking commonly associated with alcohol intake, drug use, and possibly other factors contribute to the overall result.

The Dietary Guidelines for Americans recommend that alcoholic beverages not be consumed by pregnant women (Table 17-3). For more information about fetal alcohol syndrome, visit the website www.cdc.gov/ncbddd/fasd/.

Environmental Contaminants

There is little evidence to link birth defects with the amounts of pesticides, herbicides, or other contaminants in foods or public water supplies in North America. However, evaluating such a link can be methodologically difficult and many would argue that regulations concerning contaminants in the food and water supply are too permissive. Thus, it seems prudent to take measures to decrease intake of pesticides and herbicides wherever possible. For fruits and vegetables, peeling, removing outer leaves, and/or thoroughly rinsing and scrubbing with a brush under running water will remove the majority of contaminants. In animal products, pesticides and other contaminants are most likely to accumulate in fatty tissues. Therefore, removing skin, discarding drippings, and trimming visible fat will decrease exposure from meat, poultry, and fish.

For fish, mercury is of particular concern because it can harm the nervous system of the fetus. Thus, FDA warns pregnant women to avoid swordfish, shark, king mackerel, and tile fish because of possible high mercury contamination. Largemouth bass are also implicated. In general, intake of other fish and shellfish

▶ A goal of *Healthy People 2020* is 98.3% abstinence from alcohol, cigarettes, and illicit drugs by pregnant women, a 10% improvement over current statistics.

fetal alcohol spectrum disorders (FASDs) A group of irreversible physical and mental abnormalities in the infant that result from the mother's consuming alcohol during pregnancy.

fetal alcohol syndrome (FAS) Severe form of FASD that involves abnormal facial features and problems with development of the nervous system and overall growth as a result of maternal alcohol consumption during pregnancy.

should not exceed 12 ounces per week. Canned albacore tuna is a potential mercury source, so it should not be consumed in amounts exceeding 6 ounces per week. As a rule of thumb, consuming a variety of foods minimizes risk of exposure to contaminants from the food supply.

Summing Up

Although many risk factors for birth defects are beyond our control, a woman of childbearing potential can make some wise nutrition choices to improve her chances of having a healthy baby without birth defects. A varied and balanced diet, such as the food plan for pregnant women described in this chapter, along with a daily multivitamin and mineral supplement with 400 micrograms of folic acid will ensure adequate nutrient status. It is estimated that daily use of a multivitamin and mineral supplement containing folic acid will decrease the rate of all birth defects by 50%. Discuss use of any other

dietary supplements with a physician to be sure that the fetus will not be exposed to toxic levels of vitamin A or other dangerous ingredients. Early and consistent prenatal care can help control obesity and any chronic health conditions that may complicate a pregnancy. Also, avoiding alcohol during pregnancy will eliminate any risk for fetal alcohol spectrum disorders.

Although it seems that advice for a healthy pregnancy is always directed at the mother, fathers-to-be are not off the hook. Health is a family affair, so encouraging healthy eating habits and avoiding smoking and alcohol are important for fathers, too. Less research has been done in the area, but the genetics of the baby are certainly an outcome of both parents. Indeed, inadequate supplies of zinc, folate, and vitamin C affect the quality of sperm, which may impair fertility. Considering that spermatogenesis takes approximately 70 days, the periconceptional period is a time for good nutrition and careful lifestyle practices for the father as well.

▶ In North America, maternal death as a result of childbirth is uncommon—only about 11 deaths in every 100,000 live births. The infant mortality rate, however, is much higher: for each 100,000 live births, about 600 to 700 infants die within the first year. The infant death rate among African-Americans is more than double the rates among Whites and Hispanics in the United States.

▶ Pregnant women should recognize that many cough syrups contain alcohol. Cases have been reported of infants with FASDs born to mothers who consumed generous amounts of such cough syrups but no other alcoholic beverages.

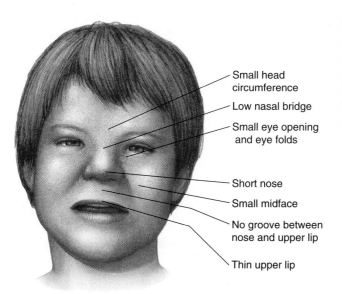

Small head circumference

Low nasal bridge

Small eye opening and eye folds

Short nose

Small midface

No groove between nose and upper lip

Thin upper lip

FIGURE 17-9 ▶ Fetal alcohol syndrome. The facial features shown are typical of affected children. Additional abnormalities in the brain and other internal organs accompany fetal alcohol syndrome but are not immediately apparent from simply looking at the child. Milder forms of alcohol-induced changes from a lower alcohol exposure to the fetus are known as alcohol-related neurodevelopmental disorders (ARNDs) and alcohol-related birth defects (ARBDs).

Case Study Preparing for Pregnancy

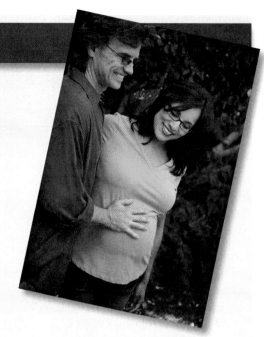

Lily and her husband have decided that they are ready to prepare for Lily's first pregnancy. She is 25 years old, weighs 135 pounds, and is 67 inches tall. Lily has been reading everything she can find on pregnancy because she knows that her prepregnancy health is important to the success of her pregnancy.

She knows she should avoid alcohol, especially because alcohol is potentially toxic to the growing fetus in the first weeks of pregnancy, and she could become pregnant and not know about it right away. Lily is not a smoker, does not take any medications, and limits her coffee intake to 4 cups a day and soft drink intake to 3 colas per day. Based on her reading, she has decided to breastfeed her infant and has already inquired about childbirth classes. She has modified her diet to include some extra protein, along with more fruits and vegetables. She has also started taking an over-the-counter vitamin and mineral supplement. Lily has always kept in good shape, and

she is admittedly worried about gaining too much weight during pregnancy. Recently, she started a running program 5 days a week, and she plans to continue running throughout her pregnancy.

Answer the following questions, and check your responses in Appendix A.

1. What recommendations do you have regarding Lily's use of dietary supplements?
2. What is Lily doing to prevent neural tube defects? What else could she do?
3. What recommendations would you make regarding Lily's caffeine consumption?
4. Lily is wise to pay attention to her protein intake to prepare for pregnancy and breastfeeding. Should she include fish as a source of protein in her diet? Why or why not?
5. Constipation is a common complaint during pregnancy. What suggestions do

you have to help Lily avoid this health concern?
6. What information would you share with Lily about appropriate weight gain during pregnancy?

Summary (Numbers refer to numbered sections in the chapter.)

17.1 The best time to prepare for pregnancy is before conception even occurs. Achieving a healthy body weight, avoiding toxic agents, correcting nutritional deficiencies, and controlling existing medical conditions will set the stage for a successful pregnancy.

17.2 Pregnancy is arbitrarily divided into three trimesters of 13 to 14 weeks each. The first trimester is characterized by a rapid increase in cell number as the zygote grows to be an embryo, then a fetus. During the first trimester, the growing organism is most susceptible to damage from exposure to toxic agents or nutrient deficiencies. By the start of the second trimester, the organs and limbs have formed and will continue to grow and develop. The third trimester is marked by rapid fetal growth and storage of nutrients in preparation for life outside the womb.

17.3 A successful pregnancy results in optimal health for both the infant and

the mother. Pregnancy success is defined as (1) gestation longer than 37 weeks and (2) birth weight greater than 5.5 pounds (2.5 kilograms). Factors that predict pregnancy success include early and regular prenatal care, maternal age within the range of 20 to 35 years, and adequate nutrition. Factors that contribute to poor pregnancy outcome include inadequate prenatal care, obesity, underweight, teenage pregnancy, smoking, alcohol consumption, use of certain prescription medications and all illicit drugs, inadequate nutrition, heavy caffeine use, and various infections, such as listeriosis.

17.4 For women with a healthy prepregnancy BMI (18.5 to 24.9), total weight gain should be within the range of 25 to 35 pounds. Underweight women and those carrying multiple fetuses should gain more; overweight and obese women should gain less. During the first trimester, although she need not increase diet

quantity, the woman should focus on diet quality to meet increased requirements for protein, carbohydrate, essential fatty acids, fiber, water, and many vitamins and minerals. A woman typically needs an additional 350 to 450 kcal per day during the second and third trimesters.

17.5 Following a plan based on the Dietary Guidelines for Americans as exemplified by MyPlate is recommended for pregnant and breastfeeding women. The mother-to-be should especially emphasize good sources of vitamin B-6, folate, iron, zinc, and calcium. Vegetarian diets are safe during pregnancy, but vegan mothers should specifically seek out good sources of vitamin B-12 and vitamin D. Prenatal multivitamin and mineral supplements are useful for meeting increased nutrient requirements during pregnancy.

17.6 Pregnancy-induced hypertension, gestational diabetes, heartburn, constipation, nausea, vomiting, edema, and anemia are all possible discomforts and complications of pregnancy. Nutrition therapy can help minimize some of these problems.

17.7 Almost all women are able to breastfeed their infants. The nutritional composition of human milk is different from that of unaltered cow's milk and is much more desirable for the infant.

For the infant, the advantages of breastfeeding over formula feeding are numerous, including fewer intestinal, respiratory, and ear infections and fewer allergies and food intolerances. Benefits for the mother include reduced risk of certain cancers, earlier recovery from pregnancy, and faster return to prepregnancy weight. For mothers who choose not to breastfeed or in medical situations that contraindicate breastfeeding (e.g., galactosemia), infants can be adequately nourished with formula.

N&YH There are several steps pregnant women can take to help prevent birth defects. Achieve a healthy body weight before pregnancy and strive to gain weight within the ranges recommended by the Institute of Medicine. Adequate intakes of folic acid, iodide, and antioxidant nutrients are essential for prevention of many types of birth defects. Excesses of vitamin A and caffeine should be avoided. There is no safe level of alcohol intake known during pregnancy. Dietary control of diseases (e.g., diabetes and PKU) will also protect the fetus.

Check Your Knowledge (Answers to the following multiple choice questions are below.)

1. The fetus is most susceptible to damage from nutrient deficiencies; teratogens; and use of certain medications, alcohol, and illicit drugs during
   a. the first trimester.
   b. the second trimester.
   c. the third trimester.
   d. labor and delivery.

2. An infant born at 38 weeks' gestation weighing 5.0 pounds can be described as
   a. preterm.   c. SGA.
   b. LBW.   d. LBW and SGA.

3. If a woman is 5′2″ and weighs 150 pounds before becoming pregnant, how much weight should she gain during pregnancy?
   a. 28 to 40 pounds (12.5 to 18 kilograms)
   b. 25 to 35 pounds (11.5 to 16 kilograms)
   c. 15 to 25 pounds (7 to 11.5 kilograms)
   d. As little as possible

4. Increased carbohydrate needs during pregnancy are set to
   a. prevent ketosis.
   b. alleviate nausea.
   c. prevent pregnancy-induced hypertension.
   d. supply adequate folate.

5. Which of the following is best paired with an iron supplement during pregnancy?
   a. skim milk
   b. orange juice
   c. coffee
   d. tea

6. A food plan for a woman in the third trimester of pregnancy differs from her prepregnancy diet in that
   a. fluid needs are higher.
   b. additional solid fats and added sugars are allowed.
   c. there are more servings from the grains group.
   d. All of the above.

7. Consuming one cup of coffee per day is associated with
   a. spontaneous abortions.
   b. LBW.
   c. birth defects.
   d. None of the above.

8. Which of the following may help to alleviate nausea during pregnancy?

   a. postponing meals until the afternoon
   b. drinking large amounts of water
   c. postponing use of iron supplements until the second trimester
   d. All of the above.

9. Which of the following conditions medically prevents a woman from breastfeeding her infant?
   a. breasts are too small
   b. infant has galactosemia
   c. inverted nipples
   d. None of the above.

10. Physiologically, milk production requires _____ kcals per day.
   a. 300
   b. 500
   c. 800
   d. 1000

Answer Key: 1. a (LO 17.2), 2. d (LO 17.2), 3. c (LO 17.3), 4. a (LO 17.1), 5. b (LO 17.5), 6. d (LO 17.4), 7. d (LO 17.2), 8. c (LO 17.6), 9. b (LO 17.7), 10. c (LO 17.4)

Study Questions (Numbers refer to Learning Outcomes)

1. Provide three key pieces of advice for parents seeking to maximize their chances of having a healthy infant. Why did you identify those specific factors? **(LO 17.2)**

2. Outline current weight-gain recommendations for pregnancy. What is the basis for these recommendations? **(LO 17.3)**

3. Identify four key nutrients for which intake should be significantly increased during pregnancy. **(LO 17.1)**

4. Describe a diet based on the Dietary Guidelines as exemplified by MyPlate that meets the increased nutrient needs of pregnancy. **(LO 17.4)**

5. Why does teenage pregnancy receive so much attention these days? At what age do you think pregnancy is ideal? Why? **(LO 17.2)**

6. Give three reasons a woman should give serious consideration to breastfeeding her infant. **(LO 17.7)**

7. Describe the physiological mechanisms that stimulate milk production and release. How can knowing about these help mothers breastfeed successfully? **(LO 17.7)**

8. Describe two nutrients that may require supplementation during pregnancy and give reasons for each. **(LO 17.5)**

9. How should the basic food plan suitable for pregnancy be modified during breastfeeding? **(LO 17.4)**

10. What nutrition advice would you give to a friend who suffers from morning sickness? **(LO 17.6)**

What Would You Choose Recommendations

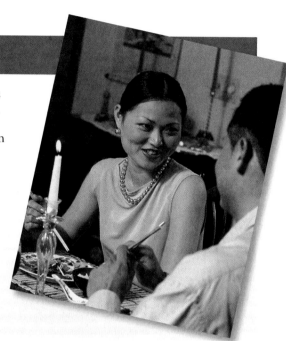

The spinach salad meal with hard-boiled egg and whole-wheat roll provides only about 2 grams of iron. It is a healthy, nutrient-dense choice that provides some protein, but does not make a significant contribution to meeting iron needs.

A hamburger is a source of iron—this meal would provide about 4.5 milligrams of iron—but it would not be a choice for a person who follows a vegetarian diet.

The bean and cheese taco option provides just as much iron (4.5 milligrams) as the hamburger meal and would be appropriate for a vegetarian.

Even though the nonheme iron in beans is not as well absorbed as the heme iron in beef, the 20 milligrams of vitamin C in the stewed tomatoes will enhance iron absorption.

All of these meals, however, pale in comparison to the iron contribution of the fortified, ready-to-eat breakfast cereal. One cup of Kellogg's Smart Start cereal provides 18 milligrams of iron, and the 72 milligrams of vitamin C in 1 cup of orange juice will enhance iron absorption. In one easy meal, any pregnant woman could obtain more than half of the 27-milligram RDA for iron during pregnancy.

Further Readings

1. AAP Committee on Genetics: Policy Statement: Maternal phenylketonuria. *Pediatrics* 122:445, 2008.

   Uncontrolled maternal phenylketonuria (PKU) leads to exposure of the fetus to elevated phenylalanine levels in the blood, which can lead to birth defects, poor physical growth, and altered brain development. All girls and women with PKU should be educated and counseled throughout life about controlling phenylalanine levels to minimize risks during pregnancy.

2. AAP Section on Breastfeeding: American Academy of Pediatrics Policy Statement: Breastfeeding and the use of human milk. *Pediatrics* 115:496, 2005.

   AAP firmly supports breastfeeding as the ideal nutrition for infants. A few contraindications to breastfeeding are discussed, such as HIV infection and galactosemia. Exclusive breastfeeding is recommended for the first 6 months of life. Breastfeeding should continue with age-appropriate introduction of complementary solid foods until 1 year of age or longer. Guidelines are provided for infant nutrient supplementation.

3. ADA Reports: Position of the American Dietetic Association: Nutrition and lifestyle for a healthy pregnancy outcome. *Journal of the American Dietetic Association* 108:553, 2008.

   The key components of a healthy lifestyle during pregnancy include appropriate weight gain; consumption of a variety of foods; appropriate and timely vitamin and mineral intake; avoidance of alcohol, tobacco, and other harmful substances; and safe food handling. Supplementation is appropriate for some nutrients.

4. James DC and others: Position of the American Dietetic Association: Promoting and supporting breastfeeding. *Journal of the American Dietetic Association* 109:1926, 2009.

   The American Dietetic Association strongly supports the breastfeeding of infants. This article discusses the benefits of breastfeeding for the mother and infant, as well as dietary considerations that need to be addressed, such as avoiding consumption of species of fish known to contain high amounts of mercury.

5. Barger MK. Maternal nutrition and perinatal outcomes. *Journal of Midwifery and Women's Health* 55:502, 2010.

   This review details the roles and requirements of various nutrients during pregnancy with an emphasis on the developmental origins of disease hypothesis. Nutritional status influences infant growth, length of gestation, and several pregnancy complications, such as gestational diabetes and preeclampsia.

6. Bodnar LM and others: Periconceptional multivitamin use reduces the risk of preeclampsia. *American Journal of Epidemiology* 164:470, 2006.

   In the Pregnancy Exposures and Preeclampsia Prevention Study, women who regularly consumed a multivitamin during the periconceptional period had a 45% lower risk of developing preeclampsia during their first pregnancy than those who did not consume multivitamins. Women with BMI less than 25 benefited most from multivitamin use.

7. Field CJ: The immunological components of human milk and their effect on immune development in infants. *Journal of Nutrition* 135:1, 2005.

   Human milk contains many factors that improve immune function in the infant. This article reviews a number of these complex factors.

8. Fraser A and others: Associations of gestational weight gain with maternal body mass index, waist circumference, and blood pressure measured 16 years after pregnancy: The Avon Longitudinal Study of Parents and Children (ALSPAC). *American Journal of Clinical Nutrition* 93:1285, 2011.

Researchers examined long-term health effects of prepregnancy weight and gestational weight gain. Mothers with high prepregnancy BMI and gestational weight gain above recommended ranges had higher BMI, waist circumference, and blood pressure measurements 16 years after pregnancy. Of interest, even among women with normal prepregnancy weight, high rates of weight gain during midpregnancy were associated with higher blood pressure later in life. The results confirm that adherence to the 2009 IOM guidelines for prepregnancy weight and weight gain during pregnancy optimizes long-term maternal health.

9. Greer FR and others: Effects of early nutritional interventions on the development of atopic disease in infants and children: The role of maternal dietary restriction, breastfeeding, timing of introduction of complementary foods, and hydrolyzed formulas. *Pediatrics* 121:183, 2008.

The American Academy of Pediatrics revised previous recommendations for prevention of atopic disease. Current evidence does not support a role of maternal dietary restrictions in prevention of atopic disease in children. The best course of action for at-risk infants is to breastfeed exclusively and delay introduction of solid foods until 4 to 6 months of age. Delaying introduction of complementary feedings beyond 6 months is not advantageous.

10. Han Z and others: Maternal underweight and the risk of preterm birth and low birth weight: A systematic review and meta-analysis. *International Journal of Epidemiology* 40:65, 2011.

Despite the increasing prevalence of overweight and obesity among women of childbearing age, maternal underweight is related to higher risk of preterm birth and low birth weight.

11. Institute of Medicine and National Research Council: *Weight gain during pregnancy: Reexamining the guidelines.* Washington, DC: The National Academies Press, 2009.

Excess maternal weight affects the health of both the fetus (size at birth, gestational age, and impact on childhood obesity) and the mother (postpartum weight retention and requirement for surgical delivery). The revised guidelines for weight gain during pregnancy recommended relatively narrow ranges based on mother's prepregnancy BMI, which was found to be an important predictor of pregnancy outcome. New guidelines for obese mothers now advise a weight gain of only 11 to 20 pounds (5 to 9 kilograms). Provisional recommendations are given for women carrying multiple fetuses.

12. Jones KL: The effects of alcohol on fetal development. *Birth Defects Research (Part C)* 93:3, 2011.

This comprehensive review traces research on fetal alcohol spectrum disorders and describes its many physiological and neurological defects with color photos. Several maternal risk factors can increase risk for FASD, including maternal age >30 years, low socioeconomic status, previous children with FASD, genetics, and malnutrition.

13. Kelly, AKW: Practical exercise advice during pregnancy. *The Physician and Sports Medicine* 33(6):24, 2005.

It is safe for pregnant women to exercise if they are experiencing uncomplicated pregnancies. Most non-weight-bearing exercises (e.g., swimming) and walking are safe for pregnant women. Women should begin with 15 minutes of exercise three times a week and progress as tolerated.

14. Lucas RM and others: Future health implications of prenatal and early-life vitamin D status. *Nutrition Reviews* 66:710, 2008.

In addition to its role in bone health, preventive effects of vitamin D on autoimmune disorders, diabetes, cancer, cardiovascular disease, osteoporosis, and psychiatric illness are mediated by the vitamin's involvement in gene expression. Maternal vitamin D supplementation could lead to widespread improvements in public health.

15. Makrides M: Outcomes for mothers and their babies: Do n-3 long-chain polyunsaturated fatty acids and seafoods make a difference? *Journal of the American Dietetic Association* 108: 1622, 2008

Omega-3 fatty acids are important for brain and eye development of the fetus and infant. These fats have been implicated in prevention of preeclampsia, preterm birth, LBW, and SGA, but current evidence does not support supplementation for these purposes. Despite the importance of n-3 fatty acids for fetal development, many women have inadequate intakes of these fats. Available data indicate that pregnant and lactating women should aim to consume at least 200 milligrams per day of omega-3 fatty acids from dietary sources, including oily fish, eggs, and lean red meats.

16. Rubin RC: Change is good—evidence to support lowering the diagnostic threshold for GDM. *Today's Dietitian* 13:10, 2011.

Gestational diabetes may lead to macrosomia, birth injuries, and postnatal hypoglycemia for infants. For mothers, GDM increases risk of type 2 diabetes later in life. The American Diabetes Association updated its guidelines on diagnosis and treatment of GDM: high-risk women should be screened for undiagnosed type 2 diabetes at their first prenatal visit; all women should undergo a standardized 75-gram oral glucose tolerance test to screen for GDM between 24 and 28 weeks of gestation; after birth, mothers with GDM should be monitored for development of type 2 diabetes.

17. Tamura T, Picciano MF: Folate and human reproduction. *American Journal of Clinical Nutrition* 83:993, 2006.

Folic acid supplementation for the prevention of megaloblastic anemia and neural tube defects represents a major public health advancement. Folate status may also be linked to placental abruption, preeclampsia, spontaneous abortion, stillbirth, low birth weight, and risk for birth defects other than neural tube defects.

18. Taylor JS and others: A systematic review of the literature associating breastfeeding with type 2 diabetes and gestational diabetes. *Journal of the American College of Nutrition* 24:320, 2005.

Breastfed infants have lower rates of obesity, type 1 diabetes, and type 2 diabetes in adulthood compared to formula-fed infants. In addition, mothers who breastfeed have improved glucose tolerance and lower risk for postpartum diabetes compared to nonlactating mothers.

19. Ward EM: Prime the body for pregnancy—preconception care and nutrition for moms-to-be. *Today's Dietitian* 10:26, 2008.

Women of childbearing potential should take steps to ensure a healthy pregnancy before becoming pregnant. The article provides practical guidelines for intakes of key nutrients (e.g., folic acid and iron), supplement use, weight management, physical activity, and caffeine and alcohol consumption.

20. Zimmerman MB: Iodine deficiency in pregnancy and the effects of maternal iodine supplementation on the offspring: A review. *American Journal of Clinical Nutrition* 89(suppl):668S, 2009.

Iodine deficiency leads to cretinism or more subtle deficits in brain function. Recently, the World Health Organization augmented recommendations for iodine deficiency during pregnancy from 200 to 250 micrograms per day. Annual supplementation with 400 milligrams of iodine in the form of iodized oil or daily supplementation with potassium iodide are effective strategies for reducing maternal iodine deficiency and associated birth defects.

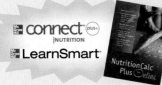

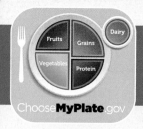

I. Targeting Nutrients Necessary for Pregnant Women

This chapter mentioned that pregnant women may have difficulty meeting their increased needs for folate, vitamin B-6, iron, and zinc. List six foods rich in each of these nutrients next to the appropriate heading. Refer to Chapter 12 if necessary.

Nutrient	Foods	Nutrient	Foods
Folate	_____	Iron	_____
	_____		_____
	_____		_____
	_____		_____
	_____		_____
Vitamin B-6	_____	Zinc	_____
	_____		_____
	_____		_____
	_____		_____
	_____		_____

1. Foods rich in more than one of these nutrients would be especially valuable for pregnant women. Write on the line any foods you listed that are good sources of more than one of these critical nutrients.

   _____

2. The needs for folate, vitamin B-6, iron, and zinc increase during pregnancy. For which of these nutrients can pregnant women usually obtain adequate intakes from dietary sources?

   _____

3. Which of these nutrients are commonly taken in supplement form during pregnancy?

   _____

   _____

4. Why might it be hard for pregnant women to meet their increased needs for these nutrients from food alone?

   _____

   _____

II. Putting Your Knowledge About Nutrition and Pregnancy to Work

A college friend, Angie, tells you that she is newly pregnant. You are aware that she usually
likes to eat the following foods for her meals:

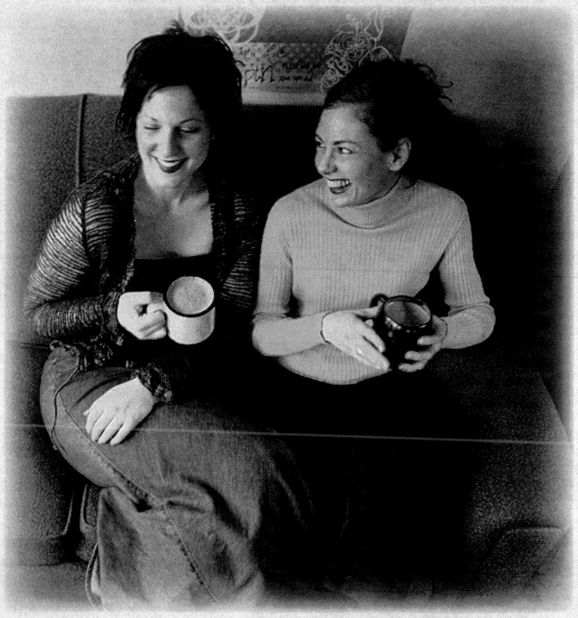

Breakfast

Skips this meal, or eats a granola bar
Coffee

Lunch

Sweetened yogurt, 1 cup
Small bagel with cream cheese
Occasional piece of fruit
Regular caffeinated soda, 12 ounces

Snack

Chocolate candy bar

Dinner

2 slices of pizza, macaroni and cheese, or 2 eggs with 2 slices of toast
Seldom eats a salad or vegetable
Regular caffeinated soda, 12 ounces

Snacks

Pretzels or chips, 1 ounce
Regular caffeinated soda, 12 ounces

1. Using NutritionCalc Plus software, evaluate Angie's diet for protein, carbohydrate, folate, vitamin B-6, iron, and zinc. How does
   her intake compare with the recommended amounts for pregnancy?

   _____

   _____

   _____

2. Now redesign her diet and make sure that her intake meets pregnancy needs for protein, carbohydrate, folate, vitamin B-6,
   and zinc. (Hint: Fortified foods, such as breakfast cereal, are generally nutrient-rich foods, which can more easily help meet
   one's needs.) Increase the iron content as well, but it still may be below the RDA for pregnancy.

   _____

   _____

   _____

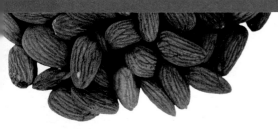

INDEX

A

ABCDE. *See* Anthropometric, Biochemical, Clinical, Dietary, and Environmental
Absorption, 82, 96
  processes, 96–97
  sites, 105t
Absorptive cells, 100, 101
Absorptive processes, types, 103f
Acceptable Daily Intake (ADI), 136
Accessory organs, 106
Acesulfame-K, 135, 136
Acetaldehyde dehydrogenase, 693
Acid-base balance (pH), 107, 320
  definition, 320
  electrolytes, importance, 319–320
  maintenance, 107
  proteins, impact, 222
  scale, 320f
Acid group, 167
Acne
  nutrition, relationship, 660
  Vitamin A analogs, usage, 359
Acquired immunodeficiency syndrome (AIDS), 538
  nutrition, relationship, 543
  worldwide impact, 542–543
Actionable health messages, usage, 56
Active absorption, 103
Activities, calorie cost approximation, 266t
Added sugars, 53, 59f, 618
  intake, limitation, 20
  sources, 149f
Additives, 569
Adenosine diphosphate (ADP), 466
Adenosine triphosphate (ATP), 86, 466
  energy form, 472
  formation, 470f
  magnesium, requirement, 401
  phosphorus component, 395
  yield, 468f
Adequate intake (AI), 48, 50f
Adipose cell, 188
Adipose tissue growth, 637
Adjustable gastric banding, 272
Adolescents
  Vitamin D ingestion, 400
  weight gain, food advertising/marketing (impact), 5
Adulthood
  Alzheimer's disease, 691
  body composition, 684
  calcium/vitamin D, impact, 682
  calories, requirement, 680–681
  carbohydrate intake, 681

carotenoid, dietary intakes, 683
chronic disease, 687
depression, 690–691
dietary recommendations, 683
diet quality, 697–699
diet recommendations, 685t
digestive system, 686–687
eating, guidelines, 698t
economic factors, 691–692
endocrine system, 687
environment, impact, 678–679
exercise guidelines, 686
fat intake, 681
folate/Vitamins B-6/B-12, role, 682
immune system, 687
iron, impact, 682
lifestyle, 678
  responses, 685t
magnesium intake, 682
medications, 688
minerals/vitamins, usage, 681–682
nervous system, 687
nutrient needs, 679–692
nutrition checklist, 680f
physiological changes, 675–679, 685t
physiological factors, 684–688
protein intake, 681
psychosocial factors, 690–692
relative nutrient requirements, 681f
skeletal system, 684, 686
Vitamin E, dietary intake, 682
water consumption, 681
zinc intake, 682
Adult obesity
  percentage, 18f
  trends, 245
Adult physical activity/exercise, *Healthy People 2010* objectives, 463
Advanced glycation endproducts (AGEs), 152
Advertising, media tool, 6
Aerobic, term (usage), 468
Aerobic glucose use, ATP yield, 468f
Aerobic process, 84
Aerobic workout, 465–466
Age groups, MyPlate calorie guidelines, 251f
Age-related macular degeneration, 362
Aging, 675
  alternative medicine, relationship, 688–689
  causes, 676
  nutritional deficiencies, 697
  physiological function, declines, 675
  process, health rating, 708
  rate, factors, 677
  success, 677
Air displacement, 254
Alcohol, 15
  absorption/metabolism, 693–694
  abuse, 693
    risks, 694, 696
  calorie content/source, 15
  consumption, nutrition implications, 692–697

dehydrogenase, 693
dependence, 694
drinking, 26
intake, limitation, 20
proof, representation, 693
release, 15
Alcoholic beverages
  alcohol/carbohydrate/calorie content, 692t
  production process, 693
Alcoholism, 694
  Vitamin B-6 deficiency, 427
Alcohol-related birth defects (ARBDs), 624
Alcohol-related neurodevelopmental disorders (ARNDs), 624
Alcohol use
  benefits/risks, 695t
  guidance, 696–697
  moderation, benefits, 694
Aldosterone, definition, 324
Allergen, 662
Allergies, 639
  prevention, 644–645
  types, 662
Almonds, choline sources, 308
Alpha-linolenic acid, 169
  DRI, 187
Alternative sweeteners, 133t, 135–136
Alzheimer's disease, 691
American Heart Association (AHA), 2006 Diet and Lifestyle Goals/Recommendations for Cardiovascular Disease Risk Reduction, 191t
Amino acids, 12, 211–213
  bonding, 12, 213–216
  B vitamin input, 308
  classification, 212t
  metabolism, 224f
    Vitamin B-6, impact, 318
  R group, 211
  supplements, 227–228, 238
Amphetamines, 270
Amylase, 99
Amylopectin, 128, 129f
Amylose, 128, 129f
Anaerobic, term (usage), 84, 468
Anaerobic glucose breakdown
  advantage, 468
  energy, 468–470
Anaerobic glucose use, ATP yield, 468f
Anaerobic metabolism, 84
Anaerobic process, disadvantages, 468
Anal canal, moisture (presence), 115
Anal sphincters, 105
Anaphylactic shock, 663
Anemia, 435–436. *See also* Iron-deficiency anemia; Physiological anemia
  case study, 453
  definition, 418f
Angular cheilitis, 421f
Animal cell, 84f
Animal food, cholesterol (presence), 173–174
Animal model, 47